Handbook of Internal Medicine

Handbook of Internal Medicine

Edited by Harriet Jacobs

hayle
medical

New York

Hayle Medical,
750 Third Avenue, 9th Floor,
New York, NY 10017, USA

Visit us on the World Wide Web at:
www.haylemedical.com

ISBN: 978-1-63241-808-1

Cataloging-in-Publication Data

Handbook of internal medicine / edited by Harriet Jacobs.
   p. cm.
Includes bibliographical references and index.
ISBN 978-1-63241-808-1
1. Internal medicine. 2. Medicine. I. Jacobs, Harriet.
RC48 .H36 2019
616--dc23

Table of Contents

Permissions

List of Contributors

Index

Preface

The main aim of this book is to educate learners and enhance their research focus by presenting diverse topics covering this vast field. This is an advanced book which compiles significant studies by distinguished experts in the area of analysis. This book addresses successive solutions to the challenges arising in the area of application, along with it; the book provides scope for future developments.

The branch of medicine dealing with the prevention, diagnosis, and treatment of adult diseases is known as internal medicine. It is also a subfield under veterinary medicine and clinical pharmacy. Doctors who have specialized in this field are called internists. They deal in the management of patients struggling with multi-system disease. They usually care for hospitalized and ambulatory patients. Internal medicine patients are mostly seriously ill and require complex investigations. Some of the main subfields of internal medicine include cardiology, critical care medicine, gastroenterology, nephrology, pulmonology, etc. This book is a compilation of chapters that discuss the most vital concepts and emerging trends in the field of internal medicine. The various advancements in this field are glanced at and their applications as well as ramifications are looked at in detail. This book includes contributions of experts and doctors, which will provide innovative insights into this medical specialty.

It was a great honour to edit this book, though there were challenges, as it involved a lot of communication and networking between me and the editorial team. However, the end result was this all-inclusive book covering diverse themes in the field.

Finally, it is important to acknowledge the efforts of the contributors for their excellent chapters, through which a wide variety of issues have been addressed. I would also like to thank my colleagues for their valuable feedback during the making of this book.

Editor

The Daily Mile makes primary school children more active, less sedentary and improves their fitness and body composition

Ross A. Chesham[1], Josephine N. Booth[2], Emma L. Sweeney[1], Gemma C. Ryde[1], Trish Gorely[1,3], Naomi E. Brooks[1] and Colin N. Moran[1*]

Abstract

Background: The Daily Mile is a physical activity programme made popular by a school in Stirling, Scotland. It is promoted by the Scottish Government and is growing in popularity nationally and internationally. The aim is that each day, during class time, pupils run or walk outside for 15 min (~1 mile) at a self-selected pace. It is anecdotally reported to have a number of physiological benefits including increased physical activity, reduced sedentary behaviour, increased fitness and improved body composition. This study aimed to investigate these reports.

Methods: We conducted a quasi-experimental repeated measures pilot study in two primary schools in the Stirling Council area: one school with, and one without, intention to introduce the Daily Mile. Pupils at the control school followed their usual curriculum. Of the 504 children attending the schools, 391 children in primary classes 1–7 (age 4–12 years) at the baseline assessment took part. The follow-up assessment was in the same academic year. Outcomes were accelerometer-assessed average daily moderate to vigorous intensity physical activity (MVPA) and average daily sedentary behaviour, 20-m shuttle run fitness test performance and adiposity assessed by the sum of skinfolds at four sites. Valid data at both time points were collected for 118, 118, 357 and 327 children, respectively, for each outcome.

Results: After correction for age and gender, significant improvements were observed in the intervention school relative to the control school for MVPA, sedentary time, fitness and body composition. For MVPA, a relative increase of 9.1 min per day (95% confidence interval or 95%CI 5.1–13.2 min, standardised mean difference SMD = 0.407, $p = 0.027$) was observed. For sedentary time, there was a relative decrease of 18.2 min per day (10.7–25.7 min, SMD = 0.437, $p = 0.017$). For the shuttle run, there was a relative increase of 39.1 m (21.9–56.3, SMD = 0.236, $p = 0.037$). For the skinfolds, there was a relative decrease of 1.4 mm (0.8–2.0 mm, SMD = 0.246, $p = 0.036$). Similar results were obtained when a correction for socioeconomic groupings was included.

Conclusions: The findings show that in primary school children, the Daily Mile intervention is effective at increasing levels of MVPA, reducing sedentary time, increasing physical fitness and improving body composition. These findings have relevance for teachers, policymakers, public health practitioners, and health researchers.

Keywords: Daily Mile, Children, Physical activity, Primary school, Fitness, Body composition

* Correspondence: colin.moran@stir.ac.uk
[1]Faculty of Health Sciences and Sport, University of Stirling, Scotland FK9 4LA, UK
Full list of author information is available at the end of the article

Background

The Daily Mile is a physical activity intervention developed at St Ninian's Primary School (Stirling, Scotland) in 2012 [1]. The initial aim was to improve the fitness of children; although, there have since been many additional benefits anecdotally reported by children, teachers and parents [1]. These include improved physical activity, sedentary time, physical fitness, body composition, sleep, diet, concentration, well-being and obesity levels. However, no objectively measured scientific evidence has yet been gathered on the validity of these reports.

The successful implementation of the Daily Mile at many schools, its continued maintenance and its increasing popularity seem to be a result of the simplicity of the activity, the autonomy given to classroom teachers over when they do it during the school day and the pupil-determined pace. Since its development, the Daily Mile has been rolled out across the country by the Scottish government [2]. It is estimated by Education Scotland that, from local authorities who responded to their query, ~ 50% of primary schools in Scotland are already doing the Daily Mile with a further 18% planning to do the Daily Mile soon (personal communication). It has also become popular in the rest of the UK with interest from the UK government [3, 4]. Additionally, it has been introduced in the Netherlands, Belgium and parts of the USA with interest from many other countries [5], despite the lack of rigorous evidence on the efficacy of taking part.

Globally, physical activity levels are low [6]. Furthermore, low physical activity levels in childhood are predictive of low physical activity levels in adulthood [7]. The World Health Organisation (WHO) considers policies and interventions to increase physical activity levels to be important in all age groups and that any potential harm of increasing physical activity is outweighed by the associated benefits [8, 9]. In a recent accelerometer study on children (2–11 years old) from eight European countries, the proportion of children achieving 60+ minutes per day (recommended for 5–18 year olds [10]) of moderate to vigorous physical activity (MVPA) ranged from 9.5% to 34.1% in boys and from 2.0% to 14.7% in girls [11]. MVPA levels generally decline with age in both genders as sedentary time increases [12]. MVPA levels are also believed to be influenced by socioeconomic status; however, systematic reviews are unclear on the consistency of this relationship and more evidence needs to be gathered [13]. School-based physical activity interventions like the Daily Mile are appealing because they include whole classes, therefore they reach many children regardless of socioeconomic status, physical activity level or fitness level. They also break up sedentary time as they occur during lessons and have the potential to reach much larger proportions of the population than opt-in groups like sports clubs. Therefore, understanding the impact of the Daily Mile on physical activity and sedentary behaviour levels is of key importance.

Overweight and obesity rates are of pandemic proportions and considered to be a key target for the WHO [8]. In Scotland, 30% of children (29% of boys and 32% of girls) aged 7–11 years were overweight or obese in 2015 [14], a figure similar to that in England [15]. At the same time, there is evidence of a decline in the performance of children in the 20-m shuttle run (an indicator of physical endurance fitness) [16]. Low fitness and low levels of physical activity in adults and children are associated with a number of risk factors for non-communicable diseases and adverse health outcomes including obesity, cardiovascular disease, diabetes, some cancers, low mood and poor cognitive function [17–21]. Additionally, both overweight and low fitness are also known to be related to lower socioeconomic status [22, 23]. Studies into the impact of the Daily Mile on fitness and body composition are important for understanding its potential to improve public health, including health inequalities, and for developing future public health policies.

The Daily Mile at least has the potential to impact on key areas of global public health. Whilst published evidence shows a positive health relationship between physical activity, particularly MVPA, and these outcomes [24], it is unknown whether 15 min of exercise, particularly with no expectation of intensity, will provide such benefits. Given the associated loss of academic classroom time (up to 75 min per week), it is paramount that evidence on the impact of the Daily Mile on each anecdotally reported benefit is gathered to ensure that government policies are appropriate. Furthermore, any associated benefits in physiological health are likely to be small [25]; thus, it is essential to use gold standard measurement techniques. Therefore, the aims of this study are to assess the anecdotally reported physiological benefits of participation in the Daily Mile. Specifically, using a repeated measures design and gold standard measurement techniques, we will assess whether the introduction of the Daily Mile into a primary school setting leads to increased MVPA, reduced sedentary time, improved fitness and improved body composition.

Methods

Study design and ethics

"Using the Daily Mile to turn the WHEEL" (Well-being, Health, Exercise, Enjoyment and Learning) is a school-based quasi-experimental study designed to assess the anecdotally reported benefits of taking part in the Daily Mile. Ethical approval was obtained from the University of Stirling, School of Sport Research Ethics Committee (reference number 760). Approval was also obtained from the Director of Children, Young People and Education at Stirling Council.

Eligibility and recruitment

State primary schools in the Stirling Council areas were eligible for inclusion. Recruiting from only one council area reduced any potential variance in the delivery of education that may have impacted on outcome measurements. Two local primary schools were identified and approached: one that was not doing the Daily Mile but was intending to introduce it (the intervention school) and one that was not doing the Daily Mile and did not intend to introduce it (the control school). Both schools had expressed a desire to introduce the Daily Mile although the control school felt that it would not be possible due to the layout of its playground. Both schools had a range of levels of deprivation, although the majority of pupils were from higher socioeconomic quintiles (Fig. 1). Participants were children in all years (age 4–12 years) at the time of recruitment.

Once the schools had agreed to participate in the study, parents and guardians of the children were sent a letter and information sheet about the study with an opt-in consent form. For children in primary classes 4–7 (age 7–12 years), an additional child consent form was included. Information sessions were held in both schools to allow parents to ask questions and see the study equipment. They were also given the opportunity to contact the research team by email or phone to discuss the study. Information about being able to withdraw from the study at any stage was given in the information sheet, consent form and verbally. All of the children were also asked to confirm verbally that they were happy to take part on each day of testing.

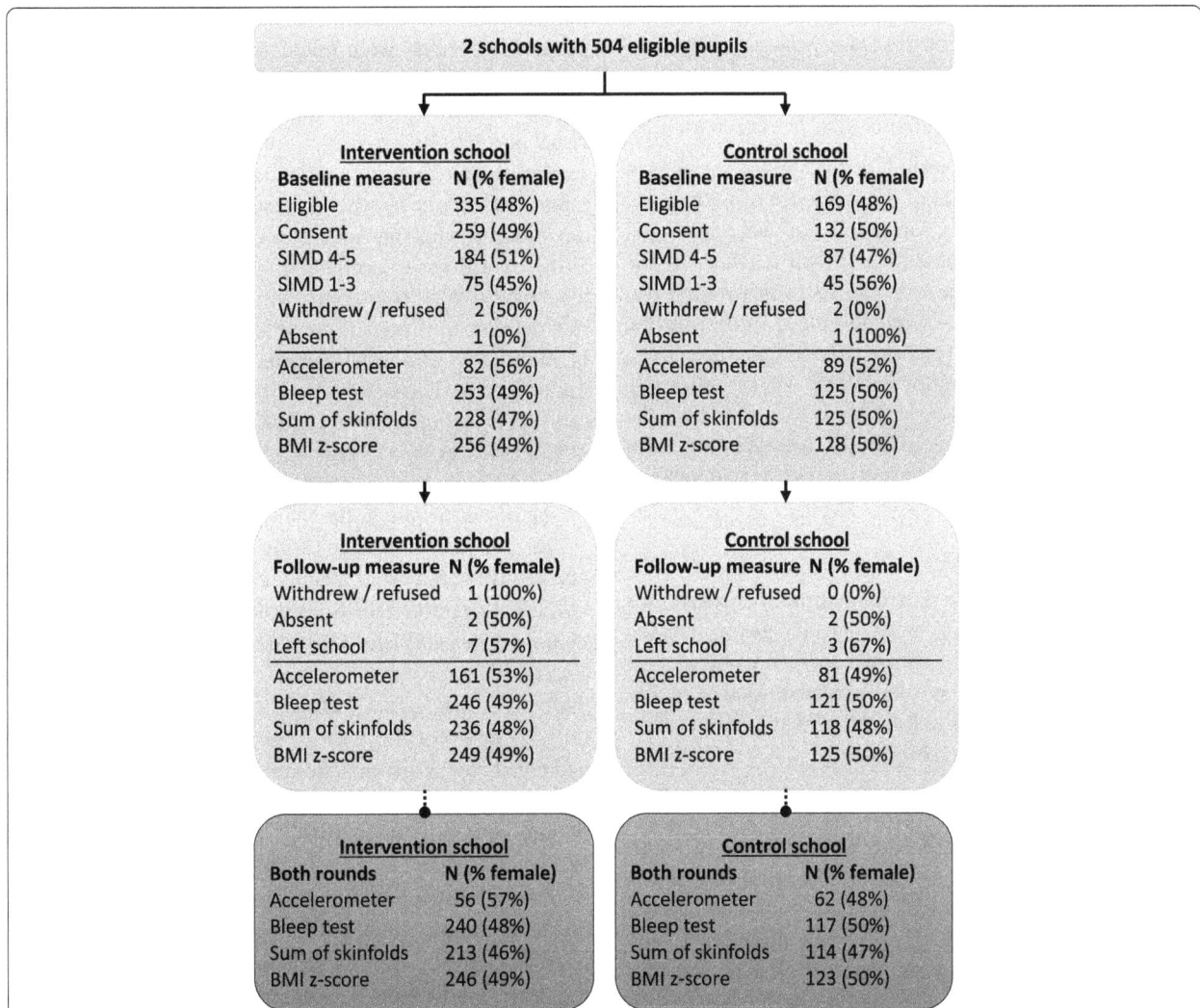

Fig. 1 Trial profile. *N* is the number of school pupil participants. The percentage of female participants for each measurement is shown in parentheses. Individual boxes show the totals for each school at baseline, or at follow-up, or the totals for participants with valid measurements in both rounds. Not all pupils with follow-up measurements had been measured at the baseline (or vice versa), since different pupils were absent at the main and follow-up assessments, some refused to complete certain measurements at each time point and some pupils left or moved between schools. BMI body mass index, SIMD Scottish Index of Multiple Deprivation

Intervention

The Daily Mile is a school-based physical activity intervention made popular by a primary school in the Stirling Council area, Scotland [1]. It involves children going outside, at a time of the classroom teacher's choosing, for ~15 min of exercise at a pace self-selected by each individual child. This is done during normal classroom time and is in addition to time spent in physical education or scheduled breaks. Typically, it involves laps of a football pitch or playground area. Children often talk as they go and perform a mixture of walking and running. Those who run the whole time will complete ~1 mile in 15 min. Children wear their normal school clothes; most wear their normal school shoes and jackets are only worn in cold or wet weather. It is completed on most days regardless of weather conditions. A leaflet produced by the originator school was given to the school implementing the Daily Mile. No additional instructions for initiation of the Daily Mile were given by the research team.

Participant involvement

The outcome measures selected for the study were chosen based on anecdotal reports of the influence of taking part in the Daily Mile. This information had been gathered from the children, their parents and their teachers by the originator school. The research question, study design and specific outcome measures were developed in part during meetings with the head teacher at the originator school, who was familiar with this information. After publication, the results from this study will be disseminated to the schools involved as copies of the manuscript and infographics, and during question and answer sessions in the schools.

Outcome measures

The primary physiology-related outcome measurements for the WHEEL project were accelerometer-assessed MVPA and sedentary time, fitness assessed using a 20-m shuttle run, and body composition assessed using skinfolds. Additional, cognitive- and well-being-related outcome measurements will be reported elsewhere.

Participant assessments

Baseline assessments (before the intervention) were carried out in October 2015 for the intervention school and March 2016 for the control school. Outcome assessments were completed in May 2016 for the intervention school and June 2016 for the control school. Identical protocols and procedures were used at both assessments. They were undertaken by trained fieldworkers. The fieldworkers worked in groups such that at least one member of each group was disclosure-checked under the Protecting Vulnerable Groups scheme [26]. Children completed tasks in a random order and were given stickers for completing each measurement type. Testing sessions lasted between 1 and 2 h and were carried out over 2 weeks, depending on class size and school timetable.

ActiGraph accelerometers were used to assess physical activity and sedentary time. Five models of accelerometer were used: ActiGraph wGT3X-BT, wGT3X+, GT3X+, GT3X and GT1M. The GT1M and GT3X monitors are comparable when classifying total time spent in specific intensity categories [27]. There is also strong agreement between the GT1M, GT3X and GT3X+ accelerometers, making it acceptable to use them in the same study [28]. The primary difference between the wGT3X-BT and GT3X+ accelerometers is the ability of the wGT3X-BT to communicate wirelessly and all measurements should function identically (personal communication from ActiGraph). Accelerometers were worn around the waist on the left side with the same orientation to standardise the position. Children were asked to wear the belt for eight consecutive days during waking hours (except when bathing or swimming). A poster and instruction sheet with visual and written prompts were provided to each child to remind them of how and when to wear the accelerometer. Upon collection by the research team, the data were downloaded with the ActiLife 6 software (ActiGraph LLC, USA). A valid measurement required at least 10 h wear for 3 days [29]. A 60-s epoch was used and non-wear time was defined as strings of consecutive zeros lasting 60 min or more [30]. The accelerometer output is in counts per minute (cpm). Evenson cut points [31] were used to define time spent being sedentary (≤ 100 cpm) and time spent in MVPA (≥ 2296 cpm). The accelerometer data were corrected for wear time in addition to gender and age in days on the day of testing in the main analysis.

The maximal multistage 20-m shuttle run test [32] was assessed using the Multistage Fitness Test CD (Sports Coach UK, UK) using the standard procedure. Cones marked shuttle boundaries and lanes. Between four (younger) and eight (older) children completed the test at the same time depending on their age group. Instructions and a demonstration of the test were provided prior to each group participating and additional verbal instructions were provided during the test as necessary. The test began at 8.5 km·h^{-1} and after each minute increased by 0.5 km·h^{-1}. When a child was unable to reach the 20-m line prior to the bleep twice in a row, they were asked to stop and their level and shuttle score was recorded. Shuttle run tests were performed outside on tarmac. Age-corrected $\dot{V}O_2$ max scores were created according to the method of [32] for comparison with other studies (Additional file 1: Tables S1–S3). However, this corrects for age in years and therefore, it was not used for the main analysis. Instead, shuttle distance corrected for gender and age in days on day of testing was used to give an improved resolution to the correction in the main analysis.

All skinfold measurements were completed with the child behind a privacy screen with at least two disclosure-checked fieldworkers present. Fieldworkers taking skinfold measurements were trained by an International Society for the Advancement of Kinanthropometry (ISAK) Level 3 instructor prior to involvement in the study and all measurements were taken according to standard ISAK procedures [33]. Triceps, biceps, iliac crest and subscapular skinfolds were measured using Harpenden skinfold callipers (Baty International, UK). All measurements were taken from the right-hand side with the child standing. Where appropriate, they stood on an anthropometric box. Skinfold measurements were summed prior to analysis to give a sum of skinfolds (in millimetres). Skinfold data were corrected for gender and age in days on day of testing in the main analysis.

Height was measured, to the nearest 1 mm, without shoes using the Leicester Height Measure (Seca, UK) according to standard ISAK procedures [33]. Body weight was measured without shoes in light clothing to the nearest 0.1 kg using electronic Sensa 804 scales (Seca, UK). Height (m) and weight (kg) were used to calculate the body mass index (BMI = weight/height^2). BMI z scores relative for age were calculated using UK 1990 reference data in the LMS Growth add-in for Microsoft Excel [34]. Healthy weight was defined as BMI z score < 1.04, overweight as BMI z score of 1.04–1.63 and obesity as BMI z score ≥ 1.64.

All anthropometric measurements were taken twice and the average taken for the analyses. Where there was a substantial difference between the two measurements, a third measurement was taken and the median value was used for the analyses.

Additional Information

Schools provided the date of birth and postcodes for all consented pupils. The date of birth allowed the analyses to be corrected for age on day of testing. The postcode allowed the assignment of the Scottish Index of Multiple Deprivation (SIMD) [35]. SIMD combines data from seven different domains of deprivation into a single score: income, employment, health, education, access to services, crime and housing. However, it should be noted that this gives a postcode-specific deprivation score that may not reflect that of an individual household.

Statistical analyses

Descriptive statistics, Pearson χ^2 and odds ratios were calculated in Excel 2013. Baseline group frequency comparisons were performed using a Pearson χ^2 test. Baseline group mean comparisons were performed using Student's t test (uncorrected) or general linear model ANOVA (corrected for age at time of testing, gender and age*gender). The main analyses were performed in SPSS Statistics (version 21.0.0.1). General linear model regression analyses with repeated measures were used to investigate the effect of doing the Daily Mile. Analyses of all outcome measures included an adjustment for the common confounders: age at time of testing, gender and age*gender. This controls for the effects of age and gender and any different effects of age in the two genders as well as any differences in length of time in the study. Analyses for MVPA and sedentary time were additionally corrected for accelerometer wear time as a covariate. Analyses were conducted first without and then with a correction for SIMD. Standardised mean differences (SMDs), or effect sizes, are calculated as a change measured in the intervention school relative to the control school as a proportion of the pooled standard deviation of the change. An SMD of 0.2–0.5 is considered to be small, an SMD of 0.5–0.8 is considered to be medium and an SMD of 0.8 or above is considered to be large [36]. No correction for multiple testing was made since all four primary outcome measures were anecdotally reported to be influenced by the Daily Mile.

Results

Figure 1 shows the study profile. Overall 77.6% of eligible pupils consented to the study (77.3% in the intervention school and 78.1% in the control school). A total of 371 pupils (247 and 124 in the intervention and control schools respectively) provided at least one measurement in both rounds of testing. All consented children, irrespective of whether they had all measurements or not, are included in Fig. 1. For each outcome measurement, the information in Tables 1 and 2 is based only on children who had measurements at both time points.

Consent for a complete set of measurements was given in the majority of cases; although, on the day of testing, some pupils did not wish to give verbal consent for skinfold measurements, had worn inappropriate clothing for some skinfold measurements or were unable to complete individual tests due to pre-existing minor injuries or ailments. In total, at both baseline and follow-up, between 84% and 94% of originally consented participants had data on fitness and body composition outcomes and the proportions were similar at both baseline and follow-up, in the intervention and control schools and in males and females (Fig. 1).

Three pupils refused to wear accelerometers. The proportion of pupils with valid accelerometer data was lower than other measurements although the proportion of males and females was similar. Only 32% of participants in the intervention school and 67% in the control school had valid accelerometer data at baseline whilst at follow-up 65% and 64% respectively had valid accelerometer data (Fig. 1). This was partially because of the requirement that wearers had at least 10 hours of valid wear time on at least 3 days [31]. However, due to a desire to start doing the Daily Mile as soon as possible in the intervention school

Table 1 Baseline characteristics of participants by study group and gender

	Total	Males	Females	Intervention vs control school (uncorrected)	Intervention vs control school (corrected)
Age (years)	8.4 ± 2.0 (379)	8.3 ± 2.0 (192)	8.4 ± 1.9 (187)	$t = 3.18$	
Intervention school	8.1 ± 2.0 (252)	8.2 ± 2.0 (129)	8.0 ± 1.9 (123)	$SMD = 0.346$	
Control school	8.8 ± 1.8 (127)	8.6 ± 1.8 (63)	9.0 ± 1.8 (64)	$p = 0.002$	
Daily MVPA (min)	55 ± 22 (118)	60 ± 20 (56)	50 ± 22 (62)	$t = 0.766$	$F = 1.982$
Intervention school	53 ± 22 (56)	53 ± 19 (24)	53 ± 24 (32)	$SMD = 0.141$	$SMD = 0.258$
Control school	56 ± 22 (62)	66 ± 19 (32)	47 ± 20 (30)	$p = 0.445$	$p = 0.162$
Daily sedentary time (min)	345 ± 74 (118)	338 ± 80 (56)	352 ± 67 (62)	$t = 1.142$	$F = 7.543$
Intervention school	337 ± 77 (56)	327 ± 84 (24)	344 ± 71 (32)	$SMD = 0.210$	$SMD = 0.493$
Control school	352 ± 71 (62)	346 ± 78 (32)	360 ± 63 (30)	$p = 0.256$	$p = 0.007$
Total shuttle distance (m)	670 ± 351 (357)	748 ± 399 (183)	589 ± 271 (174)	$t = 1.944$	$F = 0.294$
Intervention school	645 ± 351 (240)	719 ± 397 (124)	566 ± 276 (116)	$SMD = 0.219$	$SMD = 0.061$
Control school	722 ± 347 (117)	807 ± 400 (59)	635 ± 258 (58)	$p = 0.053$	$p = 0.588$
Sum of skinfolds (mm)	35.1 ± 14.7 (327)	32.6 ± 14.9 (175)	38.1 ± 13.9 (152)	$t = 2.214$	$F = 2.117$
Intervention school	33.8 ± 12.7 (213)	31.7 ± 13.5 (115)	36.4 ± 11.2 (98)	$SMD = 0.257$	$SMD = 0.169$
Control school	37.6 ± 17.6 (114)	34.4 ± 17.3 (60)	41.1 ± 17.4 (54)	$p = 0.028$	$p = 0.147$
% meeting physical activity guidelines	36.4% (118)	46.4% (56)	27.4% (62)	$\chi^2 = 4.29, p = 0.038$ OR = 2.251 (1.037–4.884), $p = 0.040$	
Intervention school	26.8% (56)	25.0% (24)	28.1% (32)		
Control school	45.2% (62)	62.5% (32)	26.7% (30)		
% overweight or obese	16.8% (369)	18.6% (188)	14.9% (181)	$\chi^2 = 0.01, p = 0.922$ OR = 1.029 (0.578–1.833), $p = 0.928$	
Intervention school	16.7% (246)	19.0% (126)	14.2% (120)		
Control school	17.1% (123)	17.7% (62)	16.4% (61)		

Values in columns 2–4 are means ± SD (*n* value) or percentage (*n* value). Comparisons are by *t* test or χ^2 and odds ratio. Corrected values are from ANOVA including correction for age, gender and age*gender. Shuttle distance is given to the nearest metre. Accelerometer minutes are given to the nearest minute. It was not possible to correct percentage values for age and gender. MVPA and sedentary time were also corrected for wear time. This table includes only participants with valid measurements both before and after the intervention

MVPA moderate to vigorous intensity physical activity, OR odds ratio, SD standard deviation, SMD standardised mean difference

and a limited number of accelerometers (117), it was possible to collect true baseline data (i.e. prior to beginning the Daily Mile) from only a portion of the intervention school participants. These participants were selected at random based on the availability of pupils for the other physiological tests.

The baseline characteristics of the participants are given in Table 1. Age was significantly higher in the control school at baseline due to the difference in the time of baseline measurements meaning that the pupils were slightly further through the academic year at the control school (Table 1). The percentage meeting the physical activity guidelines of 60+ min MVPA per day and the sum of skinfolds were both higher in the control school. However, after correction for age, gender and age*gender, only sedentary time differed significantly between the schools at baseline, suggesting that the correct confounders were accounted for in the analysis. Additionally, the intra-school differences between genders and year groups were similar (Additional file 1: Table S1).

SIMD scores were similar across schools ($\chi^2 = 1.299$, $p = 0.254$). For quintiles 4–5 (least deprived), the scores were 71% versus 65%, respectively, for the intervention school and control school. For quintiles 1–3 (most deprived), the scores were 29% versus 35%. These reflect the lower deprivation than the average across Scotland [35], since ~20% would be expected in each quintile. However, this excess of children from less deprived areas reduces the likelihood of observing an impact of the Daily Mile, rather than creating any potential artefacts, as the children are more likely to be fitter and less likely to be overweight or obese [22, 23] at baseline. Nonetheless, children from areas with lower socioeconomic scores (quintiles 1–3) had similar minutes of MVPA and sedentary time compared to those with higher socioeconomic scores (quintiles 4–5). They were also equally likely to meet the physical activity guidelines. However, they had lower shuttle distance, and a higher sum of skinfolds and rates of overweight and obesity (Table 2). A full breakdown of baseline characteristics by socioeconomic group, school and gender is given in Additional file 1: Table S2.

In the main analysis, after adjustment for the common confounders of age, gender and age*gender, significant improvements were observed in the intervention school

Table 2 Baseline characteristics of participants by study group and SIMD

	Total	SIMD 4–5	SIMD 1–3	SIMD 1–3 vs SIMD 4–5
Age (years)	8.4 ± 2.0 (379)	8.4 ± 1.9 (264)	8.4 ± 2.0 (115)	$t = 0.033$
Intervention school	8.1 ± 2.0 (252)	8.1 ± 2.0 (182)	8.2 ± 2.1 (70)	SMD = 0.004
Control school	8.8 ± 1.8 (127)	8.9 ± 1.8 (82)	8.6 ± 1.8 (45)	$p = 0.974$
Daily MVPA (min)	55 ± 22 (118)	56 ± 21 (92)	51 ± 25 (26)	$t = 1.024$
Intervention school	53 ± 22 (56)	52 ± 19 (42)	57 ± 29 (14)	SMD = 0.227
Control school	56 ± 22 (62)	60 ± 22 (50)	44 ± 17 (12)	$p = 0.308$
Daily sedentary time (min)	345 ± 74 (118)	342 ± 70 (92)	356 ± 86 (26)	$t = 0.879$
Intervention school	337 ± 77 (56)	337 ± 70 (42)	337 ± 97 (14)	SMD = 0.195
Control school	352 ± 71 (62)	346 ± 70 (50)	378 ± 70 (12)	$p = 0.381$
Total shuttle distance (m)	670 ± 351 (357)	702 ± 368 (252)	593 ± 294 (105)	$t = 2.695$
Intervention school	645 ± 351 (240)	658 ± 365 (173)	613 ± 314 (67)	SMD = 0.313
Control school	722 ± 347 (117)	800 ± 359 (79)	559 ± 255 (38)	$p = 0.007$
Sum of skinfolds (mm)	35.1 ± 14.7 (327)	32.9 ± 13.0 (229)	40.4 ± 16.9 (98)	$t = 4.350$
Intervention school	33.8 ± 12.7 (213)	32.4 ± 11.9 (154)	37.5 ± 14.0 (59)	SMD = 0.525
Control school	37.6 ± 17.6 (114)	33.8 ± 15.0 (75)	44.8 ± 20.0 (39)	$p < 0.001$
% meeting physical activity guidelines	36.4% (118)	39.1% (92)	26.9% (26)	$\chi^2 = 1.304$, $p = 0.253$
Intervention school	26.8% (56)	26.2% (42)	28.6% (14)	OR = 0.573 (0.219–1.500), $p = 0.260$
Control school	45.2% (62)	50.0% (50)	25.0% (12)	
% overweight or obese	16.8% (369)	12.4% (259)	27.3% (110)	$\chi^2 = 12.291$, $p < 0.001$
Intervention school	16.7% (246)	12.4% (178)	27.9% (68)	OR = 2.660 (1.520–4.655), $p < 0.001$
Control school	17.1% (123)	12.3% (81)	26.2% (42)	

Values in columns 2–4 are means ± SD (*n* value) or percentage (*n* value). Comparisons are by *t* test or χ^2 and odds ratio. Shuttle distance is given to the nearest metre. Accelerometer minutes are given to the nearest minute. This table includes only participants with valid measurements both before and after the intervention
MVPA moderate to vigorous intensity physical activity, *OR* odds ratio, *SD* standard deviation, *SIMD* Scottish Index of Multiple Deprivation, *SMD* standardised mean difference

relative to the control school for MVPA (+9.1 min), sedentary time (−18.2 min), fitness (+39.1 m) and body composition (−1.4 mm; Table 3). These relationships persisted after including a correction for SIMD (Table 3). Baseline values and change in BMI *z* score and age-corrected $\dot{V}O_2$ max scores are given in Additional file 1: Table S1–S3 only for comparison with other studies.

A change in MVPA predicted a change in sedentary behaviour ($r = -0.559$, $n = 118$, $p < 0.001$; Fig. 2a) but did not predict changes in other primary outcome variables. A change in shuttle distance predicted a change in sum of skinfolds ($r = -0.203$, $n = 317$, $p < 0.001$; Fig. 2b) but did not predict changes in other primary outcome variables. These correlations were not significantly altered by the

Table 3 Effect of introducing the Daily Mile on outcomes assessed immediately after the end of the intervention period

Outcome	Difference in change between schools after correction for age, gender and age*gender			Difference in change between schools after correction for age, gender, age*gender and SIMD		
	Mean (95% CI)	SMD	*p* value	Mean (95% CI)	SMD	*p* value
Mean MVPA per day (min)	9.1 (5.1 to 13.2)	0.407	0.027	9.5 (5.4 to 13.5)	0.422	0.021
Mean sedentary time per day (min)	-18.2 (−10.7 to −25.7)	0.437	0.017	-18.1 (−10.6 to − 25.6)	0.435	0.018
Total shuttle distance (m)	39.1 (21.9 to 56.3)	0.236	0.037	37.2 (20.1 to 54.3)	0.225	0.046
Sum of skinfolds (mm)	-1.4 (−2.0 to −0.8)	0.246	0.034	-1.4 (−2.0 to − 0.8)	0.258	0.026

SMD is calculated as the change in the intervention school relative to the control school as a proportion of the standard deviation of the change. Analyses were conducted using GLM-ANOVA corrected for age, gender, age*gender ± SIMD with repeated measures for the outcome. Sedentary time and MVPA were also corrected for accelerometer wear time
95% CI 95% confidence interval, *MVPA* moderate to vigorous intensity physical activity, *SIMD* Scottish Index of Multiple Deprivation, *SMD* standardised mean difference

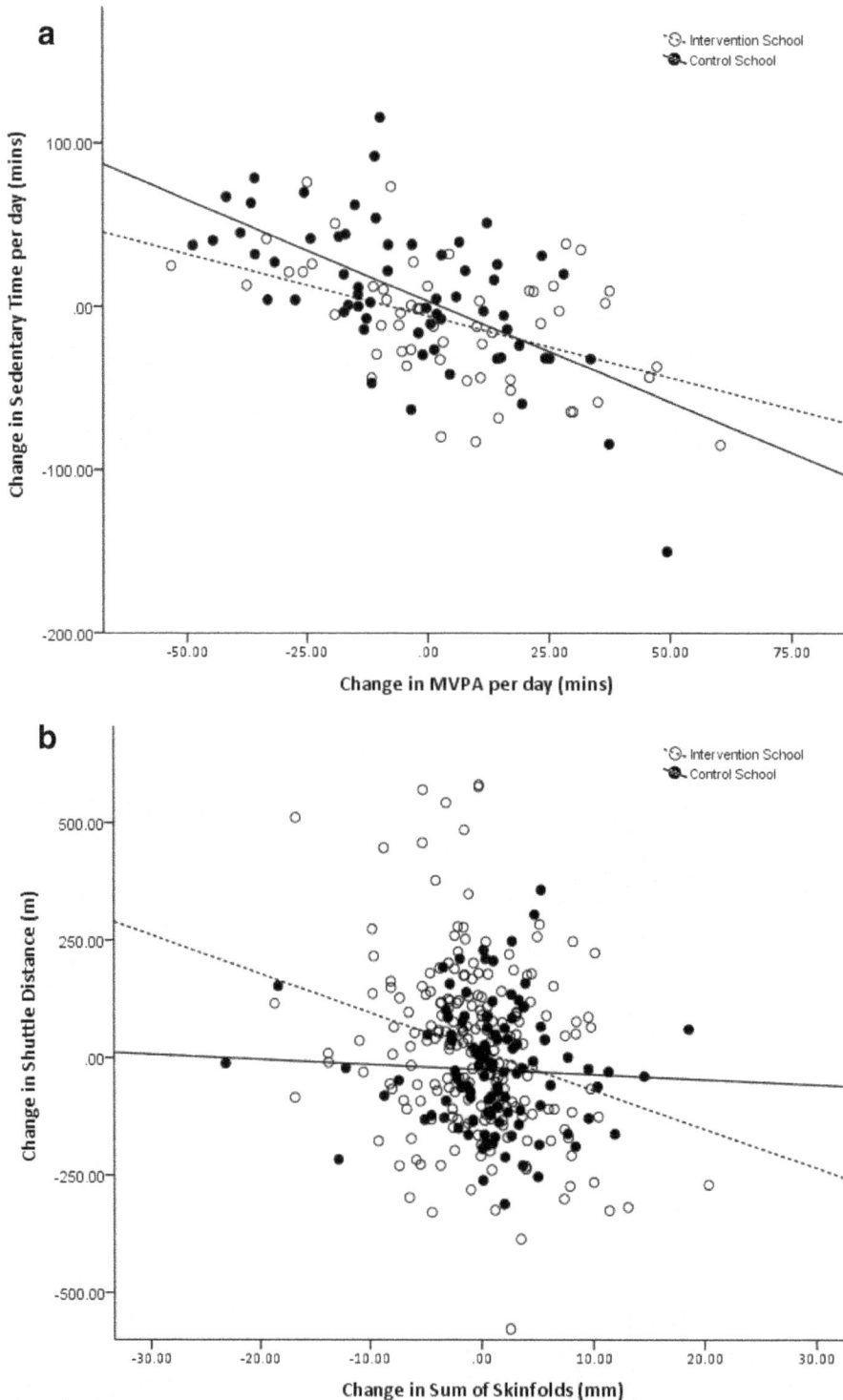

Fig. 2 Relationship between change in (**a**) MVPA and sedentary behaviour and (**b**) shuttle distance and sum of skinfolds. Both graphs are drawn after correction for gender, age in days and gender*age in days. MVPA moderate to vigorous intensity physical activity

inclusion of SIMD ($r = -0.564$ and -0.212, respectively) although a change in MVPA additionally predicted a change in shuttle distance ($r = 0.187$, $n = 115$, $p = 0.046$). However, the relationship between a change in sum of skinfolds and a change in shuttle distance differed by school (interaction $p = 0.043$). The relationship was stronger for the intervention school than the control school ($r = -0.245$ and -0.046, respectively). The relationship between a change in MVPA and a change in sedentary be-haviour was not different by school (interaction $p = 0.896$). However, it should be noted that the calculations for MVPA and sedentary time are linked by the finite number of mi-nutes in a day and a change in one is likely to result in a change in the other.

Discussion

In this primary-school-based quasi-experimental pilot study, which investigated the effects of taking part in the Daily Mile, we found evidence of a positive effect on our four primary outcomes—accelerometer-assessed time spent in MVPA, accelerometer-assessed time spent in sed-entary behaviour, physical fitness and body composition—after correcting for the common confounders of age and gender with or without socioeconomic grouping.

Comparisons with other studies

Whilst no other studies have investigated the effect of taking part in the Daily Mile, some have investigated the effect of increasing physical activity throughout the school day or introducing short physical activity breaks into the school day itself [37, 38]. On the whole, they have had mixed results, with some finding alterations in MVPA and others not. This is likely in part due to the different methods used to assess these behaviours, in part due to the different interventions involved and in part due to the different accelerometer cut-points that can be found in the literature. Additionally, some studies use self-reported physical activity measures, which although easier to ad-minister on a large scale, can lead to differing estimates in comparison to accelerometry [39]. Undoubtedly, the age and demographic of the children also has an influence and an intervention that works in one setting may not work in another.

Similarly, some studies have found changes in body composition or fitness whilst others have not [40–42]. The observed effect of the Daily Mile on fitness in the current study may be a result of the type of intervention activity involved (i.e. running) being similar to the fitness test. However, few studies have taken detailed physio-logical measurements and often assess BMI only. Changes in BMI are observed with some physical activity interven-tions but mostly in high-BMI groups. The decrease in the sum of skinfolds observed in this study without a con-comitant change in BMI z score is likely due to the higher resolution of skinfolds and its utility in assessing body fat-ness without the confounding effect of muscle mass.

Meaning of study findings

Scottish government figures suggest that 73% of children in Scotland (77% of boys and 69% of girls) meet the physical activity guidelines [14]. However, this figure is based on self-reported questionnaire results rather than

accelerometer assessment and is likely to contain bias [43, 44]. Estimates by accelerometer of the percentage of children meeting the physical activity guidelines vary across Europe, from as low as 2% to as high as 63% [11, 45]. The children in this study fall within this range and are likely typical of Scottish and European primary school children [46, 47]. Regardless of how many meet the minimum recommended guidelines (at least 60 min per day), higher levels of MVPA are generally considered to be better. This study shows that introducing the Daily Mile into a primary school setting does increase the MVPA of children by 9. 1 min (SMD = 0.407). Although the Daily Mile is a 15-min physical activity intervention, an increase of ~9 min is consistent with the pattern of running interspersed with periods of walking and chatting that is observed in children taking part (personal observations). Although the SMD would be considered to be small according to Cohen [36], small effects on a prevalent behaviour, such as physical in-activity, may have a high impact at the level of population health [48]. In addition, a change of this magnitude is close to the 10 min increase in MVPA previously associated with meaningful reductions in cardiometabolic risk in children and adolescents [49].

Sedentary time is less well studied than physical activ-ity. Nonetheless, the available evidence suggests that the children in this study are typical of European children [11, 45]. In some studies, sedentary time appears to be a predictor of chronic disease independent of physical activity levels [50]. Two aspects of sedentary behaviour appear to be key to this: total sedentary time and prolonged blocks of sedentary time. The Daily Mile is potentially able to address both these issues although the present analysis only investi-gates total sedentary time. Although children at the inter-vention school were less sedentary at the baseline (after correction for the common confounders), this would make it harder to observe a reduction in sedentary behaviour ra-ther than easier. Despite this, this study shows an ~18 min reduction (SMD = 0.437) in average daily sedentary time with the introduction of the Daily Mile. Again, this is con-sistent with a target of 15 min of physical activity since the children will at least be up from their chairs for a slightly longer period. However, if done correctly, the Daily Mile also breaks up the sedentary time, as it should happen in the middle of lessons, so that the children are likely to be sitting before and after their Daily Mile. As for MVPA, the SMD would be considered to be small but may well have significant impacts on population health due to mass participation. Additionally, the data also show a strong correlation between increasing MVPA and redu-cing sedentary time. This suggests that children are not compensating for the increase in MVPA during the Daily Mile by sitting more at other times of the day: they are re-placing sedentary time with MVPA. However, note that the calculations for MVPA and sedentary time are linked by the finite number of minutes in a day and may be more appropriately analysed in future studies using a compositional data analysis.

The children in the IDEFICS study [51] have median values of age-corrected $\dot{V}O_2$ max scores between 46.7 and 48.1 ml·kg^{-1}·min^{-1} for boys and between 45.4 and 47.4 ml·kg^{-1}·min^{-1} for girls between the ages of 6 and 9 years. Relatively, the children in the current study could be considered to have high aerobic fitness (see Additional file 1: Tables S1 and S2 for age-corrected $\dot{V}O_2$ max scores). This high baseline fitness would make it less likely that a change in fitness could be observed after a small increase in physical activity. Nonetheless, an improvement in fitness, as measured by shuttle distance (39.1 m, SMD = 0.236), was observed with the introduction of the Daily Mile. $\dot{V}O_2$ max is linked with cardiovascular health and all-cause mortality [52]. Although the SMD would be considered to be small, it may have a significant impact on a population scale. The CARDIA study in young adults suggests that having a $\dot{V}O_2$ max of 3.5 ml·kg^{-1}·min^{-1} (approximately 1 metabolic equivalent) higher gives a reduction in all-cause mortality of ~15% [53]. Whilst we only see a relative increase of ~0.35 ml·kg^{-1}·min^{-1} (Additional file 1: Table S3) with the Daily Mile, this is still predictive of an ~1.5% reduction in all-cause mortality risk. Note that the conversion from shuttle distance to $\dot{V}O_2$ max includes age in years and has, therefore, relatively lower resolution. It has also been suggested that having a higher cardiorespiratory fitness at a younger age confers the greatest survival benefit [52]. Furthermore, those with lower starting values appear likely to benefit to a greater extent [54]. This suggests that there are potentially useful health benefits associated with taking part in the Daily Mile.

The children at both schools in this study had lower rates of overweight and obesity than are typical of Scottish children. The Scottish Health Survey reports overweight and obesity rates in 7–11 year olds as 30% (29% for boys and 32% for girls) [14]. Again, this makes it less likely that a change in adiposity could be observed after a small increase in physical activity. Still, a reduction in adiposity as measured by skinfold (1.4 mm, SMD = 0.246) was observed with the introduction of the Daily Mile. Again, although the SMD would be considered to be small, at the population level it may have significant impacts on levels of adiposity. It is also possible that the impact of the Daily Mile on body composition may be larger still in children with higher rates of overweight and obesity. This intervention may be a useful component within measures designed to help tackle the obesity pandemic [8]. The strong correlation between those who reduced their skinfolds the most and those who gained the most fitness may indicate a common cause. Given that the pace each child completes the Daily Mile at is self-determined, it is possible that the children who gained the most benefits took a particular

approach to the Daily Mile. An insight into this may come when we interview the children taking part in the Daily Mile about their experiences.

Evidence linking socioeconomic status to MVPA and sedentary behaviour is unclear [13]. This is in part due to the use of different methods of capturing these outcome measures but also due to different ways of assessing socioeconomic status in different countries. Nonetheless, these outcome measures do appear to associate with specific aspects of socioeconomic status in some studies. However, clear differences between higher and lower socioeconomic groupings could be seen in the current study for fitness and body composition: children from postcodes with higher deprivation had lower levels of fitness, higher sums of skinfolds and higher rates of overweight and obesity. This is consistent with the widely recognised health inequality gap [55]. However, no differences were seen between the socioeconomic groupings in response to the introduction of the Daily Mile, suggesting that it may be beneficial to all groups regardless of background. Note that this study was not intended to investigate this, and larger more powerful studies are needed to investigate this aspect of the Daily Mile. A summary of the study and its implications can be found in Box 1.

Strengths and limitations of study

This study is the first to investigate the widely publicised and adopted Daily Mile physical activity intervention. The intervention appears to be increasingly popular and has now been maintained in the originator school for more than five years. Thus, it is undoubtedly feasible to deliver and has been adopted locally in many areas. What was unknown was the efficacy for the anecdotally reported physiological benefits of taking part in the Daily Mile. Consent rates were high (>77% in both schools) as were the number of children successfully assessed at both time points for most outcome measures. We assessed MVPA and sedentary time using the gold standard accelerometer technique, we assessed fitness using the bleep test (which has been validated in this age group) and we assessed body composition using labour-intensive skinfold assessments rather than the more straightforward but lower resolution BMI.

We acknowledge that there was a difference in sedentary time between the schools at baseline and the socioeconomic groupings were not reflective of the whole of Scotland, which are limitations of our study. However, these differences would be predicted to make any effects of the Daily Mile harder to observe, not easier. Changes were observed despite these differences. It would have been preferable to assess both the intervention and control schools at the same time of year to avoid any seasonal impact on physical activity. However, we believe that October and March should be similar enough to allow comparison [56]. Additionally, it would have been better to have had both

Box 1: What this study adds

Why was this study done?

- Low physical activity, high sedentary behaviour, declining fitness levels and high levels of overweight and obesity are global problems that have been targeted by the World Health Organisation.
- The Daily Mile is an increasingly popular school-based physical activity intervention, backed by the Scottish government, which is anecdotally reported to lead to increased physical activity, reduced sedentary time, improved fitness and improved body composition. Pupils run or walk laps of the playground at a self-selected pace for 15 min during normal classroom time. It is increasingly popular throughout the UK, in parts of Europe and some schools in the USA.
- However, these reported benefits remain anecdotal and need to be quantitatively and objectively assessed to ensure that the loss of academic classroom time is providing the reported alternative benefits.

What did the researchers do and find?

- Two schools in the Stirling Council area, Scotland, were recruited: one with intention to start the Daily Mile, the other without.
- Researchers assessed the physical activity and sedentary behaviour of children using accelerometers, their fitness using the bleep test and their body composition using skinfolds. This was done in both schools before and after the intervention school introduced the Daily Mile.
- This quasi-experimental pilot study found that, after correcting for age, gender and socioeconomic grouping, taking part in the Daily Mile did lead to an improvement in physical activity, sedentary behaviour, fitness and body composition of children in the intervention school relative to the control school.

What do these findings mean?

- This suggests that the Daily Mile is a worthwhile intervention to introduce in schools and that it should be considered for inclusion in government policy.
- This study can underpin the policy already introduced by the Scottish government and the development of future policy in other parts of the UK and abroad.

schools involved in the study for the same length of time, although, correcting for age and gender should account for this difference. It is also possible that differences in the health and well-being policies within the schools contributed to differences in the results. However, the schools were selected to be from the same local authority and to be of similar socioeconomic make-up to minimise potential differences. As predicted, changes in outcome variables had effect sizes at the smaller end of the distribution (0.2–0.5). However, given the involvement of whole classes, small effects could have an important impact on population health. To gain further confidence in the results, this study should be replicated in a larger number of schools. Furthermore, no monitoring of adherence, or level of adherence, to the intervention was carried out, although the results suggest adherence was sufficient.

Unanswered questions and future research

Additional anecdotally reported benefits to the Daily Mile (cognition, behaviour and well-being) are currently being investigated [57, 58]. It is essential that the current studies are replicated in a larger number of schools and countries to ensure that the findings are both robust and repeatable in different educational contexts. Future studies should include diet and sleep quality, which we are not yet investigating, to explore the potential mechanisms of impact. More attention should be given to when the Daily Mile is being done during the school day and whether it is breaking up sedentary time. Additionally, future studies should investigate whether MVPA and sedentary behaviour are changing on weekdays and/or weekend days.

In 2015, the Scottish government launched the Scottish Attainment Challenge with the aim of achieving equity in educational outcomes for all Scottish children [59]. Whilst the current study found no difference in the response to the Daily Mile by socioeconomic grouping, both schools were heavily weighted towards less deprived catchment areas. Furthermore, the current study was not powered to detect such a complex interaction. The Daily Mile is a free, simple intervention that can be rolled out to schools regardless of socioeconomic status. It is necessary to conduct carefully designed studies to understand the impact of the Daily Mile in different socioeconomic settings and to understand whether it can have any impact on the attainment gap.

The sample of children participating in this study included a number with challenging behaviours including autism spectrum disorders. Nonetheless, they took part in the Daily Mile and our investigations. Understanding the impact of the Daily Mile on children with differing learning needs should also be a future priority.

This study shows the value of introducing the Daily Mile into schools. Whilst the Daily Mile has been introduced as policy across Scotland, many schools do not have appropriate outdoor facilities to allow their children to take part. One of the challenges for policymakers and other stakeholders is to consider how to introduce the Daily Mile or alternative interventions that have been shown to increase MVPA and fitness into such schools or how to adapt those schools to allow the introduction of appropriate interventions.

Conclusions

In conclusion, introducing the Daily Mile to the primary school day appears to be an effective intervention for increasing MVPA and reducing sedentary time and it has measurable impacts on key aspects of metabolic health: body composition and physical fitness. This study provides the first assessment of the Daily Mile and it will allow the development of evidence-based policy around introducing the Daily Mile to more schools.

Abbreviations

95%CI: 95% confidence interval; BMI: Body mass index; cpm: Counts per minute; ISAK: International Society for the Advancement of Kinanthropometry; MVPA: Moderate to vigorous intensity physical activity; PE: Physical education; SIMD: Scottish Index of Multiple Deprivation; SMD: Standardised mean difference; WHEEL: Well-being, Health, Exercise, Enjoyment and Learning; WHO: World Health Organisation

Acknowledgements

We thank the teachers, pupils and parents of all the primary schools for taking part in this research project. We thank Stirling Council for facilitating this research project. We thank Elaine Wyllie for her advice in selecting outcome measures and in developing and facilitating the study. We thank all the volunteers involved in data collection for giving up their time: these included undergraduate students, postgraduate students, former students, academic staff from the universities and teachers and parents from the schools. We would particularly like to thank Xinming Zhang, Jack Martin, Yong Sonn Breslin and Iain Mitchell, who gave up large amounts of their time to make this research possible.

Funding

This research project was partially funded from internal sources at the University of Stirling and the University of Edinburgh. The funders had no role in study design, data collection and analysis, decision to publish or preparation of the manuscript.

Authors' contributions

JNB, GCR, TG, NEB and CNM were involved in the design of the study and in seeking funding for it. JNB, RAC, ES, NEB and CNM were responsible for conducting the study. RAC and CNM wrote the first draft of the paper, and CNM coordinated contributions from other co-authors. CNM wrote the analysis plan used for this paper, and RAC and CNM completed all analyses. JNB, RAC, NEB and CNM managed the data collection with input from other members of the study team. All authors made critical comments on drafts of the paper. CNM is the guarantor. All authors read and approved the final manuscript.

Competing interests

The authors declare that they have no competing interests.

Author details

[1]Faculty of Health Sciences and Sport, University of Stirling, Scotland FK9 4LA, UK. [2]Institute of Education, Community and Society, Moray House School of Education, University of Edinburgh, Scotland EH8 8AQ, UK. [3]Present address: School of Health, Social Care and Life Sciences, University of the Highlands and Islands, Centre for Health Sciences, Old Perth Road, Inverness IV2 3JH, UK.

References

1. Stirling Council: The Daily Mile - Health and Wellbeing for free. 2015.
2. Daily Mile roll out [https://news.gov.scot/news/daily-mile-roll-out]. Accessed 17 Apr 2018.
3. Obesity: Children: Written question - 46791 [http://www.parliament.uk/business/publications/written-questions-answers-statements/written-question/Commons/2016-10-07/46791]. Accessed 17 Apr 2018.
4. Early day motion 1074: Five Year Anniversary of Daily Mile [http://www.parliament.uk/edm/2016-17/1074]. Accessed 17 Apr 2018.
5. The Daily Mile [http://thedailymile.co.uk/]. Accessed 17 Apr 2018.
6. Kohl HW, Craig CL, Lambert EV, Inoue S, Alkandari JR, Leetongin G, Kahlmeier S. The pandemic of physical inactivity: global action for public health. Lancet. 2012;380(9838):294–305.
7. Telama R, Yang X, Viikari J, Valimaki I, Wanne O, Raitakari O. Physical activity from childhood to adulthood: a 21-year tracking study. Am J Prev Med. 2005;28(3):267–73.
8. Mendis S. Global status report on noncommunicable diseases 2014. Geneva: WHO; 2014.
9. World Health Organisation: Physical activity fact sheet. 2017.
10. Department of Health: Start active, stay active: a report on physical activity from the four home countries' Chief Medical Officers. 2011.
11. Konstabel K, Veidebaum T, Verbestel V, Moreno LA, Bammann K, Tornaritis M, Eiben G, Molnar D, Siani A, Sprengeler O, et al. Objectively measured physical activity in European children: the IDEFICS study. Int J Obes. 2014; 38(Suppl 2):S135–43.
12. Esliger D, Hall J. Health Survey for England. In: Centre TNI, editor, vol. 1. London: Department of Epidemiology and Public Health, UCL Medical School; 2008.
13. Biddle SJH, Atkin AJ, Cavill N, Foster C. Correlates of physical activity in youth: a review of quantitative systematic reviews. Int Rev Sport Exer P. 2011;4(1):25–49.
14. Brown L, Campbell-Jack D, Gray L, Hovald P, Kirkpatrick G, Knudsen L, Leyland AH, Montagu I, Rose J. The Scottish Health Survey. In. Scotland ANSPf, editor. 2016. http://www.gov.scot/Publications/2016/09/2764/0.
15. Conolly A. Health Survey for England 2015 Children's body mass index, overweight and obesity. In: Centre HaSCI, editor. London: Health and Social Care Information Centre; 2016.
16. Tomkinson GR, Leger LA, Olds TS, Cazorla G. Secular trends in the performance of children and adolescents (1980–2000): an analysis of 55 studies of the 20m shuttle run test in 11 countries. Sports Med. 2003;33(4):285–300.

17. Biddle SJ, Gorely T, Stensel DJ. Health-enhancing physical activity and sedentary behaviour in children and adolescents. J Sports Sci. 2004;22(8):679–701.

18. Lee IM, Shiroma EJ, Lobelo F, Puska P, Blair SN, Katzmarzyk PT, Lancet Physical Activity Series Working G. Effect of physical inactivity on major non-communicable diseases worldwide: an analysis of burden of disease and life expectancy. Lancet. 2012;380(9838):219–29.

19. Must A, Tybor DJ. Physical activity and sedentary behavior: a review of longitudinal studies of weight and adiposity in youth. Int J Obes. 2005;29(Suppl 2):S84–96.

20. Vos MB, Welsh J. Childhood obesity: update on predisposing factors and prevention strategies. Curr Gastroenterol Rep. 2010;12(4):280–7.

21. Weiss R, Dziura J, Burgert TS, Tamborlane WV, Taksali SE, Yeckel CW, Allen K, Lopes M, Savoye M, Morrison J, et al. Obesity and the metabolic syndrome in children and adolescents. N Engl J Med. 2004;350(23):2362–74.

22. Jimenez-Pavon D, Ortega FB, Ruiz JR, Chillon P, Castillo R, Artero EG, Martinez-Gomez D, Vicente-Rodriguez G, Rey-Lopez JP, Gracia LA, et al. Influence of socioeconomic factors on fitness and fatness in Spanish adolescents: the AVENA study. Int J Pediatr Obes. 2010;5(6):467–73.

23. Wang Y, Lim H. The global childhood obesity epidemic and the association between socio-economic status and childhood obesity. Int Rev Psychiatry. 2012;24(3):176–88.

24. Poitras VJ, Gray CE, Borghese MM, Carson V, Chaput JP, Janssen I, Katzmarzyk PT, Pate RR, Connor Gorber S, Kho ME, et al. Systematic review of the relationships between objectively measured physical activity and health indicators in school-aged children and youth. Appl Physiol Nutr Metab. 2016;41(6 Suppl 3):S197–239.

25. Foulds HJ, Bredin SS, Charlesworth SA, Ivey AC, Warburton DE. Exercise volume and intensity: a dose-response relationship with health benefits. Eur J Appl Physiol. 2014;114(8):1563–71.

26. Disclosure Scotland Website [https://www.mygov.scot/about-disclosure-scotland/]. Accessed 17 Apr 2018.

27. Hanggi JM, Phillips LR, Rowlands AV. Validation of the GT3X ActiGraph in children and comparison with the GT1M ActiGraph. J Sci Med Sport. 2013;16(1):40–4.

28. Robusto KM, Trost SG. Comparison of three generations of ActiGraph activity monitors in children and adolescents. J Sports Sci. 2012;30(13):1429–35.

29. Penpraze V, Reilly JJ, MacLean CM, Montgomery C, Kelly LA, Paton JY, Aitchison T, Grant S. Monitoring of physical activity in young children: How much is enough? Pediatr Exerc Sci. 2006;18(4):483–91.

30. Cooper AR, Goodman A, Page AS, Sherar LB, Esliger DW, van Sluijs EM, Andersen LB, Anderssen S, Cardon G, Davey R, et al. Objectively measured physical activity and sedentary time in youth: the International children's accelerometry database (ICAD). Int J Behav Nutr Phys Act. 2015;12:113.

31. Evenson KR, Catellier DJ, Gill K, Ondrak KS, McMurray RG. Calibration of two objective measures of physical activity for children. J Sports Sci. 2008;26(14):1557–65.

32. Leger LA, Mercier D, Gadoury C, Lambert J. The multistage 20 metre shuttle run test for aerobic fitness. J Sports Sci. 1988;6(2):93–101.

33. Norton K, Carter L, Olds T, Marfell-Jones M: International standards for anthropometric assessment; 2011.

34. Pan H, Cole TJ: LMSgrowth, a Microsoft Excel add-in to access growth references based on the LMS method. Version 2.74. 2011.

35. Postcode to Scottish Index of Multiple Deprivation (SIMD) rank [http://www.gov.scot/Topics/Statistics/SIMD]. Accessed 17 Apr 2018.

36. Cohen J. Statistical Power Analysis for the Behavioral Sciences. Routledge Academic: New York, NY; 1988.

37. Barr-Anderson DJ, AuYoung M, Whitt-Glover MC, Glenn BA, Yancey AK. Integration of short bouts of physical activity into organizational routine a systematic review of the literature. Am J Prev Med. 2011;40(1):76–93.

38. Norris E, Shelton N, Dunsmuir S, Duke-Williams O, Stamatakis E. Physically active lessons as physical activity and educational interventions: a systematic review of methods and results. Prev Med. 2015;72:116–25.

39. Reilly JJ, Penpraze V, Hislop J, Davies G, Grant S, Paton JY. Objective measurement of physical activity and sedentary behaviour: review with new data. Arch Dis Child. 2008;93(7):614–9.

40. Dobbins M, Husson H, DeCorby K, LaRocca RL: School-based physical activity programs for promoting physical activity and fitness in children and adolescents aged 6 to 18. Cochrane Database Syst Rev. 2013(2):CD007651. https://doi.org/10.1002/14651858.CD007651.pub2.

41. Harris KC, Kuramoto LK, Schulzer M, Retallack JE. Effect of school-based physical activity interventions on body mass index in children: a meta-analysis. CMAJ. 2009;180(7):719–26.

42. Mei H, Xiong Y, Xie S, Guo S, Li Y, Guo B, Zhang J. The impact of long-term school-based physical activity interventions on body mass index of primary school children - a meta-analysis of randomized controlled trials. BMC Public Health. 2016;16:205.

43. Ekelund U, Tomkinson G, Armstrong N. What proportion of youth are physically active? Measurement issues, levels and recent time trends. Br J Sports Med. 2011;45(11):859–65.

44. Basterfield L, Adamson AJ, Parkinson KN, Maute U, Li PX, Reilly JJ. Gateshead Millennium Study Core T: Surveillance of physical activity in the UK is flawed: validation of the Health Survey for England Physical Activity Questionnaire. Arch Dis Child. 2008;93(12):1054–8.

45. Griffiths LJ, Cortina-Borja M, Sera F, Pouliou T, Geraci M, Rich C, Cole TJ, Law C, Joshi H, Ness AR, et al. How active are our children? Findings from the Millennium Cohort Study. BMJ Open. 2013;3(8):e002893.

46. World Health Organisation. Growing up unequal: gender and socioeconomic differences in young people's health and well-being. In: Inchley J, Currie D, Young T, Samdal O, Torsheim T, Augustson L, Mathison F, Aleman-Diaz A, Molcho M, Weber M, et al., editors. Health Behaviour in School-aged Children (HBSC) study: international report from the 2013/2014 survey. Copenhagen: WHO Regional Office for Europe; 2016.

47. World Health Organisation. Adolescent obesity and related behaviours: trends and inequalities in the WHO European Region, 2002–2014. In: Inchley J, Currie D, Jewell J, Breda J, Barnekow V, editors. Observations from the Health Behaviour in School-aged Children (HBSC) WHO collaborative cross-national study. Copenhagen: WHO Regional Office for Europe; 2017.

48. Biddle SJ, O'Connell S, Braithwaite RE. Sedentary behaviour interventions in young people: a meta-analysis. Br J Sports Med. 2011;45(11):937–42.

49. Ekelund U, Luan J, Sherar LB, Esliger DW, Griew P, Cooper A, International Children's Accelerometry Database C. Moderate to vigorous physical activity and sedentary time and cardiometabolic risk factors in children and adolescents. JAMA. 2012;307(7):704–12.

50. Endorsed by The Obesity S, Young DR, Hivert MF, Alhassan S, Camhi SM, Ferguson JF, Katzmarzyk PT, Lewis CE, Owen N, Perry CK, et al. Sedentary Behavior and Cardiovascular Morbidity and Mortality: A Science Advisory From the American Heart Association. Circulation. 2016;134(13):e262–79.

51. De Miguel-Etayo P, Gracia-Marco L, Ortega FB, Intemann T, Foraita R, Lissner L, Oja L, Barba G, Michels N, Tornaritis M, et al. Physical fitness reference standards in European children: the IDEFICS study. Int J Obes. 2014;38(Suppl 2):S57–66.

52. Harber MP, Kaminsky LA, Arena R, Blair SN, Franklin BA, Myers J, Ross R. Impact of cardiorespiratory fitness on all-cause and disease-specific mortality: advances since 2009. Prog Cardiovasc Dis. 2017;60(1):11-20. https://doi.org/10.1016/j.pcad.2017.03.001.

53. Shah RV, Murthy VL, Colangelo LA, Reis J, Venkatesh BA, Sharma R, Abbasi SA, Goff DC Jr, Carr JJ, Rana JS, et al. Association of Fitness in Young Adulthood With Survival and Cardiovascular Risk: The Coronary Artery Risk Development in Young Adults (CARDIA) Study. JAMA Intern Med. 2016;176(1):87–95.

54. Kokkinos P, Myers J, Faselis C, Panagiotakos DB, Doumas M, Pittaras A, Manolis A, Kokkinos JP, Karasik P, Greenberg M, et al. Exercise capacity and mortality in older men: a 20-year follow-up study. Circulation. 2010;122(8):790–7.

55. Truesdale BC, Jencks C. The Health Effects of Income Inequality: Averages and Disparities. Annu Rev Public Health. 2016;37:413–30.

56. Atkin AJ, Sharp SJ, Harrison F, Brage S, Van Sluijs EM. Seasonal Variation in Children's Physical Activity and Sedentary Time. Med Sci Sports Exerc. 2016;48(3):449–56.

57. Booth JN, Brooks NE, Moran CN, Gallagher IJ, Ryde GC, Gorely T. Is running a mile a day associated with children's behaviour and well-being? Exploring the impact of the Daily Mile and implications for policy. In: British Psychological Society Annaul Meeting. Belfast: British Pyschological Society; 2016.

58. Brooks NE, Booth JN, Chesham R, Sweeney E, Mitchell I, Ryde GC, Gorely T, Moran CN. A feasibility study investigating body composition and physical activity levels in children taking part in the daily mile. In: Experimental Biology. vol. 30. FASEB J; 2016. p. lb669. https://www.fasebj.org/doi/abs/10.1096/fasebj.30.1_supplement.lb669.

59. The Scottish Attainment Challenge [http://www.gov.scot/Topics/Education/Schools/Raisingeducationalattainment]. Accessed 17 Apr 2018.

2

An exploratory study examining how nano-liquid chromatography–mass spectrometry and phosphoproteomics can differentiate patients with advanced fibrosis and higher percentage collagen in non-alcoholic fatty liver disease

Zobair M. Younossi[1,2,3*], Azza Karrar[1,2], Mariaelena Pierobon[4], Aybike Birerdinc[1], Maria Stepanova[1,2], Dinan Abdelatif[1,3], Zahra Younoszai[2], Thomas Jeffers[2], Sean Felix[2], Kianoush Jeiran[4], Alex Hodge[4], Weidong Zhou[4], Fanny Monge[1,3], Lakshmi Alaparthi[1,3], Vikas Chandhoke[2,4], Zachary D. Goodman[1,3] and Emanuel F. Petricoin[4]

Abstract

Background: Non-alcoholic steatohepatitis (NASH) is among the leading causes of liver disease worldwide. It is increasingly recognized that the phenotype of NASH may involve a number of different pathways, of which each could become important therapeutic targets. The aim of this study is to use high resolution mass spectrometry (MS) and phosphoproteomics techniques to assess the serum proteome and hepatic phosphoproteome in subjects with NASH-related fibrosis.

Methods: Sixty-seven biopsy-proven NAFLD subjects with frozen sera and liver tissue were included. Reverse phase protein microarray was used to quantify the phosphorylation of key signaling proteins in liver and nano-liquid chromatography (LC)-MS was used to sequence target biomarkers in the serum. An image analysis algorithm was used to quantify the percentage of collagen (% collagen) using computer-assisted morphometry. Using multiple regression models, serum proteomes and phosphorylated hepatic proteins that were independently ($p \leq 0.05$) associated with advanced fibrosis (stage ≥ 2) and higher % collagen were assessed.

Results: Phosphorylated signaling pathways in the liver revealed that apoptosis signal-regulating kinase 1, mitogen-activated protein kinase (ASK1-MAPK pathway involving ASK1 S38 ($p < 0.02$) and p38 MAPK ($p = 0.0002$)) activated by the inflammatory cytokine interleukin (IL-10) ($p < 0.001$), were independently associated with higher % collagen. LC-MS data revealed that serum alpha-2 macroglobulin (α2M) ($p = 0.0004$) and coagulation factor V ($p = 0.0127$) were independently associated with higher % hepatic collagen.

Conclusions: Simultaneous profiling of serum proteome and hepatic phosphoproteome reveals that the activation of ASK1 S38, p38 MAPK in the liver, and serum α2M and coagulation factor V are independently associated with hepatic collagen deposition in patients with NASH. These data suggest the role of these pathways in the pathogenesis of NASH-related fibrosis as a potential therapeutic target.

Keywords: NASH, Steatosis, Steatohepatitis, Reverse phase protein arrays, Mass spectrometry, Liver fibrosis

* Correspondence: zobair.younossi@inova.org
[1]Betty and Guy Beatty Center for Integrated Research, Inova Health System, 3300 Gallows Rd., Falls Church, VA, USA
[2]Department of Medicine, Inova Fairfax Hospital, Falls Church, VA, USA
Full list of author information is available at the end of the article

Background

Non-alcoholic fatty liver disease (NAFLD) is rapidly becoming the most prominent cause of chronic liver disease worldwide, with prevalence estimated at approximately 24% [1]. NAFLD is considered the hepatic manifestation of metabolic syndrome and represents a spectrum ranging from steatosis to non-alcoholic steatohepatitis (NASH) and NASH-related cirrhosis [2]. Liver biopsy data suggest that approximately 20% of subjects with NAFLD have underlying NASH [3, 4]. Furthermore, NAFLD subjects with multiple components of metabolic syndrome have an increased likelihood of having underlying NASH and advanced fibrosis [3, 5, 6]. Evidence from observational studies suggests that NASH is the subtype of NAFLD with the highest risk of progression and adverse outcomes [2, 6]. However, a small proportion of subjects whose liver biopsies indicate non-NASH NAFLD may also progress to NASH and related fibrosis [7]. Nevertheless, the exact conditions under which some of these patients' progress is still not well understood.

In addition to the clinical factors associated with adverse outcomes in NASH, a number of studies have assessed histologic features associated with mortality. In this context, the presence of histologic inflammation and ballooning degeneration of hepatocytes can be associated with advanced hepatic fibrosis in patients with NASH but not mortality [8–13]. In contrast, only hepatic fibrosis was shown to independently predict liver-related mortality [9, 12, 13]. This has prompted some experts to consider the presence of fibrosis in NASH as the most important predictor of long-term prognosis. It is important to note that, in 2017, histologic assessment remains the gold standard for diagnosing NASH and staging hepatic fibrosis [14–16]. Despite a great deal of ongoing efforts, a validated non-invasive biomarker or an effective treatment for NASH has not been approved [17–29].

Proteomics is a powerful technology that can help identify therapeutic targets and potential biomarkers in different diseases. We have utilized this high throughput technology in our previous studies of NASH in adipose tissue [21–24], where have shown that (1) NASH-specific disruption of the kinase-driven signaling cascades in visceral adipose tissue leads to detectable changes in the levels of soluble molecules released into the bloodstream, and (2) biomarkers discovered in silico could contribute to predictive models for chronic diseases.

An in-depth assessment of different proteomics platforms in patients with NASH and associated fibrosis is not available. Therefore, the present study aimed to use reverse phase protein microarray (RPMA) techniques to evaluate phosphoproteomic pathways that may be active in the hepatic tissue of patients with NASH-related fibrosis. Additionally, we aimed to use protein harvesting nanoparticles coupled with high resolution mass spectrometry (MS) to assess the serum proteome associated with NASH-related fibrosis.

Methods

Study design: study cohort, blood and liver tissue collection

The study cohort included 67 obese patients (BMI > 40 kg/m^2) who underwent a liver biopsy for clinical indications. Histological diagnosis was made by the study hepatopathologist (ZG) and patients were classified into groups as NASH NAFLD ($n = 42$) and non-NASH NAFLD (simple steatosis) ($n = 24$) or patients with fibrosis stage ≥ 2 ($n = 5$) and fibrosis stage $2 < (n = 3)$. Fibrosis was also quantified after staining for collagen type V by Sirius red staining as outlined in detail below .

Blood samples, liver tissue, and demographic and clinical data were collected at the time of liver biopsy and after obtaining informed consent. All human samples were collected according to a protocol approved by Inova Fairfax Hospital Institutional Review Board and under patient informed written consent. Consistent with the intent of the study, patients diagnosed with viral hepatitis (HCV antibody (–) and HBs Antigen (–)) or other liver diseases, hepatocellular carcinoma, and/or evidence of excessive alcohol use (≥ 10 g/d), as defined by established clinical criteria, were excluded.

Liver histological assessment and collagen quantification

All liver biopsies were stained with hematoxylin and eosin and Sirius red for steatosis and collagen quantification. All biopsies were evaluated by the study hepatopathologist for the degree of steatosis (0–3), portal inflammation (0–3), interlobular pericellular fibrosis, portal fibrosis (0–3), and the presence of bridging fibrosis and cirrhosis. The definition of NAFLD included presence of more than 5% macrovesicular hepatic steatosis. NASH diagnosis required presence of hepatic steatosis and inflammation, together with hepatocyte injury with degenerative ballooning, with or without Mallory–Denk bodies and/or pericellular fibrosis [30, 31]. Advanced fibrosis was defined as stage ≥ 2. Collagen quantification was performed following the acquisition of digitalized images of Sirius stained slides with an Aperio Scanscope XT scanner. Aperio's positive pixel count algorithm was used to quantify the percentage of stained collagen (% collagen) (Additional file 1: Figure S1). Values for % collagen were grouped into upper quartile (Q4 > 5.36% $n = 15$), middle quartiles (Q2–Q3 = 1.58–5.36, $n = 31$), and lower quartile (Q1 < 1.89%, $n = 16$).

Proteomics analysis

Serum proteome enrichment using nanoparticles

Hydrogel nanotrap particles were used to enrich for low abundance serum proteins as previously described [32]. Briefly, particles were prepared with three different affinity dyes (Trypan blue, Cibacron blue, and Bismark brown) that have been previously shown to be an optimal recipe to capture a wide range of low abundance proteins [33, 34]. Proteins were then released from the particles by elution with acetonitrile and ammonium hydroxide, followed by centrifugation.

Serum proteomics using liquid chromatography (LC) coupled with tandem MS analysis

Prior to MS analysis, nanoparticle-captured eluates were dried under compressed nitrogen and subsequently reconstituted in 8 M urea, reduced by 10 mM DTT, alkylated by 50 mM iodoacetamide, and digested by trypsin at 37 °C overnight. Tryptic peptides were further purified by Zip-Tip (Millipore, Billerica, MA, USA) and analyzed by LC coupled tandem MS (LC–MS/MS) with an LTQ-Orbitrap mass spectrometer (Thermo Fisher Scientific, Waltham, MA, USA). The reversed-phase LC column was packed with resin (Michrom BioResources, CA, USA) and then washed with 0.1% formic acid after sample injection and peptides were eluted using a linear gradient of 0% mobile phase B to 50% B to 100% B. The LTQ-Orbitrap was operated in a data-dependent mode in which each full MS scan (30,000 resolving power) was followed by eight MS/MS scans where the eight most abundant molecular ions were selected and fragmented by collision-induced dissociation using a normalized collision energy of 35%. The 'FT master scan preview mode', 'Charge state screening', 'Monoisotopic precursor selection', and 'Charge state rejection' were permitted so that only 1+, 2+, and 3+ ions were selected and fragmented by collision-induced dissociation. Tandem mass spectra data collected by Xcalibur (version 2.0.2) were examined in the NCBI human protein database using SEQUEST (Bioworks software, ThermoFisher, version 3.3.1). The SEQUEST blast search was further filtered by the criteria 'Xcorr versus charge 1.9, 2.2, 3.0 for 1+, 2+, 3+ ions; ΔCn>0.1; probability of randomized identification of peptide < 0.01'. The false discovery rate of peptides was evaluated by searching a combined forward-reversed database. The search result files from each sample were further analyzed by Scaffold (Proteome Software, Portland, OR, USA) for further comparison [34, 35]. Only proteins that were detected in at least 50% of samples were included in the analysis.

RPMA construction and analysis performed on the hepatic phosphoproteins

RPMA was performed on the liver tissue to map pathway activation as previously described [22, 24]. Whole tissue lysates were prepared directly from 8 μm cryosections using a solution of 2× tris-glycine SDS sample buffer (Invitrogen Life Technologies, Carlsbad, CA, USA) and Tissue Protein Extraction Reagent (Pierce, Rockford, IL, USA) supplemented with 2.5% β-mercaptoethanol (Sigma, St. Louis, MO, USA). Samples were boiled for 8 min and stored at – 80 °C until arrayed.

Cell lysates were printed onto nitrocellulose-coated glass slides (Grace Bio-Labs, Bend, OR, USA) using an automated arrayer system (Aushon 2470 arrayer; Aushon BioSystems, Burlington, MA, USA). Each sample was printed in triplicate alongside the reference standards as an internal quality control. To quantify the overall amount of protein in each sample, selected arrays were probed with Sypro Ruby Protein Blot Stain (Molecular Probes, Eugene, OR, USA). Prior to immunostaining, samples were incubated in Reblot Antibody Stripping solution (Chemicon, Temecula, CA, USA), washed twice in PBS, and blocked in I-Block (Applied BioSystems, Foster City, CA, USA); 150 antibodies were used to target phosphorylated, cleaved, and unmodified proteins. Detection was performed using tyramide-based Catalyzed Signal Amplification System (Dako Cytomation, Carpinteria, CA, USA) coupled with the Streptavidin-conjugated IRDye680 dye (LI-COR Biosciences, Lincoln NE, USA). Antibody specificity was validated for single band specificity by western blotting prior to use on the arrays, as described previously [36]. Antibody- and Sypro Ruby-stained slides were scanned on a Tecan laser scanner (Tecan, Mönnedorf, Switzerland) using 620 nm and 580 nm weight length channels, respectively. Array images were analyzed using MicroVigene software version 5.1.0.0, as previously described [37–40]. Briefly, the software calculates spot intensity, completes background subtraction, normalizes each sample to its matched amount of total protein, and averages the technical replicates (Vigenetech, Carlisle, MA, USA).

Statistical analysis

The clinical, demographic, and biochemical data of the study cohort groups were summarized as frequency (n), percentages (%), and mean ± standard deviation (SD). Mann–Whitney U test was used for continuous variables and χ^2 was used to compare categorical data across disease states (NASH NAFLD vs. non-NASH NAFLD or advanced fibrosis, fibrosis stage 2 ≥ vs. fibrosis stage 0–1). In the context of multiple comparisons, false discovery rates were estimated using the Benjamini–Hochberg method. Spearman's Rho (ρ) correlation analysis was performed across the detected analytes measured by MS and RPMA for patients with advanced fibrosis and higher % collagen. Correlation maps were created in Gephi version 0.8.2 for association with a correlation coefficient greater than 0.9.

Multiple regressions were built with analytes being used as predictors of the presence of significant fibrosis (logistic regression) and % collagen in liver (generalized linear model) with adjustment for demographic, clinical, and biochemical confounders (age, sex, BMI, diabetes, AST, and ALT). To limit the chance of over-fitting, the analytes were preselected at the univariate stage ($p < 0.10$ by Mann–Whitney or Spearman correlation test), and only predictors with $p < 0.05$ were left in the models after bidirectional stepwise selection. All statistical analyses were performed using statistical software JMP 9.2 (SAS Institute, Cary, NC, USA).

The open access mapping tool KEGG Pathway Painter, which uses The Kyoto Encyclopedia of Genes and Genomes (KEGG) database, was used to map the phosphoproteins determined from the multiple regression models to canonical pathways. The pathways were sorted in descending order based on number of molecules per pathway [41]. UniProt was used to manually curate the pathways and regulatory mechanisms involving the analytes found to be statistically significant in this analysis (http://www.uniprot.org/).

Results

Clinical and demographic profile of the study cohort

A total of 43 subjects with available liver tissue and serum samples met the histologic criteria for NASH and, of these, 34 had advanced fibrosis (fibrosis ≥ 2). Demographic, clinical, and histological data are summarized in Table 1, which shows the characteristics of the study cohort when divided as having NASH versus non-NASH. The p value column shows results of the χ^2 test for categorical variables and Mann–Whitney U test for continuous variables, where p values < 0.05 are considered significant.

Phosphorylated proteins in the hepatic tissue associated with advanced fibrosis and higher hepatic collagen deposition in subjects with NAFLD

The hepatic phosphoproteomic data was used for pathway activation mapping analysis. The analysis showed that 75 proteins (receptor tyrosine kinases, upstream activators, and downstream substrates) were associated with significant hepatic fibrosis (fibrosis stage ≥ 2) and higher % hepatic collagen. All significant RPMA proteomes in the liver are shown in Additional file 1: Table S1, whereas Table 2 shows the top 34 significant proteins. The false discovery rate was estimated to be 10.6%.

The phosphorylated signaling pathways from the liver tissue included the phosphoinositide 3-kinase PI3K/AKT signaling pathway, the epidermal growth factor receptor (EGF/EGFR) signaling pathway known as (ErbB1/HER1)

and, most importantly, the Apoptosis Signal-Regulating Kinase 1 (ASK1)-MAPK pathways (involving Apoptosis Signal-Regulating Kinase-1, ASK1 S83, and p38 MAPKinase; $p < 0.05$). All phosphoproteins that were significantly correlated with the presence of advanced fibrosis and higher % collagen deposition in the liver are shown in Table 2.

As depicted in the protein–protein interaction figure (Additional file 1: Figure S2), the majority of phosphoproteins relevant to advanced fibrosis in NASH are linked together to form a large interacting network. This protein–protein interaction network revealed pathways involved in the neoangiogenesis, cell motility, and immune response to be potentially playing a role in the development of advanced fibrosis and higher % collagen deposition in NASH. Furthermore, these results suggest that the proteins of fibrosis and collagen deposition network have an even more pronounced hierarchical structure than the complete network and contain a larger number of closely linked protein clusters, which could be indicative of functional protein complexes.

Serum protein profiles of LC–MS of NASH subjects with advanced fibrosis and increased hepatic collagen deposition

Important circulating proteins in sera (proteins that were detected by MS in at least 50% of NAFLD patients) were included in the further analysis. In the subsequent analysis, the strongest associations with advanced fibrosis were noted for the serum alpha-1-microglobulin/bikunin preprotein ($p = 0.0022$), the alpha-2 macroglobulin precursor ($\alpha2M$) ($p = 0.0023$), and apolipoprotein E isoform a ($p = 0.0027$) (Table 3).

On the other hand, $\alpha2M$ precursor coagulation factor V precursor and transthyretin precursor were weakly but significantly correlated with % collagen ($p < 0.05$) (Table 3). Furthermore, acute phase protein alpha-1-acid glycoprotein 1 was noted to positively correlate with % collagen while the platelet basic protein preproprotein (a chemoattractant which also functions in hyaluronic acid synthesis), histidine-rich glycoprotein isoform X1 coagulation factor V precursor, and alpha-1-microglobulin/bikunin preproprotein were all negatively correlated with % hepatic collagen deposition ($p < 0.05$) (Table 3). The false discovery rate for this round of analysis was estimated to be 28.3%.

Serum proteome and hepatic phosphoproteome independently associated with advanced hepatic fibrosis and increased hepatic collagen deposition in NASH

In a series of multivariate analyses, we assessed the independent association of these circulating serum proteins and hepatic phosphoproteins with advanced fibrosis and higher % hepatic collagen deposition (Table 4). Our

Table 1 Demographic, clinical, and biochemical characteristics of the study cohort

N	NASH	Non-NASH	All
	43	24	67
Demographic			
Male, n (%)	16 (37.2%)	6 (25.0%)	22 (32.8%)
White, n (%)	31 (77.5%)	19 (82.6%)	50 (79.4%)
Age mean ± SD	47.233 ± 10.254	45.083 ± 10.746	46.463 ± 10.403
BMI, kg/m^2	48.921 ± 10.552	48.745 ± 9.200	48.856 ± 10.001
Clinical and biochemical			
Diabetes, n (%)	28 (65.1%)	8 (33.3%)*	36 (53.7%)
Hypertension, n (%)	30 (73.2%)	14 (58.3%)	44 (67.7%)
ALT, μ/L	51.214 ± 34.985	34.042 ± 18.320*	44.970 ± 30.985
AST, μ/L	40.619 ± 24.883	23.375 ± 12.968***	34.348 ± 22.802
Bilirubin, mg/dL	0.544 ± 0.040	0.383 ± 0.034**	0.486 ± 0.030
Albumin, g/dL	4.012 ± 0.114	4.127 ± 0.067	4.052 ± 0.078
Glucose, mg/dL	125.268 ± 6.310	111.130 ± 8.946	120.188 ± 5.193
Total cholesterol, mg/dL	175.025 ± 6.628	197.000 ± 8.732	183.266 ± 5.407
LDL, mg/dL	97.811 ± 6.199	120.043 ± 8.859	106.333 ± 5.259
HDL, mg/dL	40.667 ± 1.639	47.208 ± 2.438**	43.159 ± 1.422
TGA, mg/dL	172.103 ± 13.111	161.391 ± 23.062	168.129 ± 11.788
Histological features[a]			
Fat (1,2) vs. (3,4)	14 (32.6%)	5 (20.8%)	19 (28.4%)
Inflammation			
Portal inflammation (0.1) vs. (≥ 2)	15 (34.9%)	6 (25.0%)	21 (31.3%)
Kupffer cells (0.1) vs. (≥ 2)	11 (25.6%)	1 (4.2%)*	12 (17.9%)
PMN cells (0.1) vs. (≥ 2)	5 (11.6%)	0 (0.0%)	5 (7.5%)
Lymphocytes (0.1) vs. (≥ 2)	26 (60.5%)	6 (25.0%)**	32 (47.8%)
Fibrosis			
Pericellular fibrosis (0.1) vs. (≥ 2)	28 (65.1%)	0 (0.0%)***	28 (41.8%)
Portal fibrosis (0.1) vs. (≥ 2)	28 (65.1%)	7 (29.2%)**	35 (52.2%)
Bridging fibrosis and cirrhosis	14 (32.6%)	0 (0.0%)***	14 (20.9%)
Apoptosis			
Focal necrosis (0) vs. (1,2,3)	20 (46.5%)	5 (20.8%)*	25 (37.3%)
Mallory–Denk bodies (0) vs. (1,2,3)	12 (27.9%)	0 (0.0%)**	12 (17.9%)
Ballooning degeneration (0) vs. (1,2,3)	24 (55.8%)	0 (0.0%)***	24 (35.8%)
Apoptotic bodies (0) vs. (1,2,3)	4 (9.3%)	0 (0.0%)	4 (6.0%)
Collagen percentage	4.708 ± 3.283	2.794 ± 1.736*	4.040 ± 2.970
Fat percentage	18.645 ± 8.474	12.906 ± 7.552**	16.641 ± 8.559

[a] Histopathological features were grouped by scores according to none, mild to moderate, or severe according to the hepatopathologist scoring as shown beside each variable

*p < 0.05, **p < 0.01, ***p < 0.001

ALT alanine aminotransferase, AST aspartate aminotransferase, BMI body mass index, HDL high density lipoprotein, LDL low density lipoprotein, NASH non-alcoholic steatohepatitis, PMN polymorphonuclear cells, SD standard deviation, TGA triglycerides

initial models focused on advanced fibrosis as the outcome. The first multivariate model included hepatic phosphoproteins and suggested that phosphoprotein Tyk2 as well as ALDH were the independent predictors of advanced fibrosis in NASH (Table 4). Another multivariate model using serum proteins suggested that serum Apolipoprotein C-II precursor, Apolipoprotein A-I preproprotein, and vitamin K-dependent protein S preproprotein were independently associated with advanced fibrosis in NASH (Table 4).

Table 2 Phosphorylated hepatic proteins with correlations with fibrosis and a higher percentage of collagen deposition in livers of NAFLD patients

Endpoint	Protein intensity values (mean)		
MITOGENESIS	Fibrosis (stage ≥ 2)[a,b]	Fibrosis (stage < 2)[a,b,c]	Percentage collagen ρ[c,d]
RTKS and LIGANDS			
c-Kit Y703	12,023.3253	8509.7594**	0.2727*
EGFR Y1045	7752.7248	5367.3954**	0.3061*
ErbB2 HER2 Y1248	13,638.4722	10,163.0936**	0.2544*
Met Y1234/1235	8394.0971	5442.5366***	0.4082***
Ret Y905	4840.5597	2796.3384**	0.2564*
Ron Y1353	11,455.9458	8217.8116**	0.2564*
DOWNSTREAM SUBSTRATES			
CrkII Y221	11,296.7507	7283.2336**	0.2844*
c-Myc	16,583.2182	13,624.0484*	0.2705*
ERK 1/2 TOTAL	27,683.0657	22,584.3185**	0.3574**
FRS2 alpha Y436	6745.9092	4569.8235*	0.3382**
IRS 1 S612	6603.2819	4223.5915*	0.2756*
PKA C T197	13,849.3962	11,729.8932*	0.2968*
Src Family Y416	3488.0194	1874.4209**	0.2631*
SURVIVAL			
AKT T308	19,966.2896	11,089.2265**	0.3763**
AKT TOTAL	15,739.0600	10,127.1820**	0.3282**
ASK1 S83	2072.4277	1209.4175**	0.2563*
Ephrin A3 Y779/A4 Y779/A5 Y833	10,051.2853	9008.6468*	0.3179*
PDK1 S241	13,526.9204	10,692.6456**	0.2990*
PI3K p85 Y458 p55 Y199	5930.4957	4023.6630**	0.4243***
PTEN	26,544.6698	22,904.4300*	0.2628*
PTEN S380	12,498.2321	7720.4331***	0.2677
INFLAMMATION/IMMUNE FUNCTION			
Zap 70 Y319/Syk Y352	8322.9034	4839.8932***	0.3189*
cPLA2 S505	11,697.1946	8108.4437**	0.2861*
PLCgamma1 Y783	11,995.7606	8488.3315**	0.2824*
Stat4 Y693	8407.7191	5859.6088**	0.3010*
Stat6 Y641	7840.7122	4793.4883***	0.3226*
Tyk2 Y1054/1055	8760.8030	5060.9800***	0.2955*
p38 MAPK T180/Y182	8093.9200	6807.1800	0.3901**
APOPTOSIS			
Bak	20,974.0624	18,147.0249**	0.3262**
Survivin	11,593.7421	8882.5924***	0.3180*
MOTILITY AND CELL ADHESION			
Cofilin S3	11,887.6509	2171.5929***	0.3369**
FAK Y576/577	7300.4566	5303.6335*	0.3382**
OTHERS			
ALDH	21,453.9429	26,006.4687**	−0.3009*
IL-10	1731.1300	1311.5200	0.5539***

[a] Proteins in liver tissue, detected using RPMA, that were expressed at higher and significant level in patients with fibrosis ≥ 2 compared with fibrosis < 2
[b] Non-parametric Kruskal–Wallis H test was used to identify the significantly differentially expressed proteins between the two groups
[c] Protein level correlation with % collagen tested using Spearman rank correlation test
[d] Correlation coefficient (ρ) describes the strength and direction of association between proteins and % collagen
p values < 0.05 are considered significant; *p < 0.05, **p < 0.01, ***p < 0.001

Table 3 Correlations of LC-MS serum proteomes with advanced fibrosis and a higher percentage of collagen deposition in liver

LC–MS Proteomes	Mean of protein intensity		
	Fibrosis ≥ 2 (n)[a,b]	Fibrosis < 2 (n)[a,b,c]	Percentage collagen ρ[c,d]
Protein alpha-1-microglobulin/bikunin preproprotein	0.170 ± 0.101	0.233 ± 0.091**	−0.25*
Alpha-2-macroglobulin	0.144 ± 0.144	0.060 ± 0.087**	0.32*
Apolipoprotein E isoform a	0.320 ± 0.184	0.426 ± 0.219**	−0.24
Transthyretin precursor	0.084 ± 0.056	0.053 ± 0.032**	0.26*
Vitamin K-dependent protein S preproprotein	0.057 ± 0.044	0.031 ± 0.030*	−0.06
Selenoprotein P isoform 2	0.013 ± 0.019	0.030 ± 0.044*	−0.19
Carboxypeptidase B2 isoform 2 preproprotein	0.025 ± 0.030	0.045 ± 0.042*	−0.24
Apolipoprotein C-II	0.115 ± 0.038	0.156 ± 0.093*	−0.19
Histidine-rich glycoprotein isoform X1	0.497 ± 0.252	0.619 ± 0.230*	−0.31*
Apolipoprotein B-100 isoform X1	0.250 ± 0.606	0.039 ± 0.073*	0.23
Apolipoprotein A-I preproprotein	0.753 ± 0.372	0.582 ± 0.222*	0.16
Inter-alpha trypsin inhib. hvy. ch.H4 isoform 2	0.045 ± 0.040	0.027 ± 0.030*	0.05
Coagulation factor V	0.048 ± 0.053	0.046 ±0.053	−0.36**
Alpha-1-antitrypsin	0.193 ± 0.192	0.121 ± 0.051*	0.34**
Platelet basic protein preproprotein	0.081 ± 0.053	0.100 ± 0.044	−0.33**
Vitamin D-binding protein isoform 3	0.052 ± 0.064	0.028 ± 0.037	0.28*
C4b-binding protein alpha chain	0.107 ± 0.084	0.102 ± 0.086	−0.27*
Complement C4-A isoform 1 preproprotein	0.589 ± 0.269	0.605 ± 0.212	− 0.26*
Alpha-1-acid glycoprotein 1 precursor	0.090 ± 0.062	0.065 ± 0.041	0.25*

[a] Proteins as detected by LC–MS that were expressed at higher and significant level in patients with fibrosis ≥ 2 compared with fibrosis < 2
[b] Non-parametric Kruskal–Wallis H test was used to identify the significantly differentially expressed proteins between the two groups
[c] Protein level correlation with % collagen tested using Spearman rank correlation test and the
[d] Correlation coefficient (ρ) describes the strength and direction of association between proteins and % collagen
p values < 0.05 are considered significant; *p < 0.05, **p < 0.01

The subsequent models focused on % collagen as the desired outcome. The model assessing the association of serum proteins with % collagen revealed that α2M precursor ($p = 0.0004$) and coagulation factor V ($p = 0.013$) were independently associated with increased hepatic collagen.

The last model showed that phosphoproteins, ASK1 S38 ($p = 0.02$), the receptor tyrosine kinase, Met Y1234/1235 ($p = 0.009$), p38MAPK T180/Y182 ($p = 0.0002$), LIMK1T508/LIMK2 T505 ($p = 0.004$), and tissue remodeling-related inflammatory cytokines IL-10 ($p < 0.0001$) were independently associated with a higher % collagen deposition in the liver (Table 4).

The complete list of parameters for the models also included age, gender, BMI, diabetes, AST, ALT, and the variables were then subjected to stepwise selection. The proteins included in the models (for further stepwise selection) were pre-selected at the univariate step ($p \leq 0.10$ only). In the final models, only significant associations were kept for both clinicals and proteins ($p \leq 0.05$).

Pathway analysis associated with increased hepatic collagen deposition using KEGG and Uniport

Based on the independent predictors of advanced fibrosis in NASH, the total number of pathways activated by phosphoprotein predictors is 122 (Additional file 1: Figure S3). Pathways of advanced fibrosis in NASH showed that there was an overlap of the Apolipoprotein C-II precursor, Apolipoprotein A-I preproprotein in the HDL-mediated lipid transport, and the Retinoid metabolism and transport pathways. On the other hand, Tyk2 is mapped to a total of 11 pathways, including Th1, Th2, and Th17 cell differentiation pathways (Additional file 1: Table S2).

Based on the independent predictors for increased % collagen deposition, pathway analysis revealed 173 distinct KEGG and UniProt pathways. Of these, 117 pathways involved the phosphoproteins (ASK1, Met, p38 MAPK, IL-10, LIMK1/LIMK2), 30 of which had two or more proteins per pathway. Met and p38 MAPK both mapped to the Adherens junction pathway ($n = 2$), both upstream of actin polymerization. ASK1 mapped to a total of 11 pathways, including Apoptosis, TNF, and NAFLD signaling pathways. LIMK1/LIMK2 mapped to 3 pathways, the most notable of which is the regulation of actin cytoskeleton pathway, which also includes p38MAPK. Pathways with the greatest number of convergent phosphoproteins included the Regulation of Actin Cytoskeleton ($n = 3$), Fc gamma R-mediated

Table 4 Multivariate models showing independent association of sera proteomes and phosphorylated protein in liver associated with advanced liver fibrosis and a higher percentage of collagen

Independent predictors of advanced liver fibrosis			
Predictor	Odds ratio	Lower 95% CI	Upper 95% CI
Model with RPMA proteins[a]			
AST, per 1 U/L	1.037	1.006	1.07*
Tyk2 Y1054/1055, per 1 unit	1.458	1.177	1.807***
ALDH, per 1 unit	0.873	0.783	0.973*
Model with MS proteins			
Apolipoprotein C-II precursor, per 1 unit	0.757	0.612	0.936*
Apolipoprotein A-I preproprotein, per 1 unit	1.086	1.036	1.138***
Vitamin K-dependent protein S preproprotein, per 1 unit	1.591	1.221	2.071***
Independent predictors of higher percentage collagen			
	Beta		Std. err.
Model with RPMA proteins[a]			
ASK1 S83, per 1 unit	− 0.654		0.280*
Met Y1234/1235, per 1 unit	0.450		0.167**
p38 MAPK T180/Y182, per 1 unit	0.290		0.072***
IL-10, per 1 unit	1.197		0.255***
LIMK1 T508/LIMK2 T505, per 1 unit	− 0.386		0.130**
Model with MS proteins			
Alpha-2-macroglobulin precursor, per 1 unit	0.100		0.026***
Coagulation factor V precursor, per 1 unit	− 0.159		0.062*

[a] Liver tissue RPMA proteins were divided by 1000, MS proteins multiplied by 100 for presentation purposes
$*p < 0.05$, $**p < 0.01$, $***p < 0.001$

phagocytosis ($n = 3$), TNF signaling ($n = 2$), MAPK signaling ($n = 2$), Apoptosis ($n = 2$), and EGFR tyrosine kinase inhibitor resistance ($n = 2$). Additionally, IL-10 mapped to 20 pathways and was the only protein mapping to the canonical Jak-STAT signaling pathway ($n = 1$), solidifying its role as an upstream signaling molecule (Additional file 1: Figure S3 and Table S3).

Serum analytes, α2M, and Coagulation Factor V precursor were found to be involved in a total of 25 molecular functions and biological pathways (Additional file 1: Table S2) using Uniprot manual curation. Most notably, aside from their involvement in lipid and vesicle transport, both of these analytes mapped to Platelet degranulation and Fibrin Clot Formation pathways (http://www.uniprot.org/uniprot/P12259 and http://www.uniprot.org/uniprot/P01023).

Correlations of MS proteins with independent predictors of fibrosis and higher % collagen

To investigate the relationships between the sera-derived proteins (detected by LC–MS) and tissue-derived phosphoproteins (assessed by RPMA) in the context of NASH-related fibrosis and hepatic collagen deposition, a separate analysis was performed. This analysis showed that the α2M precursor from serum was strongly and

positively correlated with the receptor tyrosine kinase Met Y1234/1235 ($\rho = 0.42$, $p = 0.0005$), as well as with the actin-binding kinase LMK1 T508/LIMK2 T505 ($\rho = 0.39$, $p = 0.001$) and, most importantly, with IL-10 ($\rho = 0.28$, $p = 0.02$) and ASK1 S83 ($\rho = 0.25$, $p = 0.04$) from liver tissue samples (Additional file 1: Figure S4). Further correlations between proteins from sera and phosphorylated proteins from liver tissue can be seen in Table 5, which shows the correlation of the independently associated serum proteins (with fibrosis and % collagen) detected by MS with the independently correlated phosphoproteins detected by RPMA (with fibrosis and % collagen) in the liver. Spearman rank correlation test was used and correlation coefficient (ρ) describes the strength and direction of association between serum and tissue proteins.

Discussion

This is the most in-depth study of patients with NASH-related fibrosis for whom liver histology, collagen quantitation by morphometry, phosphoproteomic assessment of liver by RPMA, and serum proteomic assessment by LC–MS was performed. In this combined tissue and serum proteomics study of subjects with biopsy-proven NASH/NAFLD, we identified serum

Table 5 Correlations between hepatic phosphoproteins and serum proteins in NASH with advanced fibrosis and a higher percentage of hepatic collagen deposition in the liver

Serum proteome by LC-MS	Alpha-2-macroglobulin precursor	Coagulation factor V precursor	Apolipoprotein A-I preproprotein	Apolipoprotein C-II precursor	Vitamin K-dependent protein S preproprotein
Phosphoproteins from RPMA	ρ	ρ	ρ	ρ	ρ
ASK1 S83	0.25132*	− 0.27301*	0.25187*	0.18546	− 0.004
Met Y1234/1235	0.42158***	− 0.32161**	0.3759**	0.08211	0.2009
p38 MAPK T180/Y182	0.23536*	− 0.37073**	0.814	0.22551	− 0.1066
IL-10	0.27903*	− 0.38985***	0.2616*	0.11275	− 0.859
LIMK1 T508/ LIMK2 T505	0.39353***	− 0.3773	0.3206**	0.33034**	− 0.2423*
Tyk2 Y1054/1055	0.41652***	− 0.167	0.18053	0.01864	0.0099
ALDH	− 0.07782	− 0.004	− 0.275	0.109	− 0.020

p values < 0.05 are considered significant; *p < 0.05, **p < 0.01, ***p < 0.001

proteomic profiles as well as hepatic phosphoproteomic profiles that are associated with advanced fibrosis or increased hepatic collagen deposition in NASH.

Liver tissue from this cohort was used for RPMA to assess activated (phosphorylated) proteins in the hepatic tissue of subjects with NASH and advanced fibrosis. In this context, our data shows that the phosphorylated signaling proteins in the hepatic tissue that correlate with increased collagen deposition target the ASK1-MAPK pathway. Furthermore, activation of p38 MAPK T180/Y182 members of the MAPK family was noted. Notably, phosphorylation of p38 MAPK T180/Y182 participates in a signaling cascade that controls the cellular responses to inflammatory cytokines and stress [42]. It is also important to note that ASK1 S83 is an immunoregulatory protein that plays a pivotal role in apoptosis signaling, inflammation, and fibrosis in the setting of increased oxidative stress, associated with the pathogenesis of NASH. Therefore, inhibitors of the ASK1-MAPK pathway are thought to have potential as therapeutic targets in diseases where ASK1 is activated [43–47]. Our data support the concept that ASK1 activation is a key component for NASH-related fibrosis. In fact, a phase 2 clinical trial has been reported to target ASK1 inhibition as a potential treatment option for NASH. Early data from this study reported consistent improvement of hepatic fibrosis after a short course of treatment with an investigational ASK1 inhibitor in patients with NASH and fibrosis [47]. In concordance with these findings, our proteomics data from liver tissue, representative of organ-wide signaling, provides substantial evidence for the activation of the ASK pathway in the hepatic tissue of NASH subjects with advanced fibrosis, thus yielding further support for targeting of this pathway in the treatment of NAFLD patients with fibrosis.

In addition to the ASK pathway, our study also showed that IL-10 expression in the liver was associated with the presence of higher hepatic collagen deposition in NAFLD. IL-10 is a pleiotropic anti-inflammatory cytokine with important immunoregulatory functions [42]. In fact, IL-10 signaling pathway involves the phosphorylation and activation of a number of pathways that may be important in the pathogenesis of NASH and NASH-related fibrosis. These include the ASK1-MAPK pathway, the transducer activator transcription 3 and other survival pathways (insulin receptor substrate 2 via phosphoinositide-3 kinase class IA and its downstream effectors 3-phosphoinositide dependent protein kinase-1, ribosomal protein S6 kinase polypeptide 1, and v-Akt oncogene homolog) [48]. Despite these findings, the exact role of IL-10 and these pathways requires further investigation in larger matched cohorts.

The gene expression of NAFLD and alcoholic fatty liver disease is similar not only with respect to alcohol-metabolizing genes, but also with respect to numerous other genes, as shown by the global gene expression patterns observed. The demonstration of elevated expression of alcohol-metabolizing pathways in pediatric NASH livers [49] and alcohol-producing gut microbiomes in NASH livers [50] supports the hypothesis that endogenous gut-derived alcohol microbiomes could be a potential hit in the pathogenesis of NASH. Furthermore, the same group later [51] demonstrated that, in advanced stages of NAFLD, there is less expression of the alcohol-metabolizing genes compared to in mild NAFLD. Herein, we report a similar observation, where we found the expression of ALDH in livers to be negatively correlated with % collagen in the liver and negatively associated with fibrosis. We, and others [51], think that it is unexpected that the alcohol-metabolizing molecules are not associated with severe NAFLD. One justification for why these genes were not found to be expressed by fibrotic livers from NAFLD is because most of the alcohol-metabolizing molecules are related to hepatocytes, and there is higher hepatocyte damage in fibrotic livers of NAFLD. A further support for this explanation is that, in our study, NAFLD fibrotic livers showed higher expression of the apoptosis molecules than non-fibrotic livers from NAFLD. However, in our study, phosphoproteomics was performed on whole liver tissue, making it difficult to correlate the exact phosphoproteins specific to hepatocytes.

In addition to the liver tissue, we used sera from the same patients for high resolution MS, which has excellent analytical sensitivity, coupled to nanoparticle-based protein capture technology to concentrate low abundance but clinically relevant proteins [34, 35]. Using this approach, our data shows that a total of 19 circulating proteins are associated with either advanced fibrosis (stage ≥ 2) or higher percent hepatic collagen deposition. In fact, our multivariate analysis showed that serum α2M and coagulation factor V were independently associated with a higher % hepatic collagen deposition, confirming previous data [18], which suggests their potential role in hepatic collagen deposition in NASH. Furthermore, α2M strongly correlates with the downstream transcription factors Met Y1234/1235 and LIMK1 T508/LIMK2. These hepatic phosphoproteins have been independently associated with increased hepatic collagen, further connecting serum proteome to hepatic phosphoproteome and their potential roles in collagen deposition and hepatic fibrosis. Furthermore, these data may suggest that MET and LMK can be involved in the upstream pathogenic mechanism of fibrosis and collagen deposition and therefore the interplay of these molecules should be considered for further investigation.

In addition to the above findings, our data indicates that hypercoagulable factors may also play a role in the development and progression of hepatic fibrosis. The exact mechanism of this influence is not understood, but thrombin, through its activation by coagulation factor V, may be a key component [52, 53].

Liver plays a role in regulating glucose and lipid metabolism. Glucogenesis is suppressed with insulin resistance, which may lead to hyperglycemia resulting in hepatic steatosis [1, 54]. One of the major pathways implicated in hepatic function is the JAK/STAT pathway together with IL-6-STAT3 and IL-4-STAT6 pathways. Similarly, in our studies, we have shown that IL-6 and

IL-10 were increased in patients with fibrosis, together with STAT4 and STAT6 (Additional file 1: Table S1). Previous studies have demonstrated that STAT3 absence in hepatocytes may result in insulin resistance and augmented expression of gluconeogenic genes, mediated by the dysregulation of IL-6 signaling [2, 3, 55, 56]. Taken together, this data support previous findings that STAT signaling is critical for liver metabolic functions. Dysregulation of STAT signaling pathways can result in disrupted hepatic glucose metabolism, leading to hepatic steatosis.

Finally, our systematic pathway analysis approach confirmed two key trends in the data. First, the majority of serum proteins discovered in this study seem to be best associated with the semi-quantitative assessment of advanced fibrosis by histopathology. In contrast, the phosphoproteins in the liver were more frequently associated with increased % hepatic collagen deposition as quantified by morphometry. Second, the data indicated that the proteins found to be independently associated with increased % hepatic collagen deposition are in pathways that are more intrinsically involved in the biology of fibrosis development. In contrast, proteins that are independent predictors of advanced fibrosis based on semi-quantitative assessment by histopathology are primarily involved in lipid storage and transport mechanisms. This suggests that proteins associated with increased % collagen deposition may be more sensitive markers of significant fibrosis in NASH.

The pathway distribution of IL-10 and ASK1 confirms that IL-10 is indeed upstream of the signaling activity of ASK1. It is notable that ASK1 independently mapped to both the NAFLD and apoptosis pathways (as delineated by KEGG) as this protein is known to be involved in hepatic steatosis and fibrosis [47]. In fact, when mapped to the apoptosis pathway, ASK1 is shown as upstream of pro-apoptotic genes and p38MAPK as upstream of pro-survival genes. In short, this pathway analysis confirms that ASK1 is indeed involved in the pathogenesis of hepatic fibrosis in NASH. Furthermore, the data indicates that, while IL-10 is an upstream effector, the signaling cascade does indeed pass through p38MAPK and seems to culminate with LIMK1/LIMK2 and its ability to block the stabilization of actin as seen in this composite pathway (Fig. 1).

There are some limitations to our study. First, it is an exploratory analysis of NASH and liver fibrosis processes and requires validation in a larger group of patients with NASH-related fibrosis. In fact, although in the context of multiple testing, the estimated false discovery rate was not very high; given the number of studied parameters and limited sample size, we could not rule out the risk of over-fitting for the presented models. Nevertheless, and to our knowledge, this is

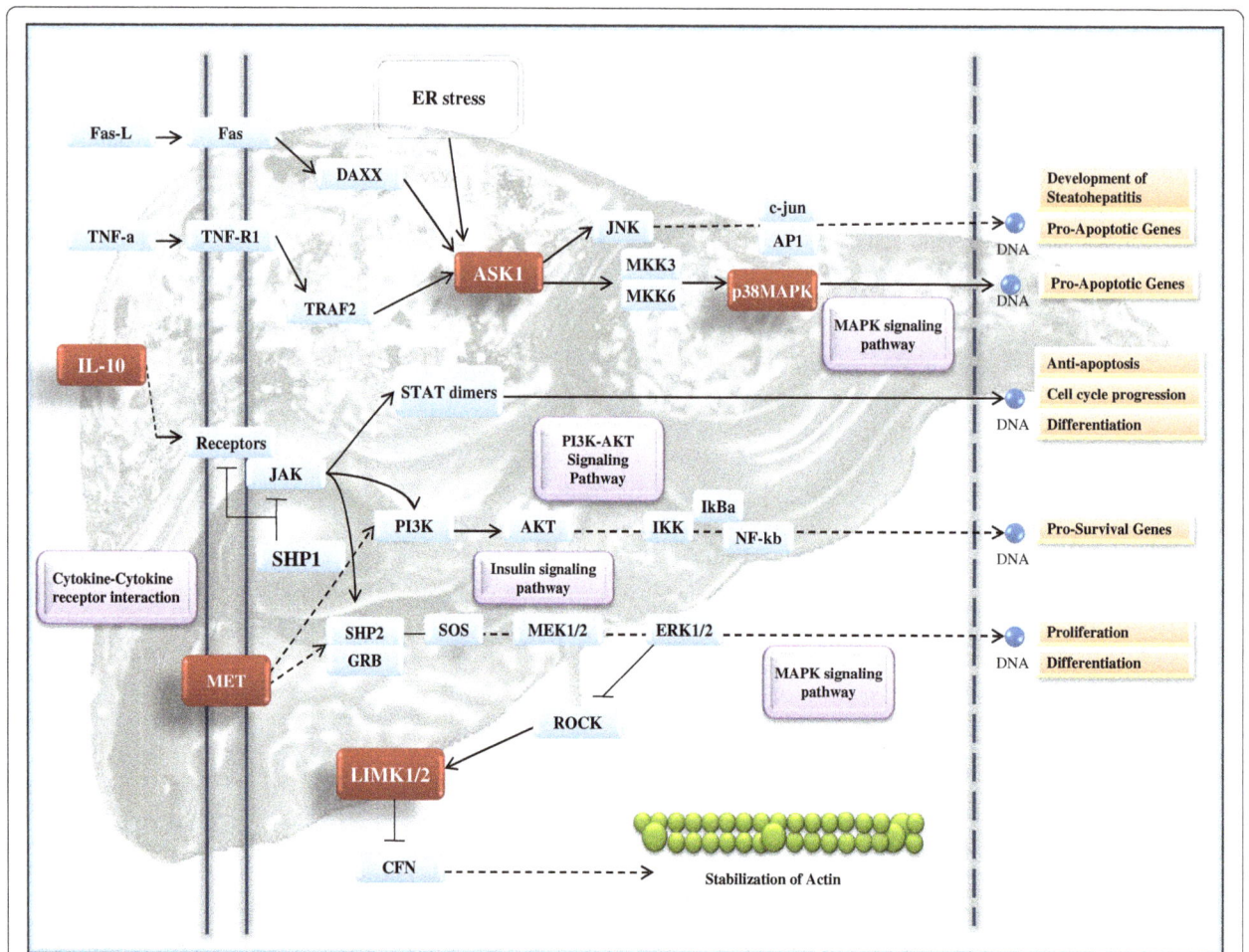

Fig. 1 Composite pathway using the KEGG pathway analysis, a composite pathway was generated based on the canonical mapping of the phosphorylated proteins independently associated with increased % collagen (red) in the liver. Canonical pathway components are also indicated (blue) as well as direct and indirect transition pathways (purple)

the first study utilizing a unique combination of tissue and serum samples coupled with proteomics analysis to identify serum proteome determined by MS- and RPMA-based protein pathway activation mapping of the liver tissue to uncover markers pertinent to fibrosis.

In summary, this study uses a very well described group of NASH subjects with advanced fibrosis with available serum and liver tissue. Our data indicates that ASK1-MAPK is the most important activated pathway in NASH subjects with advanced fibrosis. Additionally, our serum proteomic data confirms that α2M seems to have a predictive value for higher % hepatic collagen deposition in subjects with NASH. Our proteomics data (serum and hepatic) can provide guidance to investigators who are developing therapeutic targets for patients with a clinically relevant type of NAFLD, i.e., NASH with advanced fibrosis or steatofibrosis [57].

Conclusion

NAFLD is the most common liver disease worldwide. NASH is a subtype of NAFLD that may progress to cirrhosis and other liver complications. Only fibrosis can independently predict liver-related mortality. Phosphorylated signaling pathways play a role in liver fibrosis, but none has been confirmed as a pathogenic mechanism and targets for NASH treatment are still under investigation. Using simultaneous profiling of sera proteome and phosphoproteome in liver tissue reveals that ASK1 S83, p38MAPK T180/Y182, the receptor tyrosine kinase, Met Y1234/1235, LIMK1T508/LIMK2 T505, and tissue remodeling-related inflammatory cytokines IL-10 were independently associated with higher collagen deposition in subjects with NAFLD. These pathogenic mechanisms have not been previously correlated to clinical diagnostic markers. However, we were able to show that α2M (a biomarker already implemented in the Fibro Sure test) is strongly correlated to ASK1 S38 and IL-10. Although the mechanism of action of these proteins is unclear, the data suggest a potential role for these proteins in the pathogenesis of fibrosis and potential therapeutic utility in patients with NASH. The phosphorylated signaling pathways that are independently correlated to fibrosis in NASH revealed by our study might well pave the way for the revelation of more therapeutic targets and contribute to understanding the pathogenic mechanism of fibrosis in NASH. Although in the context of multiple testing, the estimated false discovery rate was not very high given the number of studied parameters and limited sample size; however, we could not rule out the risk of over-fitting for the presented models. Future validation of potential biomarkers to better define the pathogenic mechanism and stratify progression of disease in NAFLD will have great clinical significance.

Additional file

Additional file 1: Figure S1. Representative image of collagen quantification after staining with Sirius red. **Table S1.** Associations or correlations of phosphorylated hepatic proteins with fibrosis stage and higher % collagen deposition in livers of NAFLD patients. **Figure S2.** Images showing (a) advanced liver fibrosis signaling protein-protein network and (b) higher hepatic percentage collagen protein-protein network. **Figure S3.** Phosphoproteins and proteomes involved in biological processes and KEGG pathways. **Table S2.** Pathways associated with advanced fibrosis stage ≥ 2. **Table S3.** Pathways associated with higher % collagen deposition in the liver. **Figure S4.** Scatter plots of A. alpha-2 macroglobulin precursor vs. IL-10 ($\rho = 0.28$, $p = 0.02$) and ASK1 S83 ($\rho = 0.25$, $p = 0.04$). (DOCX 2995 kb)

Acknowledgements
The data used in the development of this work is the property of Inova Health System. No external funds were used in the project. All work conducted and data collected under this project remains under the ownership of Inova Health System.

Funding
The study was internally funded by Beatty Liver and Obesity and Liver Outcomes Research Funds, Inova Health System (IHS). The proteomic analysis was performed by GMU under a service contract funded by IHS.

Authors' contributions
ZY is the main supervisor and principal investigator of the study. He designed and directed the study, directed the data analysis, interpreted the study results and undertook the manuscript preparation. AK assisted with the experimental design, aims and work, data and result interpretation, and manuscript preparation. MP was responsible for the generation of the signaling network data by RPMA. MS was responsible for data management, bioinformatics and statistical analysis. ZYo, TJ, SF worked on patient' consent and specimen collection. KJ, AH, and AB assisted in pathway analysis and manuscript generation. WZ was responsible for the analysis of serum samples by mass spectrometry. ZG, FM, LA, and DA performed the pathological diagnosis, collagen quantification, and interpretation and analysis of data. EP assisted with the proteomic experimental work and data interpretation. Authors have read, accepted, and approved the final version of the manuscript.

Competing interests
The authors declare that they have no competing interests.

Author details
[1]Betty and Guy Beatty Center for Integrated Research, Inova Health System, 3300 Gallows Rd., Falls Church, VA, USA. [2]Department of Medicine, Inova Fairfax Hospital, Falls Church, VA, USA. [3]Center for Liver Diseases, Inova Fairfax Hospital, Falls Church, VA, USA. [4]Center for Applied Proteomics and Molecular Medicine, School of Systems Biology, George Mason University, Manassas, VA, USA.

References
1. Younossi ZM, Koenig AB, Abdelatif D, et al. Global epidemiology of nonalcoholic fatty liver disease-Meta-analytic assessment of prevalence, incidence, and outcomes. Hepatology. 2016;64:73–84.
2. Matteoni CA, Younossi ZM, Gramlich T, et al. Nonalcoholic fatty liver disease: a spectrum of clinical and pathological severity. Gastroenterology. 1999;116:1413–9.
3. Younossi ZM, Blissett D, Blissett R, et al. The economic and clinical burden of nonalcoholic fatty liver disease in the United States and Europe. Hepatology. 2016;64:1577–86.
4. Chalasani N, Younossi Z, Lavine JE, et al. The diagnosis and management of non-alcoholic fatty liver disease: practice Guideline by the American Association for the Study of Liver Diseases, American College of Gastroenterology, and the American Gastroenterological Association. Hepatology. 2012;55:2005–23.
5. Stepanova M, Younossi ZM. Independent association between nonalcoholic fatty liver disease and cardiovascular disease in the US population. Clin Gastroenterol Hepatol. 2012;10:646–50.
6. Hossain N, Afendy A, Stepanova M, et al. Independent predictors of fibrosis in patients with nonalcoholic fatty liver disease. Clin Gastroenterol Hepatol. 2009;7:1224–9. 9 e1–2.
7. McPherson S, Hardy T, Henderson E, et al. Evidence of NAFLD progression from steatosis to fibrosing-steatohepatitis using paired biopsies: implications for prognosis and clinical management. J Hepatol. 2015;62:1148–55.
8. Gramlich T, Kleiner DE, McCullough AJ, et al. Pathologic features associated with fibrosis in nonalcoholic fatty liver disease. Hum Pathol. 2004;35:196–9.
9. Younossi ZM, Stepanova M, Rafiq N, et al. Pathologic criteria for nonalcoholic steatohepatitis: interprotocol agreement and ability to predict liver-related mortality. Hepatology. 2011;53:1874–82.
10. Stepanova M, Rafiq N, Makhlouf H, et al. Predictors of all-cause mortality and liver-related mortality in patients with non-alcoholic fatty liver disease (NAFLD). Dig Dis Sci. 2013;58:3017–23.
11. Younossi ZM, Otgonsuren M, Venkatesan C, et al. In patients with non-alcoholic fatty liver disease, metabolically abnormal individuals are at a higher risk for mortality while metabolically normal individuals are not. Metabolism. 2013;62:352–60.

12. Dulai PS, Singh S, Patel J, Soni M, Prokop LJ, Younossi Z, Sebastiani G, Ekstedt M, Hagstrom H, Nasr P, Stal P, Wong VW, Kechagias S, Hultcrantz R, Loomba R. Increased risk of mortality by fibrosis stage in nonalcoholic fatty liver disease: Systematic review and meta-analysis. Hepatology. 2017;65(5):1557–65.

13. Ekstedt M, Hagstrom H, Nasr P, et al. Fibrosis stage is the strongest predictor for disease-specific mortality in NAFLD after up to 33 years of follow-up. Hepatology. 2015;61:1547–54.

14. Nalbantoglu IL, Brunt EM. Role of liver biopsy in nonalcoholic fatty liver disease. World J Gastroenterol. 2014;20:9026–37.

15. Kleiner DE, Bedossa P. Liver histology and clinical trials for nonalcoholic steatohepatitis-perspectives from 2 pathologists. Gastroenterology. 2015;149:1305–8.

16. Sanyal AJ, Friedman SL, McCullough AJ, et al. Challenges and opportunities in drug and biomarker development for nonalcoholic steatohepatitis: findings and recommendations from an American Association for the Study of Liver Diseases-U.S. Food and Drug Administration Joint Workshop. Hepatology. 2015;61:1392–405.

17. Degertekin B, Ozenirler S, Elbeg S, et al. The serum endothelin-1 level in steatosis and NASH, and its relation with severity of liver fibrosis. Dig Dis Sci. 2007;52:2622–8.

18. Ratziu V, Massard J, Charlotte F, et al. Diagnostic value of biochemical markers (FibroTest-FibroSURE) for the prediction of liver fibrosis in patients with non-alcoholic fatty liver disease. BMC Gastroenterol. 2006;6:6.

19. Choe YG, Jin W, Cho YK, et al. Apolipoprotein B/AI ratio is independently associated with non-alcoholic fatty liver disease in nondiabetic subjects. J Gastroenterol Hepatol. 2013;28:678–83.

20. Miller MH, Walsh SV, Atrih A, et al. Serum proteome of nonalcoholic fatty liver disease: a multimodal approach to discovery of biomarkers of nonalcoholic steatohepatitis. J Gastroenterol Hepatol. 2014;29:1839–47.

21. Younossi ZM, Baranova A, Ziegler K, et al. A genomic and proteomic study of the spectrum of nonalcoholic fatty liver disease. Hepatology. 2005;42:665–74.

22. Baranova A, Liotta L, Petricoin E, et al. The role of genomics and proteomics: technologies in studying non-alcoholic fatty liver disease. Clin Liver Dis. 2007;11:209–20. xi

23. Younossi ZM, Baranova A, Stepanova M, et al. Phosphoproteomic biomarkers predicting histologic nonalcoholic steatohepatitis and fibrosis. J Proteome Res. 2010;9:3218–24.

24. Page S, Birerdinc A, Estep M, et al. Knowledge-based identification of soluble biomarkers: hepatic fibrosis in NAFLD as an example. PloS one. 2013;8:e56009.

25. Angulo P, Hui JM, Marchesini G, et al. The NAFLD fibrosis score: a noninvasive system that identifies liver fibrosis in patients with NAFLD. Hepatology. 2007;45:846–54.

26. Guha IN, Parkes J, Roderick P, et al. Noninvasive markers of fibrosis in nonalcoholic fatty liver disease: Validating the European Liver Fibrosis Panel and exploring simple markers. Hepatology. 2008;47:455–60.

27. Rodriguez-Suarez E, Duce AM, Caballeria J, et al. Non-alcoholic fatty liver disease proteomics. Proteomics Clin applications. 2010;4:362–71.

28. Charlton M, Viker K, Krishnan A, et al. Differential expression of lumican and fatty acid binding protein-1: new insights into the histologic spectrum of nonalcoholic fatty liver disease. Hepatology. 2009;49:1375–84.

29. Shiha G, Ibrahim A, Helmy A, et al. Asian-Pacific Association for the Study of the Liver (APASL) consensus guidelines on invasive and non-invasive assessment of hepatic fibrosis: a 2016 update. Hepatol Int. 2017;11:1–30.

30. Goodman ZD. The impact of obesity on liver histology. Clin Liver Dis. 2014;18:33–40.

31. Bedossa P. Histological Assessment of NAFLD. Dig Dis Sci. 2016;61:1348–55.

32. Luchini A, Geho DH, Bishop B, et al. Smart hydrogel particles: biomarker harvesting: one-step affinity purification, size exclusion, and protection against degradation. Nano letters. 2008;8:350–61.

33. Longo C, Patanarut A, George T, et al. Core-shell hydrogel particles harvest, concentrate and preserve labile low abundance biomarkers. PloS one. 2009;4:e4763.

34. Tamburro D, Fredolini C, Espina V, et al. Multifunctional core-shell nanoparticles: discovery of previously invisible biomarkers. J Am Chem Soc. 2011;133:19178–88.

35. Zhou W, Capello M, Fredolini C, et al. Proteomic analysis of pancreatic ductal adenocarcinoma cells reveals metabolic alterations. J Proteome Res. 2011;10:1944–52.

36. Signore M, Reeder KA. Antibody validation by Western blotting. Methods Mol Biol. 2012;823:139–55.

37. Paweletz CP, Charboneau L, Bichsel VE, et al. Reverse phase protein microarrays which capture disease progression show activation of pro-survival pathways at the cancer invasion front. Oncogene. 2001;20:1981–9.

38. Einspahr JG, Calvert V, Alberts DS, et al. Functional protein pathway activation mapping of the progression of normal skin to squamous cell carcinoma. Cancer Prev Res. 2012;5:403–13.

39. Akbani R, Becker KF, Carragher N, et al. Realizing the promise of reverse phase protein arrays for clinical, translational, and basic research: a workshop report: the RPPA (Reverse Phase Protein Array) society. Mol Cell Proteomics. 2014;13:1625–43.

40. Rapkiewicz A, Espina V, Zujewski JA, et al. The needle in the haystack: application of breast fine-needle aspirate samples to quantitative protein microarray technology. Cancer. 2007;111:173–84.

41. Manyam G, Birerdinc A, Baranova A. KPP: KEGG Pathway Painter. BMC Syst Biol. 2015;9(Suppl 2):S3.

42. Vega MI, Huerta-Yepaz S, Garban H, et al. Rituximab inhibits p38 MAPK activity in 2F7 B NHL and decreases IL-10 transcription: pivotal role of p38 MAPK in drug resistance. Oncogene. 2004;23:3530–40.

43. Guo X, Harada C, Namekata K, et al. Regulation of the severity of neuroinflammation and demyelination by TLR-ASK1-p38 pathway. EMBO Mol Med. 2010;2:504–15.

44. Peifer C, Wagner G, Laufer S. New approaches to the treatment of inflammatory disorders small molecule inhibitors of p38 MAP kinase. Curr Top Med Chem. 2006;6:113–49.

45. Zhang J, Shen B, Lin A. Novel strategies for inhibition of the p38 MAPK pathway. Trends Pharmacol Sci. 2007;28:286–95.

46. Schreiber S, Feagan B, D'Haens G, et al. Oral p38 mitogen-activated protein kinase inhibition with BIRB 796 for active Crohn's disease: a randomized, double-blind, placebo-controlled trial. Clin Gastroenterol Hepatol. 2006;4:325–34.

47. Ratziu V, Sheikh MY, Sanyal AJ, et al. A phase 2, randomized, double-blind, placebo-controlled study of GS-9450 in subjects with nonalcoholic steatohepatitis. Hepatology. 2012;55:419–28.

48. Hu X, Chen J, Wang L, et al. Crosstalk among Jak-STAT, Toll-like receptor, and ITAM-dependent pathways in macrophage activation. J Leukocyte Biol. 2007;82:237–43.

49. Baker SS, Baker RD, Liu W, et al. Role of alcohol metabolism in non-alcoholic steatohepatitis. PloS One. 2010;5:e9570.

50. Zhu L, Baker SS, Gill C, et al. Characterization of gut microbiomes in nonalcoholic steatohepatitis (NASH) patients: a connection between endogenous alcohol and NASH. Hepatology. 2013;57:601–9.

51. Zhu R, Baker SS, Moylan CA, et al. Systematic transcriptome analysis reveals elevated expression of alcohol-metabolizing genes in NAFLD livers. J Pathol. 2016;238:531–42.

52. Plompen EP, Schouten JN, Janssen HL. Role of anticoagulant therapy in liver disease. Hepatol Int. 2013;7:369–76.

53. Plompen EP, Darwish Murad S, Hansen BE, et al. Prothrombotic genetic risk factors are associated with an increased risk of liver fibrosis in the general population: The Rotterdam Study. J Hepatol. 2015;63:1459–65.

54. Perry RJ, Samuel VT, Petersen KF, et al. The role of hepatic lipids in hepatic insulin resistance and type 2 diabetes. Nature. 2014;510:84–91.

55. Inoue H, Ogawa W, Ozaki M, et al. Role of STAT-3 in regulation of hepatic gluconeogenic genes and carbohydrate metabolism in vivo. Nature Med. 2004;10:168–74.

56. Moh A, Zhang W, Yu S, et al. STAT3 sensitizes insulin signaling by negatively regulating glycogen synthase kinase-3 beta. Diabetes. 2008;57:1227–35.

57. Golabi P, Stepanova M, Pham HT, Cable R, Rafiq N, Bush H, Gogoll T, Younossi ZM. Non-alcoholic steatofibrosis (NASF) can independently predict mortality in patients with non-alcoholic fatty liver disease (NAFLD). BMJ Open Gastroenterol. 2018;5(1):e000198. https://doi.org/10.1136/bmjgast-2018-000198. eCollection 2018.

3

The potential impact of the demographic transition in the Senegal-Gambia region of sub-Saharan Africa on the burden of infectious disease and its potential synergies with control programmes: the case of hepatitis B

John R. Williams[1][*][†], Piero Manfredi[2][†] and Alessia Melegaro[3]

Abstract

Background: Sub-Saharan Africa (SSA) continues to suffer high communicable disease burdens as its demographic transition (DT) proceeds. Although the consequent changes in population structures influence age-specific contact patterns relevant for transmission, the age distribution of immunity, and the disease burden, investigation of the potential of DT to affect infectious disease epidemiology in regions of SSA has hitherto been overlooked. With a substantial disease burden and complex epidemiology, hepatitis B virus (HBV) represents a prime example of an infection whose epidemiology may be significantly influenced by the DT.

Methods: An age-structured mathematical model for HBV in the Senegal and Gambia (SG) region was set within a demographic framework with varying vital rates mirroring the entire course of the DT there over 1850–2100, to investigate the effects of the DT on HBV epidemiology, with and without the combined action of vaccination. The model was run from its reconstructed *ancien régime* (old order) demo-epidemiologic equilibrium and calibrated against SG 1950 age-distribution estimates and Gambian pre-vaccination HBV age-prevalence data.

Results: The model, which reproduced well demographic and HBV age-prevalence data, predicted a complex transition of HBV epidemiology over the course of the DT. This included a prolonged epoch of expansion alongside population growth and rejuvenation until 1990–2000, followed by a dramatic retreat, mainly reflecting projected fertility decline during the twenty-first century. This transitional pattern was mostly explained by the underlying demographically driven changes in horizontal transmission resulting from the changes in the age structure of the population. During 2000–2150 the HBV burden is predicted to decline by more than 70% even in the absence of vaccination.

Conclusions: Demographic change alone may strongly affect HBV disease burden and shape HBV endemicity. The onset of the demographically driven decline in HBV prevalence, aligned with the expansion of HBV vaccination, forms a synergy potentially boosting effectiveness of control. Such a synergy currently appears to be presenting a "window of opportunity" facilitating HBV elimination which it would be important to exploit and which underlines the importance of taking demographic change into account when assessing the potential longer term impact of vaccination and other control measures.

* Correspondence: jr.williams@imperial.ac.uk
[†]John R. Williams and Piero Manfredi contributed equally to this work.
[1]Department of Infectious Disease Epidemiology, School of Public Health, Faculty of Medicine, Imperial College London, St Mary's Campus, Norfolk Place, London W2 1PG, UK
Full list of author information is available at the end of the article

Background

Sub-Saharan Africa (SSA), the world region with the highest burden from communicable diseases [1], is currently experiencing a fertility transition [2], contributing jointly with continued mortality decline and massive urbanisation, to an overall demographic transition (DT). However, an investigation of any potential effects on the epidemiology of infectious disease in areas of SSA (or indeed in the wider world) has hitherto been largely neglected.

Although demography is continually in transition, the conventional idealised picture of DT, as experienced by industrialised countries [2–4] after 1750–1800, is of an initially stationary population characterised by high mortality and fertility rates — the *ancien* or *Malthusian régime* [3] — which first experiences falling mortality rates accompanied by rapid population growth leading to a young age distribution. This mortality decline is later followed by a fertility decline with, in this idealised scenario, the eventual attainment of a *modern* stationary regime at low levels of fertility and mortality. In classical demographic and demo-economic explanations, mortality decline has been the major trigger of fertility decline, which in turn resulted as the major engine of economic development of industrialised countries [3]. The experience of industrialised countries after 1960 has shown however that replacement fertility is by no means a necessary outcome of this process, with the gradual spread of below replacement fertility, in some cases even to very low levels [5], yielding rapid population ageing.

In the different regions of SSA, the joint action of fertility and mortality decline and rapid urbanisation — not to mention HIV/AIDS — are producing marked changes in population structures, primarily in the distribution of the population by age. These changes in the population age distributions are likely to affect the proportions of people of different age groups with whom individuals come into contact day by day. Such patterns of contact by age are key determinants [6, 7] of the patterns of transmission of infectious diseases and, consequently, of the ensuing age distribution of immunity. Moreover, severity of disease can often be influenced by age at infection [6], so that the overall population burden of disease also may change as the age distribution of the population changes. For infections that are vertically transmitted, time changes in age-specific fertility, combined with an evolving female age distribution and age distribution of female immunity, will also likely have an impact on the epidemiology of the infection [6].

The aim of this work is to provide a general investigation of the overall effects that changes in population age structure associated with DT might have upon the burdens of infectious diseases with complex epidemiology, focusing on hepatitis B virus (HBV), and selecting the region of Senegal and The Gambia as our "laboratory" in

SSA. Only a few studies have so far investigated the possible effects of demographic change on infection transmission dynamics and control. Moreover, most such studies have focused on common childhood infections such as measles and varicella in view of their epidemiological characteristics, primarily a single well-identified transmission route [8–19]. The only work so far that has considered an infection with more complex epidemiology has focused on dengue [20], and that study confirmed by statistical analyses effects similar to those predicted in the aforementioned literature.

HBV infection is a major example of an infection causing a substantial continuing burden of disease worldwide [21–23], including cirrhosis and liver cancer; thus, it calls for a redoubling of efforts and prioritisation of actions aimed at elimination [22]. HBV has a complex epidemiology in which such key processes as transmission, infection, and disease development are strongly age-related [24–26]. More specifically, HBV has multiple transmission routes (see Additional file 1: Figure S3.1), with perinatal, sexual, and horizontal transmission by person-to-person contacts being most prominent in the general population. Each of these transmission routes is potentially affected by changes in the age distribution of the population. In addition, the probability, once infected, of developing persistent HBV infection is strongly age-related, being very high in infancy but declining steeply with age [25]. Given these age dependencies, it is presently unclear how the ongoing DT might affect the overall transmission and resulting disease burden of HBV. Finally, the pre-vaccination landscape of HBV exhibited a dramatic epidemiologically significant variation in prevalence worldwide [27]. In Medley et al. [28] an explanation has been proposed for this variability by the nonlinear feedback between the HBV force of infection and the age-related probability of developing HBV carriage; moreover, it was conjectured that the demographic changes along the DT might have been a major determinant of this heterogeneity.

Mathematical modelling of infectious disease transmission dynamics is a technique which naturally lends itself to the investigation of the interplay between population and infectious disease dynamics. We used an age-structured model for the transmission dynamics of HBV with realistic population dynamics parameterised with demographic (vital rates) and epidemiological data (HBV prevalence) from Senegal and The Gambia, considered here as a unique demographic entity, in an attempt to cast light on the nature and extent of the potential influence of the course of the DT on HBV epidemiology and its possible implications for the variability of HBV prevalence worldwide.

Methods

Senegal and The Gambia

Focus on Senegal and The Gambia as a unique demographic entity (denoted from now on as SG) was motivated by the fact that The Gambia, apart from its coastline (< 50 km), is entirely surrounded by Senegal, and also that there is a strong ethnic and cultural overlap between the two countries, which for a period in the 1980s together formed a loose confederation, Senegambia [29]. The Gambia itself is an exemplar of a country in SSA with good-quality data on the prevalence of pre-vaccination HBV infection by age [25]. Moreover, the two countries supplied a substantial portion of the data used previously to estimate a key function relating age and likelihood of becoming a carrier [25]. In addition, although patterns of age-specific growth rates of the small population in The Gambia are somewhat erratic, this is not the case for the much larger Senegal, which has exhibited, according to United Nations (UN) data, fairly regular patterns of DT and mortality decline since 1950, and a well-separated late onset of fertility transition (by about 1990).

Data

Data on previous experience of HBV infection by age were drawn from published work on The Gambia [30]. Plausible ranges for HBV epidemiological parameters relating to infectivity, duration of stages of infection, etc. (Additional file 1: Table S2.1) were gleaned from the literature [23]. Demographic data on fertility and mortality rates in Senegal and The Gambia were drawn from the UN 1950–2015 estimates and the subsequent 2015–2150 projections, as well as data on the population age distribution by 5-year age groups which were used for model validation [31]. In particular, data from all three main UN projections variants, namely, the "medium" one, which is the UN key variant taken as our baseline here, as well as the "high" and "low" variants, were considered. Moving averages of estimated or projected UN age-specific fertility and mortality rates in successive 5-year periods from 1950 to 1955 to 2095–2100 provided time-varying vital rates for the model over a 150-year period.

The mathematical model for population and HBV transmission/disease dynamics

The population model was age-sex structured with time-changing age-specific fertility and age- and gender-specific mortality rates to depict a realistic time course for the DT. The part of the model simulating the transmission dynamics of HBV (see the flow diagram in Fig. 1) included age dependencies in vertical, horizontal, and heterosexual modes of transmission, as well as in the probability of developing HBV carriage once infected (see

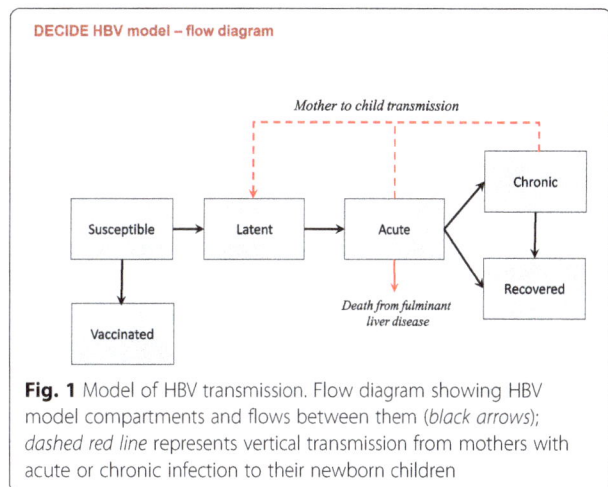

Fig. 1 Model of HBV transmission. Flow diagram showing HBV model compartments and flows between them (*black arrows*); *dashed red line* represents vertical transmission from mothers with acute or chronic infection to their newborn children

Additional file 1: Figure S3.1 and Text S2 for details including the full partial differential equations (PDEs) describing the model). A computer program designed for the purpose and coded using Fortran 77 provided for numerical solution of the model PDEs.

In the model all births to acutely and chronically HBV infected mothers were at risk of vertically transmitted HBV, acquired at a rate depending on the relative proportions of females with acute or persistent (i.e. chronic) infection in each fertile age group. A proportion of vertically infected offspring was assumed to develop chronic infection [25]. Children and adults at all ages were at risk of horizontal HBV transmission at an age-specific rate determined by an appropriately specified WAIFW (who acquires infection from whom) matrix [6] obtained by multiplying the WAIFW matrix estimated for The Gambia by Edmunds and colleagues [30] by a single scaling parameter for purposes of data fit. The influence of the evolving age distribution of the population on social contact patterns relevant for horizontal HBV transmission, and therefore on the WAIFW, was modelled in accord with previous work [10–12, 16]. Sexual transmission started at the age of sexual debut, assumed to be 15 years, at a rate dependent on (1) the rate of acquisition of new partners for each gender and age group, (2) sexual mixing matrices determining the proportion of sexual contacts to be drawn from each age group, (3) the proportion of acutely and chronically infected partners in each gender age group, and (4) the risk of transmission per acutely and chronically infected partner. The sexual mixing matrix adopted obeyed a preferred mixing rule [32] with a parameter determining the degree of age assortativeness of sexual partnerships. The underlying age-gender specific rates of sexual behaviour are kept constant during population evolution, but as male and female populations evolve separately, at each time point an adjustment is made to partner acquisition rates to ensure that male and female partnerships always balance. Note that the preferred mixing rule, in which the force of infection acting on each age-gender group explicitly depends on the proportions of the population in the various age groups, straightforwardly incorporates the feedback of the evolving age distribution of the population on sexual contact patterns.

Upon infection by any route of transmission, susceptible people moved to a latently infected but noninfectious stage and subsequently to an acutely infected and infectious stage, a small proportion of the latter being assumed to die as a result of fulminant liver disease. Following acute infection, a strongly age-dependent proportion [25] moved to a state of chronic carriage having an average duration of several decades prior to recovery, while the complementary proportion resolved the infection, moving directly into the recovered stage; for simplicity, it was assumed that there was no additional disease-specific mortality during chronic carriage and that no screening and treatment programme was in place which might hasten recovery or reduce infectivity.

The model could also be set to include HBV vaccination at birth and/or at any subsequent age point, starting from a pre-specified time point, with a vaccine assumed to have 100% efficacy and lifelong duration. Those vaccinated in the model are moved to a vaccinated and immune compartment.

Parameterisation of the demographic component

Estimated (period 1950–2015) and projected (2015–2100) mortality and fertility rates from the UN for Senegal and Gambia were pooled to obtain a unique set of rates for SG as a single entity. In order to depict the course of an entire DT for SG, from its *ancien régime* stationary demographic equilibrium, we hypothesised that SG fertility at 1950 reflected true SG fertility through its entire previous history back to when the *ancien*-demographic *régime* prevailed. We then projected mortality rates into the past to reconstruct a reasonable *ancien régime* mortality table and the related stationary population (as expected for the *ancien régime*), i.e. one characterised by a constant total population size and an invariant age distribution, (see Additional file 1: Text S1 for details). The stationarity of the *ancien régime* age distribution was ensured by requiring that the corresponding female life table once combined with SG 1950 female fertility rates promoted a net reproductive rate of the population equal to one. This equilibrium population was taken as the initial condition for the age distribution of the SG population, i.e. the one prevailing before destabilisation due to the onset of the mortality transition (Fig. 2a). Departing from the *ancien régime* equilibrium, the demographic model was then run forward in time to reproduce the DT in SG

using the pooled set of SG mortality and fertility rates. Model predictions were compared, by a least squares criterion, to the 1950 SG male-female age distribution, assuming smooth adjustment over time of *ancien régime* mortality to the 1950 UN estimate.

Parameterisation of the HBV component of the model

We assumed also that HBV was, in the demographic *ancien régime* equilibrium, at an epidemiologic equilibrium which itself was destabilised by mortality decline at onset of the DT. Based on the HBV literature, uncertainty ranges were specified for HBV epidemiological parameters in the model, and Latin hypercube sampling (LHS) was used to explore these parameter ranges (see Additional file 1: Table S2.1 for full details of HBV parameters included in the LHS procedure). By LHS we generated 24,000 sampled parameter sets. Departing from the *ancien régime* demo-epidemiologic equilibrium, the full HBV model was first run forward for each sampled parameter set until 1984 using smoothed UN-based vital rate estimates 1950–1985 [31], under the hypothesis that no interventions (vaccination, use of protection for sexual activity, etc.) were in place. Model predictions at 1984 were compared, by a least squares criterion, to Gambian early 1980s' HBV pre-vaccination age-prevalence data on both past exposure and current infection. As best fit we took the parameter combination generating the lowest value of the least squares function over the entire set of 24,000 LHS samples. In particular, the horizontal transmission WAIFW matrix was fitted to the data by adjusting the scaling factor applied to all the elements of the matrix within the overall fitting procedure. During each simulation the HBV parameters were kept constant over time, ensuring that any changes over time in results for disease prevalence arose solely from demographic change. Uncertainty bands about the best-fit set of parameters were generated by retaining the 2400 (i.e. 10% of the total) parameter sets generating the largest values of the least squares function. These uncertainty bands about parameter values were then used to generate uncertainty bands about the predicted HBV trajectories over time.

Parameterisation of HBV vaccination

Our baseline vaccination scenario was designed to approximate the Senegal situation in view of its possible larger relevance as: (1) The Gambia could be considered a special case due to the work of The Gambia Hepatitis Intervention Study [33], (2) the Senegal population is many times the size of its neighbour, (3) in common with many other countries in SSA, in Senegal the lack of availability of monovalent HBV vaccine prevented the implementation of universal vaccination at birth [34]. Thus, in our baseline scenario, vaccination is administered to children aged 3.5 months, with effective

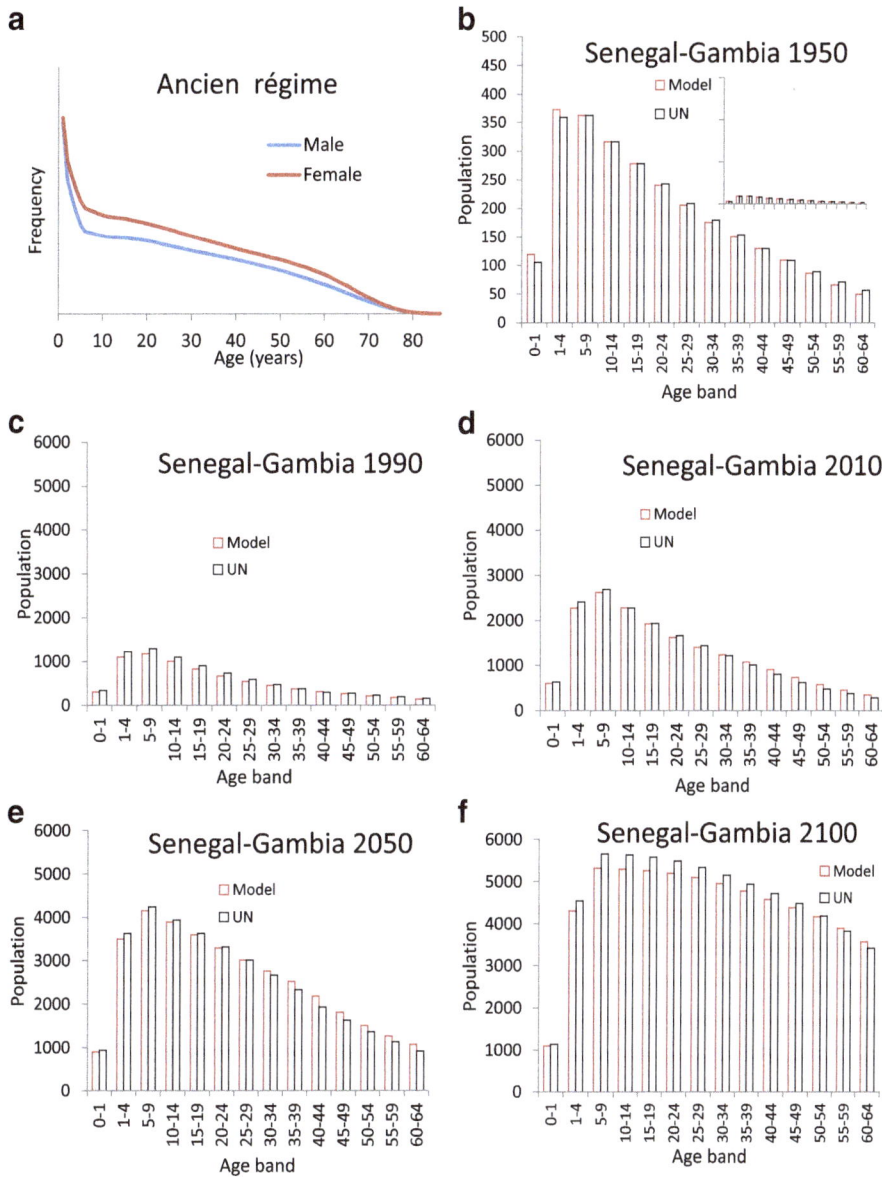

Fig. 2 Results from the demographic component of the model for the SG population. **a** Male and female age profiles of the SG population at *ancien régime* equilibrium corresponding to the years 1840–1850 in the model. **b–f** Model predictions for the age distribution by 5-year age groups up to age 65 of the SG population at specific time points compared with UN estimates 1950–2100 (note that inset in **b** has same vertical scale as **c-f**)

coverage of 46% [34] and 2005 as year of introduction of the vaccine into the Expanded Programme on Immunisation [34]. Alternative scenarios were considered including higher coverage levels (55% and 75%) as well as the possibility of vaccination at birth to prevent vertical transmission.

Prediction of the course of the demographic transition in SG

As a preliminary step, using the best demographic model, predictions for the age-sex distribution of the population for 1955–2100 were systematically compared with the corresponding UN estimates/projections, in order to ensure that the model-based prediction of the evolution of the age-sex structure depicted a course of the DT in SG always close to UN projected figures.

Prediction of the long-term transitional epidemiology of HBV

The model was then used to represent the evolving epidemiology and burden of HBV (with and without vaccination) during the entire course of the DT departing from its *ancien régime* pre-transitional epidemiological equilibrium and continuing until 2150. Extension of the horizon to 2150 (rather than 2100, which is the last year of UN projections) was carried out by freezing mortality and fertility rates for 2100–2150 at the levels projected for 2100. This was motivated by the need to explore the ultimate consequences of the demographic changes projected up to 2100, which will continue to develop for several decades further despite demographic rates having been kept constant thereafter. For the future evolution of HBV we focused — as baseline — on the UN "medium" variant, but sensitivity analyses considering the implications of the other main UN variants, namely the "high" and the "low" ones, were also undertaken, as well as a worst-case scenario where fertility is maintained constant at its maximal level (achieved during 1990–1995). This also allowed consideration of the potential long-term effects on HBV epidemiology in SSA of the eventual fall into continued below replacement fertility.

Results
Fit and reproduction of demographic and HBV data
The model identified 1840–1850 as the epoch when the *ancien regíme* equilibrium ended due to initiation of the mortality transition (Fig. 2a). Forward projections of the demographic model satisfactorily fitted the 1950 UN estimate of population age distribution for both sexes (Fig. 2b). Subsequent model-based forward projections of the age-sex distribution remained quite close to UN population estimates and projections for the entire horizon 1950–2100, as reported in Fig. 2b–f for the case of the UN "medium" projection variant. The model also reproduced quite satisfactorily the 1980s' pre-vaccination age-prevalence data for exposure to HBV (Fig. 3a) and current HBV infection (Fig. 3b).

Effects of the demographic transition on HBV epidemiology in the absence of vaccination
Figures 4 and 5 report predictions by the best model for the evolution of the natural history of HBV that would be observed in the absence of immunisation during the whole course of the DT in SG, from around 1850 (corresponding to the *ancien régime*) to 2100 according to the UN medium variant. As well summarised by the transitional trend of prevalence of exposure to HBV infection (Fig. 4a), starting from the HBV pre-transitional equilibrium profile at 1850, where prevalence by age 15 was in the region of 70%, HBV was predicted to gradually expand, reaching prevalence levels as high as 85% by age 15. Thereafter HBV entered a phase of continuing decline, returning to levels comparable to, and subsequently below, the pre-transition phase when projected fertility approached and stabilised near to replacement levels (between 2100 and 2150). At 2150, HBV prevalence (in the absence of any control measures) is predicted to settle at

25–30% by age 15. This same story is told by the other graphs of Fig. 4: in particular, the population age distribution of disease burden post-equilibrium (Fig. 4d) remained heavily skewed towards younger ages until 1950–2000 before becoming substantially more evenly distributed in later years, reflecting the changed demography.

Much of the explanation for the predicted trends lies in the dramatic changes of horizontal transmission during the DT. This is made clear by the temporal trend of the corresponding age-specific force of infection (Fig. 5a) among young individuals (aged below 15 years). Indeed, the horizontal force of infection among the youngest systematically increased during the HBV expansion phase up to levels of around 15% per year, approaching levels commonly seen for typical childhood infections such as varicella [35]. This resulted from the continued rejuvenation of the population during the major epoch of mortality decline among young individuals and persistent high fertility (roughly up to 2000). Subsequently, the horizontal force of infection among young individuals experienced continued decline, falling to very low levels — well below those of the *ancien régime* – during the major phase of fertility decline (after 2050) and corresponding progressive population ageing. This pattern arises as a consequence of the dramatic changes in the proportions of social contacts between younger and older individuals during the various stages of the DT [11, 12, 16, 17]. Notably, vertical and sexual transmission routes also showed complex patterns of evolution during the course of the DT, as signalled by the changes in route-specific incidences (Fig. 5b–d), even under the assumption of constant sexual behaviour rates. In the *ancien régime*, horizontal vs sexual transmission accounted for 85% and 8% of overall HBV incidence, respectively. During the HBV expansion phase, the two routes are predicted to diverge, with horizontal incidence growing to a maximum in the 1980s and sexual incidence declining to a minimum not long after the 1990s, when the horizontal route is predicted to account for almost 92% of total incidence. In the 1990s, after horizontal transmission has begun its long decline, sexual transmission inverts its trend, returning to *ancien régime* levels by around 2060; this pattern of incidence due to horizontal transmission is mirrored, at an order of magnitude lower, by that for vertical transmission, results well reflecting observations from The Gambia [36].

Impact of vaccination on HBV burden under different demographic transition scenarios
To separate the effects of the continuation of the DT from those of vaccination, we focus on the proportion of the overall population with persistent infection,

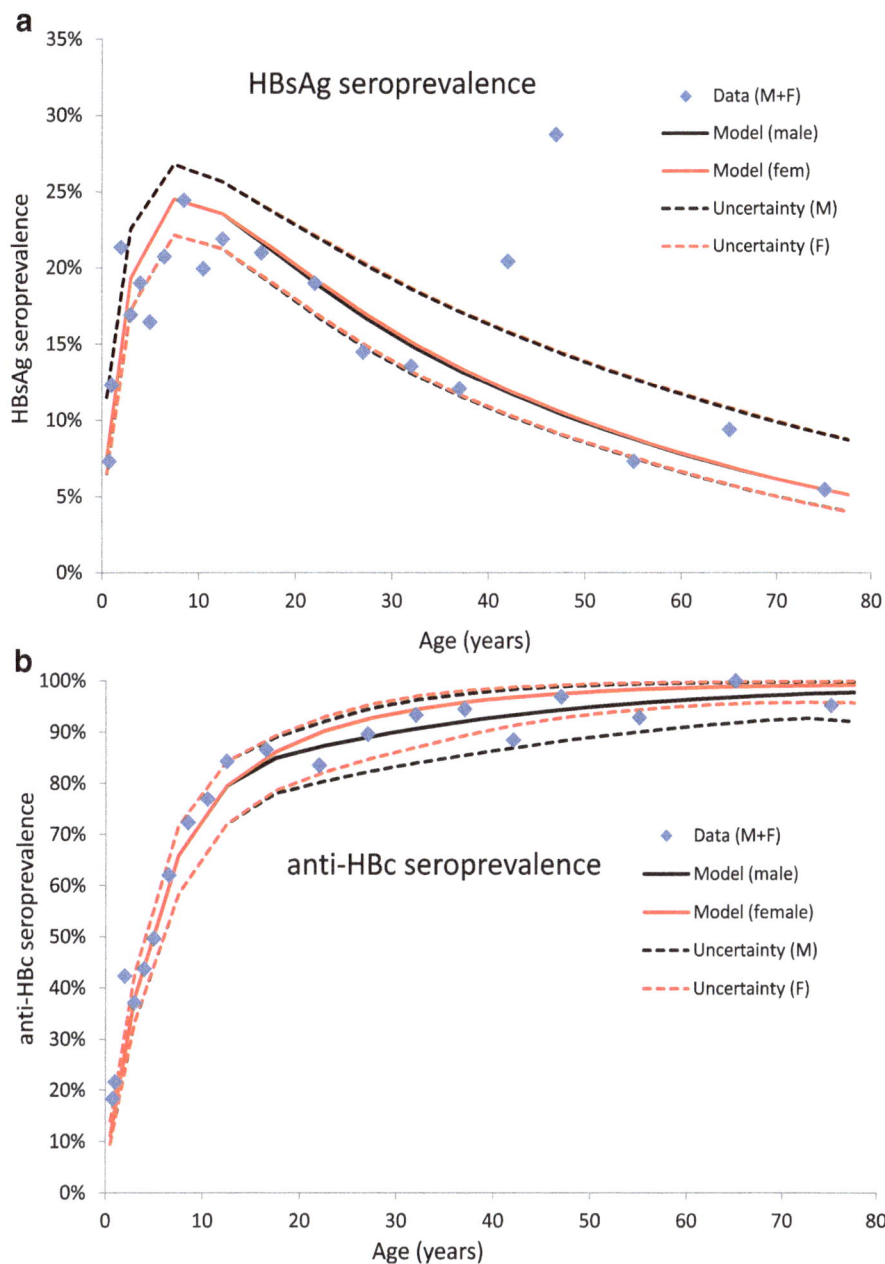

Fig. 3 Best model fit to HBV prevalence. **a** Model-predicted age-specific prevalence of exposure to HBV (represented by HBV core antibody prevalence) compared with prevalence observed in The Gambia in the early 1980s [30]. **b** Model-predicted age-specific prevalence of serological markers of persistent infection (corresponding to HBV surface antibody) compared with corresponding prevalence observed in The Gambia in 1984 [30]. Results show best-fit model results and related uncertainty bands based on those parameter constellations from LHS representing the best 10% values obtained for the least squares score function

which serves as a useful summary measure of burden of disease. Under the best model in the absence of any immunisation, this increased monotonically along the DT (in the medium variant scenario) to a peak of 17% in ~ 1992, i.e. a decade prior to the introduction of universal HBV vaccination in Senegal in 2005, before decreasing steadily thereafter (Fig. 6a, uppermost line), reaching levels as low as 5% in 2150.

Figure 6 also investigates the effects of possible vaccination programmes (all initiated in 2005) comparing our baseline DT scenario in SG (Fig. 6a) with the alternative scenario where SG total fertility is frozen at its maximal level observed in 1990–1995, namely before the fertility transition initiated (Fig. 6b), the scenario representing the worst case in terms of infection control given that it completely prevents the phase of HBV retreat. The

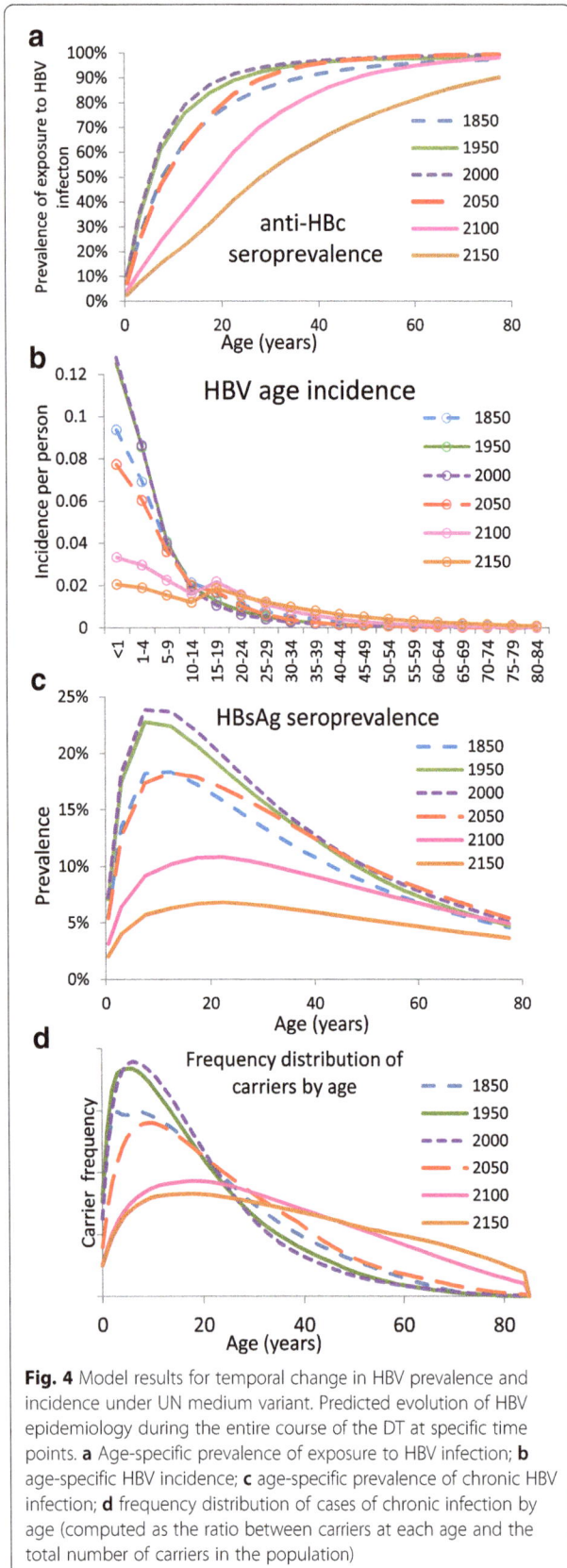

Fig. 4 Model results for temporal change in HBV prevalence and incidence under UN medium variant. Predicted evolution of HBV epidemiology during the entire course of the DT at specific time points. **a** Age-specific prevalence of exposure to HBV infection; **b** age-specific HBV incidence; **c** age-specific prevalence of chronic HBV infection; **d** frequency distribution of cases of chronic infection by age (computed as the ratio between carriers at each age and the total number of carriers in the population)

differences are stark. If fertility remains constant at its highest level, the prevalence of chronic HBV in the absence of immunisation would remain nearly constant over time at its maximum level (Fig. 6b, uppermost line). At baseline coverage (46%), chronic HBV would cease its decline at a level of around 3% prevalence, whereas coverage in excess of 75% would be effective in bringing the infection under full control.

In contrast, the onset and completion of the DT (along the medium scenario) is predicted to "sustain" immunisation by yielding a substantial decline in the prevalence of chronic HBV (down to 1% by 2150) even with the baseline coverage, and bringing it to near elimination level with a coverage just in excess of 55%. This suggests the possibility of a strong synergy between vaccination and the HBV retreat phase triggered by the DT. The impact of a hypothetical alternative programme of vaccination at birth at the same rate of 46% shows an even steeper decrease in the prevalence of chronic infection (see Additional file 1: Text S4).

Finally, the impact of different patterns of DT in the future, as embedded in the "low" and "high" variants of UN projections (in contrast to the "medium" one), and the interplay of this with vaccination are also reported (Fig. 7). The persistent fall into below replacement fertility, as hypothesised in the low variant, would made control conditions easier but only after 2050.

Discussion

Demographic change can, according to circumstances, create great challenges and opportunities. Possibly the major example in history is represented by the interplay between DT and the industrial revolution, with the acknowledged role of mortality decline as the major trigger of fertility decline, via the switch from quantity to "quality" of children, which in turn resulted as a major engine of the sustained economic development of industrialised countries [3]. Nonetheless, it has remained largely unclear where the balance may lie in terms of its effect on infectious disease epidemiology. As age distributions of infection and immunity are far from uniform, patterns of contact between different age groups are of fundamental importance for infection transmission, so that change in population age structure may strongly influence infectious disease epidemiology. It then becomes essential to attempt to understand how the two interact, especially for those world regions, such as SSA, where the burden from infectious diseases is still striking.

In SSA, although mortality decline possibly had its beginnings prior to 1900 [3], much of the process has taken place since 1950 and is still ongoing. On the other hand, the fertility transition was unexpectedly delayed and has been proceeding at a slower rate compared with other regions such as Asia and Latin America [2].

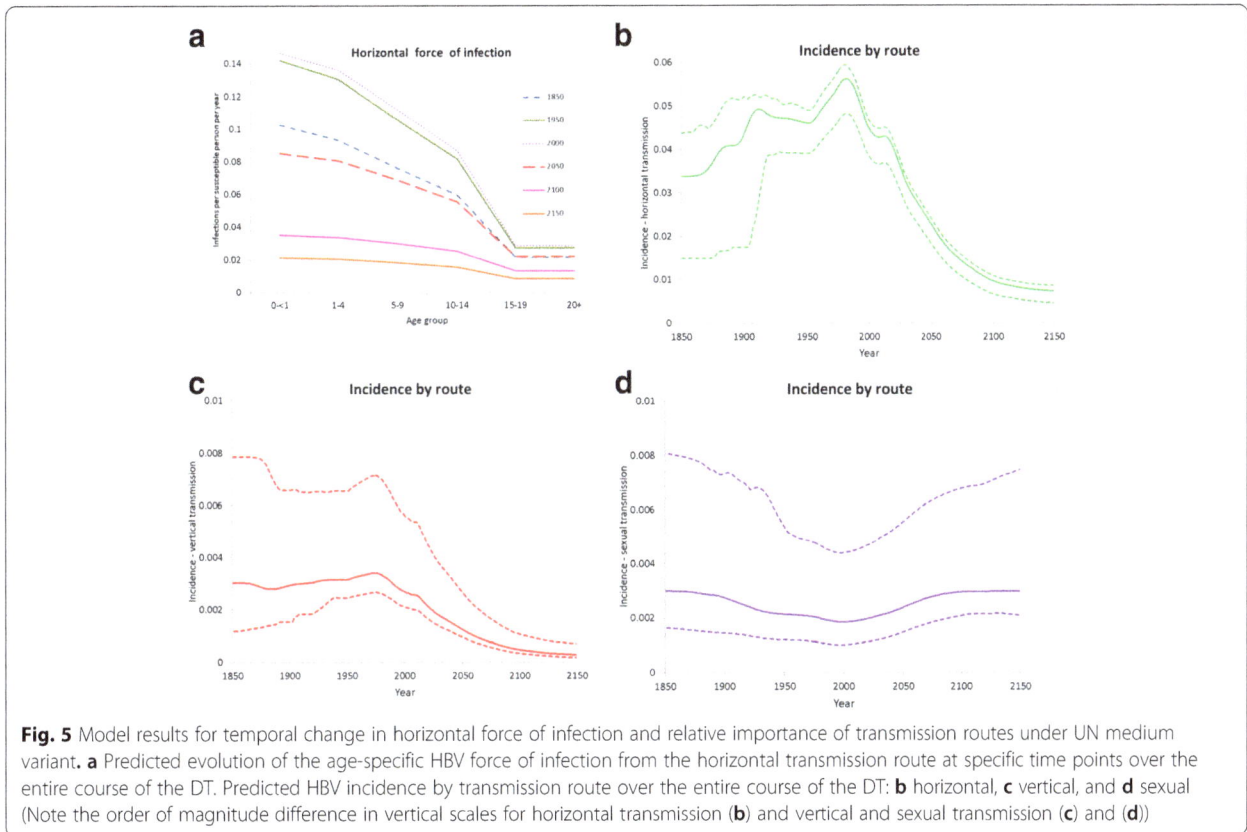

Fig. 5 Model results for temporal change in horizontal force of infection and relative importance of transmission routes under UN medium variant. **a** Predicted evolution of the age-specific HBV force of infection from the horizontal transmission route at specific time points over the entire course of the DT. Predicted HBV incidence by transmission route over the entire course of the DT: **b** horizontal, **c** vertical, and **d** sexual (Note the order of magnitude difference in vertical scales for horizontal transmission (**b**) and vertical and sexual transmission (**c**) and (**d**))

Indeed, fertility decline began, in regions such as SG, as recently as the 1990s [2] and is predicted to continue to display its effects over a span of a century or so. The resulting massive changes in the age distribution of the populations are likely to have greatest impact on those infections in which processes of transmission and disease are strongly age-related and infection may be long-lasting. HBV is one such infection and one which gives rise to a substantial burden of disease. Global mortality associated with viral hepatitis ranks equally with that from HIV/AIDS and tuberculosis, and in 2016 the World Health Assembly adopted a strategy for its global elimination [21], with HBV being responsible for the majority of deaths associated with viral hepatitis [22]. Nonetheless, the great heterogeneity in the global distribution of the burden of disease arising from HBV [27, 28] might hinder steps towards its elimination. For these reasons a mathematical modelling approach may provide a key to disentangling the mutual interplay of demographic changes and HBV epidemiology during the different phases of DT, and, by depicting an entire range of dynamic regimes, possibly offer some clues towards explaining the puzzle of the heterogeneity in HBV burden.

Using a mathematical model, we assessed the possible extent of the impact of the entire course of the DT on the transmission and burden of HBV in a region of SSA.

Our results predict that, departing from the pre-transitional demo-epidemiologic equilibrium prevailing at some time prior to 1900 and later destabilised by the onset of the mortality transition, HBV burden may have followed a complex "epidemiological transition" pattern. This pattern is initially characterised by a long epoch of expansion until ~ 2000, corresponding to the epoch of maximal population rejuvenation, and it is predicted to be subsequently followed by a dramatic "retreat" corresponding to the major epoch of fertility decline observed from 1990 onward and continuing for decades after the completion of fertility decline. This demographically driven pattern of expansion-retreat of HBV is mostly explained by the underlying dramatic changes in horizontal transmission due to the changes in the age distribution of the population. During the HBV expansion phase, this change in transmission is the consequence of the period of rejuvenation following mortality decline in young age groups while fertility remained persistently high during the first stages of the transition. During the phase of HBV retreat, the change in transmission is mostly the consequence of the decline in fertility associated with the onset and completion of the fertility transition in SG. Thereafter, between 2000 and 2150 (when below replacement fertility prevails), HBV burden is predicted to decline dramatically by around 70%.

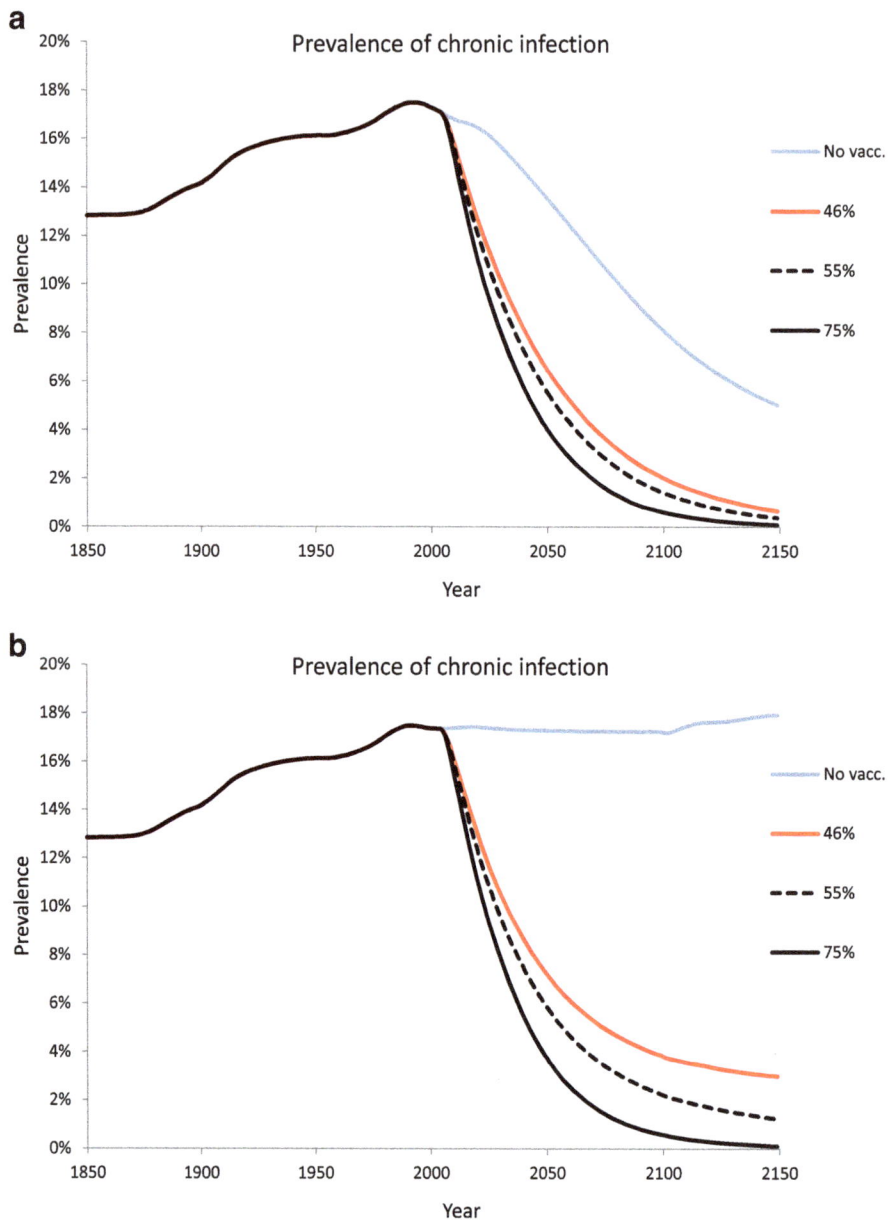

Fig. 6 Potential synergy between demographic transition and HBV vaccination under different projection variants. Reconstructed and projected overall population burden of HBV disease (over the entire course of the DT up to 2150) without and with vaccination commencing in 2005: **a** the case of UN medium variant; **b** a worst-case scenario where fertility remains constant at its maximum level. Vaccination is administered at age 3.5 months assuming 100% efficacy

These results seem to be of importance from a number of standpoints. First, they shed light on the nature, extent, and determinants of the potential influence of demographic change on the burden of HBV, and quite possibly other infections with a similarly complex epidemiology having in common age dependency in key epidemiological processes. Second, they supply a contribution to the interpretation of the long-term natural history of HBV epidemiology. Third, they provide considerable evidence in support of a conjecture formulated in [28], namely that the great variability in pre-vaccination HBV prevalence worldwide might largely be a consequence of the DT. More precisely, the present work has shown that the greatest part of this variability might result from the differences in the timing of onset and pace at which the DT was experienced in different regions of the world [2, 3]. Fourth, they indicate a precise causative role of the DT in triggering "epidemiological transitions", broadly interpreted as patterns of retreat of the burdens of disease which are a key

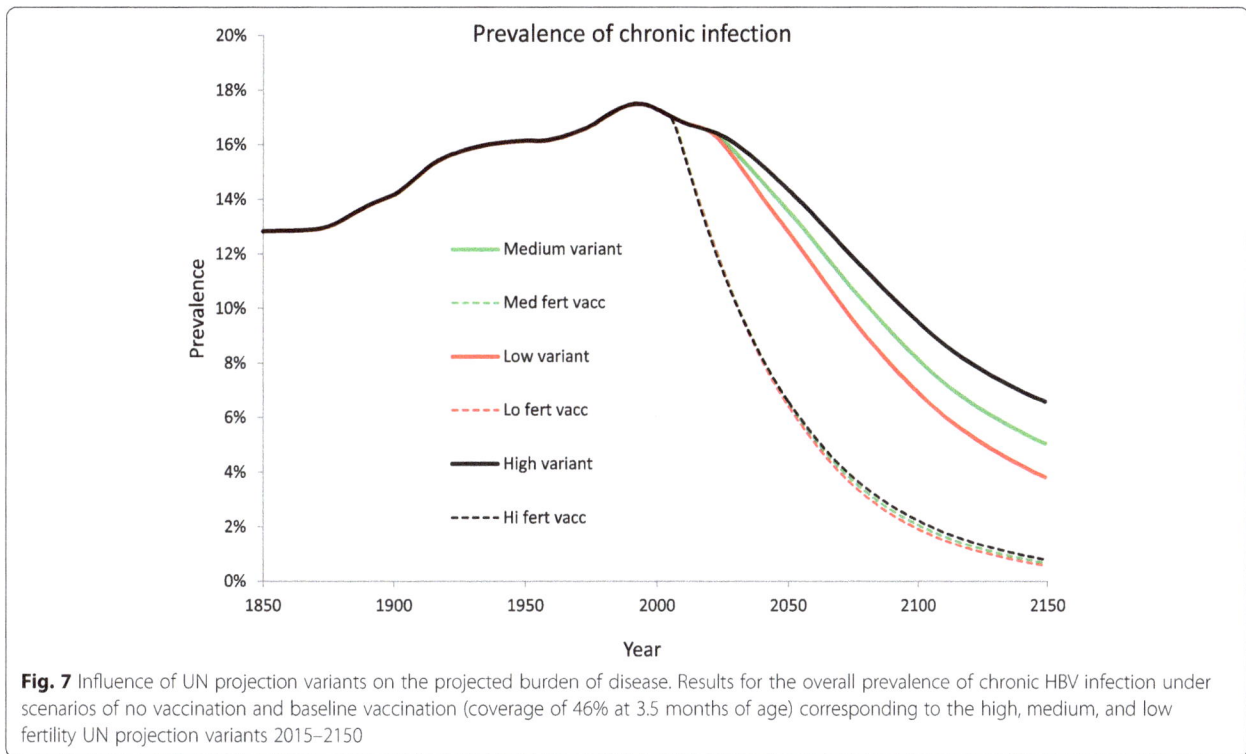

Fig. 7 Influence of UN projection variants on the projected burden of disease. Results for the overall prevalence of chronic HBV infection under scenarios of no vaccination and baseline vaccination (coverage of 46% at 3.5 months of age) corresponding to the high, medium, and low fertility UN projection variants 2015–2150

component of Omran's classical definition [37]. Last, the onset of a demographically driven decline in HBV prevalence in the model coincided with a real-world expansion of HBV vaccination, suggesting a synergy potentially boosting effectiveness of control in the decades leading up to elimination. This appears to be of fundamental importance in helping to achieve the aim of HBV global elimination [21]. Indeed, the predicted initiation of the HBV retreat phase in the last 15 years suggests that a "window of opportunity" has presented itself where fertility decline will synergistically concur with immunisation programmes to hasten the global target of HBV elimination.

Finally, although due to paucity of data our analyses focused on our characterisation of a single region of SSA, our model representations of the DT and of HBV epidemiology are fairly general. We therefore feel that a major strength of this work is that it provides a pointer for interpreting past and future long-term trends of HBV in SSA and also at the global scale.

The major limitations in studies of the impact of population change on infection transmission typically lie in the lack of availability of sufficiently long-term time series of reliable epidemiological data allowing robust estimation of the impact of demographic processes on age-related epidemiology. As here, most available studies [12, 15, 16, 18] have in common the same drawback: they have to postulate a direct influence of age-structured demographic change on transmission and typically rely on a single

age-structured infection datum (e.g. a single serological profile) to estimate transmission. However, as argued in [11], the formulation of horizontal transmission adopted here, though simple, has the advantage of potentially capturing a whole range of processes triggered by fertility decline, namely the ageing of population in the groups most involved with horizontal transmission and also the ensuing decline of family size as an engine of the decline in intra-family horizontal transmission. In this study we modelled horizontal transmission by a WAIFW matrix as previously available for the study setting [30], being obliged to do so given that direct data on social contact patterns in SSA are so far available only for Eastern Africa [38], where socio-cultural patterns are believed to be markedly different from those of Western Africa and the setting considered. The lack of direct contact data in most of Africa remains a serious limitation. Another limitation lies in the lack of precise predictions about mortality resulting from chronic HBV infection, a choice motivated by a lack of appropriate data.

To sum up, while the focus of this work has been on isolating and highlighting the impact of changing demography on the epidemiology of HBV, it is important to note that patterns of evolution of social and sexual behaviour over time will add a further layer of complexity to the resulting pattern of HBV epidemiology. More generally, it is reasonable to conclude that where processes of infection and disease or relevant behaviours display age dependencies, potential changes in age distribution associated with fertility, mortality, or migration may have a significant bearing on observed patterns of infection and should be taken into account when forward planning interventions.

Conclusions

For infections where processes of transmission, infection (including contact patterns relevant for transmission), and disease operate in an age-dependent way, demographic change can, of itself, give rise to changes in the burden of infectious disease even in the absence of changes in the processes of transmission and infection. Thus, it is clearly of importance to take account of demographic change when assessing the potential longer term impact of vaccination and other control measures focused on specific age groups.

Abbreviations

DT: Demographic transition; HBV: Hepatitis B virus; LHS: Latin hypercube sampling; PDE: Partial differential equation; SG: Senegal-Gambia; SSA: Sub-Saharan Africa; WAIFW: Who acquires infection from whom

Acknowledgements

We warmly thank the three reviewers of the journal, whose valuable comments contributed to improve the quality and exposition of the manuscript

Funding

The research leading to these results has received funding from the European Research Council (ERC) under the European Union's Seventh Framework Programme (FP7/2007–2013) and ERC Grant agreement number 283955 (DECIDE). The funder had no role in the design of the study; collection, analysis, or interpretation of data; or in writing the manuscript.

Authors' contributions

JRW and PM designed the study and analysed the results; JRW designed and implemented the model; PM undertook the analysis of demographic data; JRW and PM drafted the initial manuscript; AM acquired funding for the project. All authors provided a critical revision of the initial draft and read and approved the final manuscript.

Competing interests

All authors declare that they have no competing interests.

Author details

[1]Department of Infectious Disease Epidemiology, School of Public Health, Faculty of Medicine, Imperial College London, St Mary's Campus, Norfolk Place, London W2 1PG, UK. [2]Dipartimento di Economia e Management, University of Pisa, via Ridolfi 10, 56124 Pisa, Italy. [3]Dondena Centre for Research on Social Dynamics and Public Policy and Department of Social and Political Science, Bocconi University, Via Roentgen 1, 20136 Milan, Italy.

References

1.   Bloom DE, Canning D. The health and wealth of Africa. World Econ J. 2004; 5(2):57–81.
2.   Bongaarts J, Casterline J. Fertility transition: is sub-Saharan Africa different? Popul Dev Rev. 2012;38(Suppl 1):153–68.
3.   Livi-Bacci M. A concise history of world population growth. 6th ed. Oxford: Blackwell; 2017.
4.   Chesnais JC. The demographic transition: stages, patterns, and economic implications. Oxford: Oxford University Press; 1992.
5.   Kohler HP, Billari FC, Ortega JA. The emergence of lowest-low fertility in Europe during the 1990s. Popul Dev Rev. 2002;28(4):641–80.
6.   Anderson RM, May RM. Infectious diseases of humans: dynamics and control. Oxford: Oxford University Press; 1991.
7.   Mossong J, Hens N, Jit M, Beutels P, Auranen K, Mikolajczyk R, et al. Social contacts and mixing patterns relevant to the spread of infectious diseases. PLoS Med. 2008;5(3):e74.
8.   Meredith J A. Endemic disease in host populations with fully specified demography. Theor Popul Biol. 1990;37:455.
9.   Meredith J A. Transmission and control of childhood infectious diseases; does demography matter? Popul Studies. 1990;44:195–215.
10. Williams JR, Manfredi P. Ageing populations and childhood infections: its potential impact on epidemic patterns and morbidity. Int J Epidemiol. 2004;33:1–7.
11. Manfredi P, Williams JR. Realistic population dynamics in epidemiological models: the impact of population decline on the dynamics of childhood infectious diseases. Measles in Italy as an example. Math Biosci. 2004;192: 153–75.
12. Williams JR, Manfredi P, Ciofi degli Atti ML, Salmaso S. Measles elimination in Italy: the projected impact of the National Elimination Plan. Epidemiol Infect. 2005;133:87–97.
13. Gao L, Hethcote H. Simulations of rubella vaccination strategies in China. Math Biosci. 2006;202(2):371–85.
14. Iannelli M, Manfredi P. Demographic change and immigration in age structured epidemiological models. Math Popul Stud. 2007;14(3):169–91.
15. Merler S, Ajelli M. Deciphering the relative weights of demographic transition and vaccination in the decrease of measles incidence in Italy. Proc R Soc B. 2014;281(1777):20132676.
16. Marziano V, Poletti P, Guzzetta G, Manfredi P, Merler S. The impact of demographic changes on the epidemiology of herpes zoster: Spain as a case study. Proc R Soc Lond B. 2015;282(1804):20142509.
17. Geard N, Glass K, McCaw JM, McBryde ES, Korb KB, Keeling MJ, McVernon J. The effects of demographic change on disease transmission and vaccine impact in a household structured population. Epidemics. 2015;13:56–64.
18. Trentini F, Poletti P, Merler S, Melegaro A. Measles immunity gaps and the progress towards elimination: a multi-country modelling analysis. Lancet Infect Dis. 2017;17(10):1089–97.
19. Horn J, Damm O, Greiner W, Hengel H, Kretzschmar ME, Siedler A, et al. Influence of demographic changes on the impact of vaccination against varicella and herpes zoster in Germany — a mathematical modelling study. BMC Med. 2018;16(1):3.
20. Cummings DAT, Iamsirithaworn S, Lessler JT, McDermott A, Prasanthong R, Nisalak A, et al. The impact of the demographic transition on dengue in Thailand: insights from a statistical analysis and mathematical modeling. PLoS Med. 2009;6(9):e1000139.
21. Editorial-The Lancet. Eliminating viral hepatitis: time to match visions with action. Lancet. 2017;390(10108):2121.
22. Spearman CW, Afihene M, Ally R, et al. Hepatitis B in sub-Saharan Africa: strategies to achieve the 2030 elimination targets. Lancet Gastroenterol Hepatol. 2017;2:900–9.
23. Schweitzer A, Horn J, Mikolajczyk RT, Krause G, Ott JJ. Estimations of worldwide prevalence of chronic hepatitis B virus infection: a systematic

review of data published between 1965 and 2013. Lancet. 2015;386(10003): 1546–55.

24. Custer B, Sullivan SD, Hazlet TK, Iloeje U, Veenstra DL, Kowldey KV. Global epidemiology of hepatitis B virus. J Clin Gastroenterol. 2004;38(Suppl 3): S158–68.

25. Edmunds WJ, Medley GF, Nokes DJ, Hall AJ, Whittle HC. The influence of age on the development of the hepatitis B carrier state. Proc R Soc Lond B. 1993;253(1337):197–220.

26. Edmunds WJ, Medley GF, Nokes DJ, O'Callaghan CJ, Whittle HC, Hall AJ. Epidemiological patterns of hepatitis B virus (HBV) in highly endemic areas. Epidemiol Infect. 1996;117(2):313–25.

27. Maynard JE, Kane MA, Alter MJ, Hadler SC. Control of hepatitis B by immunisation: global perspective. In: Zuckerman AJ, editor. Viral hepatitis and liver disease. New York: Alan R. Liss; 1988. p. 967–9.

28. Medley GF, Lindop NA, Edmunds WJ, Nokes DJ. Hepatitis-B virus endemicity: heterogeneity, catastrophic dynamics and control. Nat Med. 2001;7(5):1–9.

29. Hughes A, Lewis J. Beyond Francophonie?: the Senegambia Confederation in retrospect. In: Kirk-Greene A, Bach D, e, editors. State and society in francophone Africa since independence. Oxford: St. Martin's Press; 1995.

30. Edmunds WJ, Medley GF, Nokes DJ. The transmission dynamics and control of hepatitis B virus in The Gambia. Stat Med. 1996;15:2215–33.

31. United Nations: World population prospects: the 2015 revision. 2015.

32. Garnett GP, Anderson RM. Factors controlling the spread of HIV in heterosexual communities in developing countries: patterns of mixing between different age and sexual activity classes. Philos Trans R Soc Lond Ser B Biol Sci. 1993;342(1300):137–59.

33. Viviani S, Carrieri P, Bah E, Hall A, Kirk G, Mendy M, Montesano R, Plymoth A, Sam O, Van der Sande M, et al. 20 years into the Gambia Hepatitis Intervention Study: assessment of initial hypotheses and prospects for evaluation of protective effectiveness against liver cancer. Cancer Epidemiol Biomark Prev. 2008;17(11):3216–23.

34. Bekondi C, Zanchi R, Seck A, Garin B, Giles-Vernick T, Gody JC, et al. HBV immunization and vaccine coverage among hospitalized children in Cameroon, Central African Republic and Senegal: a cross-sectional study. BMC Inf Dis. 2015;15:267.

35. Santermans E, Goeyvaerts N, Melegaro A, Edmunds WJ, Faes C, Aerts M, Beutels P, Hens N. The social contact hypothesis under the assumption of endemic equilibrium: elucidating the transmission potential of VZV in Europe. Epidemics. 2015;11:14–23.

36. Vall Mayans M, Hall AJ, Inskip HM, Chotard J, Lindsay SW, Coromina E, Mendy M, Alonso PL, Whittle H. Risk factors for transmission of hepatitis B virus to Gambian children. Lancet. 1990;336(8723):1107–9.

37. Omran AR. The epidemiologic transition: a theory of the epidemiology of population change. Milbank Mem Fund Q. 1971;49:509.

38. Melegaro A, Del Fava E, Poletti P, Merler S, Nyamukapa C, Williams J, et al. Social contact structures and time use patterns in the Manicaland province of Zimbabwe. PLoS One. 2017;12(1):e0170459.

4

Adjustment of refugee children and adolescents in Australia: outcomes from wave three of the Building a New Life

Winnie Lau[1,2*], Derrick Silove[3,4], Ben Edwards[5], David Forbes[1,2], Richard Bryant[6], Alexander McFarlane[7], Dusan Hadzi-Pavlovic[4], Zachary Steel[4,8,9], Angela Nickerson[6], Miranda Van Hooff[7], Kim Felmingham[10], Sean Cowlishaw[1,2,11], Nathan Alkemade[12], Dzenana Kartal[1,2] and Meaghan O'Donnell[1,2]

Abstract

Background: High-income countries like Australia play a vital role in resettling refugees from around the world, half of whom are children and adolescents. Informed by an ecological framework, this study examined the post-migration adjustment of refugee children and adolescents 2–3 years after arrival to Australia. We aimed to estimate the overall rate of adjustment among young refugees and explore associations with adjustment and factors across individual, family, school, and community domains, using a large and broadly representative sample.

Methods: Data were drawn from Wave 3 of the Building a New Life in Australia (BNLA) study, a nationally representative, longitudinal study of settlement among humanitarian migrants in Australia. Caregivers of refugee children aged 5–17 ($N = 694$ children and adolescents) were interviewed about their children's physical health and activity, school absenteeism and achievement, family structure and parenting style, and community and neighbourhood environment. Parent and child forms of the Strengths and Difficulties Questionnaire (SDQ) were completed by caregivers and older children to assess social and emotional adjustment.

Results: Sound adjustment according to the SDQ was observed regularly among young refugees, with 76-94% (across gender and age) falling within normative ranges. Comparison with community data for young people showed that young refugees had comparable or higher adjustment levels than generally seen in the community. However, young refugees as a group did report greater peer difficulties. Bivariate and multivariate linear regression analyses showed that better reported physical health and school achievement were associated with higher adjustment. Furthermore, higher school absenteeism and endorsement of a hostile parenting style were associated with lower adjustment.

Conclusions: This is the first study to report on child psychosocial outcomes from the large, representative longitudinal BNLA study. Our findings indicate sound adjustment for the majority of young refugees resettled in Australia. Further research should examine the nature of associations between variables identified in this study. Overall, treating mental health problems early remains a priority in resettlement. Initiatives to enhance parental capability, physical health, school achievement and participation could assist to improve settlement outcomes for young refugees.

Keywords: Mental health, Adjustment, Strengths and Difficulties Questionnaire, Psychosocial, Ecological, Refugee, Children, Adolescents, Resettlement

* Correspondence: wlau@unimelb.edu.au
[1]Phoenix Australia, Melbourne, Victoria, Australia
[2]Department of Psychiatry, University of Melbourne, Melbourne, Victoria, Australia
Full list of author information is available at the end of the article

Background

As of end-2017, 68.5 million people globally were displaced due to war and political conflict, of whom 25.4 million were recognised as refugees according to the United Nations High Commissioner for Refugees (UNHCR) (http://www.unhcr.org/en-au/figures-at-a-glance.html). More than half of all displaced people are children and adolescents. High-income countries such as Australia play important roles in the long-term resettlement of refugees, both as individuals and families (http://www.unhcr.org/en-au/figures-at-a-glance.html).

As the pressure for high-income countries to resettle greater numbers of refugees and families increases, there is a growing imperative to understand and support the well-being and emotional health of individuals and families admitted – a prerequisite for positive settlement outcomes. To date, however, there is a dearth of high quality empirical research involving representative samples that investigates the psychosocial well-being of children and adolescents within resettled families in high-income countries, and factors in the post-settlement environment associated with sound adjustment (i.e. social and emotional functioning) [1].

Prior research into the mental health and psychosocial adjustment of young refugees post-migration has yielded varying results. Systematic reviews of epidemiological studies in high-income countries estimate the prevalence of post-traumatic stress disorder, anxiety and depression to be between 19% and 54%, 33% and 50%, and 3% and 30%, respectively, among young refugees [2]. Generally, these prevalence statistics are elevated in comparison with community norms [2, 3]. The differences in prevalence of disorders across studies have been attributed to methodological variations, including sample differences (e.g. clinical, community or convenient, older vs. younger), variations in measures and diagnostic assessments (e.g. self-report vs. clinical measures, cut-off points), sampling characteristics (e.g. length of time since conflict or in resettlement) [4], cultural variations in expressions of distress [5], and specific factors relating to subsamples of refugees (e.g. higher vs. lower torture experience) [6].

The mixed findings regarding prevalence present an unresolved paradox. On the one hand, there is at least tentative consensus that the majority of refugee youth experience low level or no mental health or adjustment difficulties [7, 8]. On the other hand, it may be expected that the traumas and adversities these individuals have experienced place them at heightened risk of traumatic stress problems [9]. What is lacking from the existing body of research is a robust estimate from representative samples of how many young refugees are well adjusted and how many are not, which children will experience adjustment problems, and what factors are associated with adjustment in young refugees. Characteristics of the post-settlement environment are likely to play a key role in influencing the adjustment outcomes of refugee children and adolescents. They may also help to explain the observed variation in prevalence of psychological difficulties.

Adopting an ecological framework can assist in identifying and assessing the multiple factors that are associated with adjustment among young refugees. Bronfenbrenner's [10] original ecological framework considered child well-being within influential systems – the micro system (the day-to-day and inner relationships surrounding the child), the meso system (the network of relationships between micro systems, such as between parents and teachers), the exo system (the more remote social settings that have indirect effects on the child such as neighbourhood) and the macro system (the broader social, cultural and political beliefs, ideals, and customs that incorporate the micro, meso and exo systems) [11]. This conceptual framework has increased awareness of the risk and protective context of the child in terms of not only individual characteristics but also family, school, peer and community environments [10, 12]. In refugee populations, ecological models have been called for to improve the understanding of the health and wellbeing needs of these communities [11, 13].

The application of ecological models to young refugees suggests that a constellation of stressors from a range of domains contributes to mental health and adjustment following displacement, over and above the impact of prior war exposure [9, 13]. It is widely acknowledged that post-migration factors are important determinants of mental health outcomes in resettled adult refugee samples [14]. These can be as powerful as, or even more so, than pre-migration experiences of war-related trauma and loss in predicting mental health outcomes [15, 16]. Less is known about the significance of different post-migration environments for child and adolescent adjustment. A number of studies have suggested, however, that factors such as poor housing, insufficient financial support, language acquisition difficulties and racism, can all affect the mental health outcomes of this population [17–19].

Multiple domains have been shown to influence adjustment in young refugees, including those relating to the individual, family, school, peers and the wider community. Individual characteristics such as age, physical health and pre-migration trauma experiences are important personal and historical risk factors [16, 20]. Additionally, family factors including supportive, warm and nurturing parent-child relationships [21, 22], as well as a positive family life and unity [23], are thought to impact on the adjustment of young refugees. Among school and peer factors, support from friends and positive school experiences have been identified as indicators of adjustment among school-aged children [17], while community factors such as integration into the host society have also been associated with positive mental health outcomes among migrants and refugees [15, 16]. Consistent with this literature, one illustrative systematic review adopted an ecological model to highlight the prospective mental health risks associated with individual factors (e.g. female gender), family factors (e.g. parental mental health) and community factors (e.g. discrimination and racism) [20].

A major problem in past studies conducted with refugees relates to methodological issues associated with non-random and convenience sampling. This can result in either an under-estimation of distress (i.e. samples composed predominantly of healthy participants) or over-estimation (i.e. samples composed predominantly of individuals in need of support) [6], and limits what can be reasonably concluded and generalised about the refugee population [24]. Further evidence from representative samples is therefore required to help determine the psychosocial adjustment of refugee youth post-settlement, as well as the environmental factors that help explain or are related to these adjustment outcomes. This is particularly important given the potential for constructive screening and intervention during this crucial post-settlement period.

Post-settlement environments, including the policies and interventions in place to support refugee resettlement, vary enormously across countries. Australia for example, is highly regarded for the level of support provided to resettled humanitarian entrants (e.g. housing support, language acquisition and healthcare), but until now there has not been data available that speak to the adjustment outcomes of young refugees resettled in Australia. Gaining insight into the relative level of psychosocial adjustment in this population, and factors associated with better or poorer adjustment, is thus crucial to inform targeted policy and intervention strategies. This article is the first to report on levels of psychosocial adjustment and factors associated with optimal adjustment among a broadly representative sample of resettled child and adolescent refugees in Australia.

The aim of this study was to examine adjustment in a child and adolescent refugee cohort resettled in Australia 2 to 3 years post-migration. Specifically, we aimed to estimate the proportion of young refugees who are well/maladjusted, and to compare their adjustment with age and gender equivalent community norms. To further assist in understanding the factors associated with the observed adjustment of young refugees, a second aim was to explore the individual, familial, school, and community risk and protective factors associated with adjustment. This may then enable the identification of potential targets for intervention across these domains.

A key contribution of this study is the examination of a cohort that is broadly representative of the refugee population in Australia, allowing for a more robust examination of adjustment outcomes than has been previously possible. To enable this, we use data from the Building a New Life in Australia (BNLA) study [1]. In previous longitudinal studies that followed young refugees through to adulthood in resettled countries (the United States, Canada, Denmark, Sweden and Australia [25–30]), sample sizes were relatively small, selective or unrepresentative of contemporary youth refugee cultural groups. To our knowledge, the BNLA project is the first and largest longitudinal prospective cohort study of refugees and their families in Australia, and one of the largest in the world.

In light of the time-restricted context in which data collection in the BNLA study took place, and in the absence of available follow-up data on refugee children and adolescents at this stage (follow-up data collection is ongoing), we focus specifically on putative risk factors for early adjustment and those that are potentially modifiable (i.e. factors that fall within the remit of resettlement services in high-income countries) in the post-settlement period. The factors investigated included individual factors (age, gender, physical health and physical activity), familial factors (family structure and parenting approach), school factors (achievement and absenteeism), and community factors (extracurricular engagement, perceived support within the community, perception of safety and friendliness of the resident neighbourhood). We use the term adjustment in this study to refer to the general social and emotional functioning of young refugees.

Methods

The BNLA study and data source

The child/adolescent sample investigated in this study is derived from the BNLA study, undertaken by the Australian Government Department of Social Services and the Australian Institute of Family Studies [31]. The main BNLA study is described below, while the child and adolescent sample recruited at Wave 3 is described thereafter.

The BNLA is a population-based cohort study tracing the settlement outcomes of individuals and families over five waves, commencing from the point of being granted a permanent humanitarian visa [32]. Recruitment and Wave 1 occurred between October 2013 and February 2014, while subsequent waves of data have been collected annually. To date, four waves of data have been collected, with data from the first three waves released so far. The present data pertains to Wave 3, undertaken between October 2015 and February 2016, which was the first wave that collected information relating to children and adolescents.

BNLA sampling and participants

BNLA participants were recruited from 11 sites in Australia covering major cities and regional areas. These sites were selected to ensure an adequate sample size to allow for robust analyses, based on the concentration of eligible refugees in particular localities, appropriate geographic spread and an optimal representation of holders of different types of humanitarian visas granted in Australia. Participants in the BNLA study comprised 'principal' and 'secondary' applicants for a humanitarian visa in Australia that was granted in the period preceding the study. Principal applicants were the main applicants within a migrating unit (typically a family), whereas secondary applicants were other members of the migrating unit (e.g. child, spouse, other adult family member). Initial eligibility criteria included (1) being a 'principal applicant' for a humanitarian visa that was granted 3 to 6 months prior to the survey (i.e. May to December, 2013) and already holding a permanent protection visa (the 'offshore' group), or granted a permanent protection visa in the previous 3 to 6 months after arrival in Australia by boat or on another visa type such as a tourist visa (the 'onshore' group); and (2) being 18 years or older. Seventy-eight percent of migrating units had followed an 'offshore' pathway while the remaining 22% followed an 'onshore' pathway. During the initial recruitment phase, principal applicants provided consent for other members of their migrating unit to be contacted. These 'secondary applicants' were invited to participate if they were (1) at least 15 years of age and (2) residing with the principal applicant. Although the gender of principal and secondary applicants varied, in most cases the secondary applicant was female.

To contextualise Australia's humanitarian intake programme, those who arrive via offshore pathways typically include UNHCR identified and referred refugees, global humanitarian special programme refugees (i.e. living outside Australia and home countries but subject to gross human rights violations, nominated by a person or organisation in Australia), in-country special humanitarian cases, emergency rescue and women at risk cases, and immediate family members of people already granted protection in Australia. For those who arrive via onshore pathways (i.e. arrivals by boat or via other means such as student/tourist visas), there may be a period of waiting for an application for a humanitarian visa to be assessed. As Australia's laws require the detention of non-citizens who are in Australia without a valid visa, those who arrive via onshore pathways may spend time in community detention or immigration detention. Refugee camp experiences may vary across these humanitarian visa classes.

BNLA data collection procedures

During Wave 1 and 3, BNLA data were collected at home visits. In alternate waves, data were collected via telephone. Surveys were administered by field workers using a computer-assisted self-interview, which enabled participants to respond privately to self-report questions using a computer interface. Participants could opt instead to complete a computer-assisted personal interview, whereby field interviewers asked questions displayed on a screen and entered responses. Computer-assisted self-interviews lasted 45 minutes on average, while computer-assisted personal interviews took just over 60 minutes on average, to complete. Survey materials were available in nine languages following translation and multi-stage quality assurance review. In most cases, participants were matched with an interviewer who was a native speaker of their preferred language. Where this was not possible or desired, participants could opt to use an accredited interpreter.

BNLA Wave 3: child and adolescent sampling

Wave 3 data was collected between October 2015 and February 2016 and included interviews with 1155 principal applicants and 739 secondary applicants. For 87% of the sample, this time point corresponded to a residency period of 2 to 3 years in Australia. Nine percent of participants had spent 3 or more years living in Australia, and 4% had spent between 1 and 2 years in Australia.

Wave 3 was the first time in the BNLA study that a child module was included as a nested component of the broader study. This module targeted children and adolescents in the migrating unit aged 5 to 17 years. It incorporated two components. The first was a primary caregiver report, which was completed by participants (principal or secondary visa applicants) who identified as the primary caregiver in the migrating unit. The second component was a child self-report, which was completed by older children and adolescents (aged 11 and 17 years).

Recruitment of the child and adolescent sample purposively targeted older children (11–17 years) over younger children (5–10 years) to maximise the number of child participants able to provide self-report data. Up to two children per household were invited to participate. Initial sampling occurred by randomly selecting two children between 11 and 17 years of age in each migrating unit. In households with multiple children, but only one child between 11 and 17 years, the eldest child was recruited as well as one randomly selected younger child between 5 and 10 years. In households with exclusively younger children, two children between 5 and 10 years were randomly selected. There were no unaccompanied children in the sample. Caregivers were invited to complete the caregiver report with respect to the children selected for recruitment. Only children recruited to the study between 11 and 17 years of age were invited to complete the child self-report module, which was administered via pencil and paper.

Of the 888 eligible children, data were collected for 694 children and from 426 primary caregivers, of whom $n = 310$ were mothers (72.8%), $n = 97$ were fathers (22.8%), and $n = 19$ (4.4%) were other members of the migrating unit/household (primarily siblings). Figure 1 summarises the recruitment process, outlining the flow of participation by adults (principal and secondary applicants) recruited in Wave 1 and subsequent recruitment of caregivers and children and adolescents in Wave 3.

Measures
The child module
The child module was developed by the BNLA study team in consultation with members of the current author group, who are experts in refugee mental health and longitudinal research. The development process prioritised psychosocial factors significant to refugee settlement that could be assessed within the time available for data collection. The caregiver report component of the module was administered to caregivers of children aged 5–17 years and assessed perceptions of the child's overall physical health and activity, school participation (absenteeism) and

achievement, language use, mental health and emotional symptoms, and adjustment. It also incorporated a structured parenting questionnaire. The child self-report was administered to children aged 11–17 years and included a questionnaire assessing physical health and activity, engagement in extracurricular activities, and self-reported adjustment. The child module required 10 minutes per child to complete.

Social and emotional adjustment
Strengths and Difficulties Questionnaire (SDQ) – Parent and child form
The SDQ [33] was used to assess refugee child and adolescent adjustment. The SDQ comprises 25-items that operationalise five subscales, namely emotional symptoms, conduct problems, hyperactivity/inattention, peer problems and prosocial behaviour [33]. There are parent and child report versions available, which ask how true each item is for the nominated child (or in the case of the child version,

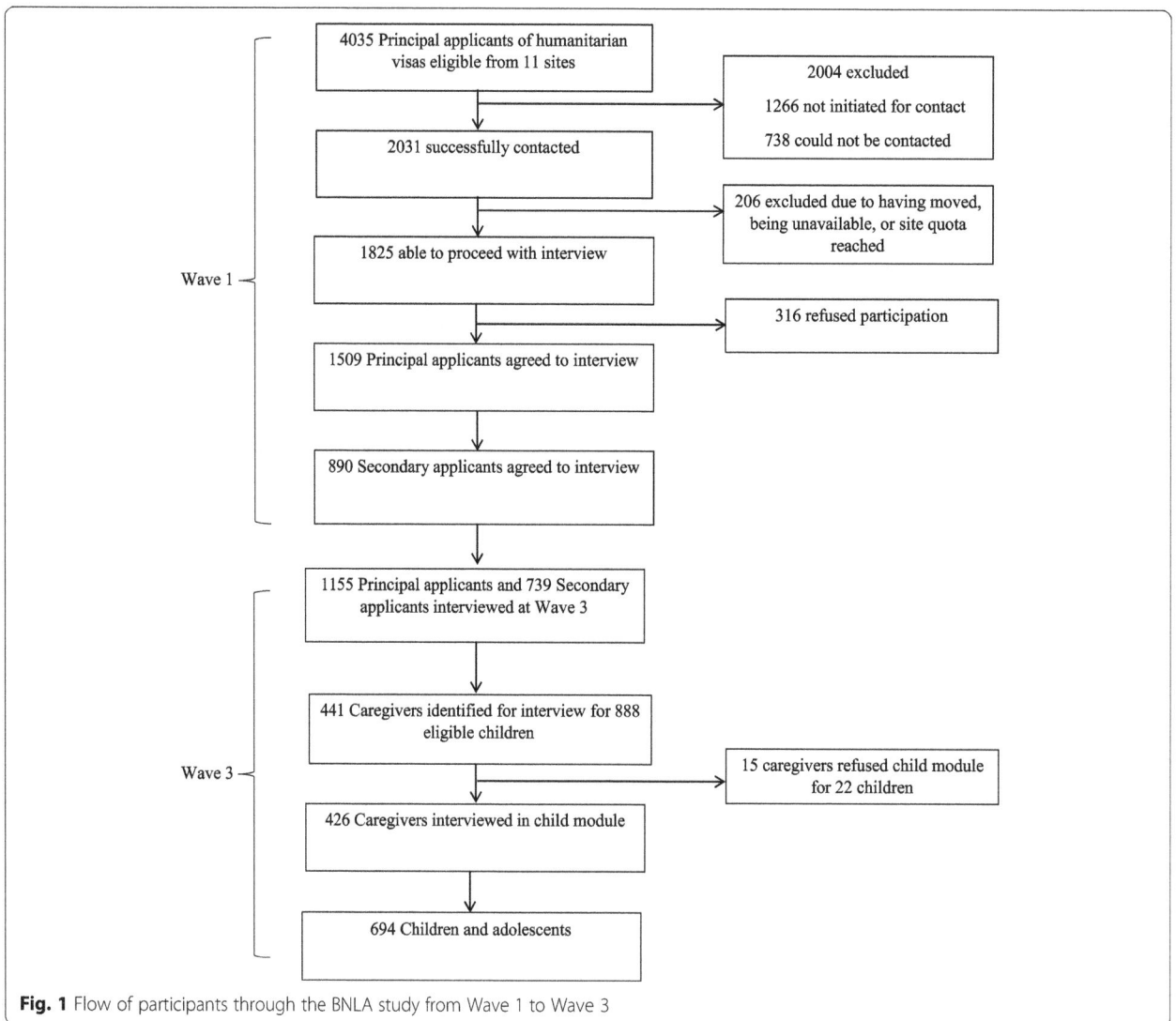

Fig. 1 Flow of participants through the BNLA study from Wave 1 to Wave 3

for him/herself) over the past 6 months. Items are scored on a 3-point Likert scale (0 = not true, 1 = somewhat true, or 2 = certainly true). With the exception of prosocial behaviour, item scores were aggregated to generate a total difficulties score (range 0–40), with higher scores indicating increased adjustment problems [34].

The SDQ is not a diagnostic measure, yet it can discriminate between children from high- and low-risk samples and screen for child psychiatric disorders, including in non-Western populations [34, 35]. The SDQ is available in more than 20 languages and is one of the most widely used dimensional assessment instruments in multicultural research [36]. It has demonstrated acceptable to strong internal consistency [37, 38] and adequate test-retest reliability [38] with refugee samples in humanitarian settings and has been used widely with child and adolescent refugees in high-income countries [30, 39–47]. Evidence for the reliability of the SDQ with refugee samples is available from Canada, where the measure demonstrated satisfactory to high internal consistency [48]. In the present study, caregivers completed the SDQ–parent form for children aged 5–17 years and children aged 11–17 completed the SDQ–child form.

For children aged 5–10 years, we analysed the SDQ caregiver report data, given that the parent/caregiver report is the most reliable index of adjustment for a younger age group [49]. For children aged 11–17, the SDQ self-report data were analysed given the increased validity of self-report data in this age group. In analysing SDQ data, children aged 5–17 were assigned to categories for 'normal', 'borderline' or 'abnormal' on subscales and total difficulties, based on the online English language cut-off scores [50]. We also compared SDQ scores of refugee children and adolescents in this sample with Australian norms. These norms (means and standard deviations), broken down by age groups, are outlined in the results section. Specifically, age groupings in this study enabled comparison to Australian norms, across three groups as follows: (1) 5–10 years old, (2) 11–13 years old and (3) 14–17 years old.

Domain measures

A summary of domains and variables examined in relation to refugee youth adjustment is presented in Fig. 2. Caregivers of refugee children and adolescents completed the following indices (except where noted as having been completed via young person self-report). Measures were also based on survey administration at Wave 3, except where specified. The origin of these questions (with exception to questions specific to refugee experience) are based

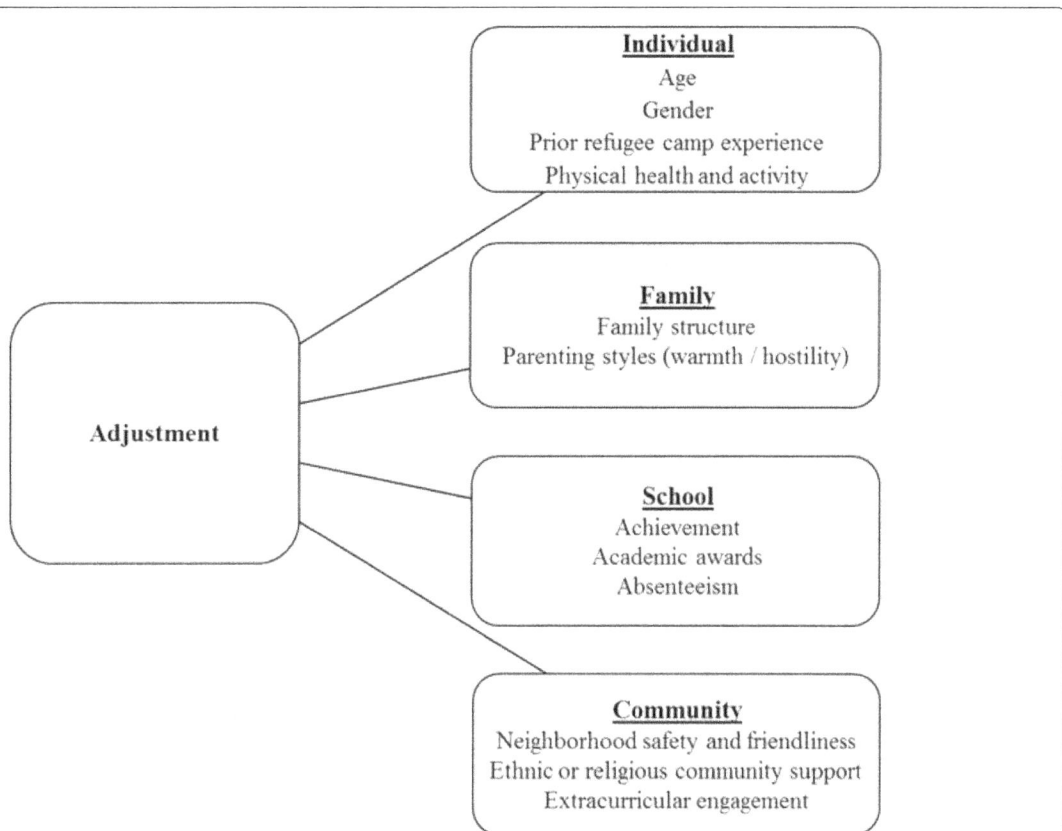

Fig. 2 Domains and corresponding variables of interest in the current study in relation to young refugees' adjustment

on the Growing Up in Australia: The Longitudinal Study of Australian Children study. This is a major longitudinal study following the development of 10,000 children and families from all areas of Australia, which includes items with origins in validated health and developmental screening measures [51].

Individual domain

Background and pre-migration experiences Sociodemographic measures were administered at Wave 1 and included items about child age and gender. During this wave, caregivers were also asked: *"Did you spend any time in a refugee camp before you came to Australia?"* If they answered yes, they were also asked: *"How long did you spend there?"*

Parent-rated child health and physical activity Parent-rated child health was measured using caregiver reports to a single-item measure: *"In general, would you say* [named child]'s *health is (1) excellent, (2) very good, (3) good, (4) fair, or (5) poor"*? Caregivers were also asked about their child's physical activity: *"In the last 7 days, how many days has* [named child] *done a total of 60 minutes or more of physical activity, which was enough to raise their breathing rate?"* The latter was scored using an open response format.

Family domain

Family structure An indicator of family structure was defined on the basis of information reported by the principal applicant, which identified the relationship of all household members to themselves (e.g. spouse, unrelated child, grandchild, biological child). This allowed for a classification of family structure in terms of whether the principal applicant was in a couple or single, and whether other family members lived in the household.

Parenting warmth and hostility Parenting warmth and hostility were measured using caregiver responses to 10 questions [52]. Examples of warmth questions included: *"How often do you have warm close times together with this child?"* and *"How often do you enjoy listening to this child and doing things with him/her?"* Examples of hostility questions included: *"I have been angry with this child"* and *"I have raised my voice"*. Responses were based on a 5-point Likert scale, with 1 = Never/Almost Never, 5 = Always/Almost always.

School domain

School achievement and absenteeism Caregivers with children who were enrolled in school were asked: *"How would you describe* [named child]'s *overall achievement at school?"* Responses were based on a 5-point Likert scale, with scores dichotomised such that 0 = Excellent/Above average/Average achievement, and 1 = Below average/Well below average achievement. School absenteeism was measured by caregiver responses to: *"During the previous four weeks of school how many days has* [named child] *been absent?"* This item was scored using an open response format.

School award Children aged 11–17 were also asked: *"In the last year, have you won any awards or been recognised for doing well in certain activities?"* Response options included (1) won an academic award, (2) received a community service award, (3) been selected to represent the school, (4) received an award in sports, or (5) received an award in music, arts, dance performance or drama.

Community domain

Extracurricular activities/engagement Children aged 11 and over were asked about participation in extracurricular activities: *"In the last 6 months, have you regularly attended any of these activities?"* Responses included (1) individual sport, (2) team sport, (3) musical instruments or singing, (4) ballet or other dance, or (5) religious group. Respondents were required to circle as many activities as were applicable.

Ethnic/religious/community support Community support was measured using caregiver responses to the following question: *"Do you feel that you have been given support/comfort in Australia from* (a) *your national or ethnic community; and* (b) *your religious community?"* Responses were measured on a 3-point scale (Yes/Sometimes/No).

Neighbourhood friendliness and safety Caregivers were asked to provide responses to statements about their neighbourhood (local area), including (1) *"The people in my neighbourhood are friendly"* and (2) *"I feel safe in my neighbourhood"*. Responses were scored on a 4-point Likert scale, with 1 = Strongly agree and 4 = Strongly disagree.

Data analysis

Data-file preparation was conducted in SPSS Version 25 and included management of data regarding children aged 5–10 years, which were obtained from caregiver reports, and regarding those aged 11–17 years, which were obtained from both caregivers and child self-report. This process was guided by the following principles (except where otherwise specified): (1) if responses from both caregiver and child reports were available (as was the case for children aged between 11 and 17 years), then self-reported data from children were used (e.g. on SDQ and SDQ subscales); (2) where data was available from child self-reports only (e.g. regarding extracurricular engagement) then this information was analysed; and (3) where information was available from caregiver reports only (e.g. about family structure) then this information was analysed.

In the first stage of analyses, descriptive statistics were produced to summarise the sociodemographic profile of the sample, as well as the distribution of measures across individual, family, school and community domains. Total and subscale scores on the SDQ were produced and reported separately for boys and girls, across three age groups (5–10, 11–13, and 14–17 years). This enabled comparison with age-equivalent Australian norms (http://www.sdqinfo.com/norms/AusNorm.html). Comparisons were based on examinations of SDQ mean scores and categorised indicators ('normal', 'borderline' or 'abnormal'), defined using the online English language cut-off scores [50], through use of independent group t tests and χ^2 tests, respectively. These were conducted in SPSS and incorporated Wave 3 cross-sectional survey weights to adjust for initial non-response and subsequent attrition, and to ensure that estimates reflected the population characteristics of refugees receiving humanitarian visas. Comparisons with age/gender equivalent community norms were analysed using SPSS modules that allowed for clustering within families (the intraclass correlation coefficient for the SDQ was 0.59).

The second stage of analyses comprised a series of regression models which examined the post-migration variables associated with children's adjustment difficulties. These models were estimated using MPlus Version 7.4, using robust maximum likelihood and multiple imputation across $k = 100$ datasets to manage item-level missing data. As such, these analyses did not incorporate information about survey weights, but did account for clustering within families using the TYPE = COMPLEX function. A series of bivariate models were estimated initially, which specified the SDQ total score as the endogenous variable, and considered exogenous independent variables across individual, family, school and community domains. Regression parameter estimates were standardised by the variance of exogenous and endogenous variables and were reported along with 95% confidence intervals. All independent variables were also entered into a single multiple regression model to examine and minimise the risk of confounded associations.

Results

Demographics

An exact breakdown of sample characteristics, including gender distributions, can be found in Table 1, for both the overall sample and by age groups. There was a fair representation of children across age groups and genders (53% male, 47% female). Most participants reported Iraq or Afghanistan as their country of origin (38.8% and 23.7%, respectively), followed by Bhutan (11.1%), Myanmar (8.1%), Iran (6.4%), or 'Other' (11.9%). Common primary languages spoken were Arabic (21.7%), Assyrian Neo-Aramaic (20.9%), Persian (13.4%), and Nepali (11.4%), followed by Dari (9.2%), Hazaraghi (9.0%), Burmese and related (6.2%), or Chaldean Neo-Aramaic (3.1%). The remaining 5.3% of the sample reported other languages. The majority of children and adolescents reported using both English and their caregivers' language, although they were more likely to use the caregivers' language at home ($\chi^2(1, N = 669) = 48.86, p < 0.001$). The majority of the sample (96%) had spent less than 12 months in Australia prior to being recruited to the study, representing a relatively early settlement group.

Descriptive findings across individual, family, school and community domains

Table 1 shows ratings provided by caregivers and older children and adolescents (age 11–17) on factors measured across domains. This information is summarised below.

Individual domain findings

As depicted in Table 1, most children had 'very good' physical health ratings (mean 4.05) and engaged in at least 1 hour of intense physical activity on average 2.5 days a week (mean 2.49). In both the 11–13 and 14–17 age groups, boys reported significantly more physical activity than girls.

Family domain findings

More than three-quarters of refugee children and adolescents were from dual caregiver households, with a high proportion also living with other family members. Due to the complexity of how responses to the relevant BNLA questions were itemised, it was not possible to state whether caregivers from dual households were both biological parents; however, it is reasonable to infer that this is likely. The composition of families was similar across Wave 1 and Wave 3, whereby 72.2% of families were in couple caregiver households and 25.9% in single caregiver households in Wave 1, compared to 71% and 28.5%, respectively, in Wave 3. In relation to caregiver parenting style, caregivers reported relatively high scores on warmth and lower scores on hostility.

School domain findings

The vast majority of caregivers reported that their children were at or above average for school achievement. Among older students, around 22.7% self-reported being the recipient of an achievement award from their school. Over half the sample (54.6%) reported no school absenteeism in the last 4 weeks, with 19.6% reporting only 1 day of absenteeism and 8.3% reporting at least 1 day per week absenteeism on average.

Table 1 Means, standard deviations and frequencies for demographic and domain (individual, family, school, community) variables investigated in this study of young refugees ($N = 694$)

	Total group	Age category		
		5–11 years	11–13 years	14–17 years
Demographics[a]				
N	597 (52.9% male)	216 (52.3% male)	169 (53.2% male)	212 (53.0% male)
Age (M, SD)	11.6 (3.6)	7.5 (1.7)	12.0 (0.81)	15.5 (1.1)
Often use carer language	69.7%	66.8%	70.7%	71.8%
Often use English	82.3%	84.8%	82.9%	79.2%
Individual domain				
Physical health[a]				
Rating of physical health (range 1–5)	4.05 (0.04)	4.08 (0.07)	4.12 (0.07)	3.96 (0.07)
Physical activity in past week (days)	2.49 (0.10)	2.61 (0.18)	2.67 (0.17)	2.27 (0.14)
Family domain				
Family structure[a]				
Couple with children under 18	45.0%	73.2%	54.0%	19.3%
Couple with children under 18 and other family	32.6%	18.3%	23.2%	47.9%
Single with children under 18	9.1%	6.7%	8.4%	11.3%
Single with children under 18 and other family	13.3%	1.7%	14.5%	21.5%
Parenting style[a]				
Parenting warmth (range 5–25)	20.42 (3.77)	21.27 (3.31)	20.30 (4.03)	19.62 (3.83)
Parenting harshness (range 5–25)	9.22 (3.72)	8.76 (3.08)	9.72 (4.27)	9.29 (3.81)
School domain				
School achievement average or above average[a]	93.9%	94.0%	94.0%	93.6%
Achievement award[b]	22.7%	–	21.2%	23.8%
Absenteeism (days per 4 weeks)[a]	1.13 (0.11)	0.87 (0.14)	0.94 (0.13)	1.45 (0.21)
Community domain				
Extracurricular engagement[b]	87.5%	–	88.2%	86.9%
Neighbourhood feels safe[a]				
Agree	96.5%	98.3%	94.7%	95.9%
Disagree	3.5%	1.7%	5.3%	4.1%
Neighbourhood friendly[a]				
Agree	96.7%	98.7%	93.4%	96.9%
Disagree	3.3%	1.3%	6.6%	3.1%
Ethnic or religious community support[a]				
Yes	32.6%	34.8%	34.5%	30.0%
Sometimes	21.9%	24.3%	19.9%	21.1%
No	45.5%	41.0%	45.6%	49.0%

Note. Values are reported in the form of either M(SD) or percentages where indicated. Based on weighted data
[a]Caregiver-reported information
[b]Child-reported information

Community domain findings

Most children aged 11 years or older reported extracurricular activities. There was a gender difference in the reporting of extracurricular activities in the 14–17 age group, where a lower proportion of girls (80.9%) reported participating in extracurricular activities compared with boys (92.2%, χ^2 (1, $N = 231$) = 6.07, $p = 0.01$). At Wave 3, most caregivers described their wider local Australian community as safe (96.5%) and friendly (96.7%). In response to questions regarding ethnic or religious community support, 32.6% of caregivers rated their ethnic or religious community as 'supportive', 21.9% as 'sometimes supportive', and 45.5% as 'not supportive'.

Adjustment outcomes
Overall adjustment
Table 2 shows findings regarding this study's main outcome of interest – social and emotional adjustment, as measured by SDQ total scores and for the five SDQ subscales. Findings are presented according to age groups (5–10, 11–13 and 14–17 years of age), as compared with mean scores of Australian age-matched norms.

Compared to Australian norms, refugee boys and girls fared comparatively well, or equivalently, on overall social and emotional functioning and subdomains, with exceptions in the 14–17 age group. Specifically, 14- to 17-year-old

refugee boys reported significantly lower SDQ total total scores (i.e. higher adjustment) than Australian norms ($p = 0.000$). In contrast, 14- to 17-year-old refugee girls reported significantly higher SDQ total scores (i.e. lower adjustment) than Australian norms ($p = 0.036$).

Significant differences across the SDQ subscale domains are described below (for a detailed overview of these comparisons refer to Table 2).

Emotional symptoms On the emotional symptoms subscale, refugee boys and girls did not differ significantly across ages or gender compared to Australian equivalent norms.

Conduct problems On the conduct problems subscale, boys aged 11–13 and 14–17 differed significantly from their Australian age matched norms on conduct problems,

Table 2 Strengths and Difficulties Questionnaire (SDQ) mean total and subscale scores for young refugees and comparison with Australian norms

	Boys			Girls		
	Parent SDQ			Parent SDQ		
	BNLA (5–10)	AUS (7 to 10)		BNLA (5–10)	AUS (7 to 10)	
Aged 5–10	n = 109	n = 160	t test p	n = 97	n = 197	t test p
Total difficulties	10.1 (0.59)	9.9 (0.51)	0.733	8.7 (0.56)	7.7 (0.41)	0.074
Emotional symptoms	2.4 (0.22)	2.3 (0.17)	0.794	2.0 (0.23)	2.3 (0.14)	0.264
Conduct problems	1.7 (0.16)	1.8 (0.13)	0.439	1.3 (0.17)	1.3 (0.11)	0.908
Hyperactivity/inattention	3.6 (0.23)	4.1 (0.21)	0.037*	3.1 (0.21)	2.6 (0.16)	0.023*
Peer problems	2.4 (0.17)	1.8 (0.16)	0.000***	2.3 (0.16)	1.5 (0.14)	0.000***
Prosocial behaviour	7.7 (0.23)	8.0 (0.14)	0.146	8.3 (0.22)	8.7 (0.11)	0.097
	Self SDQ			Self SDQ		
	BNLA (11–13)	AUS (11–13)		BNLA (11–13)	AUS (11–13)	
Aged 11 to 13	n = 86	n = 148	t test p	n = 81	n = 144	t test p
Total difficulties	8.6 (0.57)	8.8 (0.45)	0.779	8.8 (0.65)	8.0 (0.51)	0.198
Emotional symptoms	2.3 (0.21)	2.0 (0.16)	0.147	3.0 (0.26)	2.6 (0.18)	0.155
Conduct problems	1.4 (0.15)	2.0 (0.15)	0.000***	1.4 (0.22)	1.3 (0.12)	0.754
Hyperactivity/inattention	2.6 (0.21)	3.2 (0.19)	0.008*	2.3 (0.20)	2.6 (0.18)	0.179
Peer problems	2.4 (0.20)	1.7 (0.13)	0.001***	2.2 (0.19)	1.4 (0.13)	0.000***
Prosocial behaviour	8.1 (0.18)	7.8 (0.16)	0.115	8.3 (0.17)	8.6 (0.12)	0.058
	BNLA (14–17)	AUS (14–17)		BNLA (14–17)	AUS (14–17)	
Aged 14 to 17	n = 127	n = 115	t test p	n = 112	n = 144	t test p
Total difficulties	8.1 (0.41)	10.1 (0.56)	0.000***	10.3 (0.57)	9.1 (0.40)	0.036*
Emotional symptoms	2.1 (0.17)	2.1 (0.19)	0.788	3.2 (0.24)	2.9 (0.16)	0.152
Conduct problems	1.3 (0.13)	2.4 (0.18)	0.000***	1.8 (0.14)	1.7 (0.12)	0.559
Hyperactivity/inattention	2.6 (0.14)	4.0 (0.22)	0.000***	2.6 (0.16)	3.1 (0.18)	0.003*
Peer problems	2.2 (0.13)	1.6 (0.15)	0.000***	2.6 (0.17)	1.4 (0.12)	0.000***
Prosocial behaviour	7.9 (0.18)	7.3 (0.17)	0.001***	8.2 (0.16)	8.4 (0.13)	0.294

Note. Values in parentheses are standard errors due to clustering analysis. Australian normative SDs were converted to SE. SDQ Total difficulties range: 0 to 40. The five SDQ subscales range: 0 to 10
BNLA Building a New Life in Australia young refugee sample, AUS Australian norms
*$p \leq 0.05$, ***$p \leq 0.001$

wherein refugee boys reported lower levels of conduct problems ($p = 0.000$). No other significant age or gender differences emerged.

Hyperactivity/inattention symptoms On the hyperactivity/inattention subscale, refugee boys across ages reported significantly lower scores than Australian age and gender equivalent norms (5-10 age group, $p = 0.037$; 11-13 age group, $p = 0.008$; 14-17 age group, $p = 0.000$). Refugee girls aged 5–10 were found to have significantly higher levels of hyperactivity and inattention compared to Australian norms ($p = 0.023$), whereas refugee girls aged 14–17 reported significantly lower levels of hyperactivity and inattention compared with Australian norms ($p = 0.003$).

Peer problems Across all age groups, refugee boys and girls reported more peer difficulties than Australian age- and gender-matched norms (Boys: 5-10 age group, $p = 0.000$, 11-13 age group, $p = 0.001$, 14-17 age group, $p = 0.000$; Girls: 5-10 age group, $p = 0.000$, 11-13 age group, $p = 0.000$, 14-17 age group, $p = 0.000$).

Prosocial behaviours There were no significant differences for refugee boys and girls aged 5–10 and 11–13 compared to their Australian counterparts on prosocial behaviour. However, there was a significant difference for refugee boys aged 14–17 (but not girls). This group reported higher levels of prosocial behaviour compared to Australian norms ($p = 0.001$).

Percentages of normal, borderline and abnormal categories on the SDQ

Table 3 shows the proportions of boys and girls categorised in the 'Normal', 'Borderline' or 'Abnormal' ranges on the SDQ total score and subscales. Consistently, most refugee children and adolescents reported functioning in the normal ranges (SDQ total difficulties range 75.9-93.7%). Among boys and girls of all ages, the highest rates of borderline and abnormal scores were in the peer problems domain (range 0–28.4%). For boys and girls, there was an inverse pattern for peer problems with increasing age (the under 11 age group had the highest rates of elevated scores, while the 14–17 age group had the lowest rates).

Table 3 Strengths and Difficulties Questionnaire (SDQ) categorisation rates for boys and girls in the Building a New Life in Australia (BNLA) young refugee sample

	Boys			Girls		
	Normal	Borderline	Abnormal	Normal	Borderline	Abnormal
Parent-Report (5–10, $n = 216$)		($N = 109$)			($N = 107$)	
Emotional symptoms	75.2%	7.3%	17.4%	77.3%	10.3%	12.4%
Conduct problems	76.1%	9.2%	14.7%	81.4%	9.3%	9.3%
Hyperactivity symptoms	80.7%	8.3%	11.0%	88.7%	6.2%	5.2%
Peer problems	57.8%	13.8%	28.4%	62.9%	17.5%	19.6%
Prosocial behaviour	81.7%	9.2%	9.2%	91.8%	2.1%	6.2%
SDQ total difficulties	75.9%	9.3%	14.8%	84.4%	10.4%	5.2%
Self-report (11–13, $n = 170$)		($N = 88$)			($N = 82$)	
Emotional symptoms	85.1%	5.7%	9.2%	75.3%	11.1%	13.6%
Conduct problems	92.0%	3.4%	4.6%	85.2%	7.4%	7.4%
Hyperactivity symptoms	93.2%	1.1%	5.7%	96.3%	1.2%	2.4%
Peer problems	83.1%	14.5%	2.4%	86.7%	13.3%	0.0%
Prosocial behaviour	94.2%	3.5%	2.3%	95.1%	1.2%	3.7%
SDQ total difficulties	90.5%	8.3%	1.2%	90.1%	3.7%	6.2%
Self-report (14–17, $n = 243$)		($N = 128$)			($N = 115$)	
Emotional symptoms[a]	86.7%	7.0%	6.3%	68.7%	14.8%	16.5%
Conduct problems	91.4%	4.7%	3.9%	87.0%	7.0%	6.1%
Hyperactivity symptoms	97.6%	1.6%	0.8%	95.6%	4.4%	0.0%
Peer problems	77.3%	22.7%	0.0%	72.7%	25.5%	1.8%
Prosocial behaviour	89.9%	6.2%	3.9%	91.2%	3.5%	5.3%
SDQ total difficulties[a]	93.7%	6.3%	0.0%	80.4%	15.2%	4.5%

[a]Indicates significant gender differences ($p < 0.05$) based on χ^2 tests

In the 14–17 age group, there were significant gender differences in each of the three 'Total Difficulties' categories ($p = 0.004$). Inspection of the adjusted standardised residuals showed that girls were overrepresented in the 'Borderline' and 'Abnormal' categories. This suggests that more girls reported overall problems in relation to their SDQ scores compared to boys. Again, in the 14–17 age group, gender differences were evident in each of the three 'Emotional symptoms' categories, ($p = 0.002$). Inspection of the adjusted standardised residuals found that females were overrepresented in the 'Abnormal' category. This suggests more girls reported emotional problems than boys.

Predictors of adjustment

Regression analyses

A series of regression models were estimated to identify risk markers for child adjustment problems as defined by SDQ total scores. These considered the range of variables across individual, family, school and community domains that were specified as exogenous predictors of SDQ scores, with each variable considered in a separate

(bivariate) regression model in the first instance. In the context of either nominal or ordinal predictors with limited variability, or variables with highly skewed distributions, these were collapsed to form binary indicators and simplify the interpretation of effects. For example, the 5-point measure of caregiver-rated child health was collapsed to indicate good/fair/poor health = 1 (versus excellent/very good health = 0), while the continuous measure of years spent in refugee camps, which was characterised by limited variability among non-zero scores, was collapsed to form an indicator of 1 year or more spent in camps = 1 (versus no time or less than 1 year in camps = 0).

The results of these regression analyses are shown in Table 4. As can be seen, the largest effects were observed for parental hostility and subjective reports of child health, which were both associated with higher scores on the SDQ, suggesting greater adjustment difficulties. The bivariate models indicated smaller but significant effects for measures of academic achievement and absenteeism, as well as parental warmth. Table 4 shows results from a multiple regression model, which indicated that, while the association with parental warmth was reduced

Table 4 Bivariate and multiple regressions including variables from each domain as correlates of SDQ total scores

Domain/factor	n	Bivariate regression			Multiple regression		
		Estimate	95% CI		Estimate	95% CI	
			LB	UB		LB	UB
Individual							
Age	694	−0.05	−0.12	0.03	−0.11**	−0.18	−0.05
Gender (Female)[a]	694	0.02	−0.05	0.10	0.04	−0.03	0.10
Time in refugee camp (Yes)[a]	694	−0.01	−0.10	0.09	0.00	−0.08	0.08
Caregiver ratings of child health (good/fair/poor)[a]	694	0.30***	0.22	0.39	0.22***	0.14	0.29
Number of days physical activity	694	−0.07	−0.16	0.03	−0.05	−0.12	0.03
Family							
Family structure (single parent)[a]	694	0.09†	0.00	0.18	0.05	−0.03	0.13
Parental/caregiver warmth	694	−0.12*	−0.21	−0.02	−0.07†	−0.15	0.00
Parental/caregiver hostility	694	0.44***	0.34	0.53	0.39***	0.31	0.48
School							
School achievement (below average)[a]	694	0.19***	0.09	0.28	0.13**	0.05	0.21
Number of days absent	694	0.16**	0.05	0.28	0.11*	0.01	0.21
Achieved school award[b]	473	−0.02	−0.12	0.08	–	–	–
Community							
Extracurricular activities[b]	473	0.03	−0.08	0.15	–	–	–
Support from ethnic/religious community (no support)[a]	694	0.02	−0.08	0.11	0.01	−0.06	0.09
Neighbourhood feels unsafe	694	0.03	−0.05	0.11	−0.03	−0.10	0.05
People unfriendly	694	0.07	−0.03	0.18	0.03	−0.07	0.12

[a]Gender, time in refugee camp, child health, family structure, school achievement and support from ethnic/religious community were categorical variables. Their coding for the regression model is specified in brackets

[b]'Achieved school award' and 'extracurricular activities' were not included in the multiple regression model because these measures were only asked in the child self-report version (completed only by 11- to 17-year-old children), and data were thus based on a smaller sample

CI confidence interval, LB lower bound, UB upper bound

† $p < 0.10$; * $p < 0.05$; ** $p < 0.01$; *** $p < 0.001$

to marginal significance ($p < 0.10$) when controlling for other predictors, the aforementioned effects of parental hostility, caregiver-rated health, academic achievement and absenteeism were reduced but remained significant. In contrast, the effect of age was significant in the multiple regression but not in bivariate analyses. There was no evidence of associations with any variables in the community domain.

Discussion

We report herein, for the first time, psychosocial outcomes related to children and adolescents from the BNLA study – the largest, nationally representative Australian longitudinal study of resettled refugees and their families [1]. We explored the adjustment outcomes of children and adolescents 2–3 years following arrival to Australia. We were informed by an ecological framework that emphasised the individual (i.e. age, gender, physical health and activity, refugee camp experience), family (i.e. structure, parenting warmth and hostility), school (i.e. achievement, absenteeism), and community (i.e. extracurricular activity, neighbourhood friendliness and safety and ethnic/religious community support) domains.

The results indicated that refugee children and adolescents are adjusting soundly to their new lives in Australia, at a time when the acute stressors of resettlement are likely to have abated. The majority of children and adolescents were living in dual caregiver households and had adopted English in addition to using their caregivers' language at home. They reported high levels of physical health and activity and engagement in extracurricular activities (e.g. dance, sports). Notably, low levels of school absenteeism were reported, along with high ratings of school achievement and many participants (up to a quarter) reported school-based awards and achievements. These outcomes may reflect the protective acculturative factors in the post-migration period documented in the literature for refugees and migrants [7, 20].

The findings from our study show that, when considered as a group, relative to non-refugee Australians, this cohort of refugee children and adolescents were generally adjusting well. In fact, 76–94% of this sample reported functioning in the normal ranges of adjustment. Using the SDQ total scores as our indicator of adjustment, we found that refugee children and adolescents did not differ from Australian age- and gender-matched norms, with exception of 14- to 17-year-old refugee boys, who reported overall higher levels of adjustment than Australian norms. One group in which refugee children and adolescents reported lower overall adjustment than Australian peers was among 14- to 17-year-old girls. This was similarly the case across subscale measures of adjustment, including emotional difficulties, conduct problems, hyperactivity/inattention difficulties and pro-social behaviour. Refugee children and adolescents were comparable to, or had higher adjustment levels, relative to those seen in the Australian community. Among 14- to 17-year-old refugee boys in particular, a group often identified in the literature and media as at-risk for behavioural and social difficulties [16, 18], the data from this sample suggest significantly lower levels of difficulties than their Australian male counterparts. The only exception concerned 5- to 10-year-old girls, for whom caregivers reported greater levels of hyperactivity and inattention than Australian norms.

It is difficult to explicate the nuanced differences regarding gender comparisons in this study, but findings are generally consistent with prior research showing that refugee adolescent girls may be at higher risk for social and emotional difficulties than boys [20]. Although this question was not directly addressed in the current study, there are several potential reasons for such gender differences. It is possible girls may have more difficult or negative migration experiences, with a higher risk for certain traumatic events than boys (e.g. sexual violence) [45]. Further, girls may experience greater difficulties than boys in the post-migration setting, for instance, through prejudice or gender discrimination (e.g. being more identifiable as belonging to distinct cultural/religious backgrounds) [53]. Finally, adolescent girls may be more prone to internalising emotional difficulties and such risk may be particularly pronounced in refugee girls [54].

As an overall population though, refugee children and adolescents appear to be functioning soundly relative to Australian peers. This finding that young refugees function comparably despite potential adversities is suggestive of resilience among this group and might be explained in two ways. First, the positive adjustment of these young people could be related to the length of time since arriving in Australia and opportunities to acculturate within school and community contexts. This explanation is consistent with longitudinal studies that show decreases in the experience of mental health problems among resettled refugees over time [25, 55] and studies examining acculturative processes in refugees [56]. As Wave 3 represents the 2- to 3-year period following being granted a visa, it is plausible that acute social stressors, such as housing and accommodation concerns, language acquisition and school integration, are stabilised, which may have helped to promote the overall adjustment in these young people. This study did not measure the impacts of these acute stressors so careful interpretation is required, though our data support an explanation of stabilisation in the latter stages of early resettlement. The finding that the majority of refugee children and adolescents did not endorse emotional difficulties is also consistent with a multitude of adult and child studies that suggest the majority of refugees do not have psychological disorders [57].

A second possible explanation is that positive adjustment outcomes of this cohort reflect the screening and selection processes that Australia engages in, particularly in their 'offshore' humanitarian migration pathway. For example, the majority of young refugees in this sample had not arrived as asylum seekers, had not spent time in multiple refugee camps, and arrived accompanied. This explanation is further supported by the finding that most children in this sample were living in relatively intact dual caregiver households, which may be somewhat higher than that seen in other studies. These factors may have contributed to a better adjusted sample generally. Additionally, once granted a humanitarian visa, Australia has a well-established and often enviable Humanitarian Settlement Service programme that provides assistance to refugees with accommodation, as well as information and access to food, education, language and health services. The positive adjustment seen in these young people could be a reflection of the successes of policies and services offered as part of Australia's settlement programme.

Notwithstanding the overall adjustment of young refugees in this sample, as a whole, they did report significantly higher levels of peer problems than comparative Australian norms. This was a consistent finding across all age groups and genders and may in part have driven the increased risk seen in the subgroup of 14- to 17-year-old refugee girls. Peer difficulties measured by the SDQ concern problems with peer interactions, forming friendships, being generally liked, picked on, and preference for being on one's own or with adults. While difficulties with peers among young refugees was consistent, it is not clear what the conditions of such problems are, or indeed, whether these problems are in themselves a risk for, cause of adjustment difficulty or consequence of other factors (e.g. peer difficulties as an outcome of multiple school transitions or social exclusion, or an outcome of mental health problems).

Although further investigation is required to examine the nature of peer difficulties among this group of young refugees, the findings could suggest a number of relevant contextual factors. The development and maintenance of friendships, particularly in the adolescent period, is critical to social and emotional development [58]. The peer difficulties relative to Australian norms in this sample of young refugees could reflect an amplification of acculturative stress around forming and maintaining supportive peer relations (e.g. language difficulties as barriers, navigating customs around interacting with peers), as well as experiences of social exclusion, including isolation, prejudice, racism or discrimination. This is supported by studies showing that social exclusion and lack of belonging are risk factors for poor wellbeing in refugee youth [26], as well as evidence from school and community-based programmes which show that promoting social networks can enhance adjustment [59].

In addition to examining how young refugee children and adolescents compare to Australian norms, we also examined a range of individual, familial, school and community factors associated with adjustment as indicated by total SDQ scores. While existing research has identified a range of putative risk and protective factors, our study extended previous work by measuring factors systematically to assess their associations with a global assessment of functioning in young people, rather than mental health difficulties specifically. The results indicated that higher adjustment was associated with ratings of better physical health and school achievement, while poorer adjustment was associated with school absenteeism and a hostile parenting style.

Although the causal nature of these relationships cannot be established at this stage, and work is required to examine causal relationships and interactions within and across time for young refugees, these early findings suggest that certain factors can contribute to an understanding of young refugees' adjustment during the early settlement period. Collectively, the findings suggest that risk and protective factors most proximal to the child (e.g. in what Bronfenbrenner describes as the microsystem – individual, family, school and peer networks) may play critical roles in the adjustment of young refugees in the post-migration period. From a health and settlement policy perspective, our findings suggest that individual factors, including physical health, family factors such as hostile parenting styles, and school factors such as absenteeism and achievement, may inform prevention, screening and intervention efforts (e.g. strategies to improve physical health, parenting strategies that focus on decreasing hostility and enhancing warmth and nurturance, and strategies to encourage school participation and recognise achievement). Further, our gender-specific findings regarding adjustment point to value from more focused strategies (i.e. targeting adolescent girls, and hyperactivity and inattention difficulties among younger girls, 5 to 10 years old).

Strengths and limitations

This is the first large and broadly representative study of refugee children and adolescents resettled in Australia, which provides robust indications of adjustment among resettled young refugees. As such, the study has helped to bridge some of the disparate findings concerning mental health and well-being in prior studies. However, these findings should be considered in light of limitations. As with all cross-cultural studies, transcultural bias and translation non-equivalence associated with measures developed in western cultural settings may have affected responses. Social desirability may have also influenced reporting of positive adjustment (for example, there were only 6.1% of parents who reported overall school achievement as being 'below or well below average'). This desire to respond with socially appropriate answers may have differentially affected refugees given the public discourse surrounding refugee resettlement in Australia. Unfortunately, investigation of culturally specific idioms of distress (e.g. somatic complaints) were beyond the scope of this study but future directions could involve mapping these findings onto culturally specific expressions of adjustment. In some instances, single item tools were the only measures available to assess some domains (e.g. physical health). Whilst this study did use reports from either caregivers or children themselves, where available or appropriate (older children as more reliable self-reporters), these are not necessarily interchangeable. Given constraints on primary data collection, information obtained directly from schools (for example, regarding school achievement) were also not available. Obtaining these may help future research validate relevant findings. Finally, our statistical analyses incorporated adjustments for clustering within families, but were unable to model clustering within schools or neighbourhoods. While multilevel frameworks provide enhanced correspondence with ecological models, the current approach was 'single-level' and may be characterised by underestimates of standard errors (e.g. due to non-independence of families within neighbourhoods). The bivariate regression analyses were accompanied by a multiple regression model that included predictor variables simultaneously. This was intended to minimise the risk of confounded associations, but should be viewed cautiously given limitations in hypotheses regarding causal structures. Until more accurate predictive models can be determined, it is important to recognise these individual factors as conferring risk or protection rather than being a necessary condition for good or poor adjustment [60–62].

Conclusions

This was the first study to report outcomes for children and adolescents from the longitudinal BNLA study. Generally, refugee children and adolescents in the study reported adjusting soundly in the 2 to 3-year period after arrival in Australia. While it cannot be ignored that refugee children and adolescents do experience vulnerability on account of pre- and post-migration adversities, we present preliminary evidence suggesting that parental capability, physical health, school participation and achievement may be linked to improved settlement outcomes for this population. Further research may seek to replicate these findings and examine the nature of peer difficulties to inform how these are linked to adjustment outcomes. Contextual factors, including the settlement policies of host countries and the host country itself, should also be considered when assessing post-settlement adjustment outcomes in young refugees.

Acknowledgements

We acknowledge the funders of the Building a New Life in Australia (BNLA) project, the Australian Government Department of Immigration and Border Protection (DIBP), and the Australian Government Department of Social Services, which administer the BNLA project. We also acknowledge the Australian Institute of Family Studies, which undertook the design, administration and fieldwork of the BNLA project. We also acknowledge the support of the NHMRC programme grant (#1073041) in funding the child component of BNLA Wave 3. We acknowledge the assistance of Carolina Barbosa, Dr Sonia Terhaag, Kari Gibson and Dr Ellie Brown who helped edit this manuscript. We acknowledge the participants of the BNLA study who shared their time and experiences to inform this project.

Funding

This work was supported by the NHMRC programme grant (#1073041). The funding sources had no involvement in the study design, the collection, analysis and interpretation of data, writing of the report, and the decision to submit the article for publication.

Authors' contributions

WL, MO, DS, RB, AM and ZS designed the study and interpreted the findings. WL and MO drafted and revised the manuscript. DHP and NA conducted the statistical analyses and SC provided statistical advice. DS, BE, DF, RB, AM, DHP, ZS, AN, MVH, KF, SC, NA and DK each contributed expert advice to the study, interpretation of findings, and revisions to the manuscript. All authors approved the final version published.

Competing interests

The authors declare that they have no competing interests.

Author details

[1]Phoenix Australia, Melbourne, Victoria, Australia. [2]Department of Psychiatry, University of Melbourne, Melbourne, Victoria, Australia. [3]Liverpool Hospital, Sydney, NSW, Australia. [4]School of Psychiatry, University of New South Wales, Sydney, NSW, Australia. [5]ANU Centre for Social Research and Methods, Australian National University, Canberra, Australian Capital Territory, Australia. [6]School of Psychology, University of New South Wales, Sydney, NSW, Australia. [7]Centre for Traumatic Stress Studies, University of Adelaide, Adelaide, SA, Australia. [8]Black Dog Institute, Sydney, NSW, Australia. [9]St John of God Hospital Richmond, Sydney, Australia. [10]Melbourne School of Psychological Sciences, University of Melbourne, Melbourne, Victoria, Australia. [11]Population Health Sciences, Bristol Medical School, University of Bristol, Bristol, UK. [12]Monash Health, Melbourne, Victoria, Australia.

References

1. Jenkinson R, Silbert M, De Maio J, Edwards B. Building a New Life in Australia: Settlement experiences of recently arrived humanitarian migrants. J Home Econ Inst Aust. 2015;22(3):22–8.
2. Bronstein I, Montgomery P. Psychological distress in refugee children: a systematic review. Clin Child Fam Psychol Rev. 2011;14(1):44–56.

3.	Copeland WE, Keeler G, Angold A, Costello E. Traumatic events and posttraumatic stress in childhood. Arch Gen Psychiatry. 2007;64(5):577–84.

4.	Fazel M, Wheeler J, Danesh J. Prevalence of serious mental disorder in 7000 refugees resettled in western countries: a systematic review. Lancet. 2005;365(9467):1309–14.

5.	Bhui K, Warfa N, Edonya P, McKenzie K, Bhugra D. Cultural competence in mental health care: a review of model evaluations. BMC Health Serv Res. 2007;7(1):15.

6.	Steel Z, Chey T, Silove D, Marnane C, Bryant RA, van Ommeren M. Association of torture and other potentially traumatic events with mental health outcomes among populations exposed to mass conflict and displacement: a systematic review and meta-analysis. JAMA. 2009;302(5):537–49.

7.	Lustig SL, Kia-Keating M, Knight WG, Geltman P, Ellis H, Kinzie JD, Keane T, Saxe GN. Review of child and adolescent refugee mental health. J Am Acad Child Adolesc Psychiatry. 2004;43(1):24–36.

8.	Steel Z, Silove D, Brooks R, Momartin S, Alzuhairi B, Susljik I. Impact of immigration detention and temporary protection on the mental health of refugees. Br J Psychiatry. 2006;188(1):58–64.

9.	Miller K, Rasmussen A. The mental health of civilians displaced by armed conflict: an ecological model of refugee distress. Epidemiol Psychiatr Sci. 2017;26(2):129–38.

10.	Bronfenbrenner U, Morris PA. The ecology of developmental process. In R. M. Lerner & W. Damon (Eds.), Handbook of child psychology: Theoretical models of human development (5th ed). New York: John Wiley; 1998. p. 993–1028.

11.	Paat Y-F. Working with immigrant children and their families: an application of Bronfenbrenner's ecological systems theory. J Hum Behav Soc Environ. 2013;23(8):954–66.

12.	Bronfenbrenner U, Morris PA. The Bioecological Model of Human Development. In R. M. Lerner & W. Damon (Eds.), Handbook of child psychology: Theoretical models of human development (6th ed). Hoboken: Wiley; 2006. p. 793–828.

13.	Miller KE, Rasco LM (Eds.) The mental health of refugees: ecological approaches to healing and adaptation. Mahwah: Erlbaum; 2004.

14.	Li SS, Liddell BJ, Nickerson A. The relationship between post-migration stress and psychological disorders in refugees and asylum seekers. Curr Psychiatry Rep. 2016;18(9):82.

15.	Ellis BH, MacDonald HZ, Lincoln AK, Cabral HJ. Mental health of Somali adolescent refugees: the role of trauma, stress, and perceived discrimination. J Consult Clin Psychol. 2008;76(2):184.

16.	Heptinstall E, Sethna V, Taylor E. PTSD and depression in refugee children. Eur Child Adolesc Psychiatry. 2004;13(6):373–80.

17.	Goosen S, Stronks K, Kunst AE. Frequent relocations between asylum-seeker centres are associated with mental distress in asylum-seeking children: a longitudinal medical record study. Int J Epidemiol. 2014;43:94–104.

18.	Colic-Peisker V. 'At least you're the right colour': identity and social inclusion of Bosnian refugees in Australia. J Ethn Migr Stud. 2005;31(4):615–38.

19.	Bhui KS, Lenguerrand E, Maynard MJ, Stansfeld SA, Harding S. Does cultural integration explain a mental health advantage for adolescents? Int J Epidemiol. 2012;41(3):791–802.

20.	Fazel M, Reed RV, Panter-Brick C, Stein A. Mental health of displaced and refugee children resettled in high-income countries: risk and protective factors. Lancet. 2012;379(9812):266–82.

21.	Barber BK. Adolescents and War: How Youth Deal with Political Violence. New York: Oxford University Press; 2008.

22.	Barber BK, Stolz HE, Olsen JA, Collins WA, Burchinal M. Parental support, psychological control, and behavioral control: assessing relevance across time, culture, and method. Monogr Soc Res Child Dev. 2005;70(4):1–137.

23.	Al-Sabah R, Legerski J, Layne CM, Isakson B, Katalinski R, Pasalic H, Bosankic N, Pynoos RS. Adolescent adjustment, caregiver-adolescent relationships, and outlook towards the future in the long-term aftermath of the Bosnian war. J Child Adolesc Trauma. 2015;8(1):45–60.

24.	Jacobsen K, Landau LB. The dual imperative in refugee research: some methodological and ethical considerations in social science research and forced migration. Disasters. 2003;27(3):186–206.

25.	Beiser M. Resettling refugees and safeguarding their mental health: lessons learned from the Canadian refugee resettlement project. Transcult Psychiatry. 2009;46(4):539–83.

26.	Correa-Velez I, Gifford SM, McMichael C. The persistence of predictors of wellbeing among refugee youth eight years after resettlement in Melbourne, Australia. Soc Sci Med. 2015;142:163–8.

27.	Hjern A, Angel B. Organized violence and mental health of refugee children in exile: a six-year follow-up. Acta Paediatr. 2000;89(6):722–7.

28.	Montgomery E. Long-term effects of organized violence on young middle eastern refugees' mental health. Soc Sci Med. 2008;67(10):1596–603.

29.	Sack WH, Him C, Dickason D. Twelve-year follow-up study of Khmer youths who suffered massive war trauma as children. J Am Acad Child Adolesc Psychiatry. 1999;38(9):1173–9.

30.	Zwi K, Woodland L, Williams K, Palasanthiran P, Rungan S, Jaffe A, Woolfenden S. Protective factors for social-emotional well-being of refugee children in the first three years of settlement in Australia. Arch Dis Child. 2018;103(3): 261–8.

31.	Australian Institute of Family Studies. Buliding a New Life in Australia: The Longitidinal Study of Humanitarian Migrants. Overview of Waves 1, 2 and 3; Considerations for Main Wave 4 and Wave 5. In: Edited by Australian Government DoSS. Victoria: Australian Government, Department of Social Services; 2016.

32.	Edwards B, Smart D, De Maio J, SIlbert M, Jenkinson R. Cohort profile: building a new life in Australia BNLA): the longitudinal study of humanitarian migrants. Int J Epidemiol. 2018;47(1):20–28h.

33.	Goodman R. Psychometric properties of the strengths and difficulties questionnaire. J Am Acad Child Adolesc Psychiatry. 2001;40(11):1337–45.

34.	Goodman R, Ford T, Simmons H, Gatward R, Meltzer H. Using the strengths and difficulties questionnaire (SDQ) to screen for child psychiatric disorders in a community sample. Br J Psychiatry. 2000;177(6):534–9.

35.	Mullick MSI, Goodman R. Questionnaire screening for mental health problems in Bangladeshi children: a preliminary study. Soc Psychiatry Psychiatr Epidemiol. 2001;36(2):94–9.

36.	Achenbach TM, Becker A, Dopfner M, Heiervang E, Roessner V, Steinhausen H-C, Rothenberger A. Multicultural assessment of child and adolescent psychopathology with ASEBA and SDQ instruments: research findings, applications, and future directions. J Child Psychol Psychiatry. 2008;49(3):251–75.

37.	Shehadeh A, Loots G, Vanderfaeillie J, Derluyn I. The impact of parental detention on the psychological wellbeing of Palestinian children. PLoS One. 2015;10(7):1–11.

38.	Panter-Brick C, Grimon M-P, Eggerman M. Caregiver-child mental health: a prospective study in conflict and refugee settings. J Child Psychol Psychiatry. 2014;55(4):313–27.

39.	Dalgaard NT, Todd BK, Daniel SI, Montgomery E. The transmission of trauma in refugee families: associations between intra-family trauma communication style, children's attachment security and psychosocial adjustment. Attach Hum Dev. 2016;18(1):69–89.

40.	Dura-Vila G, Klasen H, Makatini Z, Rahimi Z, Hodes M. Mental health problems of young refugees: duration of settlement, risk factors and community-based interventions. Clin Child Psychol Psychiatry. 2013;18(4):604–23.

41.	Vaage AB, Thomsen PH, Rousseau C, Wentzel-Larsen T, Ta TV, Hauff E. Paternal predictors of the mental health of children of Vietnamese refugees. Child Adolesc Psychiatry Mental Health. 2011;5:2.

42.	Vaage AB, Tingvold L, Hauff E, Van Ta T, Wentzel-Larsen T, Clench-Aas J, Thomsen PH. Better mental health in children of Vietnamese refugees compared with their Norwegian peers - a matter of cultural difference? Child Adolesc Psychiatry Mental Health. 2009;3:34.

43.	Daud A, Rydelius P-A. Comorbidity/overlapping between ADHD and PTSD in relation to IQ among children of traumatized/non-traumatized parents. J Atten Disord. 2009;13(2):188–96.

44.	Daud A, Af Klinteberg B, Rydelius P-A. Resilience and vulnerability among refugee children of traumatized and non-traumatized parents. Child Adolesc Psychiatry Mental Health. 2008;2:7.

45.	Derluyn I, Broekaert E. Different perspectives on emotional and behavioural problems in unaccompanied refugee children and adolescents. Ethn Health. 2007;12(2):141–62.

46.	Leavey G, Hollins K, King M, Barnes J, Papadopoulos C, Grayson K. Psychological disorder amongst refugee and migrant schoolchildren in London. Soc Psychiatry Psychiatr Epidemiol. 2004;39(3):191–5.

47.	O'Shea B, Hodes M, Down G, Bramley J. A school-based mental health service for refugee children. Clin Child Psychol Psychiatry. 2000;5(2):189–201.

48.	Rousseau C, Benoit M, Lacroix L, Gauthier M-F. Evaluation of a sandplay program for preschoolers in a multiethnic neighborhood. J Child Psychol Psychiatry. 2009;50(6):743–50.

49.	Mellor D. Furthering the use of the strengths and difficulties questionnaire: reliability with younger child respondents. Psychol Assess. 2004;16(4):396.

50.	Scoring the SDQ. http://www.sdqinfo.com/py/sdqinfo/c0.py. Accessed 11 Aug 2017.

51. Gray M, Sanson, A. Growing up in Australia: The longitudinal study of Australian children. Family Matters. 2005; 72:4–9.
52. Edwards B, Gray M, Wise S, Hayes A, Katz I, Muir K, Patulny R. Early impacts of communities for children on children and families: findings from a quasi-experimental cohort study. J Epidemiol Community Health. 2011;65(10):909–14.
53. Ellis BH, MacDonald HZ, Klunk-Gillis J, Lincoln A, Strunin L, Cabral HJ. Discrimination and mental health among Somali refugee adolescents: the role of acculturation and gender. Am J Orthopsychiatry. 2010;80(4):564–75.
54. Hodes M, Jagdev D, Chandra N, Cunniff A. Risk and resilience for psychological distress amongst unaccompanied asylum seeking adolescents. J Child Psychol Psychiatry. 2008;49(7):723–32.
55. Sack W, Clarke G, Him C, Dickason D, Goff B, Lanham K, Kinzie JD. A 6-year follow-up study of Cambodian refugee adolescents traumatized as children. J Am Acad Child Adolesc Psychiatry. 1993;32:431–7.
56. Liebkind K. Acculturation and stress Vietnamese refugees in Finland. J Cross-Cult Psychol. 1996;27(2):161–80.
57. Liddell BJ, Nickerson A, Sartor L, Ivancic L, Bryant RA. The generational gap: mental disorder prevalence and disability amongst first and second generation immigrants in Australia. J Psychiatr Res. 2016;83:103–11.
58. Viner RM, Ozer EM, Denny S, Marmot M, Resnick M, Fatusi A, Currie C. Adolescence and the social determinants of health. Lancet. 2012; 379(9826):1641–52.
59. Fazel M, Doll H, Stein A. A school-based mental health intervention for refugee children: an exploratory study. Clin Child Psychol Psychiatry. 2009;14(2):297–309.
60. Cicchetti D, Blender JA. A multiple-levels-of-analysis perspective on resilience. Ann N Y Acad Sci. 2006;1094(1):248–58.
61. Luthar SS, Cicchetti D, Becker B. Research on resilience: response to commentaries. Child Dev. 2000;71(3):573–5.
62. Masten AS. Ordinary magic: resilience processes in development. Am Psychol. 2001;56(3):227.

5

Do healthcare services behave as complex systems? Analysis of patterns of attendance and implications for service delivery

Christopher Burton[1]*(iD), Alison Elliott[2,4], Amanda Cochran[2] and Tom Love[3]

Abstract

Background: The science of complex systems has been proposed as a way of understanding health services and the demand for them, but there is little quantitative evidence to support this. We analysed patterns of healthcare use in different urgent care settings to see if they showed two characteristic statistical features of complex systems: heavy-tailed distributions (including the inverse power law) and generative burst patterns.

Methods: We conducted three linked studies. In study 1 we analysed the distribution of number of contacts per patient with an urgent care service in two settings: emergency department (ED) and primary care out-of-hours (PCOOH) services. We hypothesised that these distributions should be heavy-tailed (inverse power law or log-normal) in keeping with typical complex systems. In study 2 we analysed the distribution of bursts of contact with urgent care services by individuals: correlated bursts of activity occur in complex systems and represent a mechanism by which overall heavy-tailed distributions arise. In study 3 we replicated the approach of study 1 using data systematically identified from published sources.

Results: Study 1 involved data from a PCOOH service in Scotland (725,000) adults, 1.1 million contacts) and an ED in New Zealand (60,000 adults, 98,000 contacts). The total number of contacts per individual in each dataset was statistically indistinguishable from an inverse power law ($p > 0.05$) above 4 contacts for the PCOOH data and 3 contacts for the ED data. Study 2 found the distribution of contact bursts closely followed a heavy-tailed distribution ($p < 0.008$), indicating the presence of correlated bursts. Study 3 identified data from 17 studies across 8 countries and found distributions similar to study 1 in all of them.

Conclusions: Urgent healthcare use displays characteristic statistical features of large complex systems. These studies provide strong quantitative evidence that healthcare services behave as complex systems and have important implications for urgent care. Interventions to manage demand must address drivers for consultation across the whole system: focusing on only the highest users (in the tail of the distribution) will have limited impact on efficiency. Bursts of attendance — and ways to shorten them — represent promising targets for managing demand.

Keywords: Health services research, Emergency department, Primary care, Complex systems, Complexity, Frequent attendance

Abbreviations: CDF, Cumulative distribution function; CI, Confidence interval; ED, Emergency Department; KS, Kolmogorov Smirnoff; NHS, (UK) National Health Service; NHS24, NHS Scotland Primary Care Out of Hours Service; PCOOH, Primary Care Out of Hours Service

---

* Correspondence: Chris.burton@sheffield.ac.uk
[1]Academic Unit of Primary Medical Care, University of Sheffield, Samuel Fox House, Northern General Hospital, Sheffield S5 7AU, UK
Full list of author information is available at the end of the article

Background

Managing demand for healthcare is a global problem. The science of complex systems [1, 2] has been proposed as a way of understanding health services [3, 4], but there has been little quantitative evidence to support this notion. The idea that healthcare services can be considered as complex systems is not new [4–7] and remains current [3, 8], but it has rarely been tested, particularly in ways that use large-scale data. Healthcare self-evidently possesses many of the characteristics of a complex system [1, 2, 5] in that there are many component parts (patients, clinicians, services) with many interactions (consultations) which occur in the context of prevailing social attitudes and norms (e.g. ideas about when it is appropriate to seek healthcare). Because of the interactions and the way that characteristics of the system emerge from these interactions, complex systems are different from conventional systems in several ways [1, 9]. Some of these differences are listed in Table 1. Much current health services research and innovation addresses healthcare as a conventional system rather than as a complex one, with important implications for the development and implementation of complex interventions to change health and healthcare [1, 3, 9, 10].

Despite the resemblance of healthcare to a complex system and the wide recognition that complex systems display characteristic statistical properties [11, 12], there have been very few studies which have sought to test this by comparing the statistical properties of healthcare use with known properties of complex systems [13–15]. However, robust methods are available for this [11] which have been widely used in many other areas of science (examples include the size distributions of avalanches, forest fires and human settlements and patterns of Internet activity) [16].

One aspect of healthcare which is well suited to being examined as a complex system is the use of urgent care [17, 18]. Urgent care (emergency department (ED) and primary care out-of-hours (PCOOH) services) represents a relatively open system in which use is driven by patients rather than controlled by the service. It also includes the particular problem of high-using, or frequently attending, patients [17]. These patients take up a disproportionate amount of resources including professional time and treatment costs and are frequently portrayed as problematic individuals for whom initiatives are developed to identify and manage individual frequent attenders [19, 20]. This action at the level of the individuals carries the implication that tackling these extreme cases will resolve the pressure on urgent care services [21]. However, frequent attenders comprise a very heterogeneous group [22], including both patients who appear to need multiple attendances because of severe or complex medical conditions and others who attend for conditions that could be managed elsewhere [23] or to an extent which is disproportionate to their medical conditions [19, 24–26]. While interventions to tackle specific problems for some frequent attenders are successful at the individual level, there is little evidence that they lead to a substantial reduction in overall demand.

In contrast to the view of frequent attendance as a problem of a few individuals, a complex system perspective could argue that (1) frequent attenders might represent the "black swans [27]" occurring in the natural heavy-tailed distribution of events [11], (2) patterns of consultation by individuals over time should show the bursts typically seen in complex systems [12] and (c) there should be plausible social mechanisms which drive the behaviour of individuals across all levels of attendance from least to most frequent. While social mechanisms have been documented in several qualitative studies of healthcare seeking [28–32], there have been no studies, to our knowledge, which have examined the statistical properties of complex systems in urgent healthcare use. The closest to this have been some reports of the overall population distribution of urgent

Table 1 Comparison of features between a complex system and a conventional system

	Conventional system	Complex system
Relationship of individual to system	System comprises discrete individuals, who are considered as distinct and statistically independent from each other, but who share the system environment	System comprises individuals, each interacting with others in the system; characteristics of the whole system emerge from these interactions
Context and culture	Context or culture seen as separate from the individuals and may be externally directed or imposed. Treated as a confounder or covariate in analysis	Context or culture seen as emergent properties of the system. In turn, these properties condition the interactions of individuals within the system
Predictability of response to events	Multiple independent responses to change produce a coherent average value response and an approximately normal distribution	Changes to the system are usually buffered by local interaction (so have minimal effect), but sometimes events spread through the system with unexpectedly large effects
Statistical Distributions	Normal distribution for continuous measures, Poisson distribution for events	Heavy-tailed distributions for events: typically inverse power law or log-normal

care use which described non-normal distributions [33, 34]; however, none have carried out more detailed statistical analyses.

In this study we tested the hypothesis that patterns of attendance at urgent care services should display two typical statistical characteristics of complex systems. Specifically we hypothesised first, that the overall distribution of consultations per individual would follow a power law [2, 11] and second, that individuals' consultations would occur in correlated bursts (sequences of consultations clustered in time), with the distribution of burst lengths also approximating to a power law [12]. The implication of these hypotheses is that if urgent care services do behave as complex systems, then interventions to influence their use need to act in a system-wide fashion rather than focus on problematic individuals.

Methods
We conducted three linked studies to compare the statistical properties of urgent healthcare use with the typical properties of a complex system. First, we defined the total number of contacts per person and compared this to two heavy-tailed distributions, the inverse power law and the log-normal. Second, we used the same data to examine the pattern of bursts of attendance. Third, we conducted a systematic search for and analysis of reports, from other centres, of the distribution of number of contacts per person to compare these results with the findings from our primary data sources.

Data sources
We analysed primary data from two sources: PCOOH data from a study of NHS 24, the service which provides out-of-hours primary care services throughout Scotland (population 5.6 million (M)) [35] and ED data supplied by Canterbury District Health Board in New Zealand. The data was for the ED of Christchurch Hospital, serving a population of approximately 500,000 people. Both datasets were derived from routine management data and thus included all cases handled by the respective services.

In the PCOOH service, all calls were initially managed through a nurse-based triage system with a range of options including telephone advice by the nurse, consultation with a general practitioner (GP), either at a treatment centre or in the patient's home, and direct ambulance transfer to an ED. The data included all calls to the NHS 24 service throughout 2011. We excluded calls during office hours (08.00 to 18.00 weekdays except public holidays) because the vast majority of urgent care requests during these hours go directly to the patient's GP practice. All data was anonymised and handled under a data-sharing agreement between the University of Aberdeen and NHS 24; as no patient-identifiable data

was involved, additional research ethical permission was not required. The ED data comprised anonymised data of adult attendance for the period July 2011 to June 2013. Since no identifying patient information was involved, research ethical permission was not required under New Zealand's Standard Operating Procedures for Health and Disability Ethics Committees.

Definitions of attendance
For both datasets, the unit of analysis was a contact — defined as one or more attendances or phone calls with the service on a given day. While some patients had more than one attendance or call on the same day, we limited data to one contact per day, since most repeated calls on the same day related to the same episode of care (e.g. escalation of a contact from telephone advice to consultation). PCOOH contacts included episodes of care which were managed by telephone, in the urgent care department or at home, and by any healthcare professionals. ED contacts included emergency attendances by any route.

Heavy-tailed statistical distributions and correlated bursts of activity
Heavy tails are a feature of a number of statistical distributions, including the inverse power law and the log-normal, which have been repeatedly observed in large, naturally occurring systems [11]. The term refers to the long, or thick, "tail" of the distribution, in contrast to the shorter tails of distributions such as the normal, where data points cluster close to the mean (and almost always within a few standard deviations of it). One of the first described heavy-tailed distributions was the Pareto principle whereby 80% of the wealth is held by 20% of the population (and of that wealth, 80% is held by only 20% of the 20%, and so on) [16]. This observation is mathematically related to the inverse power law. The result of such a distribution is that the range of wealth from poorest to richest is much greater than would occur if individuals were normally distributed around a mean. While plots of the normal distribution produce the familiar bell curve, conventional plots of heavy-tailed distributions are difficult to interpret because of the much larger range of values. A simple solution to this is to plot cumulative distributions with logarithmic axes. Using this format an inverse power law will describe a straight line (from top left to bottom right). Heavy-tailed distributions are typically seen in theoretical complex systems and have been held to be a typical feature, or fingerprint, of complex systems [11].

While there are many possible explanations for the occurrence of heavy-tailed distributions [36], and their presence alone is not proof of the presence of a complex system, the more recent description of correlated bursts of activity within a complex system leading to heavy-tailed overall distributions [12] means that identifying both in the same data strengthens the evidence for the presence of a complex system. Correlated bursts of activity represent clusters of activity in time, with the distribution of burst lengths also following a heavy-tailed distribution [12]. This distribution of bursts means that long bursts arise more often than would occur by chance, and furthermore that bursts undergo a kindling process, whereby the longer a burst has gone on, the more likely it is to continue.

Study 1: analysis of total contacts per patient

We conducted this analysis using the total number of contacts per patient in 1 year of data from each dataset. We plotted the complementary cumulative distribution function (CDF), defined as the proportion of patients whose total number of contacts was equal to or greater than each number of contacts between 1 and the largest recorded. This is preferable to plotting the probability distribution function, as the CDF is more robust against fluctuations in the tail of the distribution due to finite sample sizes [11]. Plots of the CDF were made with logarithmic axes, on which a power law distribution displays a straight line. The slope of this line is equal to one minus the scaling parameter of the power law distribution (for example, a scaling parameter of 3 produces a slope of − 2). We fitted inverse power law and log-normal functions to each dataset using maximum likelihood fitting with the poweRlaw package in R 3.3.2. We examined the closeness of fit of the data to a power law distribution, using the Kolmogorov-Smirnoff (KS) test. Where data was deemed different from a power law distribution (p value < 0.05) we examined whether the data was closer in fit to a power law or log-normal distribution using the Vuong test for non-nested distributions [37] at a significance level of 0.01. As naturally occurring distributions often include a power law only above a certain threshold [11], we repeated this analysis with a range of minimum values for the number of contacts per patient.

Subgroup and sensitivity analysis

We conducted a subgroup analysis of the PCOOH data with data split by sex and by age using the median value. For each subgroup we repeated the plotting and model-fitting procedure described above, with the addition of 95% confidence intervals (CIs) derived from a non-parametric bootstrapping procedure (1000 iterations). We did not conduct a subgroup analysis of the ED data because of the smaller number of patients.

We conducted two post hoc sensitivity analyses to test for artefacts arising from the fact that each dataset contained a calendar year but that patients might have their first consultation at any point during the year and thus have different durations of follow-up. In the first sensitivity analysis we limited data to patients consulting within the first half of the year and censored each patient's data 6 months after their first contact. In the second sensitivity analysis we considered that some patients consulting in the first few weeks of the year would be doing so within a burst of contacts. We thus split the PCOOH data into patients whose first contact was before the 15th day of the time period and those whose first contact was on or after the 15th day. In each of the sensitivity analyses we used the same method for plotting and analysing distributions as described for the whole dataset.

Study 2: analysis of bursts of contacts

We examined bursts of contacts using the method developed by Karsai [12]. We defined a burst as a sequence of contacts in which the interval between each pair of consecutive contacts is less than a specified time window Δt. We used a range of values for Δt of 4 and 7 days for the PCOOH data and 4, 7 and 10 days for the ED data. For each burst we counted the number of contacts within the burst. We pooled the burst patterns across all individuals and limited the analysis to patients with between 4 and 52 contacts in order to exclude data with too few contacts to display bursts, or so many contacts that bursts were inevitable because the PCOOH data comprised only 1 year. We conducted the burst analysis on the PCOOH dataset (1 year) and on the whole ED dataset (2 years).

For each dataset and value of Δt we plotted the CDF. As for the distribution of total contacts, we plotted the CDFs using logarithmic axes, so that an inverse power law would display as a straight line. In order to assess whether the burst patterns could have arisen by chance, we conducted a bootstrapping procedure in which we compared the actual data with a set of surrogate datasets in which the temporal structure of bursts was broken by randomly allocating the number of contacts for each patient to dates within the time between their first contact and the end of the study period. These surrogate datasets were thus identical to the original dataset except that the bursts they contained arose at random. We conducted this bootstrapping procedure with 250 iterations, meaning that the probability of any observed distribution lying wholly above the bootstrapped range by chance was less than 0.008.

Study 3: review of data from published reports

We systematically identified papers reporting numbers of patients attending EDs, using a structured search of the MEDLINE and Embase databases (Table 2 lists the search terms). Titles, abstracts and full manuscripts were screened by two authors independently to identify usable

Table 2 Search terms

Emergency department

1) Emergency Service, Hospital/

2) ((emergency or casualty) adj1 department).mp.

3) (accident adj2 emergency).mp.

4) 1 or 2 or 3

5) (frequen$ adj2 attend$).mp.

6) "high use$".mp.

7) (hig$ adj (utiliz$ or utilis$)).mp.

8) "frequent flier".mp.

9) (frequen$ adj3 use$).mp.

10) 5 or 6 or 7 or 8 or 9

11) 4 and 10

Primary care out-of-hours service

1) General Practice/

2) Primary Health Care/

3) "General Practi$".mp.

4) "GP".mp.

5) "primary care".mp.

6) 1 or 2 or 3 or 4 or 5

7) (out adj2 hours).mp.

8) "out-of-hours".mp.

9) "unscheduled".mp.

10) 7 or 8 or 9

11) (frequen$ adj2 attend$).mp.

12) "high use$".mp.

13) (hig$ adj (utiliz$ or utilis$)).mp.

14) "frequent flier".mp.

15) (frequen$ adj3 use$).mp.

16) 11 or 12 or 13 or 14 or 15

17) 6 and 10 and 16

data. We followed references from, and citations of, eligible papers to identify additional studies.

Inclusion and exclusion criteria

We included studies which reported urgent care attendance data either in EDs or PCOOH services. We required reports to include all of the following: setting (time and place), an unselected population (e.g. "all attenders" or "all adults", but not "adults with asthma") and a continuous or categorical (binned) distribution of individual patient attendances over 1 year which included all attenders. We excluded studies which reported less than four categories or where the lower threshold of the highest category was less than 10 episodes of care, in order to ensure a spread of data points and include at least one order of magnitude for the number of episodes of care. Where a study reported

more than 1 year or more than one site for care separately, we used the most recent year or the largest site. Where studies reported several sites together, we did not attempt to separate them. Studies varied in the categories they used to report attendance (individual numbers of attendances, ranges of attendances or a mixture of the two). In most cases we kept data in the original format; where studies reported many categories, each with small numbers (< 10) of individuals, we aggregated them into category ranges containing 10 or more individuals. We did not restrict studies on the basis of healthcare system or level of economic development.

Quality assessment of included studies

All studies were observational studies describing similar retrospective data collection of a complete sample. Provided studies met our stringent inclusion and exclusion criteria we did not apply further quality assessments, as the topics for evaluation in common tools (e.g. completeness of sample, sources of bias, etc.) are designed for studies which make inferences based on samples from populations, whereas the studies we included reported on counts of attendance for entire services.

Distributions of attendance per patient in review data

For each study we plotted the complementary CDF: the proportion of patients whose total number of attendances was equal to or greater than the lower boundary of each category. Plots used logarithmic axes to facilitate the display of heavy-tailed data. We plotted data for ED and PCOOH studies separately. In addition, we selected a subset of studies which contained at least 8 data bins, with the highest data bin threshold set ≥ 20. As most studies provided heavily aggregated data with wide categories, we did not attempt to fit distributions to this data.

Results

Analysis of total contacts per patient

Primary data was available from 724,921 PCOOH patients (1,085,796 contacts) and 60,106 ED patients (98,228 contacts). The age and sex characteristics and number of contacts per patient are listed in Table 3.

Plots of total number of contacts per individual are shown in Fig. 1a (PCOOH data) and 1b(ED data). Both plots show a heavy-tailed distribution, which approximates to an inverse power law (straight line) for the whole distribution in the ED data and from approximately 5 contacts to 30 contacts in the PCOOH data. Above 30 contacts in the PCOOH data (Fig. 1a) the tail of the distribution can be seen to deviate from the power law; there were more patients than expected with very high numbers of contacts: 225 patients (0.03%) had more than 30 contacts. This represents approximately

Table 3 Characteristics of patients in PCOOH and ED datasets

	PCOOH patients (N = 724,921)	%	ED patients (N = 60,106)	%
Age				
<=5	119,611	16.5	7482	14.5
6–17	78,757	10.9	6414	12.4
18–45	263,234	36.3	17,905	34.6
46–70	154,826	21.4	12,361	23.9
71+	108,486	15.0	7524	14.6
Not recorded	7	–	8420	–
Sex				
Female	420,663	58.0	–	–
Male	304,258	42.0	–	–
Number of contacts				
1	532,807	73.5	40,011	66.6
2–5	181,906	25.1	18,965	31.6
6–10	8105	1.1	951	1.6
11–50	2002	0.3	177	0.3
51–100	79	0.01	2	0.003
101+	22	0.003	0	–

twice as many as would have been expected if the data followed a power law distribution. This pattern is suggestive of more than one overlapping distribution. Figure 1c shows the result of the sensitivity analysis in which the PCOOH data was split into patients whose first contact occurred within the first 14 days of the year and those whose first contact came later. The rationale was that patients consulting in the first 14 days might be within a burst of consultations at the start of the data collection and thus might be more likely to have repeat consultations than those starting their first burst after at least 14 days of no contact. The two resulting distributions in Fig. 1c both showed close approximation to a power law. Finally, Fig. 1d shows the analysis repeated with censoring of data at 6 months after the first consultation, indicating that this had no adverse influence on the observed distribution's approximation to a power law.

Statistical model fitting

Table 4 lists the statistical parameters from the fitting of inverse power law and log-normal distributions to the data. Values for PCOOH (first contact after the first 14 days) and ED data were broadly similar, and for patients with 5 or more contacts both distributions showed good fit to a power law (KS test p value > 0.05) with similar exponents of 3.8 and 3.7.

The good fit of the power law (and log-normal) distributions to the whole population supports the hypothesis that urgent healthcare systems show one of the typical statistical characteristics of complex systems. Despite the

occurrence of extreme frequent attenders (the maximum number of contacts was 266 and 94 in the PCOOH and ED data respectively), the proximity of these extreme points to the fitted curves shows that these events occurred with the expected frequency for their respective distributions. This suggests that frequent attenders are indeed the "black swans" which naturally occur in complex systems [27].

Subgroup analysis

The subgroup analysis, by age and sex, is reported in Table 5 and Fig. 2. The figures and data indicate that the distributions were heavy-tailed in each subgroup, but that the scaling parameter was larger (a steeper gradient on the plots) in younger than older adults. There was less difference between the sexes.

Analysis of bursts of contacts

Plots of the distribution of burst length are shown in Fig. 3a and b for both the PCOOH data and ED data. Both plots use a 7-day window for inclusion of contacts within bursts. Both distributions are clearly heavy tailed, approximating to a straight line indicative of an inverse power law. None of the 250 surrogate datasets, in which the temporal structure of bursts was disrupted, showed this distribution, suggesting that it was unlikely to have arisen in the data by chance. Similar patterns were seen from the PCOOH data with a 4-day window (Fig. 3c) and from the ED data with 4- and 10-day windows (Fig. 3d). This similarity across different time windows makes it unlikely that the observed results were due to an

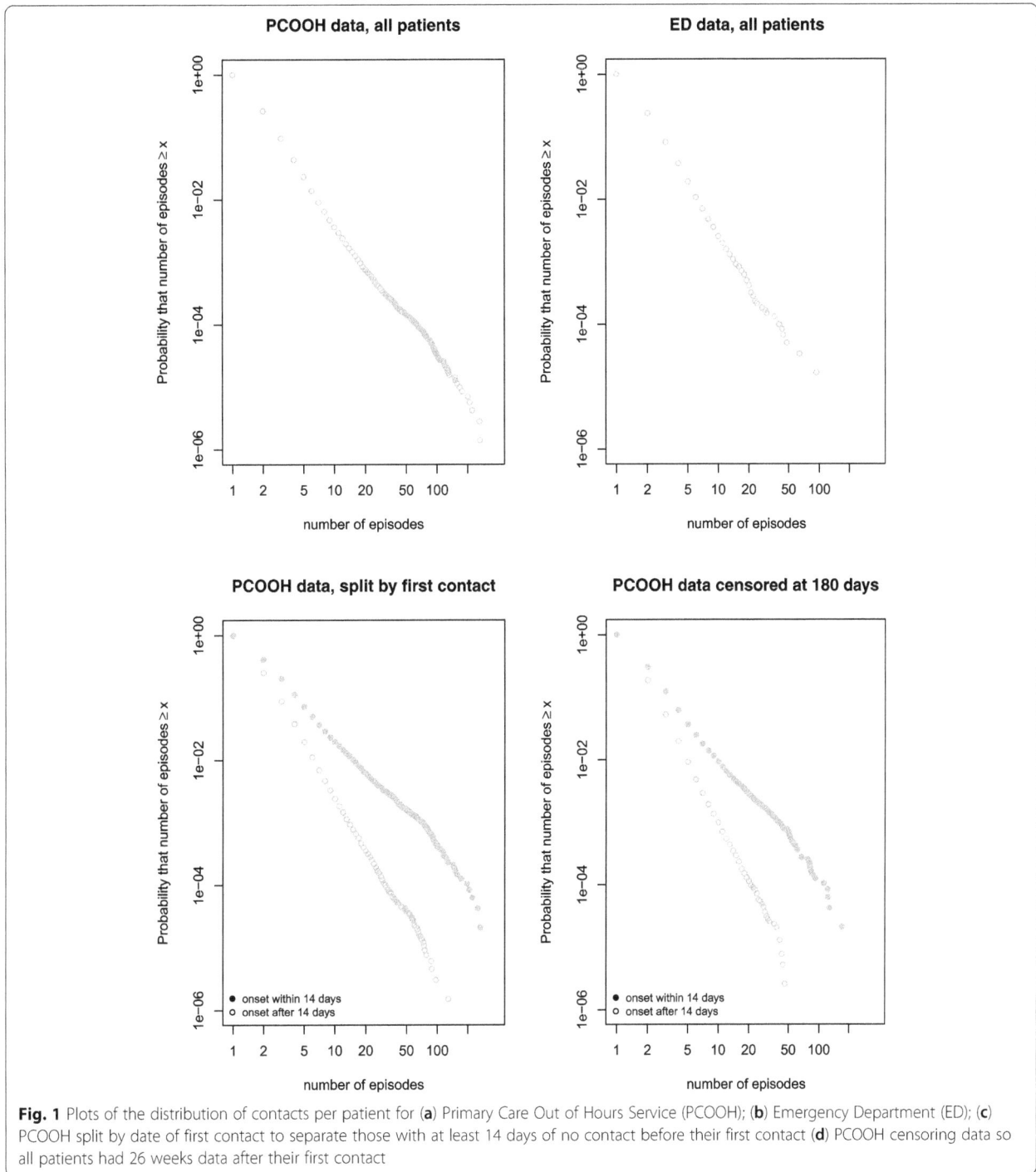

Fig. 1 Plots of the distribution of contacts per patient for (**a**) Primary Care Out of Hours Service (PCOOH); (**b**) Emergency Department (ED); (**c**) PCOOH split by date of first contact to separate those with at least 14 days of no contact before their first contact (**d**) PCOOH censoring data so all patients had 26 weeks data after their first contact

artefact of the measurement parameters and more likely that these new findings represent real phenomena present in the data.

Systematic analysis of data from published reports
Included studies
We identified 883 titles from the search of ED attendance, from which 15 studies contained data suitable for analysis. We also identified 25 titles relating to out-of-hours primary care, resulting in two studies with data suitable for analysis. Flowcharts of the selection process are shown in Fig. 4. Characteristics of the included studies are summarised in Table 6. Briefly, studies dated from between 1999 and 2015. Eight were from single EDs (range of sample size 22,492–95,170) [19, 33, 38–43]; six from multiple departments in the same city

Table 4 Power Law scaling parameter and tests of fit for selected distributions by minimum value of contacts included in analysis

Data	Measure	Minimum number of contacts per individual for inclusion				
		3	4	5	6	8
PCOOH	Alpha	3·45	3·5	3·46	3·38	3·23
all patients	KS p-value	<.001	<.001	<.001	<.001	<.001
	Vuong p-value	<.001	<.001	<.001	<.001	<.001
ED	Alpha	3·54	3·71	3·72	3·59	3·55
all patients	KS p-value	<·001	0·23	0·07	0·93	0·89
	Vuong p-value	0.44	0.67	0.10	0.92	0.97
PCOOH	Alpha	2·75	2·76	2·71	2·66	2·6
Contact in	KS p-value	0·02	0·004	0·01	0·07	0·53
first 14 days	Vuong p-value	0.32	<0.001	0.001	0.01	0.69
PCOOH: 1st	Alpha	3·63	3·77	3·8	3·8	3·76
contact after	KS p-value	<0.001	0.001	0.40	0.32	0.19
first 14 days	Vuong p-value	0.001	0.15	0.26	0.12	0.08

PCOOH primary care out-ofhours (service), *ED* emergency department
Alpha represents the scaling parameter of the power law probability distribution $p(x) \propto x^{-\alpha}$
KS Kolmogorov-Smirnoff test for fit of data to power law, reported as *p* value (value > 0·05 indicates no difference between data and power law)
Vuong Better fitting distribution to the data by Vuong test (*p* values in blue indicate that the power law was the better fitting distribution, *p* values in red that the log-normal was the better fit

(range 13,959–212,959) [34, 44–48]; and one from a network of departments (N = 930,712) [49]. Eight ED studies were from the USA [39, 40, 42, 43, 46–49], two from the UK [19, 33] and one each from Canada [45], Australia [44], Singapore [41], the Netherlands [34] and Ireland [38]. One PCOOH study was from the Netherlands (44,953 patients) [50] and one from Italy (17,657) [51].

Distribution of contacts per patient from included studies

Figure 5 shows data from the 15 ED studies. In each plot, the distribution was typical of a heavy-tailed distribution, and for all but one study (which included pooled patient data from multiple sites [49]) followed an approximately straight line above 3 episodes, suggesting a power law. Figure 6a shows a subset of four

studies which met more stringent criteria of reporting at least 8 data bins and with a threshold for the highest bin of at least 20 attendances. These studies all show distributions similar to those in our primary data. Finally, Fig. 6b shows the two primary care studies.

The similarity of the distributions across location, healthcare type (free at the point of delivery, paid/insured) and time (almost 20 years) suggests that the patterns we observed are consistently present and represent a characteristic property of urgent care systems. While we did not fit statistical models to the data (because the effect of binning meant that the data was too sparse), the data in Fig. 6 can be compared with the more detailed data in Fig. 1. Simple visual comparison of the plots indicates that for the ED data in Fig. 1b, 1 in

Table 5 Power law scaling parameter (alpha) by minimum value of contacts included in analysis in subgroups of patients split by sex and by median age

Inclusion	Subgroup	Minimum number of contacts per individual for inclusion			
		Minimum 3 contacts		Minimum 5 contacts	
		Alpha	95% CI	Alpha	95% CI
	Younger male	3.35	3.28–3.41	3.05	2.94–to 3.16
All patients	Younger female	3.42	3.38–3.46	3.29	3.21–3.38
	Older male	3.13	3.09–3.17	3.31	3.22–3.39
	Older female	3.19	3.15–3.22	3.24	3.17–3.31
Patients with first contact after 14th day	Younger male	3.60	3.52–3.67	3.42	3.28–3.57
	Younger female	3.62	3.57–3.67	3.65	3.55–3.75
	Older male	3.30	3.26–3.35	3.64	3.54–3.74
	Older female	3.37	3.34–3.41	3.58	3.50–3.67

Alpha: scaling parameter of the power law probability distribution $p(x) \propto x^{-\alpha}$
95% confidence intervals (CIs) derived by non-parametric bootstrapping with 1000 iterations

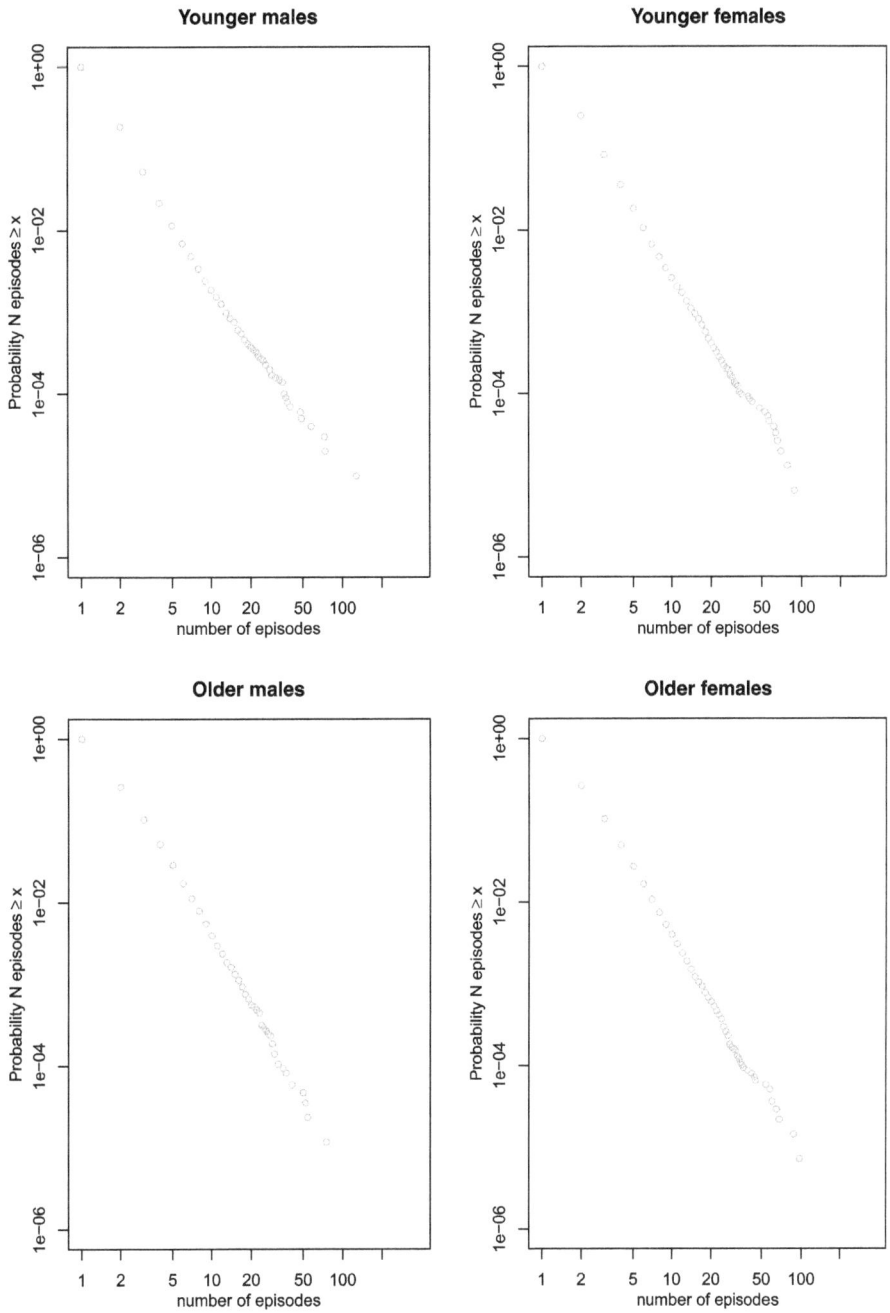

Fig. 2 Plots of the distribution of contacts per patient for primary care out of Hours by age and sex subgroups

10,000 patients ($y = 10^{-4}$) had 30 or more contacts, whereas in Fig. 6a, a similar proportion had between 20 + and 30+ more contacts. This suggests that our detailed dataset was broadly comparable to the other published but less detailed series.

Discussion

This data provides original and robust evidence that patients using urgent care do so in patterns typical of individuals within a complex system. This evidence is present in both the distribution of bursts of contacts by individuals and in the overall distribution of contacts per individual. Finding both features together is important, as bursts of contact are a plausible generative mechanism for the overall distribution [12]. Frequent attenders occurred with a frequency which was in keeping with the hypothesised statistical distributions.

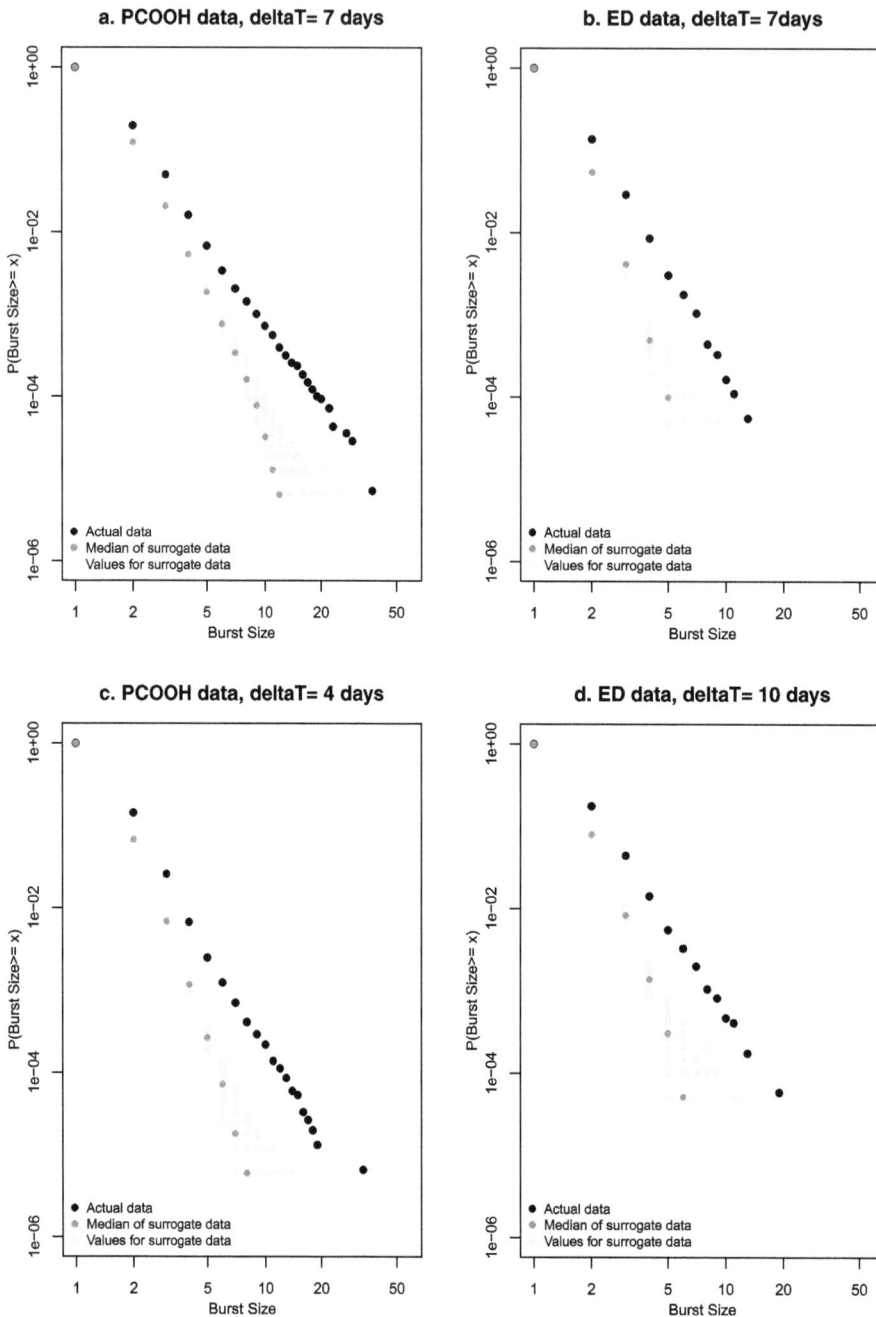

Fig. 3 Distribution of burst lengths in original data and in bootstrapped surrogate data (250 iterations): (**a**) Primary Care Out of Hours (PCOOH) data with time window Δt = 7 days; (**b**) Emergency Department (ED) data with Δt = 7 days; (**c**) PCOOH data with Δt = 4 days; and (**d**) ED data with Δt = 10 days

Strengths and limitations

This study used large, recent and complete datasets from two different urgent care settings in different healthcare systems. The analysis used established techniques for burst estimation [12] and model fitting [11]. We also adjusted for different lengths of follow-up by censoring data and found it had no influence on the findings. Examining the combination of both burst analysis and overall distribution analysis is important, as bursts have been identified as a generative mechanism for power laws in other systems. Furthermore, bursts have been identified in other healthcare research, such as the tendency of exacerbations of chronic obstructive pulmonary disease to cluster in time [52].

While the ED data showed a close fit to a power law across the whole range of contact numbers, there was

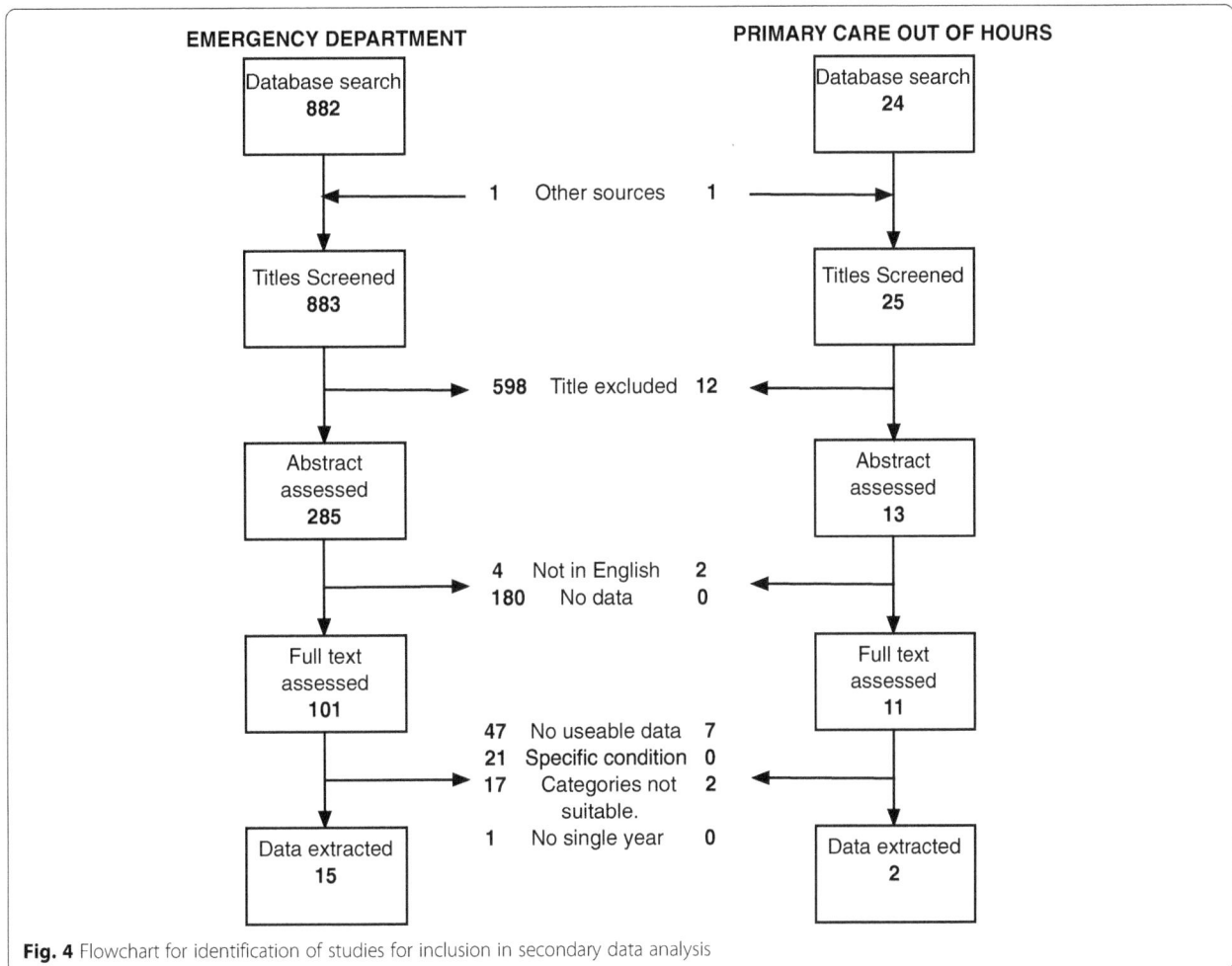

Fig. 4 Flowchart for identification of studies for inclusion in secondary data analysis

some evidence that the PCOOH data contained more very frequent attenders (above 30 contacts) than expected from the best fitting model. This may indicate some excessive or inappropriate use, but the absolute number of patients was small. When we restricted the analysis to patients who did not use the service in the first 2 weeks of the year (and so who were not currently in a burst of consultations), the observed data showed a closer fit to an inverse power law.

The inclusion of the systematic identification of secondary data adds strength to our findings of overall distributions, as heavy-tailed distributions of use, similar to those seen in our primary data, were observed across very different healthcare settings, with generally similar parameters for the proportion of frequent consultation. We were not able to conduct statistical analysis on these secondary sources of data, as they did not have sufficient detail.

Relationship to other research

While complex systems have been hypothesised as a way of describing healthcare services [3–5, 7, 13], this is the first large-scale empirical examination of whether urgent healthcare displays the typical statistical properties of a complex system. No previous studies have reported the population distribution of urgent care attendance in detail; however, non-normal distributions of use have been previously noted but not analysed in the ways we have used in this study [33, 34].

To be plausible, our finding of the typical statistical properties of a complex system must be compatible with real-life mechanisms, which in modelling of social systems can be considered as rules [5, 53]. Qualitative studies have already suggested candidate rules: patients simultaneously seek to balance being a prudent user of services [29] with being "better safe than sorry" [30], and this balance is influenced by societal processes and norms [31, 32]. In turn, these rules may be mediated through processes such as candidacy (seeing oneself as an appropriate user of services) and recursivity (a tendency to repeat patterns of help-seeking which have been successful) [28]. Together, these processes — which are socially mediated — can be seen as comprising system-wide mechanisms which drive, and restrain, urgent care use by individuals.

Table 6 Characteristics of studies included in secondary data analysis

Author	Year	Location	Number of departments	Study Population	Total patients	Attendance categories	Highest category
Emergency department							
Van der Linden [34]	2014	Netherlands	2 ·	All	51,272	14	34
Billings [48]	2013	USA	Multiple	Medicaid, ages 18–62	212,259	7	15+
Capp [47]	2013	USA	1 + satellites	Medicaid, all ages	13,959	4	18+
Doran [49]	2013	USA	Network	Veterans, Veterans Health Administration insurance	930,712	5	26+
Liu [43]	2013	USA	1	All	65,201	4	19+
Martin [42]	2013	USA	1	All	95,170	5	20+
Minassian	2013	USA	2	All	39,249	20	41+
Doupe [45]	2012	Canada	6	Age 18+	105,688	12	18+
Paul [41]	2010	Singapore	1	All — if has not attended the ED in past 12 months	82,172	6	10+
Moore [19]	2009	UK	1	All	82,812	6	10+
Locker [33]	2007	UK	1	All	75,141	16	16+
Jelinek [44]	2008	Australia	9	Age 15+	186,069	6	40+
Ruger [40]	2004	USA	1	All	50,850	5	21+
Riggs [39]	2003	USA	1	All	22,492	17	35
Murphy [38]	1999	Ireland	1	All	34,908	13	21+
Primary care out of hours							
Buja [51]	2015	Italy	1	All	17,657	11	11+
Den Boer-Wolters [50]	2010	Netherlands	1	All	44,953	10	10+

Frequent attendance is commonly regarded as abnormal and taken to be a sign of an inefficient system, however many frequent attenders appear to use healthcare appropriately [17], suggesting the system may in fact be operating efficiently. Recent work in information theory suggests that power law distributions may represent an optimal configuration for a system to meet very variable demands [54]: in the case of urgent care, systems must deal with many patients with minor problems while retaining the capacity to handle a few with intensive ones. Heavy-tailed distributions of attendance may be a feature of well-optimised urgent care rather than a sign that something is wrong.

Implications for policy, practice and research

Our findings of striking similarity between data from urgent care use and statistical features of typical complex systems support the argument that services need to engage more with a complex systems approach [3]. This means there should be a greater focus on contextual matters across the whole system and a recognition that the mechanisms driving processes such as demand both arise from, and influence, many individual interactions. In turn, this means there is a need for interventions to influence these mechanisms, which are social, both through information channels and media, and through creating and sharing positive patient experiences. A second general consequence of considering healthcare systems as complex is that interventions to change services must recognise that complex systems respond unpredictably to interventions to change them [3, 5, 15], and that what works in one setting will not necessarily work in another. This dependence on context is still under-acknowledged in the development of "complex interventions" [3], which should be viewed as "interventions in complex systems" [55].

In practice, the implication of our findings for front-line care is that there must be a partial shift in thinking from individual frequently attending patients to the workings of the whole system. While each frequently attending individual is unique, the consistent and mathematically predictable frequency with which they occur is highly suggestive of overall system effects. In theoretical models of complex systems, this dependence on system effects means that even if extreme outliers (such as individual frequent attenders) are removed (representing action on individuals), new ones will arise to fill their place [56]. This phenomenon can be seen in waiting lists — whereby initiatives to shorten them (by bringing forward treatment of individuals) generally lead to them rapidly re-growing through system effects [57, 58].

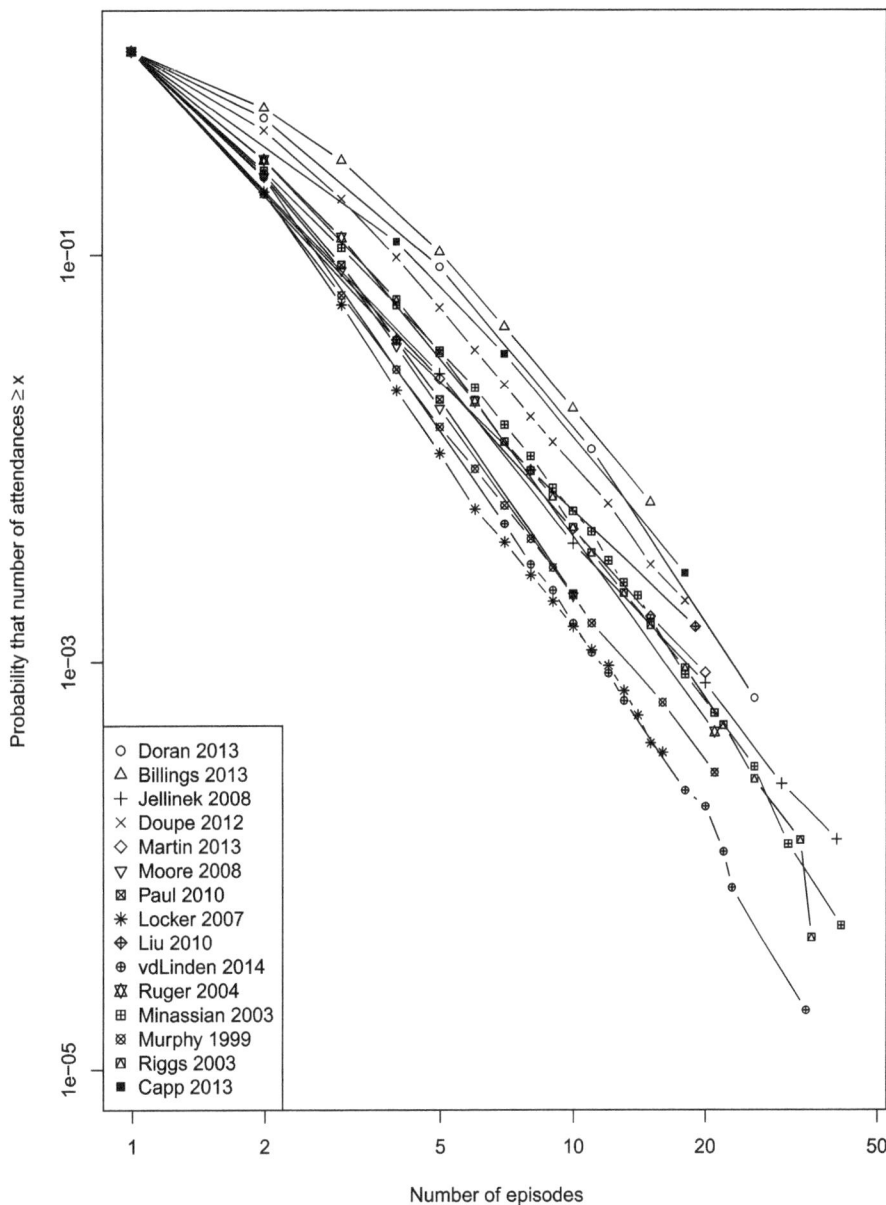

Fig. 5 Cumulative distribution function of urgent care episodes per patient in individual study reports: all emergency department studies

Services thus need to provide care which is simultaneously person-centred and system-aware.

For research, our identification of bursts represents a potential target for interventions to identify and respond to individuals with high need. Interventions should be developed to prevent, or shorten, bursts. These interventions must be safe, while addressing the mechanisms by which patients rationalise decisions to consult, such as candidacy and recursivity [28]. This may involve forms of explanation or sign-posting which make patients more likely to use alternative management the next time a situation occurs rather than more likely to re-attend

the urgent care service, as currently happens. A focus on recognising bursts at an early stage may also permit identification of individuals at high risk of frequent attendance. In our ED data, among people who attended at least four times in a year, a burst of 3 consultations each separated by no more than 7 days represented only 1% of bursts. In the PCOOH setting, bursts of 4 consultations each separated by no more than 7 days accounted for 1% of bursts. These may represent useful "early warnings" of emerging problems, and these and other potential signals of ongoing high use should be tested in further analyses.

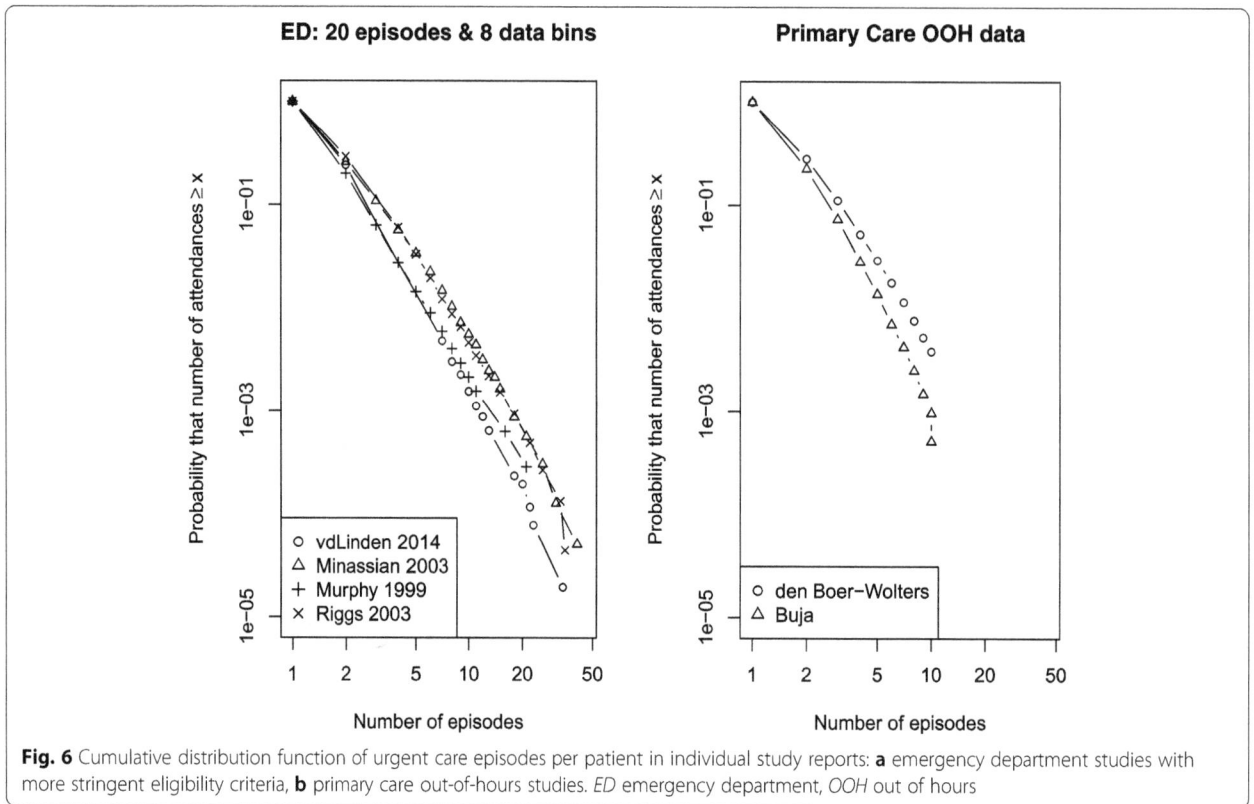

Fig. 6 Cumulative distribution function of urgent care episodes per patient in individual study reports: **a** emergency department studies with more stringent eligibility criteria, **b** primary care out-of-hours studies. *ED* emergency department, *OOH* out of hours

Conclusions

We have demonstrated new and widespread evidence of typical complex system behaviour in urgent care use, particularly in the links between bursts of attendance and overall demand. Interventions to address demand must reflect this, by addressing systemic processes across all levels of use and by safely reducing re-attendance to shorten bursts of contacts which act as a major driver of heavy use.

Authors' contributions

The study was conceived by CB and TL and developed jointly with AE and AC. AE and TL were responsible for primary data provision and preparation; CB and TL conducted the primary analysis. AC and CB extracted data and conducted the secondary analysis of published data. CB drafted the manuscript, and AE, AC and TL all contributed to its revision. All authors contributed to the writing and revision of the manuscript and approve its content. CB is guarantor for the study.

Competing interests

All authors have completed the International Committee of Medical Journal Editors (ICMJE) uniform disclosure form at http://www.icmje.org/conflicts-of-interest/ and declare the following: no support from any organisation for the submitted work; no financial relationships with any organisations that might have an interest in the submitted work in the previous 3 years; no other relationships or activities that could appear to have influenced the submitted work.

Author details

[1]Academic Unit of Primary Medical Care, University of Sheffield, Samuel Fox House, Northern General Hospital, Sheffield S5 7AU, UK. [2]University of Aberdeen, Aberdeen, UK. [3]University of Otago, Wellington, New Zealand. [4]Abertay University, Dundee, UK.

References

1. Byrne DS. Complexity theory and the social sciences : the state of the art, first edition. Oxford: Routledge; 2014.
2. Newman MEJ. Complex systems: a survey. Am J Phys. 2011;79:800–10.
3. Hawe P. Lessons from complex interventions to improve health. Annu Rev Public Health. 2015;36:307–23.
4. Plsek PE, Greenhalgh T. Complexity science: The challenge of complexity in health care. BMJ. 2001;323(Generic):625–8.
5. Lipsitz LA. Understanding health care as a complex system: the foundation for unintended consequences. JAMA. 2012;308(3):243–4.

6.　Rouse WB. Health care as a complex adaptive system: implications for design and management. Bridge. 2008;38(1):17.

7.　Resnicow K, Page SE. Embracing chaos and complexity: a quantum change for public health. Am J Public Health. 2008;98(8):1382–9.

8.　Mahajan A, Islam SD, Schwartz MJ, Cannesson M. A hospital is not just a factory, but a complex adaptive system—implications for perioperative care. Anesth Analg. 2017;125(1):333–41.

9.　Cilliers P: Complexity and postmodernism. Abingdon-on-Thames: Routledge; 1998.

10.　Sterman JD. Learning from evidence in a complex world. Am J Public Health. 2006;96(3):505–14.

11.　Clauset A, Shalizi CR, Newman MEJ. Power-law distributions in empirical data. SIAM Rev. 2009;51:661–703.

12.　Karsai M, Kaski K, Barabasi A, Kertacsz J. Universal features of correlated bursty behaviour. SciRep. 2012;2:397.

13.　Love T, Burton C. General practice as a complex system: a novel analysis of consultation data. Fam Pract. 2005;22(Generic):347–52.

14.　Bar-Yam Y. Improving the effectiveness of health care and public health: a multiscale complex systems analysis. Am J Public Health. 2006;96(3):459–66.

15.　Burton C. Heavy tailed distributions of effect sizes in systematic reviews of complex interventions. PLoS One. 2012;7(3):34222.

16.　Newman MEJ. Power laws, Pareto distributions and Zipf's law. Contemp Phys. 2005;46(5):323–51.

17.　Mason SM. Frequent attendance at the emergency department is a symptom but not a disease. Emerg Med J. 2014;31(7):524–5.

18.　Pines JM, Hilton JA, Weber EJ, Alkemade AJ, Al Shabanah H, Anderson PD, Bernhard M, Bertini A, Gries A, Ferrandiz S, et al. International perspectives on emergency department crowding. Acad Emerg Med. 2011;18(12):1358–70.

19.　Moore L, Deehan A, Seed P, Jones R. Characteristics of frequent attenders in an emergency department: analysis of 1-year attendance data. Emerg Med J. 2009;26(4):263–7.

20.　Vedsted P, Olesen F. Frequent attenders in out-of-hours general practice care: attendance prognosis. Fam Pract. 1999;16(3):283–8.

21.　Mason S, Mountain G, Turner J, Arain M, Revue E, Weber EJ. Innovations to reduce demand and crowding in emergency care; a review study. Scandinavian J Trauma Resuscitation Emerg Med. 2014;22(1):55.

22.　Pines JM, Asplin BR, Kaji AH, Lowe RA, Magid DJ, Raven M, Weber EJ, Yealy DM. Frequent users of emergency department services: gaps in knowledge and a proposed research agenda. Acad Emerg Med. 2011;18(6):e64–9.

23.　Fielding S, Porteous T, Ferguson J, Maskrey V, Blyth A, Paudyal V, Barton G, Holland R, Bond CM, Watson MC. Estimating the burden of minor ailment consultations in general practices and emergency departments through retrospective review of routine data in North East Scotland. Fam Pract. 2015;32(2):165–72.

24.　Vedsted P, Fink P, Sorensen HT, Olesen F. Physical, mental and social factors associated with frequent attendance in Danish general practice. A population-based cross-sectional study. Soc Sci Med (1982). 2004;59(4):813–23.

25.　Neal RD, Heywood PL, Morley S. Frequent attenders' consulting patterns with general practitioners. Br J Gen Pract. 2000;50(461):972–6.

26.　Pines JM, Buford K. Predictors of frequent emergency department utilization in southeastern Pennsylvania. J Asthma. 2006;43(3):219–23.

27.　Taleb NN. The black swan: The impact of the highly improbable, vol. 2. London: Random house; 2007.

28.　Hunter C, Chew-Graham C, Langer S, Stenhoff A, Drinkwater J, Guthrie E, Salmon P. A qualitative study of patient choices in using emergency health care for long-term conditions: the importance of candidacy and recursivity. Patient Educ Couns. 2013;93(2):335–41.

29.　Adamson J, Ben-Shlomo Y, Chaturvedi N, Donovan J. Exploring the impact of patient views on 'appropriate' use of services and help seeking: a mixed method study. Br J Gen Pract. 2009;59(564):e226–33.

30.　Houston AM, Pickering AJ. 'Do I don't I call the doctor': a qualitative study of parental perceptions of calling the GP out-of-hours. Health Expect. 2000;3(4):234–42.

31.　O'Cathain A, Goode J, Luff D, Strangleman T, Hanlon G, Greatbatch D. Does NHS Direct empower patients? Soc Sci Med (1982). 2005;61(8):1761–71.

32.　Hanlon G, Goode J, Greatbatch D, Luff D, O'Cathain A, Strangleman T. Risk society and the NHS—from the traditional to the new citizen? European Critical Accounting Symposium: Leicester Special Issue. 2006;17(2–3):270–82.

33.　Locker TE, Baston S, Mason SM, Nicholl J. Defining frequent use of an urban emergency department. Emerg Med J. 2007;24(6):398–401.

34.　Van Der Linden MC, Van Den Brand CL, Van Der Linden N, Rambach AH, Brumsen C. Rate, characteristics, and factors associated with high emergency department utilization. Int J Emerg Med. 2014;7:9.

35.　Elliott AM, McAteer A, Heaney D, Ritchie LD, Hannaford PC. Examining the role of Scotland's telephone advice service (NHS 24) for managing health in the community: analysis of routinely collected NHS 24 data. BMJ Open. 2015;5(8):e007293.

36.　Adamic L. Complex systems: unzipping Zipf's law 1. Nature. 2011;474:164–5.

37.　Vuong QH. Likelihood ratio tests for model selection and non-nested hypotheses. Econometrica. 1989;57(2):307–33.

38.　Byrne M, Murphy AW, Plunkett PK, McGee HM, Murray A, Bury G. Frequent attenders to an emergency department: a study of primary health care use, medical profile, and psychosocial characteristics. Ann Emerg Med. 2003; 41(3):309–18.

39.　Riggs JE, Davis SM, Hobbs GR, Paulson DJ, Chinnis AS, Heilman PL. Association between early returns and frequent ED visits at a rural academic medical center. Am J Emerg Med. 2003;21(1):30–1.

40.　Ruger JP, Richter CJ, Spitznagel EL, Lewis LM. Analysis of costs, length of stay, and utilization of emergency department services by frequent users: implications for health policy. Acad Emerg Med. 2004;11(12):1311–7.

41.　Paul P, Heng BH, Seow E, Molina J, Tay SY. Predictors of frequent attenders of emergency department at an acute general hospital in Singapore. Emerg Med J. 2010;27(11):843–8.

42.　Martin GB, Stokes-Buzzelli SA, Peltzer-Jones JM, Schultz LR. Ten years of frequent users in an urban emergency department. Western J Emerg Med. 2013;14(3):243–6.

43.　Liu SW, Nagurney JT, Chang Y, Parry BA, Smulowitz P, Atlas SJ. Frequent ED users: are most visits for mental health, alcohol, and drug-related complaints? Am J Emerg Med. 2013;31(10):1512–5.

44.　Jelinek GA, Jiwa M, Gibson NP, Lynch AM. Frequent attenders at emergency departments: a linked-data population study of adult patients. Med J Aust. 2008;189(10):552–6.

45.　Doupe MB, Palatnick W, Day S, Chateau D, Soodeen RA, Burchill C, Derksen S. Frequent users of emergency departments: developing standard definitions and defining prominent risk factors. Ann Emerg Med. 2012;60(1):24–32.

46.　Minassian A, Vilke GM, Wilson MP: Frequent emergency department visits are more prevalent in psychiatric, alcohol abuse, and dual diagnosis conditions than in chronic viral illnesses such as hepatitis and human immunodeficiency virus. J Emerg Med 2013, 45(4):520–525.

47.　Capp R, Rosenthal MS, Desai MM, Kelley L, Borgstrom C, Cobbs-Lomax DL, Simonette P, Spatz ES. Characteristics of Medicaid enrollees with frequent ED use. Am J Emerg Med. 2013;31(9):1333–7.

48.　Billings J, Raven MC. Dispelling an urban legend: frequent emergency department users have substantial burden of disease. Health Aff. 2013; 32(12):2099–108.

49.　Doran KM, Raven MC, Rosenheck RA. What drives frequent emergency department use in an integrated health system? National data from the veterans health administration. Ann Emerg Med. 2013;62(2):151–9.

50.　den Boer-Wolters D, Knol MJ, Smulders K, de Wit NJ. Frequent attendance of primary care out-of-hours services in the Netherlands: characteristics of patients and presented morbidity. Fam Pract. 2010;27(2):129–34.

51.　Buja A, Toffanin R, Rigon S, Sandona P, Carraro D, Damiani G, Baldo V. Out-of-hours primary care services: demands and patient referral patterns in a Veneto region (Italy) Local Health Authority. Health Policy (Amsterdam, Netherlands). 2015;119(4):437–46.

52.　Hurst JR, Donaldson GC, Quint JK, Goldring JJ, Baghai-Ravary R, Wedzicha JA. Temporal clustering of exacerbations in chronic obstructive pulmonary disease. Am J Respir Crit Care Med. 2009;179(5):369–74.

53.　Ostrom E. Background on the institutional analysis and development framework. Policy Stud J. 2011;39(1):7–27.

54.　Baek SK, Bernhardsson S, Minnhagen P. Zipf's law unzipped. New J Phys. 2011;13(4):043004.

55.　Shiell A, Hawe P, Gold L. Complex interventions or complex systems? Implications for health economic evaluation. BMJ. 2008;336(7656):1281–3.

56.　Bak P. How nature works: the science of self-organised criticality. London: Oxford University Press; 1996.

57.　Newton JN, Henderson J, Goldacre MJ. Waiting list dynamics and the impact of earmarked funding. BMJ. 1995;311(7008):783–5.

58.　Smethurst DP, Williams HC. Self-regulation in hospital waiting lists. J R Soc Med. 2002;95(6):287–9.

6

Developing a measure of polypharmacy appropriateness in primary care

Jenni Burt[1][*] [iD], Natasha Elmore[1], Stephen M. Campbell[2], Sarah Rodgers[3], Anthony J. Avery[4] and Rupert A. Payne[5]

Abstract

Background: Polypharmacy is an increasing challenge for primary care. Although sometimes clinically justified, polypharmacy can be inappropriate, leading to undesirable outcomes. Optimising care for polypharmacy necessitates effective targeting and monitoring of interventions. This requires a valid, reliable measure of polypharmacy, relevant for all patients, that considers clinical appropriateness and generic prescribing issues applicable across all medications. Whilst there are several existing measures of potentially inappropriate prescribing, these are not specifically designed with polypharmacy in mind, can require extensive clinical input to complete, and often cover a limited number of drugs. The aim of this study was to identify what experts consider to be the key elements of a measure of prescribing appropriateness in the context of polypharmacy.

Methods: Firstly, we conducted a systematic review to identify generic (not drug specific) prescribing indicators relevant to polypharmacy appropriateness. Indicators were subject to content analysis to enable categorisation. Secondly, we convened a panel of 10 clinical experts to review the identified indicators and assess their relative clinical importance. For each indicator category, a brief evidence summary was developed, based on relevant clinical and indicator literature, clinical guidance, and opinions obtained from a separate patient discussion panel. A two-stage RAND/UCLA Appropriateness Method was used to reach consensus amongst the panel on a core set of indicators of polypharmacy appropriateness.

Results: We identified 20,879 papers for title/abstract screening, obtaining 273 full papers. We extracted 189 generic indicators, and presented 160 to the panel grouped into 18 classifications (e.g. adherence, dosage, clinical efficacy). After two stages, during which the panel introduced 18 additional indicators, there was consensus that 134 indicators were of clinical importance. Following the application of decision rules and further panel consultation, 12 indicators were placed into the final selection. Panel members particularly valued indicators concerned with adverse drug reactions, contraindications, drug-drug interactions, and the conduct of medication reviews.

Conclusions: We have identified a set of 12 indicators of clinical importance considered relevant to polypharmacy appropriateness. Use of these indicators in clinical practice and informatics systems is dependent on their operationalisation and their utility (e.g. risk stratification, targeting and monitoring polypharmacy interventions) requires subsequent evaluation.

Trial registration: Registration number: PROSPERO (CRD42016049176).

Keywords: Inappropriate prescribing, polypharmacy, medication errors, multimorbidity, primary care, consensus methods, systematic review

* Correspondence: jenni.burt@thisinstitute.cam.ac.uk
[1]THIS Institute (The Healthcare Improvement Studies Institute), University of Cambridge, Cambridge Biomedical Campus, Clifford Allbutt Building, Cambridge CB2 0AH, UK
Full list of author information is available at the end of the article

Background

The use of multiple medications in a single individual (polypharmacy) is a global phenomenon, creating new challenges for many health services [1], driven by increasing levels of multimorbidity [2] and a culture of single-condition guideline-based prescribing [3].

Polypharmacy is associated with several undesirable consequences [4–8]. However, we have previously demonstrated that the association between polypharmacy and adverse outcomes is attenuated in the most multimorbid individuals [9]. This suggests that overly simplistic analyses of polypharmacy, relating simple medication counts to adverse outcomes, may be misleading [9, 10]. Polypharmacy is typically measured using arbitrary numeric thresholds, but these fail to capture medication appropriateness; therefore, more sophisticated approaches accounting for clinical context are required.

A number of prescribing indicators that assess medication appropriateness are considered to have face validity [11], and may have value in improving quality and reducing adverse outcomes [12]. However, such indicators generally do not account for multiple drug use and do not measure polypharmacy per se. In addition, explicit 'drug specific' indicators (e.g. Beers criteria [13]) do not apply to all patients, and implicit measures (e.g. the Medication Appropriateness Index [14]) require time consuming input from an experienced clinician.

There is therefore a need to develop a valid and reliable means of measuring polypharmacy that takes account of clinical appropriateness. Further, a framing of polypharmacy appropriateness (rather than appropriate or inappropriate polypharmacy) acknowledges a spectrum of prescribing within the context of polypharmacy, including the need to support individualised prescribing approaches where potentially risky (or 'inappropriate') combinations may be fitting for a particular patient. To be usable in clinical practice, this measure should ideally focus on generic prescribing issues (to ensure relevance to all patients, and avoiding simply focusing on a finite number of medications, i.e. implicit indicators), whilst still permitting automation as part of a computerised clinical system. We anticipate that this measure of polypharmacy appropriateness would enable more effective targeting and evaluation of medication optimisation interventions. Used as a first step in identifying which patients may be at risk of inappropriate prescribing, such a measure could facilitate targeted conversations with patients to subsequently ascertain their views on the appropriateness of their current medication regimen.

Methods

The aim of this study was to identify the key elements of a measure of prescribing appropriateness in the context of polypharmacy. We conducted a systematic review and RAND/UCLA Appropriateness Method consensus study, as outlined below. Whilst our aim was to develop a measure of polypharmacy appropriateness, the orientation of most measures to date has been one of inappropriate prescribing, and we therefore adopt that terminology when referencing existing approaches.

Systematic review of indicators of polypharmacy appropriateness

To locate and derive implicit indicators of polypharmacy appropriateness for consideration by the expert panel, an initial systematic review was undertaken. The protocol was prospectively registered with PROSPERO (registration number CRD42016049176) [15, 16] and the manuscript was written in accordance with the PRISMA statement [17].

Search strategy

We searched Embase, MEDLINE (Ovid), PsycINFO, CINAHL, Health Management Information Consortium, Cochrane Library, Web of Science, the Trip and NHS Evidence databases, from 1992 (the year the Medication Appropriateness Index was first published [14]) until October 10, 2016. Search terms were developed in collaboration with an experienced medical librarian. We used exploded MeSH terms (e.g. inappropriate prescribing) and combinations of relevant keywords and their variants (e.g. medication, drug therapy, drug utilisation, drug utilisation review, prescribing). We adapted our initial MEDLINE search strategy (Box 1) to run in the additional databases, and to perform a review of reviews to identify any previous reviews in this field (Box 2). Further relevant publications were identified by a manual search of references and citations of included papers.

Inclusion criteria

Articles were eligible for inclusion if they reported the use of a specific tool to assess polypharmacy or inappropriate prescribing, including both implicit and explicit indicators. We defined 'implicit' (or 'generic') indicators as judgement-based indicators that facilitate the consideration of the whole patient, rather than having a narrow focus on specific drugs or diseases [11]. We defined 'explicit' indicators as criterion-based indicators that assess specific drug-based or disease-based prescribing against specific standards derived from guidelines or expert opinion [11].

Box 1 MEDLINE search strategy

(exp Inappropriate prescribing/ or exp. polypharmacy/ or exp. medication errors/ or exp. Potentially Inappropriate Medication List/ or (polypharmacy or underprescrib* or under-prescrib* or over-prescrib* or mis-prescrib* or overprescrib* or misprescrib* or (beer* adj criteri*) or (pim adj list*)).ti,ab. or ((prescrib* or prescript* or medicat* or medicin* or drug* or pharm*) adj2 (sub-optimal or suboptimal or optim* or appropriat* or inappropriat* or unaccept* or accept* or underus* or under-us* or over-us* or overus* or underutili* or under-utili* or malpractice* or safe* or unsafe* or danger* or error* or mistak* or (adverse* adj (event* or effect* or react*)) or harm* or omiss* or omit* or problem*)).ti,ab.) AND (((exp "Surveys and Questionnaires"/ or exp. guideline/ or exp. quality assurance, health care/) and ((updat* or develop* or valid* or creat* or design* or consensus* or Delphi or rand* or reliab* or interrat* or inter-rate* or (inter adj rate*) or (appropriate* adj method*)).ti,ab.) or (((score* or index* or scale* or survey* or questionnaire* or instrument* or outcome* or tool* or indicat* or measur* or screen* or criteri* or (quality adj2 assur*) or (patient adj2 experience*)) adj4 (updat* or develop* or valid* or creat* or design* or consensus* or Delphi or rand* or reliab* or interrat* or inter-rate* or (inter adj rate*) or (appropriate* adj method*))).ti,ab.))

Box 2 MEDLINE search strategy for review of reviews

1. ((exp Inappropriate prescribing/ or exp. polypharmacy/ or exp. medication errors/ or exp. Potentially Inappropriate Medication List/ or (polypharmacy or underprescrib* or under-prescrib* or over-prescrib* or mis-prescrib* or overprescrib* or misprescrib* or (beer* adj criteri*) or (pim adj list*)).ti,ab.) Or ((prescrib* or prescript* or medicat* or medicin* or drug* or pharm*) adj2 (sub-optimal or suboptimal or optim* or appropriat* or inappropriat* or unaccept* or accept* or underus* or under-us* or over-us* or overus* or underutili* or under-utili* or malpractice* or safe* or unsafe* or danger* or error* or mistak* or (adverse* adj (event* or effect* or react*)) or harm* or omiss* or omit* or problem*)).ti,ab.) And ((exp "Surveys and Questionnaires"/ or exp. guideline/ or exp. quality assurance, health care/) or (score* or index* or scale* or survey* or questionnaire* or instrument* or outcome* or tool* or indicat* or measur* or screen* or criteri* or (quality adj2 assur*) or (patient adj2 experience*)).ti,ab.) and ((updat* or develop* or valid* or creat* or design* or consensus* or Delphi or rand* or reliab* or interrat* or inter-rate* or (inter adj rate*) or (appropriate* adj method*)).ti,ab.)

2. ((exp Inappropriate prescribing/ or exp. polypharmacy/ or exp. medication errors/ or exp. Potentially Inappropriate Medication List/ or (polypharmacy or underprescrib* or under-prescrib* or over-prescrib* or mis-prescrib* or overprescrib* or misprescrib* or (beer* adj criteri*) or (pim adj list*)).ti,ab.) Or ((prescrib* or prescript* or medicat* or medicin* or drug* or pharm*) adj2 (sub-optimal or suboptimal or optim* or appropriat* or inappropriat* or unaccept* or accept* or underus* or under-us* or over-us* or overus* or underutili* or under-utili* or malpractice* or safe* or unsafe* or danger* or error* or mistak* or (adverse* adj (event* or effect* or react*)) or harm* or omiss* or omit* or problem*)).ti,ab.) And ((exp "Surveys and Questionnaires"/ or exp. guideline/ or exp. quality assurance, health care/) or (score* or index* or scale* or survey* or questionnaire* or instrument* or outcome* or tool* or indicat* or measur* or screen* or criteri* or (quality adj2 assur*) or (patient adj2 experience*)).ti,ab.) and ((updat* or develop* or valid* or creat* or design* or consensus* or Delphi or rand* or reliab* or interrat* or inter-rate* or (inter adj rate*) or (appropriate* adj method*)).ti,ab.) AND ((systematic adj (review$1 or overview$1)).tw.)
2 not 1

The decision to include both implicit and explicit indicators at full-text screening, rather than including only articles stating the focus was on implicit indicators, was based on our observation that implicit indicators were not always clearly identified as such. For example, a single implicit indicator may be embedded within instruments labelled as explicit indicators, as is the case with the guidelines developed by Basger et al. [18, 19] in the Australian context. We excluded papers describing non-instrument based medication reviews, educational interventions, validation studies of previously published tools, general guidelines and recommendations relating to assessing inappropriate prescribing, and articles not published in English.

Screening

Publications were assessed for eligibility by title and abstract screening. An initial random sample of 100 titles/abstracts was triple screened to refine the application of inclusion and exclusion criteria. A single reviewer (NE) subsequently screened all titles/abstracts, with a 10% random sample screened by two additional reviewers (JB, RP). Any disagreements were resolved by discussion between the three reviewers. Articles included for full text screening were retrieved and reviewed against the inclusion criteria by two reviewers (NE and JB) independently, with discrepancies resolved by discussion with RP.

Extraction of indicators

All full-text papers meeting the inclusion criteria were reviewed to find implicit indicators of polypharmacy or inappropriate prescribing. Indicators were extracted and subjected to qualitative content analysis to identify categories into which they could be grouped [20]. Two authors (JB and RP) independently reviewed all indicators and generated a coding framework, which was refined through consensus discussions to produce a final set of indicator categories. Indicators that, on further scrutiny, were deemed not to be truly implicit were excluded at this stage. All indicators, within their categories, were subsequently taken forward for expert review in a consensus panel.

Quality assessment of indicators

Where stated, the development method for the identified indicators was extracted, and its strengths and limitations were assessed with reference to the Joanna Briggs Institute critical appraisal checklist for text and opinion [21].

Expert consensus process

The two-stage RAND/UCLA Appropriateness Method was employed to reach consensus on indicators of prescribing considered by experts to be key to a measure of polypharmacy appropriateness. The RAND/UCLA Appropriateness Method is a well-established approach for systematically generating expert consensus by combining scientific evidence with expert opinion, and subsequently aggregating individual opinions into a single perspective [22].

Patient views

We convened a panel of five patient representatives from a local 'patient and public involvement in research' group to gather their views on which aspects of polypharmacy and prescribing identified by the systematic review were of particular relevance and concern to them. The panel meeting was facilitated by a general practitioner (RP), with support from a specialist Patient and Public Involvement coordinator responsible for facilitating patient involvement in research [23]. The categories of polypharmacy or inappropriate prescribing into which the identified indicators had been grouped were presented to the panel, and discussion encouraged around the particular importance or relevance of this area to the patient experience. Patient representatives were asked, in particular, to reflect on the relevance and importance of each prescribing indicator category, whether doing something about it would make a difference, the potential challenges of measuring it,

and whether they would prioritise one or more categories. Field notes were taken during the conduct of the panel meeting and key points across each category were summarised. A synopsis of the patient views in relation to each category was presented in narrative form in the evidence summaries supplied to the expert panel (see below).

Evidence summaries

For each indicator category, the research team developed a corresponding brief evidence summary. These summaries drew upon clinical and academic literature, and addressed the importance and relevance of the issue in relation to polypharmacy, the potential consequences for patients, and how the indicators had been developed and evaluated. As outlined above, patient views were also incorporated based on the earlier patient panel discussion. Evidence summaries were then presented to panel members to support discussions as part of the RAND/UCLA Appropriateness Method consensus exercise; these included a brief summary of the strengths and weaknesses of the approach to deriving each included indicator, as derived from the quality assessment of indicators.

Expert panel members

We undertook a snowball approach to recruit expert panel members, aiming to include a range of professions and levels of experience. We particularly focused on individuals immersed in the general prescribing process and those who regularly dealt with polypharmacy; we therefore targeted general practice, pharmacy, pharmacology, and geriatric medicine. We therefore approached relevant professional organisations, including the Royal College of General Practitioners, Royal Pharmaceutical Society, British Pharmacological Society, and additional known contacts of the research team. Our final ten-member panel consisted of four general practitioners, two pharmacists, three geriatricians, and one clinical pharmacologist; RAND/UCLA approaches typically include anything from 7 to 15 members in a panel [22]. Panel members were not involved in the systematic review itself.

First stage assessment

In stage one, we asked panel members to participate in an online survey to evaluate the implicit indicators of inappropriate prescribing or polypharmacy identified through the systematic review. Panel members were sent a personalised link to complete the first stage of ratings using the survey software, Qualtrics (https://www.qualtrics.com). Indicators were presented to panel members in their category groupings. Panel members were asked to review the indicators within each category and score each indicator in turn in relation to (1) its clinical importance with regards to polypharmacy and (2) its clarity, using a rating scale numbered 1 to 9, where a score of 1 meant the indicator was extremely unimportant (or unclear) in evaluating polypharmacy appropriateness, and a score of 9 meant the indicator was extremely important (and clear). Consensus classifications for each indicator were established using a series of rules, outlined in Table 1.

Second stage assessment

In stage two, we convened a face-to-face meeting of all panel members to further review and discuss indicators and their scores. The meeting was facilitated by an experienced RAND/UCLA Appropriateness Method facilitator (SC) with input from a general practitioner with expertise in polypharmacy (RP). Anonymised frequency distributions and median scores for the clinical importance rating of every stage one indicator were provided to each panel member at the start of the meeting, alongside the scores they had themselves assigned to every indicator. Categories of indicator were discussed, in turn, with panel members given the opportunity to suggest changes to the wording of the indicators; the wording of all new variations of indicators needed to be agreed by all panellists. At the end of discussions around each category, panel members were asked to rate each indicator again, including new variations, in relation to their clinical importance to polypharmacy.

Table 1 Rules used to determine consensus classification for panel ratings

Median panel score	Criteria for:		
	Disagreement	Equivocal	Agreement
		> 20% of individual scores equal to:	20% of individual scores equal to:
1		4–9	4–9
2		5–9	5–9
3		6–9	6–9
4	≥ 33% of individual scores equal to 1–3 AND ≥ 33% of individual scores equal to 7–9	1, 7–9	1, 7–9
5		1, 2, 8, 9	1, 2, 8, 9
6		1–3, 9	1–3, 9
7		1–4	1–4
8		1–5	1–5
9		1–6	1–6

Application of final decision rules

As indicators considered by the panel were presented in categorical groupings, many indicators, whilst drawn from different sources, were closely related. To ensure our final indicator set was a non-duplicative measure of polypharmacy appropriateness, we took the following steps. First, in order to decide which of the highest scoring indicators within each category to take forward to the final set, two members of the research team (JB and RP) independently coded indicators within each category grouping to identify sub-category groupings, which were further refined through discussion with two other team members (AA and SR). The highest scoring indicator from each sub-category grouping was subsequently taken forward; all such indicators scored a minimum of 7. Where more than one indicator in each sub-category had the same highest score, the decision as to which indicator to select was made within the research team through discussion and consideration of the likely feasibility of the operationalisation of that indicator in primary care. We then applied the following decision rules to the remaining indicators:

1. Able to be applied at the level of individual drugs
2. Not overlapping with or duplicating another indicator

The final suggested list was circulated to the panel members for any last comments and review.

Results
Systematic review

Our review identified 20,879 papers for title/abstract screening, from which 273 full-text papers were identified for review (Fig. 1). Double screening of a 10% random sample of all citations had a 97% consensus rate, with both reviewers making the same decision. Following full text screening, we selected 17 papers that included either all implicit or a mixture of implicit and explicit indicators. A further five papers were identified through forward and backward citation searching of the 17 papers. From the resulting 22 papers (Appendix 1), we identified 189 potential implicit indicators of polypharmacy or inappropriate prescribing. On further scrutiny, 29 indicators did not meet our inclusion criteria. The remaining 160 indicators (Additional file 1) were placed into 18 categories derived through content analysis (Box 3). The wording of each indicator remained unchanged from its original source and thus, at this stage, categories could contain similar

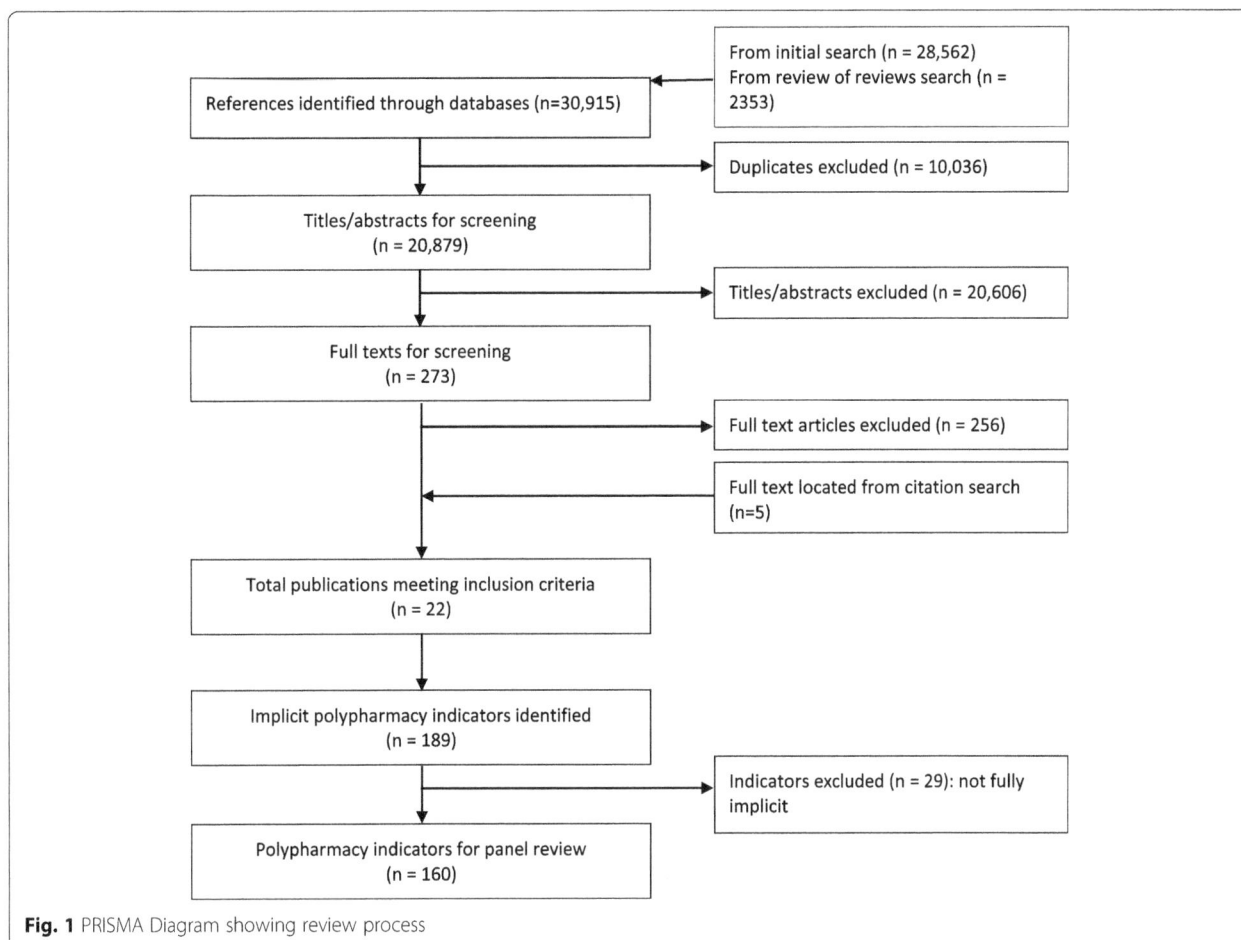

Fig. 1 PRISMA Diagram showing review process

Box 3 Prescribing indicator categories, derived from content analysis of identified indicators

1. Adherence
2. Adverse drug reactions
3. Drug-drug interactions
4. Medication review
5. Contraindication (drug-disease interactions)
6. Alternatives to current therapy
7. Clinical efficacy
8. Complexity of medication
9. Compliance with guidance
10. Cost-effectiveness
11. Directions
12. Dosage/duration
13. Duplication
14. Other inappropriate prescribing
15. Indication
16. Under-prescribing
17. Specific safety issues
18. General indicators

indicators varying only slightly in their wording or grammatical construction.

Patient panel
Although patient representatives discussed all of the prescribing indicator categories, they prioritised adherence, drug–drug interactions and clinical efficacy as fundamental to polypharmacy appropriateness. They raised concerns about how feasible it was to evaluate adherence, but felt it was a central issue for patients managing complex medication regimens. The avoidance of adverse drug–.drug interactions was also seen as vital; the patient panel stated that they looked to clinical expertise to evaluate and avoid these risks for patients. Finally, discussions on the role of clinical efficacy focused on how specific this was to the individual, and patient representatives voiced concerns raised about how clinicians could evaluate and optimise the overall efficacy of a complex medical regimen for each patient. Cost-effectiveness was seen as relevant but not a core consideration, although patient representatives

agreed with the prescribing of generic medications where possible.

RAND/UCLA Appropriateness Method

In stage one, the 160 indicators identified from the systematic review were presented to the panel for consideration and rating. In the stage two face-to-face meeting, panel discussions led to the introduction of 18 re-worded or new indicators, giving a total pool of 178 indicators for consideration. There was panel consensus that 134 indicators were of clinical importance (scoring a median rating of 7 or above); for a further 5 indicators, the panel was equivocal as to clinical importance. The panel agreed that 19 indicators were not of clinical importance, and they did not reach consensus about the importance of 20 indicators. There was a notable lack of prioritisation of, and consensus around, indicators relating to cost-effectiveness, and all indicators in this group were eliminated at this stage.

The remaining 134 indicators represented 17 categories, from which we derived 29 sub-categories. Application of the agreed decision rules led to a final listing of 12 indicators (Table 2 and Box 4), which,

---

Box 4 Final indicators as agreed by expert panel

Implicit indicators of polypharmacy appropriateness

For this specific drug:

1. The indication for the drug is recorded in the medical record

2. There are no effective non-pharmacological alternatives available

3. Drug selection is consistent with established clinical practice

4. There are no clinically significant drug-drug interactions (including duplication of therapy)

5. If the drug is contraindicated, the prescriber gives a valid reason

6. The drug is effective in this patient for this indication

7. The drug, as currently prescribed, is not likely to be sub-therapeutic or toxic, based on the dose, route and dosing interval for the age, renal and hepatic status of the patient

8. The drug regimen cannot be simplified

9. The patient/caregiver is clear about the drug regimen

10. The patient adheres to the drug schedule

11. The drug treatment is reviewed by an appropriate clinician at least once per year, or more frequently if in accordance with best clinical practice

12. If an adverse drug reaction occurs, there are details given of the reaction and recommended future monitoring in the medical record

---

in consultation with the panel, were re-worded to be consistent in the use of terminology (e.g. 'drug' rather than 'medication'), grammar (e.g. statements rather than questions) and positive-versus-negative framing. These came from nine previously developed indicator lists (one indicator from each of seven existing lists [14, 24–29] and two indicators each from a further two lists [30, 31]). The panel introduced one entirely new indicator during stage two discussions. The final suggested list was circulated to the panel members for final comment and agreement; minor rewording was suggested and agreed for three indicators as a result (indicators 2, 7, and 11), most notably the insertion of 'hepatic status' into indicator 7 (the drug as currently prescribed is not likely to be sub-therapeutic or toxic, based on the dose, route and dosing interval for the age, renal and hepatic status of the patient).

Discussion

We have identified a set of 12 indicators of prescribing appropriateness suitable for use in the context of a patient with polypharmacy. We are currently operationalising these indicators for use in clinical practice and informatics systems, with the aim of facilitating risk stratification, and the targeting and monitoring of polypharmacy interventions.

Our review identified a proliferation of implicit indicators of inappropriate prescribing; our final set of 12 indicators of polypharmacy appropriateness originated from nine different existing measures, including the influential Medication Appropriateness Index (MAI) [14, 32]. The MAI is comprised of 10 questions, completed by a pharmacist or physician in order to assess the appropriateness of a drug. It has been widely used as an outcome measure in randomised trials of interventions to improve prescribing; however, its authors specifically state that, whilst it is suited to identifying instances of potentially inappropriate prescribing, it was not developed to identify sub-optimal prescribing in the context of polypharmacy [32]. Whilst only one of our indicators was directly derived from those within the MAI, it is important to note that our final list overlaps with the MAI in many ways, suggesting both that a number of core constructs of inappropriate polypharmacy (including indication, effectiveness and interactions) were captured well by this measure, and that subsequent measures of inappropriate prescribing may have been replicating much of the original MAI work.

However, areas of clinical importance not captured by the MAI were also selected by our expert panel, reflecting our particular focus on the context of

Table 2 Origination, panel rating and wording of final agreed indicators

Indicator group	Original indicator wording	Source	Method of development	Revised wording suggested in stage two	Median score	Final revised wording agreed with panel
Adherence	Does the patient adhere to his/her medication schedule?	Drenth-van Maanen, 2009 [24]	- Literature based - Research team - Developed by the research team on basis of literature review		8.5	The patient adheres to the drug schedule
Adverse effect	If a [type A/B] drug reaction occurs, there are details given of the reaction and recommended future monitoring in the patient medical record	Tully, 2005 [30]	- Literature based - Nominal Group Technique (NGT) - Domains of appropriate prescribing established using NGT - Indicators based on this and previously published indicators; refined through cyclical operationalisation in UK hospital setting		9	If an adverse drug reaction occurs, there are details given of the reaction and recommended future monitoring in the medical record
Alternatives to current therapy	Non-pharmacological	Lenaerts, 2013 [25]	- Not stated - No details in source of how indicators were developed	Are there non-pharmacological alternatives?	8.5	There are no effective non-pharmacological alternatives available
Clinical response	Is the drug effective for this indication?	Lara, 2012 [26]	- Literature based - Expert panel - Developed from literature review and a two-stage consensus process with panel of 11 multidisciplinary experts		8.5	The drug is effective in this patient for this indication
Interaction	Are there clinically significant drug–drug interactions?	Hanlon, 1992 [14]	- Literature based - Expert review - Developed from literature review; clinical pharmacist and internist-geriatrician identified key elements to derive criteria		9	There are no clinically significant drug–drug interactions (including duplication of therapy)
Complexity of medication	Could the drug regimen be simplified?	Newton, 1994 [31]	- Expert panel - Two geriatric internists discussed medications of four elderly patients; further internist recorded implicit rules used - Initial algorithm developed and reviewed by panel of 5 internists; final algorithm tested in a hospital outpatient clinic		9	The drug regimen cannot be simplified
Compliance with guidance	Medication selections are consistent with established clinical practice guidelines	Bergman-Evans, 2006 [27]	- Literature based - Research team - Developed by the research team on basis of literature review/evidence synthesis of previously published indicators		8	Drug selection is consistent with established clinical practice
Adequate directions	Is the patient/caregiver unclear about the medication regimen?	Newton, 1994 [31]	- Expert panel - Two geriatric internists discussed medications of four elderly patients; further internist recorded implicit rules used	Is the patient/caregiver clear about the medication regimen?	9	The patient/caregiver is clear about the medication regimen

Table 2 Origination, panel rating and wording of final agreed indicators *(Continued)*

Indicator group	Original indicator wording	Source	Method of development	Revised wording suggested in stage two	Median score	Final revised wording agreed with panel
			- Initial algorithm developed and reviewed by panel of five internists; final algorithm tested in a hospital outpatient clinic			
Contraindication	If the drug is contraindicated, the prescriber gives a valid reason	Cantrill, 1998 [28]	- Nominal group technique - Delphi survey - NGT (panel of nine multidisciplinary experts) convened to derive potential indicators - Two-round Delphi (100 GPs and 100 community pharmacists) used to assess face validity and content validity and develop consensus		8	If the drug is contraindicated, the prescriber gives a valid reason
Indication available	The indication for the drug is recorded in the discharge summary	Tully, 2005 [30]	- Literature based - NGT - Domains of appropriate prescribing established using NGT - Indicators based on this and previously published indicators; refined through cyclical operationalisation in UK hospital setting		8.5	The indication for the drug is recorded in the medical record
Review	The drug treatment is reviewed by an appropriate clinician at least once per year in accordance with best clinical practice	NEW	- Expert panel - Proposed by expert panel during stage 2 discussions		9	The drug treatment is reviewed by an appropriate clinician at least once per year, or more frequently if in accordance with best clinical practice
Dose/route/ formulation/frequency	Is the drug as currently given likely to be sub-therapeutic or toxic, based on the dose, route and dosing interval for the age and renal status of the patient?	Hamdy, 1995 [29]	- Research team - Developed by the research team, based on guidelines from drug-regimen review criteria used by consultant pharmacists		8	The drug as currently prescribed is not likely to be sub-therapeutic or toxic, based on the dose, route and dosing interval for the age, renal and hepatic status of the patient

multiple medications. These included patient adherence, the complexity of the medication regimen and the availability of non-pharmacological alternatives. Determinants of patient adherence are complex; specific factors, including frequent dosing, longer duration of treatment and the presence of adverse effects, may all decrease adherence [33]. Medication regimen complexity is negatively associated with levels of adherence in patients, and medications become increasingly complex with increasing levels of polypharmacy [34]. Increased toxicity as a consequence of multiple medicines [35] may be reduced by using other treatment options. Lifestyle measures and non-pharmacological treatments are key alternative therapeutic options for a range of clinical conditions commonly found in patients with polypharmacy, including depression and cardiovascular risk management [36, 37].

The importance of a regular full review of prescribed medications was formulated as a new indicator specifically following panel discussion. Systematically conducted medication reviews have been shown to be of particular importance to patients with polypharmacy [38] and have been recommended for those over 75 taking multiple drugs. Not conducting regular medication reviews, particularly for those prescribed multiple drugs, places patients at greater risk of potential harm [39]. However, current evidence is limited on the clinical effectiveness of systematically conducted medication review for reducing the suboptimal use of medicines and improving patient-reported outcomes [40].

Cost-effectiveness was included in a number of identified instruments, including the MAI, but discarded by our panel. Their view was that cost-effectiveness in prescribing (typically defined as ensuring that medication is both clinically and economically appropriate for the conditions [41]) was not, in itself, a marker of polypharmacy appropriateness; instead, they viewed cost-effectiveness as a potentially positive consequence of patient-centred medicines optimisation. Our patient panel, too, echoed this opinion, agreeing simply that the prescribing of generic drugs, when available and when cheaper than branded products, was a sensible approach.

A number of strengths and limitations of this study are worth acknowledging. We have conducted a large-scale systematic review, supported by an experienced medical librarian, and followed a well-established consensus method with a diverse expert panel. As polypharmacy is relevant to all ages, we placed no restrictions on age in our analyses in order to ensure the generalisability of the findings. To locate all potentially relevant indicators,

we used a high sensitivity, low precision search strategy; we acknowledge the subsequent high citation screening workload (with only 10% double screening) may have therefore resulted in important relevant citations being missed. Most of the indicators located, reviewed and evaluated for clinical importance had previously been subject to robust development processes, increasing our confidence in their face and content validity. However, we note that it is possible we missed additional relevant indicators if they were not readily identifiable as implicit measures of appropriate prescribing or polypharmacy. Whilst we recruited a wide range of experts to the panel, they may not be representative of all healthcare professionals involved in caring for patients with polypharmacy. The lack of international perspectives on the panel, which was convened only from UK participants, may reduce the applicability of our findings to other contexts. Following our stage two panel meeting, we developed and applied additional decision rules to produce a non-duplicative and coherent indicator list; whilst this was done in consultation with the panel, we acknowledge that other research teams may have made different decisions about which indicators to retain. Additional work will be necessary to explore the acceptability and operationalisation of the chosen indicators within clinical systems, and to ascertain their utility for risk stratification, targeting and monitoring of polypharmacy interventions. This work will additionally consider issues such as whether indicators should be weighted in an assessment of polypharmacy appropriateness. Finally, we note that this approach does not by itself facilitate the inclusion of patient perspectives of polypharmacy appropriateness. Whilst our proposed measure, when operationalised, may highlight patients where there are clinical concerns about medication regimen, it cannot offer a holistic assessment of the appropriateness of the regimen, where the patients' perspectives must be central to any decisions about care.

Conclusions

This study has integrated and adapted existing indicators of appropriate prescribing, and introduced a new one, to produce a short, yet comprehensive list of 12 indicators suitable to the assessment of prescribing appropriateness in a patient with polypharmacy. Use of these indicators in clinical practice and informatics systems is dependent on their operationalisation, and their utility (e.g. risk stratification, targeting and monitoring polypharmacy interventions) requires subsequent evaluation.

Appendix 1

Table 3 Table of included studies

Authors and year	Country	Setting	Development of indicators	Name of instrument	Number of indicators	Implicit only or mixed (explicit/implicit) indicators	Example indicator
Basger et al., 2008 [18]	Australia	Primary care	Literature review and expert discussions to develop indicators	Australian prescribing indicators for commonly occurring conditions in patients aged > 65 years	48	Mixed	Patient has no significant medication interactions (agreement between two medication interaction databases)
Basger et al., 2012 [19]	Australia	Primary care	Literature review and expert discussions to develop indicators RAND/UCLA Appropriateness Method to refine indicators	Validated prescribing appropriateness criteria for older Australians (≥ 65 years) for commonly used medications and medical condition	41	Mixed	Patient has no clinically significant medication interactions (agreement between two medication interaction databases)
Bergman-Evans, 2006 [27]	USA	Not confined to one setting	Literature review to develop indicators	Medication Management Outcomes Monitor	18	Implicit	Medications prescribed match established diagnosis
Buetow et al., 1996 [42]	UK	Primary care	Nominal group technique to develop indicators Indicators applied to studies located through systematic review	Dimensions and indicators of prescribing appropriateness	19	Implicit	The formulation and route and method of delivery are designed to maximise compliance for an individual patient
Cantrill et al., 1998 [28]	UK	Primary care	Nominal Group Technique to develop indicators Delphi method to assess validity of indicators	Indicators of appropriateness of prescribing	9	Mixed	If a potentially hazardous drug–drug combination is prescribed, the prescriber shows knowledge of the hazard
Caughey et al., 2014 [43]	Australia	Primary care	Literature review and review of clinical indicators to identify existing indicators and develop new ones Modified RAND appropriateness method to assess validity of indicators	Australian medication-related indicators of potentially preventable hospitalisations	29	Mixed	Use of two or more agents with anticholinergic activity OR use of an agent with high anticholinergic activity
Drenth-van Maanen et al., 2009 [24]	The Netherlands	Primary care	No detail on how indicators developed	Prescribing Optimization Method	6	Implicit	Which adverse effects are present?
Fried et al., 2016 [44]	USA	Not confined to one setting	Literature review and expert discussions to develop indicators Modified Delphi method to refine indicators	Strategies for addressing problems with medication regimens	10	Mixed	It is reasonable to undertake dose reduction or discontinuation of medications associated with both benefits and side effects if the patient views the side effects as more important than the benefits
Gazarian et al., 2006 [45]	Australia	Not confined to one setting	Expert working party using consensus-based approaches to develop decision algorithm	Assessing appropriateness of off-label medicines use	Not available – decision algorithm with accompanying	Implicit	Will this medicine be used according to a registered indication, age, dose and route?

Table 3 Table of included studies (*Continued*)

Authors and year	Country	Setting	Development of indicators	Name of instrument	Number of indicators (explanatory notes)	Implicit only or mixed (explicit/implicit) indicators	Example indicator
Hamdy et al., 1995 [29]	USA	Care homes	Literature review to develop indicators	Criteria for medication profile review	5	Implicit	Are any significant drug–drug or drug–disease interactions present?
Hanlon et al., 1992 [14]	USA	Internal medicine	Literature review and expert discussions to develop indicators	Medication Appropriateness Index	10	Implicit	Is the dosage correct?
Hassan et al., 2010 [46]	Malaysia	Not confined to one setting	Literature review and expert discussions to develop indicators Modified Delphi method to assessing validity of indicators	Prescription Quality Index	22	Implicit	Is there unnecessary duplication with other drug(s)?
Johnson et al., 1995 [47]	USA	Pharmacy	Literature review and expert discussions to develop indicators	–	10	Implicit	Interaction: drug–drug
Lara et al., 2012 [26]	Spain	Not confined to one setting	Literature review to identify indicators Delphi method to refine indicators	–	12	Implicit	Is there a lack of diagnoses or symptoms recorded in the medical history that do not have drug treatments but could have it?
Lenaerts et al., 2013 [25]	Belgium	Primary care	No detail on how indicators developed	Appropriate Medication for Older people-tool	8	Implicit	Are dosage and dosage form adapted to the patient?
Newton et al., 1994 [31]	USA	Primary care	Expert discussions to develop indicators	The Geriatric Medication Evaluation Algorithm	10	Implicit	Is the patient/caregiver unclear about the medication regimen?
O'Mahoney et al., 2014 [48]	Europe	Not confined to one setting	Literature review and expert consultation to review existing indicators and propose new ones Two-round Delphi method to refine and validate indicators	STOPP/START	114 (80 STOPP; 34 START)	Mixed	Any drug prescribed without an evidence-based clinical indication
Stange et al., 2010 [49]	Germany	Not confined to one setting	Forward and backward translation of the English version of the MCRI	Medication Regimen Complexity Index – German	1	Implicit	Not available: three sections (Section A: dosage forms; Section B: dosage frequency; Section C: additional instructions) to compute a score indicating the complexity of a given pharmacotherapeutic regimen
Tommelein et al., 2015 [50]	Belgium	Primary care	Literature review and two-round RAND/UCLA Appropriateness method to develop indicators	Ghent Older People's Prescriptions community Pharmacy Screening (GheOP^{3}S) tool	83	Mixed	Polypharmacy patients (chronically taking five or more drugs) were not questioned about whether a clear medication scheme was available to them

Table 3 Table of included studies *(Continued)*

Authors and year	Country	Setting	Development of indicators	Name of instrument	Number of indicators	Implicit only or mixed (explicit/implicit) indicators	Example indicator
Tully et al., 2005 [30]	UK	Secondary care	Literature review and expert discussions to develop indicators Pre- and pilot-testing on patient records, and expert panel, to assess validity of indicators	Appropriateness of long-term prescribing commenced in hospital practice	14	Implicit	Hazardous drug–drug combination
van Dijk et al., 2003 [51]	The Netherlands	Primary care	Does not state how indicators developed	Evaluation of drug use in nursing homes	6	Mixed	More than one drug from same drug class
Winslade et al., 1997 [52]	Canada	Pharmacy	Expert discussions and application in practice to revise two previous sets of indicators	Pharmacist management of drug-related problems	8	Implicit	The patient is taking/receiving a drug for which there is no valid indication

Acknowledgements

We would like to thank Isla Kuhn for her expert assistance with developing and conducting database searches in the systematic review. We are deeply grateful to all the panel members and patients who contributed to this study.

Funding

This paper presents independent research funded by the National Institute for Health Research School for Primary Care Research (NIHR SPCR) (Ref. SPCR-2014-10043). The views expressed are those of the authors and not necessarily those of the NHS, the NIHR or the Department of Health.

Authors' contributions

JB designed the study, oversaw the systematic review, drafted the evidence summaries, helped convene the RAND/UCLA Appropriateness Method consensus panel, oversaw the development of the final set of indicators and drafted the paper. NE conducted the systematic review, drafted the evidence summaries, organised the RAND/UCLA Appropriateness Method consensus panel, and reviewed the final draft of the paper. SC contributed to the design of the study, chaired the RAND/UCLA Appropriateness Method consensus panel, and reviewed the final draft of the paper. SR contributed to the design of the study, gave advice on the development of the indicators, and reviewed the final draft of the paper. AA contributed to the design of the study, gave advice on the development and categorisation of the indicators, and reviewed the final draft of the paper. RAP designed the study, oversaw the systematic review, drafted the evidence summaries, helped convene the RAND/UCLA Appropriateness Method consensus panel, oversaw the development of the final set of indicators, and drafted the paper. All authors read and approved the final manuscript.

Competing interests

The authors have no competing interests to declare.

Author details

[1]THIS Institute (The Healthcare Improvement Studies Institute), University of Cambridge, Cambridge Biomedical Campus, Clifford Allbutt Building, Cambridge CB2 0AH, UK. [2]NIHR Greater Manchester Patient Safety Translational Research Centre, Division of Population Health, HSR & Primary Care, School of Health Sciences, Faculty of Biology, Medicine and Health, University of Manchester, Manchester, UK. [3]Division of Primary Care, University of Nottingham, Room 1312, Tower Building, University Park, Nottingham NG7 2RD, UK. [4]Division of Primary Care, School of Medicine, University of Nottingham, Dean's Office, B Floor, Medical School, Queens Medical Centre, Nottingham NG7 2UH, UK. [5]Centre for Academic Primary Care, Population Health Sciences, Bristol Medical School, University of Bristol, Canynge Hall, 39 Whatley Road, Bristol BS8 2PS, UK.

References

1. Duerden M, Avery T, Payne R, et al. Polypharmacy and Medicines Optimisation: Making it Safe and Sound. London: King's Fund; 2013.
2. Barnett K, Mercer SW, Norbury M, et al. Epidemiology of multimorbidity and implications for health care, research, and medical education: a cross-sectional study. Lancet. 2012;380:37–43.
3. Boyd CM, Darer J, Boult C, et al. Clinical practice guidelines and quality of care for older patients with multiple comorbid diseases: implications for pay for performance. JAMA. 2005;294:716–24. https://doi.org/10.1001/jama.294.6.716.
4. Avery AJ, Ghaleb M, Barber N, et al. The prevalence and nature of prescribing and monitoring errors in English general practice: a retrospective case note review. Br J Gen Pract. 2013;63:e543–53. https://doi.org/10.3399/bjgp13X670679.
5. Dequito AB, Mol PGM, van Doormaal JE, et al. Preventable and non-preventable adverse drug events in hospitalized patients. Drug Saf. 2011;34:1089–100. https://doi.org/10.2165/11592030-000000000-00000.
6. Fincke BG, Miller DR, Spiro A. The interaction of patient perception of overmedication with drug compliance and side effects. J Gen Intern Med. 1998;13:182–5. https://doi.org/10.1046/j.1525-1497.1998.00053.x.
7. Vik SA, Maxwell CJ, Hogan DB. Measurement, correlates, and health outcomes of medication adherence among seniors. Ann Pharmacother. 2004;38:303–12. https://doi.org/10.1345/aph.1D252.
8. Jyrkkä J, Enlund H, Korhonen MJ, et al. Polypharmacy status as an indicator of mortality in an elderly population. Drugs Aging. 2009;26:1039–48. https://doi.org/10.2165/11319530-000000000-00000.
9. Payne RA, Abel GA, Avery AJ, et al. Is polypharmacy always hazardous? A retrospective cohort analysis using linked electronic health records from primary and secondary care. Br J Clin Pharmacol. 2014;77:1073–82. https://doi.org/10.1111/bcp.12292.
10. Appleton SC, Abel GA, Payne RA. Cardiovascular polypharmacy is not associated with unplanned hospitalisation: evidence from a retrospective cohort study. BMC Fam Pract. 2014;15:58. https://doi.org/10.1186/1471-2296-15-58.
11. Spinewine A, Schmader KE, Barber N, et al. Appropriate prescribing in elderly people: how well can it be measured and optimised? Lancet. 2007;370:173–84.
12. Hill-Taylor B, Walsh KA, Stewart S, et al. Effectiveness of the STOPP/START (Screening Tool of Older Persons' potentially inappropriate Prescriptions/Screening Tool to Alert doctors to the Right Treatment) criteria: systematic review and meta-analysis of randomized controlled studies. J Clin Pharm Ther. 2016;41:158–69. https://doi.org/10.1111/jcpt.12372.
13. American Geriatrics Society 2015 Beers Criteria Update Expert Panel. American Geriatrics Society 2015 updated Beers criteria for potentially inappropriate medication use in older adults. J Am Geriatr Soc. 2015;63:2227–46. https://doi.org/10.1111/jgs.13702.
14. Hanlon JT, Schmader KE, Samsa GP, et al. A method for assessing drug therapy appropriateness. J Clin Epidemiol. 1992;45:1045–51.
15. Elmore N, Burt J, Payne R, et al. Developing and Evaluating a Measure of Inappropriate Polypharmacy in Primary Care. PROSPERO 2016 CRD42016049176. PROSPERO. http://www.crd.york.ac.uk/PROSPERO/display_record.php?ID=CRD42016049176. Accessed 9 Mar 2018.
16. Burt J, Elmore N, Rodgers S, et al. Developing and Evaluating a Measure of Inappropriate Polypharmacy in Primary Care. Cambridge: Primary Care Unit, University of Cambridge; 2016. http://www.crd.york.ac.uk/PROSPEROFILES/49176_PROTOCOL_20160910.pdf
17. Preferred Reporting Items for Systematic Reviews and Meta-Analyses: The PRISMA Statement. http://journals.plos.org/plosmedicine/article?id=10.1371/journal.pmed.1000097. Accessed 9 Mar 2018.
18. Basger BJ, Chen TF, Moles RJ. Inappropriate medication use and prescribing indicators in elderly Australians: development of a prescribing indicators tool. Drugs Aging. 2008;25:777–93.
19. Basger BJ, Chen TF, Moles RJ. Validation of prescribing appropriateness criteria for older Australians using the RAND/UCLA appropriateness method. BMJ Open. 2012;2:e001431. https://doi.org/10.1136/bmjopen-2012-001431.
20. Hsieh H-F, Shannon SE. Three approaches to qualitative content analysis. Qual Health Res. 2005;15:1277–88. https://doi.org/10.1177/1049732305276687.

21. Joanna Briggs Institute. Critical Appraisal Tools - JBI. http://joannabriggs.org/research/critical-appraisal-tools.html. Accessed 16 Mar 2018.
22. Fitch K, Bernstein SJ, Aguilar MD, et al. The RAND/UCLA Appropriateness Method User's Manual. Santa Monica, CA: RAND Corporation; 2001. https://www.rand.org/pubs/monograph_reports/MR1269.html
23. INVOLVE. Public Involvement in Research: Values and Principles Framework – INVOLVE. Southampton (UK): INVOLVE 2015. http://www.invo.org.uk/posttypepublication/public-involvement-in-researchvalues-and-principles-framework/. Accessed 16 Mar 2018.
24. Drenth-van Maanen AC, van Marum RJ, Knol W, et al. Prescribing optimization method for improving prescribing in elderly patients receiving polypharmacy: results of application to case histories by general practitioners. Drugs Aging. 2009;26:687–701. https://doi.org/10.2165/11316400-000000000-00000.
25. Lenaerts E, De Knijf F, Schoenmakers B. Appropriate prescribing for older people: a new tool for the general practitioner. J Frailty Aging. 2013;2:8–14. https://doi.org/10.14283/jfa.2013.2.
26. Alfaro Lara ER, Vega Coca MD, Galván Banqueri M, et al. Selection of tools for reconciliation, compliance and appropriateness of treatment in patients with multiple chronic conditions. Eur J Intern Med. 2012;23:506–12. https://doi.org/10.1016/j.ejim.2012.06.007.
27. Bergman-Evans B. Evidence-based guideline. Improving medication management for older adult clients. J Gerontol Nurs. 2006;32:6–14.
28. Cantrill JA, Sibbald B, Buetow S. Indicators of the appropriateness of long-term prescribing in general practice in the United Kingdom: consensus development, face and content validity, feasibility, and reliability. Qual Health Care QHC. 1998;7:130–5.
29. Hamdy RC, Moore SW, Whalen K, et al. Reducing polypharmacy in extended care. South Med J. 1995;88:534–8.
30. Tully MP, Javed N, Cantrill JA. Development and face validity of explicit indicators of appropriateness of long term prescribing. Pharm World Sci PWS. 2005;27:407–13. https://doi.org/10.1007/s11096-005-0340-1.
31. Newton PF, Levinson W, Maslen D. The geriatric medication algorithm: a pilot study. J Gen Intern Med. 1994;9:164–7.
32. Hanlon JT, Schmader KE. The Medication Appropriateness Index at 20: where it started, where it has been, and where it may be going. Drugs Aging. 2013;30:893–900. https://doi.org/10.1007/s40266-013-0118-4.
33. Kardas P, Lewek P, Matyjaszczyk M. Determinants of patient adherence: a review of systematic reviews. Front Pharmacol 2013;4:91. https://doi.org/10.3389/fphar.2013.00091.
34. Lam PW, Lum CM, Leung MF. Drug non-adherence and associated risk factors among Chinese geriatric patients in Hong Kong. Hong Kong Med J. 2007;13:284.
35. Juurlink DN, Mamdani M, Kopp A, et al. Drug-drug interactions among elderly patients hospitalized for drug toxicity. JAMA. 2003;289:1652–8. https://doi.org/10.1001/jama.289.13.1652.
36. Dirmaier J, Steinman MA, Krattenmacher T. Non-pharmacological treatment of depressive disorders: a review of evidence-based treatment options. Rev Recent Clin Trials. 2012;7:141–9.
37. NICE. Cardiovascular Disease: Risk Assessment and Reduction, Including Lipid Modification. NICE; 2016. https://www.nice.org.uk/guidance/CG181. Accessed 1 June 2018.
38. Krska J. Pharmacist-led medication review in patients over 65: a randomized, controlled trial in primary care. Age Ageing. 2001;30:205–11. https://doi.org/10.1093/ageing/30.3.205.
39. Sorensen L, Stokes JA, Purdie DM, et al. Medication reviews in the community: results of a randomized, controlled effectiveness trial. Br J Clin Pharmacol. 2004;58:648–64. https://doi.org/10.1111/j.1365-2125.2004.02220.x.
40. NICE. Medicines Optimisation: The Safe and Effective Use of Medicines to Enable the Best Possible Outcomes. NICE 2015. https://www.nice.org.uk/guidance/ng5/resources/medicines-optimisation-the-safe-and-effective-use-of-medicines-to-enable-the-best-possible-outcomes-51041805253. Accessed 30 Nov 2016.
41. Whitburn S. Prescribing the Cost-effective Way. GP. 2007; http://www.gponline.com/prescribing-cost-effective/article/662699. Accessed 1 Dec 2016
42. Buetow SA, Sibbald B, Cantrill JA, et al. Prevalence of potentially inappropriate long term prescribing in general practice in the United Kingdom, 1980–95: systematic literature review. BMJ. 1996;313:1371–4. https://doi.org/10.1136/bmj.313.7069.1371.
43. Caughey GE, Ellett LMK, Wong TY. Development of evidence-based Australian medication-related indicators of potentially preventable hospitalisations: a modified RAND appropriateness method. BMJ Open. 2014;4:e004625. https://doi.org/10.1136/bmjopen-2013-004625.
44. Fried TR, Niehoff K, Tjia J, et al. A Delphi process to address medication appropriateness for older persons with multiple chronic conditions. BMC Geriatr 2016;16:67. https://doi.org/10.1186/s12877-016-0240-3.
45. Gazarian M, Kelly M, McPhee JR, et al. Off-label use of medicines: consensus recommendations for evaluating appropriateness. Med J Aust. 2006;185:544–8.
46. Hassan NB, Ismail HC, Naing L, et al. Development and validation of a new Prescription Quality Index: Prescription quality. Br J Clin Pharmacol. 2010;70:500–13. https://doi.org/10.1111/j.1365-2125.2009.03597.x.
47. Johnson KA, Nye M, Hill-Besinque K, et al. Measuring the impact of patient counseling in the outpatient pharmacy setting: development and implementation of the counseling models for the Kaiser Permanente/USC Patient Consultation Study. Clin Ther. 1995;17:988–1002.
48. O'Mahony D, O'Sullivan D, Byrne S, et al. STOPP/START criteria for potentially inappropriate prescribing in older people: version 2. Age Ageing. 2015;44(2):213–8. https://doi.org/10.1093/ageing/afu145.
49. Stange D, Kriston L, Langebrake C, et al. Development and psychometric evaluation of the German version of the Medication Regimen Complexity Index (MRCI-D): Medication Regimen Complexity Index - German translation and evaluation. J Eval Clin Pract. 2012;18:515–22. https://doi.org/10.1111/j.1365-2753.2011.01636.x.
50. Tommelein E, Petrovic M, Somers A, et al. Older patients' prescriptions screening in the community pharmacy: development of the Ghent Older People's Prescriptions community Pharmacy Screening (GheOP^{3}S) tool. J Public Health. 2016;38:e158–70. https://doi.org/10.1093/pubmed/fdv090.
51. van Dijk KN, Pont LG, de Vries CS, et al. Prescribing indicators for evaluating drug use in nursing homes. Ann Pharmacother. 2003;37:1136–41.
52. Winslade NE, Bajcar JM, Bombassaro AM, et al. Pharmacist's management of drug-related problems: a tool for teaching and providing pharmaceutical care. Pharmacotherapy. 1997;17:801–9.

7

Iron deficiency during pregnancy is associated with a reduced risk of adverse birth outcomes in a malaria-endemic area in a longitudinal cohort study

Freya J. I. Fowkes[1,2,3,4*], Kerryn A. Moore[1,3], D. Herbert Opi[1,5], Julie A. Simpson[3], Freya Langham[1,2], Danielle I. Stanisic[6], Alice Ura[7], Christopher L. King[8], Peter M. Siba[7], Ivo Mueller[9,10], Stephen J. Rogerson[11] and James G. Beeson[1,4,11*]

Abstract

Background: Low birth weight (LBW) and preterm birth (PTB) are major contributors to infant mortality and chronic childhood morbidity. Understanding factors that contribute to or protect against these adverse birth outcomes is an important global health priority. Anaemia and iron deficiency are common in malaria-endemic regions, but there are concerns regarding the value of iron supplementation among pregnant women in malaria-endemic areas due to reports that iron supplementation may increase the risk of malaria. There is a lack of evidence on the impact of iron deficiency on pregnancy outcomes in malaria-endemic regions.

Methods: We determined iron deficiency in a cohort of 279 pregnant women in a malaria-endemic area of Papua New Guinea. Associations with birth weight, LBW and PTB were estimated using linear and logistic regression. A causal model using sequential mediation analyses was constructed to assess the association between iron deficiency and LBW, either independently or mediated through malaria and/or anaemia.

Results: Iron deficiency in pregnant women was common (71% at enrolment) and associated with higher mean birth weights (230 g; 95% confidence interval, CI 118, 514; $p < 0.001$), and reduced odds of LBW (adjusted odds ratio, aOR = 0.32; 95% CI 0.16, 0.64; $p = 0.001$) and PTB (aOR = 0.57; 95% CI 0.30, 1.09; $p = 0.089$). Magnitudes of effect were greatest in primigravidae (birth weight 351 g; 95% CI 188, 514; $p < 0.001$; LBW aOR 0.26; 95% CI 0.10, 0.66; $p = 0.005$; PTB aOR = 0.39, 95% CI 0.16, 0.97; $p = 0.042$). Sequential mediation analyses indicated that the protective association of iron deficiency on LBW was mainly mediated through mechanisms independent of malaria or anaemia.

Conclusions: Iron deficiency was associated with substantially reduced odds of LBW predominantly through malaria-independent protective mechanisms, which has substantial implications for understanding risks for poor pregnancy outcomes and evaluating the benefit of iron supplementation in pregnancy. This study is the first longitudinal study to demonstrate a temporal relationship between antenatal iron deficiency and improved birth outcomes. These findings suggest that iron supplementation needs to be integrated with other strategies to prevent or treat infections and undernutrition in pregnancy to achieve substantial improvements in birth outcomes.

Keywords: Iron deficiency, Low birth weight, Preterm birth, Malaria, Anaemia, Pregnancy, *Plasmodium falciparum*

* Correspondence: freya.fowkes@burnet.edu.au; beeson@burnet.edu.au
[1]Burnet Institute, Maternal and Child Health Program, Life Sciences and Public Health, Melbourne, VIC 3004, Australia
Full list of author information is available at the end of the article

Background

Low birth weight (LBW; birth weight < 2500 g) and pre-term birth (PTB; <37 weeks gestation) are major contributors to infant mortality and chronic childhood morbidity. LBW is associated with >80% of infant deaths [1]. Understanding factors that moderate or exacerbate the burden of LBW and PTB is, therefore, an important global health priority. Poor nutrition, anaemia and infectious diseases are common among pregnant women globally, particularly in resource-limited settings, and are important contributors to LBW. Iron deficiency (defined by the World Health Organisation [WHO] as ferritin < 15 µg/L [2]) is a common feature of undernutrition and a major cause of anaemia and it contributes to an estimated global burden of 600,000 perinatal and 100,000 maternal deaths per year [3]. Many regions with a high burden of undernutrition and anaemia are also endemic for malaria and approximately 125 million women living in malaria-endemic areas become pregnant each year [4, 5]. Malaria contributes to anaemia by causing haemolysis and dyserythropoiesis and it is also a major cause of LBW and PTB [6, 7].

Despite the high prevalence of undernutrition and anaemia among pregnant women in resource-limited and malaria-endemic settings, there is limited knowledge on the contribution of iron deficiency and other specific preventable deficiencies to LBW and poor pregnancy outcomes. To reduce the burden of anaemia and poor pregnancy outcomes, the WHO recommends that all pregnant women receive daily iron and folate supplements (30–60 mg of elemental iron plus 400 µg of folic acid), in addition to "measures to prevent, diagnose and treat malaria" in malaria-endemic areas [8]. However, there are concerns regarding the value of antenatal iron supplementation in malaria-endemic areas due to reports of harmful interactions between iron and malaria [9]. Moreover, the link between iron deficiency and poor pregnancy outcomes in malaria-endemic and tropical regions, and the value of iron supplementation on improving birth outcomes, is unclear.

Iron deficiency has been associated with reduced high-density *Plasmodium falciparum* parasitaemia, associated clinical symptoms of malaria and reduced placental *P. falciparum* infection in case–control and cross-sectional studies of pregnant women living in malaria-endemic areas [10]. Iron supplements given to children in malaria-endemic areas have been associated with increased parasitaemia, risk of clinical malaria and risk of severe illness and death (not specific to malaria) in some controlled trials [11, 12]. However, clinical trials have shown inconsistent associations between daily iron supplementation and risk of peripheral or placental *P. falciparum* infection in Africa [10, 13–15]. One study reported an increased risk of *P. vivax* after supplementation in Asia [10]. There is also no clear evidence for the association between iron supplementation and birth outcomes in pregnant women living in areas where they are at risk of malaria [10, 13–16]. A recent trial in west African pregnant and non-pregnant women found an increased rate of adverse events among those receiving iron supplementation [17]. These issues are compounded by a lack of understanding of how iron deficiency, anaemia and malaria may interact to influence birth outcomes. This knowledge is essential to the evidence base of iron supplementation programmes in malaria-endemic and resource-limited settings where there is a high burden of infectious diseases and poor nutrition.

The objectives of this study were to determine the association between iron deficiency and birth outcomes, and to quantify how malaria mediated these associations, in a longitudinal study of pregnant women in a malaria-endemic area of Papua New Guinea (PNG), which has the largest population at risk of anaemia, undernutrition malaria and poor birth outcomes in the South-West Pacific region.

Methods

Study design

Pregnant women ($n = 470$) were enrolled into a longitudinal study of malaria in pregnancy in Madang Province, PNG, conducted through the PNG Institute of Medical Research (Additional file 1: Methods) [18]. Briefly, study participation occurred in parallel with clinic attendance at the first antenatal visit, at 30–34 weeks' gestation and at delivery. Pregnant women were enrolled at their first antenatal consultation at Alexishafen Health Centre between September 2005 and October 2007. At enrolment and delivery, 5 ml of peripheral blood was collected, and stored at -20 °C or -70 °C. Gestational age at enrolment was estimated from fundal height (cm) and haemoglobin was measured using a HemoCue haemoglobinometer (Hemocue, Ängelholm, Sweden). Women with haemoglobin concentrations < 5 g/dL were referred for appropriate care and were not enrolled in the study. All women were prescribed ferrous sulfate 270 mg and folic acid 0.3 mg daily, according to local policy; women with Hb 5–7 g/dL were prescribed two tablets daily. Intermittent preventative treatment in pregnancy with sulfadoxine-pyrimethamine (IPTp-SP; 1500 mg/75 mg respectively) was recommended to all women according to national guidelines. At delivery, intervillous placental blood and placental tissue samples were collected. Birth weight was measured using SECA baby scales and gestational age was estimated from Ballard scores performed by the study nurse, following training by a paediatrician [18]. Ethical approval was granted by the PNG Medical Research Advisory Council and the Alfred Health Human Research Ethics Committee, and written informed consent was obtained from all study participants. Of the 470 women enrolled into the initial study [18], 376 women completed follow-up to delivery and 97 women were excluded from the current analysis (5 multiple births; 43 newborns were not seen within 3 days after delivery; 1 data entry error; 31 with insufficient blood sample; and 17 women with missing birth outcome data) (Additional file 1). Therefore, 279 women were included in this analysis (Table 1). Included and excluded women did not differ in the distribution of enrolment variables (Additional file 1: Table S1).

Exposures and outcomes

Exposures of interest were iron stores (ferritin) and iron deficiency (ferritin < 15 μg/L) at enrolment. Birth outcomes of interest were birth weight (grams), LBW (<2500 g) and PTB (<37 weeks gestation). Malaria outcomes of interest were peripheral *P. falciparum or P. vivax* spp. infection [by polymerase chain reaction (PCR) or light microscopy] and placental *P. falciparum* infection (detected by light microscopy or placental histology).

Laboratory procedures

Peripheral and placental *Plasmodium* spp. infection was determined by light microscopy of Giemsa-stained thick and thin blood films, and PCR, as previously described [18]. Among women who completed follow-up to delivery, ferritin concentrations were measured in serum samples (collected at enrolment) by established ELISA with reference controls (Immunology Consultants Laboratory Immunoperoxidase Assay). C-reactive protein (CRP) levels were determined using established ELISA kits with reference controls (Elisakit). The ferritin and CRP intra-assay and inter-assay coefficients of variation were all <10%.

Statistical analysis

Changes in *Plasmodium* spp. prevalence and haemoglobin within an individual woman between enrolment and delivery were quantified using McNemar's chi-square test or Student's paired *t*-test, respectively. Associations between ferritin (transformed to log base 2) and iron deficiency and birth outcomes (birth weight, LBW and PTB) were estimated using multivariable linear and logistic regression, respectively. Confounding variables identified a priori [gravidity, maternal education, maternal mid upper arm circumference (MUAC) at enrolment (as a marker of undernutrition), maternal smoking and gestational age] were adjusted for in multivariable regression models. Red blood cell genetic polymorphisms (SAO, CR1 and α-thalassaemia) were not included in the models, as we have previously shown in this cohort that they are not associated with risk of *Plasmodium* infection or birth weight [18]. Newborn sex, a predictor of birth outcomes, was also included in the multivariable linear regression models to potentially reduce the residual standard deviation, and thus increase the precision

Table 1 Participant characteristics, malaria parameters, iron markers and delivery outcomes

Variable	Mean [SD], range; or median {IQR}, range; or N (%)
Participant characteristics at enrolment[1]	
Maternal age, years (N = 268)	24 [17], 16–49
Mid upper arm circumference, cm (N = 270)	22.4 [1.8], 12–30
Primigravidae	106/279 (38)
Estimated gestational age, weeks (N = 276)	25.3 [4.2], 7–36
Education	
None or primary	154/275 (56)
Secondary+	121/275 (44)
Current smoker (yes)	56/278 (20)
Used bed net last night (yes)	200/264 (76)
Clinical history of fever, chills or headache in past 7 days (yes)	67/276 (24)
Palpable spleen (yes)	51/262 (19)
Malariometrics and iron status at enrolment	
Plasmodium spp. infection detectable by PCR	185/279 (66)
Plasmodium spp. infection[2]	98/279 (35)
P. falciparum	93/279 (33)
P. vivax	9/279 (3)
Haemoglobin, g/dL (N = 279)	8.5 [1.4], 5.3–12.8
Ferritin, μg/L (N = 279)	8.2 {4.6–17.5}, 2.4–121.3
Iron deficient (ferritin < 15 μg/L)	199/279 (71)
CRP, mg/L (N = 258)[3]	5.15 {1.80–11.72}, 0.18–255.65
High CRP (> 10 mg/L)	90/279 (32)
Malariometric and birth outcomes at delivery	
Placental *Plasmodium* spp. infection[2]	39/223 (17)
P. falciparum	34/223 (15)
P. vivax	6/223 (3)
Plasmodium spp. infection[2]	37/274 (13)
P. falciparum	31/274 (11)
P. vivax	6/274 (2)
Haemoglobin, g/dL (N = 270)	9.2 [1.7], 4.7–14.2
Birth weight, grams (N = 279)	2857 [452], 1400–4500
Low birth weight (< 2500 g)	47/279 (17)
Gestational age at delivery, weeks (N = 279)	38 {37–40}, 28–42
Preterm birth (<37 weeks gestation)	62/279 (22)

[1]N = 279
[2]*Plasmodium* spp. infection detectable by light microscopy of Giemsa-stained thick and thin blood films, unless otherwise specified. Four women had a mixed infection at enrolment (*P. falciparum* and *P. vivax*), one woman had mixed placental infection and one woman had mixed peripheral infection at delivery
[3]21 measurements were outside the assay standard curve so were excluded from the CRP concentration descriptive analysis but classified as >10 mg/L for high CRP descriptive analysis
CRP C-reactive protein, *IQR* interquartile range, *PCR* polymerase chain reaction, *SD* standard deviation

of our parameter estimates for iron exposures. Effect modification by gravidity (primigravid/multigravid) was investigated by including an interaction term between iron exposures and gravidity; *p* values for interactions were derived from likelihood ratio tests comparing models including and excluding interaction terms. We performed sequential mediation analyses to estimate marginal natural direct and indirect effects for the association between iron deficiency and LBW mediated through: (1) peripheral infection detected by light microscopy or PCR, (2) placental *P. falciparum* infection detected by light microscopy or histology, and (3) anaemia, by calculating potential outcomes from logistic models with inverse probability weighting to achieve balance in the iron deficiency groups in terms of the confounders (gravidity, maternal education, maternal mid-upper arm circumference at enrolment, gestational age). We obtained 95% confidence intervals (CIs) for marginal natural direct effects and marginal natural indirect effects by bootstrapping using the percentile method and 1000 replications. All statistical analyses were performed using Stata Version 13 (StataCorp, College Station, TX, USA).

Results

Iron deficiency and malaria in the study population

At enrolment (first antenatal visit), the median maternal age was 24 years (interquartile range, IQR 21–28), the mean estimated gestational age was 25 weeks (standard deviation, SD 4.2) and 62% of women were multigravidae. Reported use of a bed net (to prevent malaria) during the night before enrolment was 76%. For clinical symptoms, 24% of women had a history of fever, headache or chills within the 7 days prior to enrolment, and 19% had a palpable spleen (Table 1). *Plasmodium* spp. infection at enrolment was common; 35% and 66% of women had peripheral *Plasmodium* spp. parasitaemia detectable by light microscopy and PCR, respectively. The majority (95%) of infections were *P. falciparum.*

At enrolment, haemoglobin levels were generally very low (mean 8.5 g/dL, SD 1.4) and the prevalence of anaemia was very high. Overall, 95% (266/279) of women had anaemia (Hb < 11 g/dL), 61% (171/279) had moderate anaemia (Hb < 9 g/dL) and 12% (33/279) had severe anaemia (Hb < 7 g/dL). Furthermore, ferritin concentrations were low (median 8.2 µg/L; IQR 4.6–17.5) and iron deficiency (defined as ferritin < 15 µg/L according to the WHO) was present in 71% of women at enrolment (Table 1). The prevalence was 62% and 77% in primigravid and multigravid women respectively. Elevated CRP can be a marker of an acute phase response that may also raise ferritin levels and potentially lead to misclassification of iron-deficient women as iron-replete. In our study, elevated CRP (>10 mg/L) was found in 46 (57%)

iron-replete women and 44 (22%) iron-deficient women ($p < 0.001$). When potentially misclassified women were excluded (women with raised CRP and ferritin > 15), the prevalence of iron deficiency was 85%. Ferritin and CRP levels were only weakly correlated (Spearman's rho, $\rho = 0.245$; 95% CI 0.127, 0.357; $p < 0.001$). There was no correlation between haemoglobin at enrolment and ferritin at enrolment ($\rho = 0.035$; 95% CI −0.083, 0.152; $p = 0.562$), and no association between iron deficiency and anaemia at enrolment, suggesting that multiple factors contributed to anaemia, aside from iron deficiency. We found that 96% (77/80) of iron-replete and 95% (189/199) of iron-deficient women were anaemic ($p = 0.648$), 69% (55/80) of iron-replete and 58% (116/199) of iron-deficient women had moderate anaemia ($p = 0.105$), and 9% (7/80) of iron-replete and 13% (26/199) of iron-deficient women had severe anaemia ($p = 0.313$).

At delivery, 13% of women had peripheral parasitaemia detectable by light microscopy (a significant decrease from enrolment, $p < 0.001$), and mean haemoglobin was 9.2 g/dL (SD 1.7), a significant increase from enrolment, with a mean difference of −0.66 (95% CI −0.86, − 0.45; $p < 0.001$) (Table 1). Placental parasitaemia was present in 17% by light microscopy (18% and 17% in primigravidae and multigravidae, respectively) (Table 1).

Associations between iron deficiency and birth outcomes

Mean birth weight in the cohort was 2857 g (SD 452 g) and median (IQR) gestational age was 38 weeks (37–40 weeks). Poor pregnancy outcomes were common, with 17% being LBW and 22% of babies born preterm (<37 weeks estimated gestation) (Table 1). Surprisingly, lower ferritin levels and iron deficiency were associated with higher mean birth weights in multivariable regression analyses (Table 2). For every twofold increase in ferritin, the estimated adjusted mean decrease in birth weight was −63 g (95% CI −103, −123; $p = 0.002$), and iron-deficient women gave birth to newborns that were 230 g heavier than newborns of iron-replete women (95% CI 118, 342; $p < 0.001$; Table 2). There was evidence of effect modification by gravidity, whereby the reduction in mean birth weight associated with higher iron stores was greatest in primigravidae (Table 2). Among primigravidae, birth weight was 351 g higher among iron-deficient (95% CI 188, 514), compared to iron-replete women ($p < 0.001$), whereas among multigravidae, birth weight was 125 g higher among iron-deficient women (95% CI −28, 277; $p = 0.108$; Table 2).

Iron deficiency was associated with a 68% reduction in the odds of LBW (adjusted odds ratio, aOR = 0.32; 95% CI 0.16, 0.64; $p = 0.001$), and a 43% reduction in the odds of preterm birth, although the association with PTB had weak statistical significance (aOR = 0.57; 95% CI 0.30,

Table 2 Associations between iron deficiency and birth outcomes and effect modification by gravidity

Birth weight (grams)			
Iron stores	Unadjusted mean difference (95% CI); p	Adjusted mean difference (95% CI); p	
Ferritin, µg/L ($\log_2$)[1]	−72 (−113, −30); 0.001	−63 (−103, −23); 0.002	
		Primigravid	Multigravid
		−114 (−173, −55); <0.001	−20 (−74, 33); 0.457
Iron deficiency			
Iron replete	Reference group	Reference group	
Iron deficient	204 (89, 320); 0.001	230 (118, 342); <0.001	
		Primigravid	Multigravid
		351 (188, 514); <0.001	125 (−28, 277); 0.108
Low birth weight (<2500 g)			
Iron stores	Unadjusted OR (95% CI); p	Adjusted OR (95% CI); p	
Iron deficiency			
Iron replete	Reference group	Reference group	
Iron deficient	0.34 (0.18, 0.65); 0.001	0.32 (0.16, 0.64); 0.001	
		Primigravid	Multigravid
		0.26 (0.10, 0.66); 0.005	0.42 (0.15, 1.20); 0.105
Preterm birth (<37 weeks)			
Iron stores	Unadjusted OR (95% CI); p	Adjusted OR (95% CI); p	
Ferritin, µg/L ($\log_2$)[1]	1.13 (0.91, 1.41); 0.254	1.06 (0.84, 1.35); 0.605	
		Primigravid	Multigravid
		1.20 (0.86, 1.66); 0.280	0.93 (0.65, 1.33); 0.681
Iron deficiency			
Iron replete	Reference group	Reference group	
Iron deficient	0.60 (0.33, 1.10); 0.098	0.57 (0.30, 1.09); 0.089	
		Primigravid	Multigravid
		0.39 (0.16, 0.97); 0.042	0.86 (0.32, 2.30); 0.767

Multivariable models including confounding variables (gravidity, gestational age, education, mid-upper arm circumference and smoking), and sex of the newborn (linear models only). [1]Ferritin transformed to log base 2 due to positively skewed distribution; coefficients are, therefore, for the absolute or relative change in outcome associated with each twofold increase in ferritin concentration. p values for gravidity interaction parameters are 0.019 (ferritin, birth weight), 0.042 (iron deficiency, birth weight), 0.500 (iron deficiency, LBW), 0.299 (ferritin, PTB) and 0.236 (iron deficiency, PTB)
CI confidence interval, *LBW* low birth weight, *OR* odds ratio, *PTB* preterm birth

1.09; $p = 0.089$). An analysis of effect modification also showed that the magnitudes of effect between iron deficiency and LBW were highly significant and greater in primigravidae (LBW aOR 0.26; 95% CI 0.10, 0.66; $p = 0.005$) than in multigravidae (LBW aOR 0.42; 95% CI 0.15, 1.20; $p = 0.105$; Table 2). An analysis of effect modification also showed that the association between iron deficiency and PTB was restricted to primigravidae (aOR 0.39; 95% CI 0.16, 0.97; $p = 0.042$) compared to multigravidae (aOR 0.86; 95% CI 0.32, 2.30; $p = 0.767$; Table 2). Additionally, we performed analyses excluding iron-replete women who had evidence of inflammation (ferritin >15 µg/ml and CRP > 10 mg/L), that is women who may have been misclassified as iron replete due to elevated ferritin resulting from an acute phase response. This did not alter our results and a similar association between iron deficiency and birth weight was found (Additional file 1).

Investigating iron deficiency, malaria and anaemia as causes of LBW using mediation analyses

To investigate the causes of the association between iron deficiency and LBW further, we explored the association between iron deficiency and anaemia (Hb < 9 g/dL), peripheral malaria infection and placental malaria and whether these variables mediated the association between iron deficiency and LBW. Iron deficiency was associated with a 48% reduction in moderate anaemia at enrolment (aOR 0.52; 95% CI 0.27, 0.97; $p = 0.040$, adjusted for gravidity, education, smoking, MUAC and gestational age), reflective of multiple contributors to anaemia in the study population. Iron deficiency was also associated with a 56% reduction in peripheral blood parasitaemia at enrolment as detected by light microscopy (aOR = 0.44; 95% CI 0.25, 0.79; $p = 0.006$) and a 67% reduction in PCR-detected infection (aOR 0.33; 95%

CI 0.17, 0.67; $p = 0.002$), but no association was found with placental malaria (aOR = 0.85; 95% CI 0.38, 1.90; $p = 0.695$). However, these associations were confounded by women potentially misclassified as iron replete. After excluding these potentially misclassified women, there were no significant protective associations between iron deficiency and anaemia (aOR = 0.77; 95% CI 0.33, 1.79; $p = 0.543$), peripheral parasitaemia (light microscopy aOR 1.47; 95% CI 0.59, 3.68; $p = 0.406$; PCR aOR 0.66; 95% CI 0.28, 1.56; $p = 0.343$) or placental malaria (aOR = 1.60; 95% CI 0.43, 5.87; $p = 0.480$).

We used sequential mediation analyses to assess the effects of iron deficiency on LBW, either directly or mediated through placental *P. falciparum* malaria, anaemia or peripheral malaria at enrolment. Sequential mediation analyses were performed to quantify the proportion of the observed protective effect of iron deficiency on LBW that was mediated through malaria and anaemia, accounting for potential confounders (maternal education, MUAC, gravidity, smoking and gestational age) (Table 3). The mediators were malaria at enrolment by light microscopy, moderate to severe anaemia at enrolment (Hb < 9 g/dL), placental malaria at delivery by light microscopy (directed acyclic graph shown in Fig. 1). The mediation analyses are sequential because there were multiple mediators that are not independent of each other (Fig. 1). In sequential mediation analyses, mediation through placental malaria only can be determined as it immediately precedes the outcome (LBW). Malaria detected at enrolment precedes other mediators of interest (anaemia and placental malaria) and therefore, mediation solely through malaria detected at enrolment cannot be determined, only what is mediated through malaria at enrolment *and* anaemia *and* placental malaria.

Interestingly, there was evidence for a substantial direct protective effect of iron deficiency on risk of LBW that was not mediated through protection against placental malaria, anaemia or malaria present in peripheral blood (risk ratio = 0.44; 95% CI 0.25, 0.79). In contrast, only 7% of the association between iron deficiency and LBW was mediated through placental *P. falciparum* malaria and only 12% was mediated through pathways that included peripheral malaria infection, which included indirect pathways via anaemia and placental malaria (Table 3). Similar effects were seen in sensitivity analyses whereby women with raised CRP levels who may have been misclassified as iron replete (ferritin >15 µg/ml and CRP > 10 mg/L) were excluded from analyses (Table 3). Furthermore, similar associations were found in analyses investigating the mediation through malaria and anaemia detected at the second antenatal visit (30–34 weeks gestation) and/or placental malaria defined by placental histology (Additional file 1). In summary, these analyses suggest that the protective association of iron deficiency on LBW is largely mediated through mechanisms independent of malaria and anaemia.

Discussion

LBW and PTB are major risk factors for infant morbidity and mortality and identifying factors that contribute to these risks, or protect against them, is crucial for advancing child health globally. Furthermore, concerns regarding potentially harmful malaria–iron interactions have raised questions about the appropriateness of antenatal iron supplementation for anaemia in malaria-endemic populations [9]. Here, we provide the first evidence of a protective association of maternal iron deficiency on LBW, and to a lesser extent PTB, in a malaria-endemic area where iron deficiency and anaemia are common, and elucidated the potential effect of malaria–iron interactions on birth outcomes. Iron deficiency was associated with substantially reduced risks of LBW, and this beneficial effect appeared largely mediated through mechanisms that are independent of an interaction between iron deficiency and malaria. The apparent protective effect of iron deficiency was greatest in primigravid women, a high-risk

Table 3 Mediation of association between iron deficiency and low birth weight

Mediating variables	Natural direct effect, risk ratio (95% CI)	Natural indirect effect, risk ratio (95% CI)	Proportion indirect
All women			
Placental malaria only	0.47 (0.25, 0.83)	0.92 (0.63, 1.25)	7%
Anaemia and placental malaria	0.45 (0.25, 0.79)	0.88 (0.60, 1.18)	10%
Malaria, anaemia and placental malaria	0.44 (0.25, 0.79)	0.87 (0.69, 1.39)	12%
Sensitivity analyses*			
Placental malaria only	0.34 (0.17, 0.79)	1.09 (0.67, 1.80)	4%
Anaemia and placental malaria	0.33 (0.17, 0.78)	1.07 (0.63, 1. 86)	4%
Malaria, anaemia and placental malaria	0.33 (0.17, 0.78)	1.06 (0. 65, 1.84)	3%

Numbers are risk ratios (95% confidence interval). Natural direct effect is the effect of iron deficiency on birth outcome, not mediated through the specified mediators. Natural indirect effect is the effect of iron deficiency on birth outcome, mediated through the specified mediator.
CI confidence interval
*Women potentially misclassified as iron deficient (ferritin > 15 and C-reactive protein > 10) are excluded from analysis ($N = 46$)

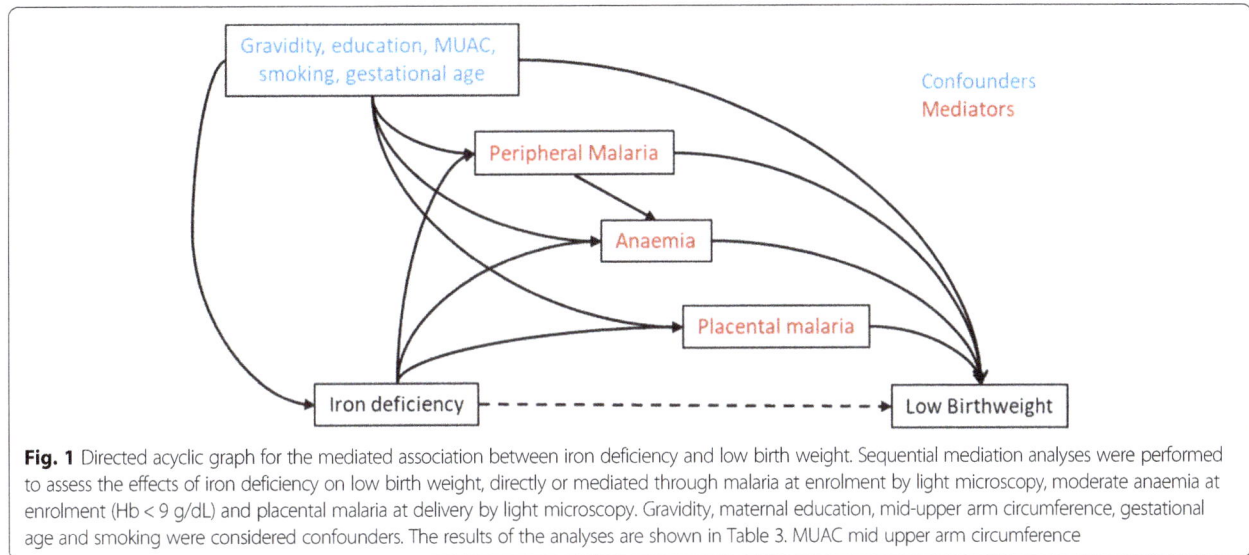

Fig. 1 Directed acyclic graph for the mediated association between iron deficiency and low birth weight. Sequential mediation analyses were performed to assess the effects of iron deficiency on low birth weight, directly or mediated through malaria at enrolment by light microscopy, moderate anaemia at enrolment (Hb < 9 g/dL) and placental malaria at delivery by light microscopy. Gravidity, maternal education, mid-upper arm circumference, gestational age and smoking were considered confounders. The results of the analyses are shown in Table 3. MUAC mid upper arm circumference

group who are more susceptible to, and more severely affected by, a range of infectious diseases [19].

We demonstrated that the associations between iron deficiency and malaria infection were confounded by the presence of an acute phase response (raised CRP). Iron deficiency was associated with reduced malaria infection when the analysis included all women. However, when women who were potentially misclassified as iron replete (ferritin> 15 but raised CRP levels) were excluded, no protective association was found. Women with malaria are more likely to have raised CRP and therefore, more likely to be misclassified as iron replete. As a result, the analyses would more likely demonstrate an apparent protective effect of iron deficiency unless these effects are considered in analyses. Previously published analyses of cross-sectional and case–control studies of associations between iron deficiency and peripheral and placental *P. falciparum* infection of women [10] have included these potentially misclassified women, which may have biased results towards finding an association between iron deficiency and reduced malaria risk, or increased the magnitude of the protective effect. There is some biological plausibility to protective associations of iron deficiency, as in vitro studies have shown that iron deficiency can limit the development of blood-stage infection by starving the parasite of exoerythrocytic forms of iron [20–23], impair merozoite invasion and propagation [24], or increase the immune-mediated clearance of infected erythrocytes [25, 26]. However, a direct causal mechanism between iron deficiency and placental malaria independent of the aforementioned reductions in peripheral infection is yet to be proposed and we found no association between iron deficiency and placental malaria in this study.

A strength of our study is that we used sequential mediation analysis as a valuable approach to estimate the contribution of potential causal relationships. This is the first analysis to quantify the mediation of the effect of iron deficiency on birth outcomes through malaria (both peripheral and placental) and anaemia. This is also the first mediation analysis of the effect of iron deficiency on birth outcomes to account for both exposure-outcome and mediator-outcome confounders, which is a source of bias in traditional mediation analysis [27]. Importantly, we found that only 12% of the protective effect of iron deficiency on LBW was mediated through malaria or anaemia. Iron deficiency was not significantly associated with anaemia or peripheral or placental malaria, which are key determinants of LBW and PTB in this population [18]. This may explain the lack of mediation through placental malaria in this cohort study and further studies using sequential mediation analyses are warranted in other populations. After accounting for mediation through peripheral *Plasmodium* spp. infection and placental *P. falciparum* infection, we found that iron deficiency was still associated directly with a >50% reduction in the odds of LBW. Host iron is essential to a range of other bacteria, parasites and viruses, and iron deficiency may also inhibit the development of these pathogens [28–30]. Therefore, reductions in infectious pathogens due to iron deficiency may explain the association between iron deficiency and improved birth outcomes in our study. In PNG, there is a high burden of disease from bacterial and viral pathogens, including respiratory, gastrointestinal and sexually transmitted infections [31], that may be influenced by iron status [30]. In PNG, a higher prevalence of these infections is also found in primigravid compared to multigravid women [32], which may also explain why larger magnitudes of the effect of iron deficiency on birth outcomes were observed in high risk primigravid women. Other infections may also be important. A recent study of iron supplementation in non-pregnant African women found higher rates of treatment for gastrointestinal infections in women receiving iron [17]. Further studies are needed to understand the mechanisms by which iron deficiency leads to improved birth weight, and this knowledge would help identify appropriate strategies to reduce LBW while also reducing the burden of iron deficiency and anaemia. Examining the effects of iron deficiency on other infectious pathogens common in pregnancy, together with their interactions with malaria and anaemia, is a priority for future studies.

This study is the first longitudinal study globally to demonstrate a temporal relationship between antenatal iron deficiency and birth outcomes, and together with the sequential mediation analyses, provides significant causal evidence for the associations observed. In PNG, malaria transmission is high and both *P. falciparum* and *P. vivax* are endemic. The majority of infections (>95%) in our study were *P. falciparum* and therefore, our findings may be more broadly applicable to other high *P. falciparum* transmission areas, such as sub-Saharan Africa. However further studies are required to determine the consistency of our findings and the effect size across areas of varying prevalence of iron deficiency, malaria and other infections and in areas where the relative contribution of the multiple factors that cause iron deficiency differs. Research that identifies populations or settings where iron deficiency associations with birth weight are strongest would be valuable in guiding public health policy. In our study, we experienced a ~40% loss to follow-up; however, given that the characteristics of the women lost to follow-up did not differ from those of the included women (Additional file 1), the loss is unlikely to have affected the internal validity of the study. While the specific causes of iron deficiency have not been defined, these are likely to include low dietary intake as well as infections such as hookworm and malaria that can impact iron absorption or utilisation.

Iron deficiency was defined according to the WHO standard definition (ferritin < 15 μg/L for non-pregnant women) [2]. Ferritin is also an acute phase protein that may increase during inflammation independently of iron stores [33]. Previous cross-sectional and case–control studies of iron deficiency and malaria in pregnancy either did not measure inflammation or reported that a proportion of women had inflammation and their reported associations may have been confounded [34, 35]. In our study, we performed sensitivity analyses to show that the protective associations observed between iron deficiency and birth weight were not confounded by the presence of inflammation. In the absence of bone marrow biopsies, ferritin remains the gold standard to assess iron deficiency [36], and although other markers of iron

deficiency have been explored, such as the soluble transferrin receptor, they currently lack established definitions for iron deficiency in pregnancy. Any potential bias associated with misclassification of true iron status with the use of ferritin for defining iron deficiency is unlikely to change the conclusions of this study given the magnitude and statistical strength of the observed associations and the biological plausibility.

Conclusions

Our findings show that iron deficiency in pregnancy is associated with a reduced risk of LBW and PTB that is not simply explained by a potential protective effect against malaria. The mechanism(s) underlying this paradox in malaria-endemic and resource-limited settings with high burdens of infectious diseases and poor nutrition are not yet well understood but are essential to elucidate given the importance and scale of this global public health issue and that LBW and PTB are important determinants of poor infant outcomes. Our results highlight that it is essential to provide both supplementation for anaemia and effective malaria prophylaxis during pregnancy, and future implementation trials to improve the uptake of these interventions as well as trials of integrated interventions for nutrition, malaria and other infections linked with LBW and PTB are warranted. Integration of screening and prophylaxis for other infectious diseases and poor nutrition, alongside current interventions in antenatal care, may be needed to achieve substantial improvements in birth and infant outcomes.

Abbreviations
aOR: Adjusted odds ratio; CI: Confidence intervals; CRP: C-reactive protein; Hb: Haemoglobin; IQR: Inter-quartile range; LBW: Low birthweight; MUAC: Mid upper arm circumference; OR: Odds Ratio; PCR: Polymerase chain reaction; PNG: Papua New Guinea; PTB: Pre-term birth; SD: Standard deviation; WHO: World Health Organization

Acknowledgements
We thank all the study participants, Francesca Baiwog and the staff of the Alexishafen Health Centre under the direction of Sister Valsi Kurian for their enthusiastic cooperation with the study, and the staff of the PNG Institute of Medical Research for assistance with microscopy, data entry and study administration.

Funding
Funding was provided by the Australian Research Council (future fellowship to FJIF), the National Health and Medical Research Council, Australia (program grant and senior research fellowship to JGB and JAS). The Burnet Institute is supported by the Independent Research Institutes Infrastructure Support Scheme of the National Health and Medical Research Council and a Victoria State Government Operational Infrastructure Support grant. Funding bodies had no role in the design of the study, the collection, analysis and interpretation of the data or in writing the manuscript.

Authors' contributions

FJIF, FL, DHO and JGB performed and interpreted the iron-deficiency assays. CLK, PMS, IM, SJR and JGB conceived and designed the cohort study. DIS and AU performed the fieldwork. FJIF, KAM and JAS analysed the data and drafted the report. All authors approved the final report.

Competing interests

The authors declare that they have no competing interests.

Author details

[1]Burnet Institute, Maternal and Child Health Program, Life Sciences and Public Health, Melbourne, VIC 3004, Australia. [2]Department of Epidemiology and Preventive Medicine, Monash University, Melbourne, VIC 3008, Australia. [3]Centre for Epidemiology and Biostatistics, Melbourne School of Population and Global Health, The University of Melbourne, Melbourne, VIC 3010, Australia. [4]Department of Infectious Diseases, Central Clinical School, Monash University, Melbourne, VIC 3004, Australia. [5]Department of Immunology, Monash University, Central Clinical School, Melbourne, VIC 3004, Australia. [6]Institute for Glycomics, Griffith University, South Brisbane, QLD 4101, Australia. [7]Papua New Guinea Institute of Medical Research, Goroka, EHP, Papua New Guinea. [8]Center for Global Health and Diseases, Case Western Reserve University, Cleveland, OH, USA. [9]Walter and Eliza Hall Institute of Medical Research, Parkville, VIC 3050, Australia. [10]Department of Parasites and Insect Vectors, Institut Pasteur, 75015 Paris, France. [11]Department of Medicine (RMH), The University of Melbourne, Parkville, VIC 3010, Australia.

References

1. Lawn JE, Cousens S, Zupan J. 4 million neonatal deaths: when? Where? Why? Lancet. 2005;365(9462):891–900.
2. WHO. Serum ferritin concentrations for the assessment of iron status and iron deficiency in populations, vol. 2011. Geneva; 2011. p. 1–5.
3. Are We Making Progress on Reducing Anemia in Women? Cross-country Comparison of Anemia Prevalence, Reach, and Use of Antenatal Care and Anemia Reduction Interventions. A2Z: The USAID Micro-nutrient and Child Blindness Project. http://www.a2zproject.org/pdf/ReducingAnemia_low_res_06212011.pdf.
4. Desai M, Kuile FO, Nosten F, Mcgready R, Asamoa K, Brabin B, Newman RD. Epidemiology and burden of malaria in pregnancy. Lancet Infect Dis. 2007;7:93–104.
5. Dellicour S, Tatem AJ, Guerra CA, Snow RW, ter Kuile FO. Quantifying the number of pregnancies at risk of malaria in 2007: a demographic study. PLoS Med. 2010;7(1):e1000221.
6. Guyatt HL, Snow RW. Impact of malaria during pregnancy on low birth weight in sub-Saharan Africa. Clin Microbiol Rev. 2004;17(4):760–9. table of contents
7. Walker PG, ter Kuile FO, Garske T, Menendez C, Ghani AC. Estimated risk of placental infection and low birthweight attributable to Plasmodium falciparum malaria in Africa in 2010: a modelling study. Lancet Glob Health. 2014;2(8):e460–7.
8. WHO. Guideline: Daily iron and folic acid supplementation in pregnant women, vol. 2012. Geneva; 2012.
9. Schumann K, Solomons NW. Can iron supplementation be reconciled with benefits and risks in areas hyperendemic for malaria? Food Nutr Bull. 2013; 34(3):349–56.
10. Sangaré L, van Eijk AM, Ter Kuile FO, Walson J, Stergachis A. The association between malaria and iron status or supplementation in pregnancy: a systematic review and meta-analysis. PLoS One. 2014;9:e87743.
11. Oppenheimer S, Gibson F, Macfarlane S, et al. Iron supplementation increases prevalence and effects of malaria: report on clinical studies in Papua New Guinea. Trans R Soc Trop Med Hyg. 1986;80:603–12.
12. Sazawal S, Black RE, Ramsan M, Chwaya HM, Stoltzfus RJ, Dutta A, Dhingra U, Kabole I, Deb S, Othman MK, et al. Effects of routine prophylactic supplementation with iron and folic acid on admission to hospital and mortality in preschool children in a high malaria transmission setting: community-based, randomised, placebo-controlled trial. Lancet. 2006; 367:133–43.
13. Mwangi MN, Roth JM, Smit MR, Trijsburg L, Mwangi AM, Demir AY, Wielders JP, Mens PF, Verweij JJ, Cox SE, et al. Effect of daily antenatal Iron supplementation on Plasmodium infection in Kenyan women: a randomized clinical trial. JAMA. 2015;314(10):1009–20.
14. Etheredge AJ, Premji Z, Gunaratna NS, Abioye AI, Aboud S, Duggan C, Mongi R, Meloney L, Spiegelman D, Roberts D, et al. Iron supplementation in Iron-replete and nonanemic pregnant women in Tanzania: a randomized clinical trial. JAMA Pediatr. 2015;169(10):947–55.
15. Pena-Rosas JP, De-Regil LM, Garcia-Casal MN, Dowswell T. Daily oral iron supplementation during pregnancy. Cochrane Database Syst Rev. 2015;7: CD004736.
16. Pena-Rosas JP, De-Regil LM, Gomez Malave H, Flores-Urrutia MC, Dowswell T. Intermittent oral iron supplementation during pregnancy. Cochrane Database Syst Rev. 2015;10:Cd009997.
17. Brabin L, Roberts SA, Gies S, Nelson A, Diallo S, Stewart CJ, Kazienga A, Birtles J, Ouedraogo S, Claeys Y, et al. Effects of long-term weekly iron and folic acid supplementation on lower genital tract infection - a double blind, randomised controlled trial in Burkina Faso. BMC Med. 2017;15(1):206.
18. Stanisic DI, Moore KA, Baiwog F, Ura A, Clapham C, King CL, Siba PM, Beeson JG, Mueller I, Fowkes FJ, et al. Risk factors for malaria and adverse birth outcomes in a prospective cohort of pregnant women resident in a high malaria transmission area of Papua New Guinea. Trans R Soc Trop Med Hyg. 2015;109(5):313–24.
19. Jamieson DJ, Theiler RN, Rasmussen SA. Emerging infections and pregnancy. Emerg Infect Dis. 2006;12(11):1638–43.
20. Raventos-Suarez C, Pollack S, Nagel RL. Plasmodium falciparum: inhibition of in vitro growth by desferrioxamine. Am J Trop Med Hyg. 1982;31(5):919–22.
21. Ferrer P, Tripathi AK, Clark MA, Hand CC, Rienhoff HY Jr, Sullivan DJ Jr. Antimalarial iron chelator, FBS0701, shows asexual and gametocyte Plasmodium falciparum activity and single oral dose cure in a murine malaria model. PLoS One. 2012;7(5):e37171.
22. Pollack S. Effects of iron and desferrioxamine on the growth of Plasmodium falciparum in vitro. Br J Haematol. 1987;65(2):256–7.
23. Pollack S, Rossan RN, Davidson DE, Escajadillo A. Desferrioxamine suppresses Plasmodium falciparum in Aotus monkeys. Proc Soc Exp Biol Med. 1987; 184(2):162–4.
24. Clark MA, Goheen MM, Fulford A, Prentice AM, Elnagheeb MA, Patel J, Fisher N, Taylor SM, Kasthuri RS, Cerami C. Host iron status and iron supplementation mediate susceptibility to erythrocytic stage Plasmodium falciparum. Nat Commun. 2014;5:4446.
25. Matsuzaki-Moriya C, Tu L, Ishida H, Imai T, Suzue K, Hirai M, Tetsutani K, Hamano S, Shimokawa C, Hisaeda H. A critical role for phagocytosis in resistance to malaria in iron-deficient mice. Eur J Immunol. 2011;41(5):1365–75.
26. Weiss G, Werner-Felmayer G, Werner ER, Grunewald K, Wachter H, Hentze MW. Iron regulates nitric oxide synthase activity by controlling nuclear transcription. J Exp Med. 1994;180(3):969–76.
27. Richiardi L, Bellocco R, Zugna D. Mediation analysis in epidemiology: methods, interpretation and bias. Int J Epidemiol. 2013;42(5):1511–9.
28. Skaar EP. The battle for iron between bacterial pathogens and their vertebrate hosts. PLoS Pathog. 2010;6(8):e1000949.
29. Noinaj N, Buchanan SK, Cornelissen CN. The transferrin-iron import system from pathogenic Neisseria species. Mol Microbiol. 2012;86(2): 246–57.
30. Cross JH, Bradbury RS, Fulford AJ, Jallow AT, Wegmuller R, Prentice AM, Cerami C. Oral iron acutely elevates bacterial growth in human serum. Sci Rep. 2015;5:16670.

31. Vallely A, Page A, Dias S, Siba P, Lupiwa T, Law G, Millan J, Wilson DP,
     Murray JM, Toole M, et al. The prevalence of sexually transmitted infections
     in Papua New Guinea: a systematic review and meta-analysis. PLoS One.
     2010;5(12):e15586.
32. Vallely LM, Toliman P, Ryan C, Rai G, Wapling J, Tomado C, Huliafi S,
     Munnull G, Rarau P, Phuanukoonnon S, et al. Prevalence and risk factors of
     chlamydia trachomatis, Neisseria gonorrhoeae, trichomonas vaginalis and
     other sexually transmissible infections among women attending antenatal
     clinics in three provinces in Papua New Guinea: a cross-sectional survey. Sex
     Health. 2016;13(5):420–7.
33. Gabay C, Kushner I. Acute-phase proteins and other systemic responses to
     inflammation. N Engl J Med. 1999;340(6):448–54.
34. Senga EL, Harper G, Koshy G, Kazembe PN, Brabin BJ. Reduced risk for
     placental malaria in iron deficient women. Malar J. 2011;10:47.
35. Kabyemela ER, Fried M, Kurtis JD, Mutabingwa TK, Duffy PE. Decreased
     susceptibility to Plasmodium falciparum infection in pregnant women with
     Iron deficiency. J Infect Dis. 2008;198:163–6.
36. Wheeler S. Assessment and interpretation of micronutrient status during
     pregnancy. Proc Nutr Soc. 2008;67(4):437–50.

8

Infectious disease testing of UK-bound refugees

Alison F. Crawshaw[1], Manish Pareek[2], John Were[1], Steffen Schillinger[3], Olga Gorbacheva[4], Kolitha P. Wickramage[3], Sema Mandal[5], Valerie Delpech[6], Noel Gill[6], Hilary Kirkbride[1] and Dominik Zenner[7,8*] (iD)

Abstract

Background: The UK, like a number of other countries, has a refugee resettlement programme. External factors, such as higher prevalence of infectious diseases in the country of origin and circumstances of travel, are likely to increase the infectious disease risk of refugees, but published data is scarce. The International Organization for Migration carries out and collates data on standardised pre-entry health assessments (HA), including testing for infectious diseases, on all UK refugee applicants as part of the resettlement programme. From this data, we report the yield of selected infectious diseases (tuberculosis (TB), HIV, syphilis, hepatitis B and hepatitis C) and key risk factors with the aim of informing public health policy.

Methods: We examined a large cohort of refugees ($n = 18,418$) who underwent a comprehensive pre-entry HA between March 2013 and August 2017. We calculated yields of infectious diseases stratified by nationality and compared these with published (mostly WHO) estimates. We assessed factors associated with case positivity in univariable and multivariable logistic regression analysis.

Results: The number of refugees included in the analysis varied by disease (range 8506–9759). Overall yields were notably high for hepatitis B (188 cases; 2.04%, 95% CI 1.77–2.35%), while yields were below 1% for active TB (9 cases; 92 per 100,000, 48–177), HIV (31 cases; 0.4%, 0.3–0.5%), syphilis (23 cases; 0.24%, 0.15–0.36%) and hepatitis C (38 cases; 0.41%, 0.30–0.57%), and varied widely by nationality. In multivariable analysis, sub-Saharan African nationality was a risk factor for several infections (HIV: OR 51.72, 20.67–129.39; syphilis: OR 4.24, 1.21–24.82; hepatitis B: OR 4.37, 2.91–6.41). Hepatitis B (OR 2.23, 1.05–4.76) and hepatitis C (OR 5.19, 1.70–15.88) were associated with history of blood transfusion. Syphilis (OR 3.27, 1.07–9.95) was associated with history of torture, whereas HIV (OR 1521.54, 342.76–6754.23) and hepatitis B (OR 7.65, 2.33–25.18) were associated with sexually transmitted infection. Syphilis was associated with HIV (OR 10.27, 1.30–81.40).

Conclusions: Testing refugees in an overseas setting through a systematic HA identified patients with a range of infectious diseases. Our results reflect similar patterns found in other programmes and indicate that the yields for infectious diseases vary by region and nationality. This information may help in designing a more targeted approach to testing, which has already started in the UK programme. Further work is needed to refine how best to identify infections in refugees, taking these factors into account.

Keywords: Refugees, Refugee health, Health assessment, Infectious diseases, Migrant health

* Correspondence: dominik.zenner@ucl.ac.uk
[7]TB Screening Unit, National Infection Service, Public Health England, 61 Colindale Avenue, London NW9 5EQ, UK
[8]Institute for Global Health, Faculty of Population Health Sciences, University College London, Gower Street, London WC1E 6BT, UK
Full list of author information is available at the end of the article

Background

International migration has increased significantly (by 41%) since 2000. In 2015, it was estimated that there were 244 million international migrants globally, the majority (151 million) with destination countries in Europe and Asia [1]. In many recipient countries, international migration is becoming an increasingly important determinant of population change. For instance, in January 2016, it was estimated that 35 million residents (approximately 6.9% of the European Union (EU) population) in the EU were born outside of the EU, in addition to 19.3 million persons who were living in a different EU Member State from the one in which they were born [2, 3]. Forcible displacement, as a result of conflict, persecution, violence or human rights violations, has also reached a record-high, with an estimated 21.3 million refugees globally in 2015; an increase of 55% since year-end 2001. This is largely attributable to the ongoing civil conflict in the Syrian Arab Republic [4].

A number of countries have official resettlement programmes for refugees, including the USA, Canada, Australia, New Zealand, the UK and many others [5–7]. The UK government accepts refugees under four different schemes, namely the Gateway Protection Programme, the Mandate Resettlement Scheme, the Syrian Vulnerable Persons Resettlement Scheme (VPRS) and the Vulnerable Children Resettlement Scheme (VCRS) (hereafter collectively the 'UK programme'). The Gateway Protection Programme has committed to resettle approximately 750 refugees per year on the basis of their refugee status and need for resettlement [8]. The Mandate Resettlement Scheme is much smaller, and applicable only to individuals who have been granted refugee status by the United Nations High Commissioner for Refugees (UNHCR) and who have close ties[1] to the UK. The VPRS and VCRS, on the other hand, represent specific resettlement schemes that the UK has devised to offer protection to people on a larger scale in times of crisis [9]. For this reason, and due to its recent rapid expansion, the VPRS is probably the most high-profile of the UK schemes.

The VPRS was established by the UK Government in January 2014 in response to the Syrian crisis [10]. It aims to enable vulnerable Syrians and other nationalities affected by the conflict to settle in the UK, prioritising those who meet the UNHCR vulnerability criteria, including women and children at risk, survivors of violence or torture, refugees with legal or physical protection needs, medical needs or disabilities, children and adolescents at risk, and refugees with family links in resettlement countries [10]. Initially small, and with no fixed quota, it has increased in prominence following a pledge by the UK Government in September 2015 to resettle up to 20,000 people from the Syrian region by 2020 [11]. This has attracted heightened media coverage

and public interest (Additional file 1: Appendix III).[2] Subsequently, the VCRS was established in January 2016 to support and resettle up to 3000 vulnerable and refugee children and their families affected by the conflict [12]. As of the last quarter of 2016, 20,878 refugees had been resettled through the entire UK programme [13].

Under these schemes,[3] refugees are referred by the UNHCR and reviewed by UK authorities for resettlement in the UK. Prior to departure, a detailed health assessment (HA) is performed by the International Organization for Migration (IOM). The aim of the HA is to facilitate early integration of the refugee, promoting individual health, protecting public health where relevant and linking individual needs with appropriate health and social services in the UK. The UK HA protocol has recently been reviewed and updated with this in mind, to align it more closely with UK public health policy and best practice [14]. The components of the HA are briefly outlined in Table 1.

There is evidence that most migrants in Europe, at least initially, are relatively healthy compared to the host population, although migrants do face specific health challenges and may experience a deterioration in health over time in the host country [15, 16]. It is possible that refugees, including those resettled through international resettlement schemes, may be at slightly higher risk of infectious diseases due to a higher prevalence of these diseases in their country of origin, specific circumstances of their residency and travel, and programme selection criteria which favour vulnerable migrants. However, there is limited information available on the exact epidemiology of infectious diseases in these groups. Therefore, there is a need to analyse these data and compare

Table 1 Components of the standardised pre-entry health assessment for refugee applicants

Standardised pre-entry health assessment components	
General assessment	Medical history
	Physical examination (vital signs, assessment of systems, oral and dental examination, skin examination, developmental milestones for children)
	Routine laboratory and radiological examinations, including urinalysis and chest x-ray
Testing for specific conditions	Tuberculosis (according to the UK tuberculosis technical instructions [38]) HIV Syphilis Other sexually transmitted infections Hepatitis B and C Helminthic infection (as appropriate, according to protocol) Malaria (as appropriate, according to protocol)
Immunisation	According to the UK immunisation schedule [39]
Additional clinical assessments	Relating to other chronic, physical, psychosocial or mental health issues, as appropriate

them with other sources of prevalence figures to ensure that appropriate public health measures, including HA, can be applied to these population groups most at risk and that individuals can be thus linked early to appropriate healthcare services in the UK.

This paper aims to analyse and describe, for the first time, data on the prevalence of all infectious diseases (tuberculosis (TB), HIV, syphilis, hepatitis B and hepatitis C) from a large cohort of refugees who underwent comprehensive pre-entry health assessments as part of the UK resettlement programme. It compares the recorded prevalence against published estimates in order to assess whether moving to risk-based testing would be feasible.

Methods

Study design, participants and consent

We undertook a population-based cross-sectional study of all refugees included in the UK programme ($n = 18,418$) who had a complete HA conducted by IOM between March 2013 and August 2017. Applicants whose HA was not completed were excluded ($n = 686$). Additional exclusion criteria were applied during analysis (Fig. 1). In general, the subjects included versus those excluded were similar in their demographic characteristics (Additional file 1: Appendix IV). The reporting of this study conforms to the STROBE statement (Additional file 1: Appendix V). As part of the testing process, applicants consented for their data to be used by the relevant UK authorities and agencies.

Data sources

Data were collected from all 22 IOM clinics enrolled in the UK pre-entry migration HAs in 14 countries,

according to a standardised pro forma.[4] Laboratory/radiology services were performed by IOM or contracted providers where local clinic capacity did not permit carrying out these services in house.

Data were entered directly into the electronic form by the examining physician/nurse at the time of examination, and any additional hand-written notes incorporated into qualitative fields. All information was entered into the medical module of IOM's electronic database system, the Migrant Management Operational System Application (MiMOSA), which has a set of data validation rules in place, and further data validation was done by the IOM medical department using statistical and database functions. Data was saved as a transactional database using the Microsoft SQL Server.

Data were extracted for the current study on demographics (sex, age, nationality, country of examination, position in family) and infectious disease testing results (HIV serology, syphilis testing, other sexually transmitted infection (STI) testing, TB chest x-ray, TB clinical signs and symptoms, TB culture, TB smear, hepatitis B serology (hepatitis B surface antigen and any additional markers) and hepatitis C serology (hepatitis C antibody, anti-hepatitis C antibody, and hepatitis C virus RNA)). All cases were classified using pre-defined case definitions and further corroborated against the physician's notes and/or laboratory notes to ensure rigour. Active TB cases were identified in a two-step process. First, suspected cases were identified from clinical and radiological database variables. These were then individually verified by each IOM clinic and categorised as active TB on the basis of culture confirmation. Further

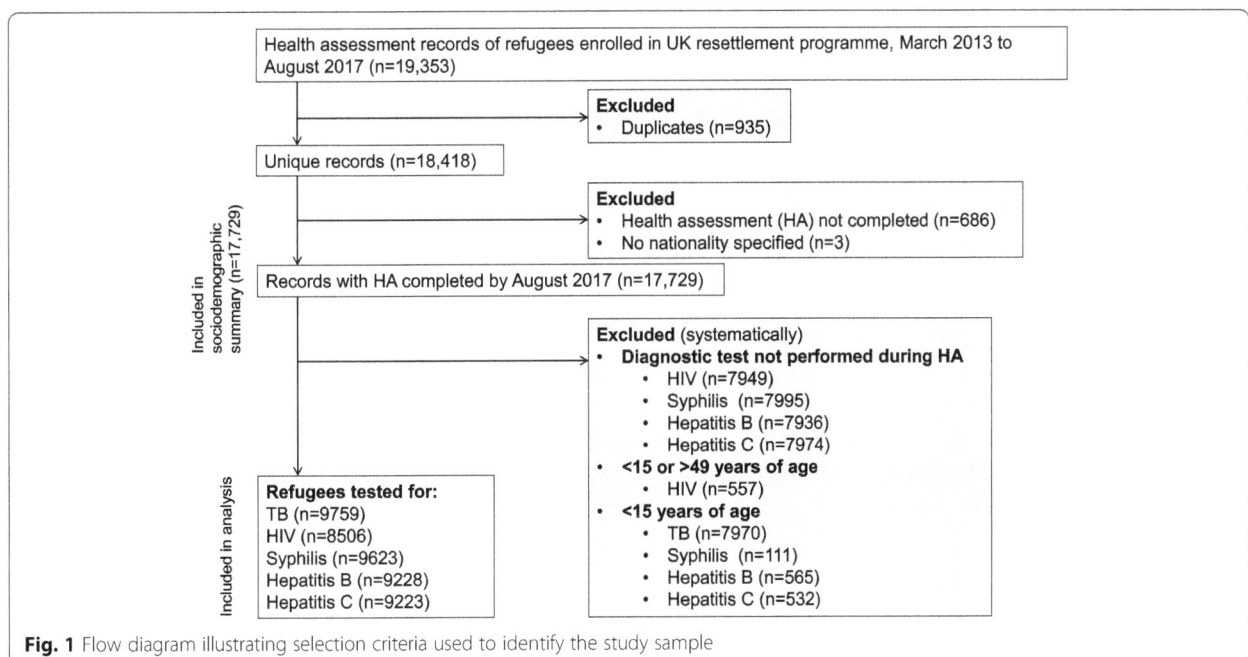

Fig. 1 Flow diagram illustrating selection criteria used to identify the study sample

information on testing cohorts and case definitions are included in Additional file 1: Appendix I.

Country-specific prevalence estimates for the infectious diseases of interest were also extracted from annual World Health Organization (WHO) country reports and/or the literature [17–22].

Data management and statistical analysis

Data cleaning and analyses were carried out using Stata version 13.1 [23]. All tests were two-tailed and p values less than 0.05 were regarded as significant. A full description of the data management, variable classifications and definitions is provided in Additional file 1: Appendix I.

Briefly, data analysis was undertaken in several steps. We first described the demographics of applicants tested, and summarised continuous data with median and interquartile range and described categorical responses as a simple descriptive percentage, with (95% confidence interval (CI)), and comparisons made using Pearson's χ^2 test.

For each of the infectious diseases of interest we calculated the absolute numbers of positive test results, the proportion positive (number of individuals testing positive divided by the number of eligible applicants tested; this was the testing yield or positivity rate of the individual diseases in the cohort), stratified by nationality.

We calculated testing yield of the different diseases, stratified by nationality, and presented these next to published disease-specific country level prevalence rates.

Univariable and multivariable logistic regression analyses were conducted to assess factors associated with case positivity. The model was built in stepwise forward fashion evaluating each variable for inclusion using likelihood ratio tests. Age, sex, world region of nationality, exam year and history of displacement were adjusted for in each multivariable model as well as additional variables specific to each outcome (Additional file 1: Appendix II). Interaction was only tested where biologically plausible. Certain variables were removed from the final model to reduce collinearity (Additional file 2: Tables S1–S5). Cluster analysis was performed to account for correlation that may occur between individuals of the same immediate family, based on their resettlement case number.[5] For TB, we restricted all analyses to confirmed cases of active TB, but repeated multivariable analysis with suspected cases (Additional file 1: Appendix VI). The limited number of events in the confirmed case analysis limits statistical certainty for that analysis.

Results

Demographics of cohort

Between March 2013 and August 2017, 18,418 applicants for resettlement in the UK were screened by IOM in clinics in 14 different countries. Of these, 17,729

(96.3%) applicants had undergone at least one complete pre-entry HA at the time of data extraction (August 2017) and were included in the analysis. The majority of applicants (16,055, 90.6%) were nationals of the WHO Eastern Mediterranean Region[6] and the African Region[7] (AFR; 1608, 9.1%), representing 29 countries. Just over half were male (51.2%) and median age was 18 years (interquartile range 7–33 years). There were 4665 (26.3%) principal applicants,[8] whilst the majority (12,943, 73.0%) of applicants were their family or dependents (defined as immediate family, i.e. spouse/civil partner, children, parents/step-parents, siblings). The mean family size was estimated at 3.8 persons.

Infectious disease yield and exposure factors identified

The number of refugees included in the yield calculation and logistic regression analysis varied by disease and ranged from 8506 to 9759 (Fig. 1). Of the five infectious diseases of interest, the most commonly identified infections were hepatitis B (188 cases out of 9228 tested). Relatively fewer cases of hepatitis C (38/9223), HIV (35/8506), syphilis (23/9623) and active TB (9/9759) were identified.

The magnitude of overall testing yields for hepatitis B (2.04%, 95 % CI 1.77–2.35%) were particularly high. Testing yields for the other infections remained under 1.0% but varied widely by nationality.

A total of 4 applicants with coinfections were identified: HIV-syphilis ($n = 2$) and HIV-hepatitis B ($n = 2$). No applicant had more than 2 concurrent infections.

Active TB

Of 9 active TB cases, 6 (67%) were male and 7 (78%) were aged 25–49. Cases came from the Democratic Republic of Congo (DRC), Ethiopia, Somalia and Syria. The total testing yield for active TB was 92 (95% CI 48–177) cases per 100,000 but varied widely by nationality from 42 (13–129) per 100,000 for Syria to 526 (170–1621) per 100,000 for DRC. The testing yields in this study were relatively consistent with WHO prevalence rates (last available data 2014) for those nationalities with positive cases; however, a number of nationalities of countries with high TB prevalence also yielded zero positive cases, mostly because of low screening throughput (Table 2).

Additional file 2: Table S1 presents details of the univariable and multivariable regression analyses for active TB ($n = 9$). On multivariable analysis, the adjusted odds of active TB remained significantly higher for applicants who had a past history of TB infection (adjusted odds ratio (aOR) 145.53, 95% CI 25.99–814.84, $p < 0.001$) after adjusting for age, sex, WHO region of nationality, year of examination and history of displacement. The confirmed case analysis was limited by the low number of events for some variables, so we carried out an additional analysis with suspected cases ($n = 134$)

Table 2 Active tuberculosis (TB) yield per 100,000 population among tested applicants compared to WHO country TB prevalence estimates per 100,000 population (reference year 2014), by country of nationality

Country of nationality	Number screened (n)	Number of cases detected (%)	TB yield per 100,000 among tested applicants (95% CI)[a]	WHO country prevalence per 100,000 (95% CI), 2014 reference year [22]
Afghanistan	63	0	0	340 (178–555)
Democratic Republic of Congo	570	3 (0.53)	526 (170–1621)	532 (282–859)
Eritrea	59	0	0	123 (63–203)
Ethiopia	290	1 (0.34)	345 (48–2414)	200 (161–243)
Iran	15	0	0	33 (17–55)
Iraq	540	0	0	67 (35–111)
Palestine	28	0	0	N/A
Somalia	562	2 (0.36)	356 (89–1413)	491 (254–805)
South Sudan	40	0	0	319 (139–572)
Sudan	369	0	0	151 (67–267)
Syria	7195	3 (0.04)	41 (13–129)	19 (6.2–39)
Uganda	2	0	0	159 (87–253)
Other AFR[b]	8	0	0	
Other EMR[c]	9	0	0	
Other EUR[d]	5	0	0	
Other[e]	4	0	0	
Total	9759	9 (0.09)	92 (48–177)	

[a]TB yield was calculated on adults aged > 15 for ethical reasons and consistency
[b]Other AFR included Burundi, Congo, Rwanda, Cameroon, Nigeria
[c]Other EMR included Jordan, Lebanon, Djibouti, Yemen, Pakistan
[d]Other EUR included UK, St Helena, Switzerland, Turkey
[e]Other included Solomon Islands, China, Taiwan or applicants with no nationality specified
CI confidence interval

(Additional file 1: Appendix VI). This showed similar findings, albeit with slightly changed effect sizes (notably, aORs of suspected TB were significantly higher with increasing age and among applicants who were examined in 2014, had past history of TB and had a household member with history of TB).

HIV

Of 35 HIV cases, 7 (20%) were male and 31 (89%) cases were aged between 15 and 49 years. The overall HIV positivity rate among adults aged 15–49 years was 0.36% (0.25%–0.50%). The rate ranged by nationality, from 0.6% (0.2%–1.8%) among nationals from Somalia to 3.6% (2.3%–5.6%) among nationals from the DRC. Compared to WHO prevalence estimates, rates were generally higher (by up to 5 times among DRC nationals) (Table 3).

On multivariable analysis, those who remained with significantly higher odds of being HIV positive included women from the AFR region (aOR 51.72, 95% CI 20.67–129.39, $p < 0.001$), aged 35–49 (5.76, 2.05–16.22, $p = 0.001$) and with past history of STI (aOR 1521.54, 342.76–6754.23, $p < 0.001$). Those who remained with significantly lower odds of HIV included males (0.18, 0.07–0.50, $p = 0.001$) who were examined in 2014–2016

(2014: 0.11, 0.02–0.55, $p = 0.007$; 2015: 0.28, 0.08–0.97, $p = 0.043$; 2016: 0.35, 0.13–0.97, $p = 0.043$) (Additional file 2: Table S2).

Syphilis

Of 23 cases, 14 (61%) were male and 18 (78%) were aged between 15 and 49 years. The overall syphilis testing yield among adults aged 15 years and older was 0.24% (0.15–0.36%). The lowest non-zero yield was among Syrian nationals at 0.06% (0.02–0.15%) and the highest yield 3.33% (1.90–5.78%) among Sudanese nationals. Yields were generally lower in the screened cohort compared to WHO country prevalence estimates (Table 4).

In the multivariable analysis, those who remained at significantly higher odds for syphilis included those from AFR (aOR 4.24, 95% CI 1.21–24.82, $p = 0.024$), 35 years of age and older (35–49 years: 11.97, 1.45–99.22, $p = 0.021$; 50+ years: 12.15, 1.38–106.65, $p = 0.024$), HIV positive (10.27, 1.30–81.40, $p = 0.027$) and with a history of torture (3.27, 1.07–9.95, $p = 0.037$). Those examined in 2015–2016 remained at significantly lower odds for syphilis (2015: 0.15, 0.03–0.86, $p = 0.033$; 2016: 0.26, 0.09–0.72, $p = 0.009$) (Additional file 2: Table S3).

Table 3 HIV yield (%)[a] among tested applicants aged 15–49 years, compared to WHO country HIV prevalence estimates (%) in adults aged 15–49 years (reference year 2016), by nationality

Country of nationality	Number screened (n)	Number of cases detected (%)	HIV positivity rate in 15–49 year olds in tested cohort, % (95% CI	Estimated country prevalence, 15–49 year olds, 2016, % (95% CI) [18]
Afghanistan	56	0	0.0	< 0.1 (< 0.1 to < 0.1)
Democratic Republic of Congo	504	18 (3.57)	3.6 (2.3–5.6)	0.7 (0.6–0.9)
Eritrea	52	0	0.0	0.6 (0.4–0.9)
Ethiopia	259	4 (1.54)	1.5 (0.6–4.0)	1.1 (0.8–1.3)
Iran	14	0	0.0	0.1 (< 0.1–0.2)
Iraq	462	1	0.0	No data
Palestine	25	0	0.0	No data
Somalia	499	3 (0.60)	0.6 (0.2–1.8)	0.4 (0.2–0.5)
South Sudan	35	0	0.0	2.7 (1.7–4.0)
Sudan	329	5 (1.52)	1.5 (0.6–3.6)	0.2 (0.1–0.4)
Syria	6245	0	0.0	No data
Uganda	1	0	0.0	6.5 (6.1–7.0)
Other AFR[b]	8	0	0.0	4.2 (3.7–4.8)[f]
Other EMR[c]	8	0	0.0	0.1 (< 0.1–0.2)[f]
Other EUR[d]	4	0	0.0	0.4 (0.4–0.4)[f]
Other WPR[e]	4	0	0.0	0.1 (< 0.1–0.2)
Total	8506	31 (0.36)	0.4 (0.3–0.5)	

[a] HIV yield was calculated on adults aged 15–49 for ethical reasons and for ease of comparison to reference ranges from WHO
[b] Other AFR included Burundi, Congo, Rwanda, Cameroon, Nigeria
[c] Other EMR included Jordan, Lebanon, Djibouti, Yemen, Pakistan
[d] Other EUR included UK, St Helena, Switzerland, Turkey
[e] Other WPR included Solomon Islands, China, Taiwan or applicants with no nationality specified
[f] Regional prevalence comparisons for AFR, EMR, EUR and WPR are based on estimates from WHO Member States
CI confidence interval

Hepatitis B

Of 188 cases of hepatitis B, 130 (69%) were male and 132 (70%) were aged between 25 and 49 years. The overall testing yield for hepatitis B was 2.04% (1.77%–2.35%) and ranged by nationality from 0.58% (0.19%–1.79%) for Iraq to 12.50% (5.24%–26.96%) for South Sudan. Testing yields from Somali, Sudanese and Syrian nationals were lower than the available WHO estimates (Table 5).

Those who remained at significantly higher odds for hepatitis B in the multivariable analysis included men (aOR 2.66, 95% CI 1.92–3.69, $p < 0.001$), aged 25 years and older (25–34 years: 2.83, 1.69–4.77, $p < 0.001$; 35–49 years: 3.86, 2.32–6.41, $p < 0.001$; 50+: 4.07, 2.34–7.09, $p < 0.001$), from AFR (4.37, 2.91–6.55, $p < 0.001$), with a history of STI (7.65, 2.33–25.18, $p = 0.001$) and blood transfusion (2.23, 1.05–4.76, $p = 0.038$) (Additional file 2: Table S4).

Hepatitis C

Of 38 cases of hepatitis C, 19 (50%) were male and 17 (45%) were aged 50 years and over. The overall testing yield for hepatitis C was 0.41% (0.30%–0.57%) and ranged by nationality from 0.26% (0.04–1.84%) for Somalia to 7.14% (0.92–38.84%) for Iran (Table 6).

Table 3 presents details of the univariable and multivariable regression analysis for hepatitis C. In the multivariable analysis, applicants aged 50 and older (6.71, 2.67–16.87, $p < 0.001$) with a history of blood transfusion (5.19, 1.70–15.88, $p = 0.004$) remained at significantly higher odds for hepatitis C infection (Additional file 2: Table S5).

Discussion

This is the first study which reports on, and compares findings of, medical HAs for infectious diseases among a UK-bound refugee population. We found higher diagnostic yields than expected for a number of diseases, including hepatitis B.

For TB, testing yields broadly mirror WHO-estimated prevalence figures [24]. The UK programme is particularly focussed on resettlement of vulnerable refugees and, whilst the possibility of testing bias cannot be ruled out (see below), it is likely this refugee population significantly differs from the general population of the respective country. In addition, the limitations of WHO prevalence estimates have been well recognised [25] even in politically stable countries, and these limitations may be increased by political unrest present in many of the sender countries [26].

Table 4 Syphilis yield (%)[a] in tested applicants ≥15 years of age compared to WHO syphilis seropositivity among antenatal care attendees, by country of nationality (reference year 2015 unless otherwise stated)

Country of nationality	Number screened (n)	Number of cases detected (%)	Yield in tested cohort, % (95% CI)	Syphilis seropositivity among antenatal care attendees, 2015, % [17][b]
Afghanistan	60	0	0.0	0.6
Democratic Republic of Congo	570	2 (0.35)	0.35 (0.09–1.39)	1.9
Eritrea	55	0	0.0	0.6
Ethiopia	277	3 (1.08)	1.08 (0.35–3.31)	1.1
Iran	15	0	0.0	0.0[g]
Iraq	538	1 (0.19)	0.19 (0.03–1.31)	0.0[h]
Palestine	28	0	0.0	N/A
Somalia	554	0	0.0	5.9
South Sudan	39	1 (2.56)	2.56 (0.35–16.44)	5.6[i]
Sudan	360	12 (3.33)	3.33 (1.90–5.78)	2.3
Syria	7100	4 (0.06)	0.06 (0.02–0.15)	N/A
Uganda	1	0	0.0	6.4
Other AFR[c]	8	0	0.0	
Other EMR[d]	9	0	0.0	
Other EUR[e]	5	0	0.0	
Other WPR[f]	4	0	0.0	
Total	9623	23 (0.24)	0.24 (0.15–0.36)	

[a]Syphilis yield was calculated on adults aged 15 years and older, for ethical reasons and for ease of comparison to reference ranges from WHO
[b]No confidence intervals provided for WHO data
[c]Other AFR included Burundi, Congo, Rwanda, Cameroon, Nigeria
[d]Other EMR included Jordan, Lebanon, Djibouti, Yemen, Pakistan
[e]Other EUR included UK, St Helena, Switzerland, Turkey
[f]Other WPR included Solomon Islands, China, Taiwan or applicants with no nationality specified
[g]2011 data
[h]2010 data
[i]2013 data
CI confidence interval

TB testing results among refugees have been highly variable. Active TB yields for German-bound Syrian asylum seekers range between 93 and 153 per 100,000 [27, 28], with some authors estimating significantly higher estimates [29]. However, other countries found significantly lower yields, as illustrated by the Dutch (22 per 100,000) [30]. Where reported in comparable pre-entry testing programmes, refugees tend to have higher TB testing yield than other migrants [5].

In our analysis of confirmed cases of TB, we demonstrated an association between active TB disease and history of TB. This is not unexpected and could reflect recurrence or reinfection and the larger proportion of cases in this cohort that came from high TB burden countries, who may have been previously exposed to TB or not completed treatment. Based on the analysis of suspected cases (Additional file 1: Appendix VI), there is additional evidence that a number of other factors may be associated with TB, including increasing age and the presence of previous household contact with TB cases. Whilst these are largely expected findings [31], they are important to help inform testing policy and guide clinical practice on the ground.

As with TB, HIV prevalence rates generally mirrored WHO figures, although we found that overall yields were higher than those that would be predicted by WHO figures. This may reflect a more vulnerable, high-risk population than expected based on the resettlement criteria of the UK programme. Among refugees from DRC, for example, HIV testing yield was five times higher than the WHO prevalence estimate, at 3.6% (2.3–5.6%) compared to the WHO estimate of 0.7% (0.6–0.9%). Overall, however, the prevalence of HIV was still relatively low (0.3%) but varied significantly between countries. Sub-Saharan African countries accounted for the majority of cases of HIV infection in this cohort, reflecting the higher prevalence rates of HIV in this region. On the other hand, the generally low prevalence seen among refugees from the Eastern Mediterranean region compared to those from sub-Saharan Africa suggests a potential practical advantage of applying a risk algorithm for determining which individuals should be tested.

Our analysis identified a number of factors, both demographic and behavioural, which increased the odds of HIV infection, including being female between the

Table 5 Hepatitis B yield (%) in tested applicants compared to estimated prevalence of chronic HBV infection (reference years 1965–2013), by country of nationality

Country of nationality	Number screened (n)	Number of cases detected	Yield in tested cohort, % (95% CI)[a]	Estimated prevalence of chronic HBV infection (HBsAg seroprevalence), 1965–2013, % (95% CI) [21]
Afghanistan	57	1	1.75 (0.24–11.61)	1.62 (1.29–2.03)
Democratic Republic of Congo	499	29	5.81 (4.07–8.24)	5.99 (5.68–6.31)
Eritrea	54	0	0.0	2.49 (2.32–2.67)
Ethiopia	251	12	4.78 (2.73–8.24)	6.03 (5.77–6.31)
Iran	14	0	0.0	0.96 (0.95–0.96)
Iraq	514	3	0.58 (0.19–1.79)	0.67 (0.65–0.70)
Palestine	28	0	0.0	1.80 (1.07–3.02)
Somalia	384	13	3.39 (1.97–5.75)	14.77 (13.77–15.84)
South Sudan	40	5	12.50 (5.24–26.96)	22.38 (20.10–24.84)
Sudan	361	21	5.82 (3.82–8.76)	9.76 (9.03–10.54)
Syria	6996	102	1.46 (1.20–1.77)	2.62 (2.17–3.17)
Uganda	2	0	0.0	9.19 (8.65–9.77)
Other AFR[b]	8	1	12.50 (1.50–57.31)	8.83 (8.82–8.83)
Other EMR[c]	9	0	0.0	3.01 (3.01–3.01)
Other EUR[d]	5	1	20.00 (2.11–74.35)	2.06 (2.06–2.06)
Other WPR[e]	3	0	0.0	5.26 (5.26–5.26)
Total	9228	188	2.04 (1.77–2.35)	

[a]Yield was calculated on adults aged 15 years and older, for ethical reasons and consistency
[b]Other AFR included Burundi, Congo, Rwanda, Cameroon, Nigeria
[c]Other EMR included Jordan, Lebanon, Djibouti, Yemen, Pakistan
[d]Other EUR included UK, St Helena, Switzerland, Turkey
[e]Other WPR included Solomon Islands, China, Taiwan or applicants with no nationality specified
CI confidence interval

ages of 35–49, of sub-Saharan African nationality and with a history of STI. The increased vulnerability of women to HIV infection stemming from biological, social, behavioural and structural risk factors is well recognised [32, 33]. The finding of syphilis being associated with a reported history of torture is interesting, however perhaps not surprising given that more than half (12/23; 5 female, 7 male) of syphilis cases are from Sudan, where experiences of torture were generally more prevalent (reported in 21.43% of Sudanese applicants). The higher odds of syphilis among individuals with HIV are not unexpected and again reflect the biological mechanisms and similar risk factors which facilitate transmission.

A large number of refugees were identified to have hepatitis B infection in this cohort. Overall prevalence was over 2% but, as with other infections, we found that prevalence varied substantially between countries and with respect to WHO estimates. Whilst sub-Saharan African countries had particularly high prevalence, Syrian refugees accounted for most cases. In particular, testing yields for refugees from Somalia (3.39%, 1.97–5.75%), Sudan (5.82%, 3.82–8.76%) and South Sudan (12.50%, 5.24–26.96%) were noticeably lower compared to prevalence estimates (Table 5), which could reflect the limitations of prevalence estimates from these countries, but

also that the refugee population may be different to the general population. An additional consideration is that these countries may have WHO-recommended universal and selective hepatitis B vaccination programmes, although vaccine coverage is unlikely to be optimal in countries with fragile infrastructures and during conflicts. The disparity between observed testing yield and country prevalence estimates therefore needs to be explored further. The high yield from the other European region category (20.00%, 2.11–74.35) reflects higher rates associated with refugees from Turkey [34, 35], an intermediate endemicity country, but the low numbers are noted [36].

We demonstrated that a number of factors are associated with increased odds of hepatitis B infection, including being male, increasing age, sub-Saharan African nationality and a history of STI and blood transfusion. It is likely that male predominance may be due to adult exposures more associated with males, and should be explored further.

Hepatitis C testing yield was considerably lower (0.41%) than seen for hepatitis B, although again this varied by nationality and in comparison with prevalence estimates, likely reflecting different risk exposure. We demonstrated that the main factors associated with increased odds of hepatitis C were older age (> 50 years)

Table 6 Hepatitis C yield in tested applicants compared to country prevalence estimates, where available, by country of nationality

Country of nationality	Number screened (n)	Number of cases detected (%)	Yield in tested cohort, % (95% CI)	Estimated prevalence, % (95% CI) [19, 20][a]
Afghanistan	57	1 (1.75)	1.75 (0.24–11.61)	1.1 (0.40–1.92)
Democratic Republic of Congo	499	4 (0.80)	0.80 (0.30–2.12)	4.3 (3.2–13.7)[b]
Eritrea	54	0	0.0	N/A
Ethiopia	250	1 (0.40)	0.40 (0.06–2.79)	0.96 (0.60–1.20)
Iran	14	1 (7.14)	7.14 (0.92–38.84)	0.5 (0.20–1.00)
Iraq	517	0	0.0	0.40 (0.30–0.50)
Palestine	28	0	0.0	N/A
Somalia	382	1 (0.26)	0.26 (0.04–1.84)	N/A
South Sudan	40	0	0.0	N/A
Sudan	361	1 (0.28)	0.28 (0.04–1.94)	N/A
Syria	6994	29 (0.41)	0.41 (0.29–0.60)	2.80 (0.60–)
Uganda	2	0	0.0	N/A
Other AFR[c]	8	0	0.0	
Other EMR[d]	9	0	0.0	
Other EUR[e]	5	0	0.0	
Other WPR[f]	3	0	0.0	
Total	9223	38 (0.41)	0.41 (0.30–0.57)	

WHO regional estimates: AFR: 1.0% (0.7–1.6%); EMR: 2.3% (1.9–2.4%); EUR: 1.5% (1.2–1.5%); WPR: 0.7% (0.6–0.8%) [40]

[a]Data from Polaris Observatory HCV Collaborators, 2017 [20] unless otherwise stated. Yield was calculated on adults aged 15 years and older, for ethical reasons and consistency

[b]Data source from Gower et al. 2014 [19]

[c]Other AFR included Burundi, Congo, Rwanda, Cameroon, Nigeria

[d]Other EMR included Jordan, Lebanon, Djibouti, Yemen, Pakistan

[e]Other EUR included UK, St Helena, Switzerland, Turkey

[f]Other WPR included Solomon Islands, China, Taiwan or applicants with no nationality specified

CI confidence interval

and history of blood transfusion, yet unlike hepatitis B, there was no association with geographic region. The strong association with blood transfusion particularly among the older age groups likely reflects the lack of routine blood-borne virus testing in many low- and middle-income countries, possible iatrogenic transmission through reusing of needles and medical equipment, and potentially chronic infection in some cases. It is interesting, although not totally surprising, that illicit drug use was not reported, considering the high prevalence of this exposure in some countries; however, this is not necessarily a dominant risk factor in those countries from which the majority of screened refugees originate.

The current HA programme run by IOM undertakes a significant number of tests in this vulnerable refugee population. Our novel work highlights that prevalence of infectious diseases varies widely, raising the possibility of changing testing from a blanket modality to a more nuanced, risk-based model that targets those at highest risk. Our findings also demonstrate that refugees are not a homogeneous group and provides a baseline for further evaluation of the effectiveness of the HA in facilitating initial linkages with primary care and in the years following resettlement.

Given that the primary aim of the UK programme and HA is to facilitate early integration and linkage of the refugee to appropriate health and social services in the UK, it is important that the HA is tailored with this end goal in mind and conducted according to what is appropriate for the individual, performed with the voluntarily provided informed consent of the individual. Informed consent is a key element in the protocol [14], yet it is important to be conscious that resettlement circumstances may potentially affect the freedom of consent.

Our study benefits from a large, well completed and comprehensive dataset of UK-bound refugee testing. Nevertheless, these observational data have a number of limitations, including data recording issues with potential for incomplete data or misclassification. Whilst the dataset was not subject to the routine IOM validation process, there has been rigorous data cleaning and validation before analysis to minimise such issues and it is therefore likely that the potential for misclassification is small and occurring at random. For active TB, IOM provided a rigorous case ascertainment exercise which verified status according to culture confirmation with the attending physicians in the field for all suspected cases.

Detecting diseases depends on the availability and quality of testing sites and it is possible that this may lead to testing bias. Most diseases require confirmatory tests and we employed very robust algorithms for case definition, so any testing bias would likely lead to case under-ascertainment. We have analysed the impact of assessment site on disease prevalence and think that these effects are likely minimal. For active TB, there is a possibility of confirmed case under-ascertainment owing to the methodology used.

Detected disease yields in our study are often similar, but sometimes different compared with WHO-estimated disease prevalence. It is expected that infectious disease risk and prevalence in this refugee population is different from the general population, not least because of differences in socioeconomic circumstances, access to care and/or accommodation, including overcrowding and camp conditions, which would minimise the generalisability of our yield as disease prevalence for the specific countries. Likewise, our study population is generalisable to UK-bound refugee populations and likely to refugee populations to other destination countries with similar programmes (e.g. USA, Canada, Australia, New Zealand). However, the generalisability of our results to other migrant or asylum seeker populations is limited due to differences in epidemiological profiles, socioeconomic status and possible selection bias (e.g. due to different selection criteria of resettlement programmes). Nevertheless, our findings provide an important snapshot into infectious disease risk of UK-bound refugees and yields important lessons to inform public health measures in this vulnerable population.

The limitations in self-reporting of risk factors, particularly if potentially considered criminal or stigmatising in the country of origin, should also be considered here. Whilst the null report of illicit drug use among hepatitis C cases may be real, it could also reflect lack of disclosure in response to fear of stigma or legal implications affecting rights to resettlement.

A further limitation is that the data recorded provided disease prevalence on a select group of refugees, predominantly from Africa and the Middle East, with fewer from Asia, who may have had a different infectious disease profile.

Conclusions
Our paper compares the findings of systematic infectious disease testing within the UK refugee programme with WHO prevalence estimates and comparable testing programmes, and elicits factors associated with case positivity. Whilst the magnitude of infectious disease findings was unexpected for some diseases in some settings, most of our study corroborates findings from similar programmes [5, 7, 31]. There are a number of important lessons, most notably the geographical variation of testing yields, which

may help design a more targeted approach to testing. It is worth noting, for example, that HIV and syphilis rates tend to be very low in the Eastern Mediterranean Region, as expected on the basis of WHO rates, and this fact could help inform testing policies, which currently do not take country-level disease prevalence into consideration in their advice. The most recent iteration of the UK HA protocol [14] has made progress in this regard, tailoring testing policies for hepatitis B and C on the basis of personal risk factors and prevalence in the area of origin, which has also been suggested in the literature [37]. These findings provide evidence to potentially support a similar approach for other infectious diseases in some settings. Further evaluation of the utility of the HA in linking refugees with primary care and social services on resettlement in the UK would also be a valuable next step in informing policy. Our paper is the first exploration of such issues and further, more detailed analysis is needed to guide best practice in refugee health and infectious disease testing in particular.

Endnotes
[1]Close family members or, in some cases, history of time spent in the UK.

[2]Google searches in the UK for 'refugees' increased nearly 100-fold between March and September 2015 and peaked in September 2015 over a 5-year period, Additional file 1: Appendix III.

[3]All cases, under all UK resettlement programmes, are subject to health assessments according to UK protocol [41].

[4]Protocol jointly developed by the UK Home Office, Public Health England and IOM, and updated on an ad hoc basis, as appropriate. Most recently updated in July 2017. The data analysed in this study were collected according to pre-2015 versions of the protocol.

[5]Note that, whilst refugees with the same case number belong to the same immediate family, refugees with different case numbers may still be related. That is, they may be members of the same extended family (IOM, personal communication). It was not possible to account for correlation that may occur between individuals of the same extended family in the cluster analysis.

[6]WHO EMR: Afghanistan, Iran, Iraq, Jordan, Lebanon, Somalia, Sudan, Syria, Djibouti, Yemen, Pakistan.

[7]WHO AFR: Burundi, Congo, Democratic Republic of Congo, Eritrea, Ethiopia, Rwanda, South Sudan, Uganda, Cameroon, Nigeria.

[8]UNHCR conducts a Refugee Status Determination interview individually with each asylum seeker. According to the UNHCR Procedural Standards for Refugee Status Determination under UNHCR's mandate (2005), each accompanying adult family member/dependent should have an individual and confidential Registration Interview [42].

Additional files

Additional file 1: Supplementary material. (DOCX 69 kb)

Additional file 2: Supporting tables: logistic regression analysis. **Table S1.** Testing yield and logistic regression analysis of the TB test cohort[†] (outcome = active TB). **Table S2.** Testing yield and logistic regression analysis of the HIV test cohort[†] (outcome = HIV positive). **Table S3.** Testing yield and logistic regression analysis of the syphilis test cohort[†] (outcome = syphilis positive). **Table S4.** Testing yield and logistic regression analysis of the hepatitis B test cohort[†] (outcome= hepatitis B positive). **Table S5.** Testing yield and logistic regression analysis of the hepatitis C test cohort[†] (outcome: hepatitis C positive). (DOCX 62 kb)

Abbreviations
AFR: WHO African Region; aOR: adjusted odds ratio; CI: confidence interval; DRC: Democratic Republic of Congo; EU: European Union; HA: health assessment; HIV: Human immunodeficiency virus; IOM: International Organization for Migration; OR: odds ratio; STI: sexually transmitted infection; TB: Tuberculosis; UNHCR: United Nations High Commission for Refugees; VCRS: Vulnerable Children Resettlement Scheme; VPRS: Vulnerable Persons Resettlement Programme; WHO: World Health Organization

Funding
This study was internally funded by Public Health England. MP is supported by the National Institute for Health Research (NIHR Post-Doctoral Fellowship, Dr. Manish Pareek, PDF-2015-08-102). The views expressed in this publication are those of the authors and do not necessarily reflect those of the affiliated organisations, including Public Health England, the International Organization for Migration, the NHS, the National Institute for Health Research or the Department of Health and Social Care.

Authors' contributions
DZ conceptualised the initial hypothesis and idea for the study and provided overall supervision. AC did the data cleaning, analyses, drafted the introduction, methods and results, and prepared the manuscript for publication. DZ, MP, OG and AC agreed to case definitions and drafted the discussion and conclusions. SS supported the TB case ascertainment exercise. JW provided technical oversight to the quantitative methodology and data management process. All authors contributed to the interpretation and contextualisation of findings, and read and approved the final manuscript.

Competing interests
DZ is head of the Tuberculosis Screening Unit at Public Health England and has shared responsibilities for quality assurance within the UK pre-entry screening programme and contributes to the UK refugee programmes. SM reports funding for commissioned surveillance reports from a drug manufacturer (Gilead), outside the submitted work. MP reports an institutional grant (unrestricted) for project related to blood-borne virus testing from Gilead Sciences outside the submitted work.

Author details
[1]Travel and Migrant Health Section, National Infection Service, Public Health England, 61 Colindale Ave, London NW9 5EQ, UK. [2]Department of Infection, Immunity and Inflammation, University of Leicester, Leicester, UK. [3]International Organization for Migration (IOM), Citibank Center, 28th Floor, 8741, Paseo de Roxas, Makati, 1200 Metro Manila, Philippines. [4]International Organization for Migration (IOM), 17 Route des Morillons, 1218 Grand-Saconnex, Switzerland. [5]Immunisation, Hepatitis and Blood Safety, National Infection Service, Public Health England, 61 Colindale Ave, London NW9 5EQ, UK. [6]HIV and STI Department, National Infection Service, Public Health England, 61 Colindale Ave, London NW9 5EQ, UK. [7]TB Screening Unit, National Infection Service, Public Health England, 61 Colindale Avenue, London NW9 5EQ, UK. [8]Institute for Global Health, Faculty of Population Health Sciences, University College London, Gower Street, London WC1E 6BT, UK.

References
1. United Nations, Department of Economic and Social Affairs PD. International Migration Report 2015: Highlights. 2016. http://www.un.org/en/development/desa/population/migration/publications/migrationreport/docs/MigrationReport2015_Highlights.pdf. Accessed 25 July 2018.
2. Eurostat. Migration and Migrant Population Statistics. 2017. http://ec.europa.eu/eurostat/statistics-explained/index.php/Migration_and_migrant_population_statistics. Accessed 25 July 2018.
3. Eurostat. Population and Population Change Statistics. 2017. http://ec.europa.eu/eurostat/statistics-explained/index.php/Population_and_population_change_statistics. Accessed 25 July 2018.
4. International Organization for Migration. Global Migration Trends Factsheet. IOM's Global Migration Data Analysis Centre (GMDAC). 2015;13:45. http://gmdac.iom.int/global-migration-trends-factsheet. Accessed 25 July 2018.
5. Liu Y, Weinberg MS, Ortega LS, Painter JA, Maloney SA. Overseas screening for tuberculosis in U.S.-bound immigrants and refugees. N Engl J Med. 2009; 360:2406–15.
6. Aldridge RW, Yates TA, Zenner D, White PJ, Abubakar I, Hayward AC. Pre-entry screening programmes for tuberculosis in migrants to low-incidence countries: a systematic review and meta-analysis. Lancet Infect Dis. 2014;14:1240–9.
7. Pareek M, Baussano I, Abubakar I, Dye C, Lalvani A. Evaluation of immigrant tuberculosis screening in industrialized countries. Emerg Infect Dis. 2012;18:1422–9.
8. UK Visas and Immigration. Guidance: Gateway Protection Programme. 2010. https://www.gov.uk/government/publications/gateway-protection-programme-information-for-organisations/gateway-protection-programme. Accessed 25 July 2018.
9. Refugee Council. Refugee Resettlement: The Facts. 2017. https://www.refugeecouncil.org.uk/what_we_do/refugee_services/resettlement_programme/refugee_resettlement_the_facts. Accessed 25 July 2018.
10. UK Home Office. Syrian Vulnerable Persons Resettlement Scheme (VPRS) Guidance for Local Authorities and Partners. 2017. Available online: https://www.gov.uk/government/publications/syrian-vulnerable-person-resettlement-programme-fact-sheet. Accessed 25 July 2018.
11. National Audit Office. The Syrian Vulnerable Persons Resettlement Programme. 2016. https://www.nao.org.uk/wp-content/uploads/2016/09/The-Syrian-Vulnerable-Persons-Resettlement-programme.pdf. Accessed 25 July 2018.
12. Home Office, The Rt Hon James Brokenshire MP and RHM. New Scheme Launched to Resettle Children at Risk. 2016. https://www.gov.uk/government/news/new-scheme-launched-to-resettle-children-at-risk. Accessed 25 July 2018.
13. UK Home Office. National Statistics: Asylum. Immigration Statistics 2017. https://www.gov.uk/government/publications/immigration-statistics-october-to-december-2016/asylum#data-tables. Accessed 25 July 2018.
14. UK Visas and Immigration. Health protocol: pre-entry health assessments for UK-bound refugees. Published 18 September 2017. Available from: https://www.gov.uk/government/publications/pre-entry-health-assessments-guidance-for-uk-refugees. Accessed 25 July 2018.
15. Rechel B, Mladovsky P, Ingleby D, Mackenbach JP, McKee M. Migration and health in an increasingly diverse Europe. Lancet. 2013;381:1235–45.
16. Norredam M, Agyemang C, Hoejbjerg Hansen OK, Petersen JH, Byberg S, Krasnik A, et al. Duration of residence and disease occurrence among

refugees and family reunited immigrants: test of the "healthy migrant effect" hypothesis. Trop Med Int Heal. 2014;19:958–67. http://doi.wiley.com/10.1111/tmi.12340

17. World Health Organization. Antenatal Care Attendees who were Positive for Syphilis, Data by Country. 2016. http://apps.who.int/gho/data/node.main.A1359STI?lang=en. Accessed 25 July 2018.

18. World Health Organization. Prevalence of HIV Among Adults Aged 15–49, Estimates by Country. 2015. http://apps.who.int/gho/data/view.main.22500?lang=en. Accessed 25 July 2018.

19. Gower E, Estes C, Blach S, Razavi-Shearer K, Razavi H. Global epidemiology and genotype distribution of the hepatitis C virus infection. J Hepatol. 2014;61:S45–57.

20. Polaris Observatory HCV Collaborators. Global prevalence and genotype distribution of hepatitis C virus infection in 2015: a modelling study. Lancet Gastroenterol Hepatol. 2017;2:161–76.

21. Schweitzer A, Horn J, Mikolajczyk RT, Krause G, Ott JJ. Estimations of worldwide prevalence of chronic hepatitis B virus infection: a systematic review of data published between 1965 and 2013. Lancet. 2015;386:1546–55.

22. World Health Organization. WHO TB Prevalence Estimates. 2014. http://www.who.int/tb/country/data/download/en/. Accessed 20 Jul 2016.

23. StataCorp. Stata Statistical Software: Release 13. College Station, TX: StataCorp LP; 2013.

24. Cookson ST, Abaza H, Clarke KR, Burton A, Sabrah NA, Rumman KA, et al. Impact of and response to increased tuberculosis prevalence among Syrian refugees compared with Jordanian tuberculosis prevalence: case study of a tuberculosis public health strategy. Confl Health. 2015;9:18.

25. World Health Organization. Global Tuberculosis Report 2016. World Health Organization. 2016. Available at: http://apps.who.int/medicinedocs/documents/s23098en/s23098en.pdf. Accessed 25 July 2018.

26. Ismail SA, Abbara A, Collin SM, Orcutt M, Coutts AP, Maziak W, et al. Communicable disease surveillance and control in the context of conflict and mass displacement in Syria. Int J Infect Dis. 2016;47:15–22. https://doi.org/10.1016/j.ijid.2016.05.011.

27. Meier V, Artelt T, Cierpiol S, Gossner J, Scheithauer S. Tuberculosis in newly arrived asylum seekers: A prospective 12 month surveillance study at Friedland, Germany. Int J Hyg Environ Health. 2016;219:811–5. https://doi.org/10.1016/j.ijheh.2016.07.018.

28. Kortas AZ, Polenz J, von Hayek J, Rüdiger S, Rottbauer W, Storr U, et al. Screening for infectious diseases among asylum seekers newly arrived in Germany in 2015: a systematic single-centre analysis. Public Health. 2017;153:1–8.

29. Mockenhaupt FP, Barbre KA, Jensenius M, Larsen CS, Barnett ED, Stauffer W, et al. Profile of illness in Syrian refugees: a GeoSentinel analysis, 2013 to 2015. Euro Surveill. 2016;21:1–5.

30. de Vries G, Gerritsen RF, van Burg JL, Erkens CGM, van Hest NA, Schimmel HJ, van Dissel JT. Tuberculosis among asylum-seekers in the Netherlands: a descriptive study among the two largest groups of asylum-seekers. Ned Tijdschr Geneeskd. 2016;160:D51. https://www.ncbi.nlm.nih.gov/pubmed/26980468. Accessed 25 July 2018.

31. Aldridge RW, Zenner D, White PJ, Williamson EJ, Muzyamba MC, Dhavan P, et al. Tuberculosis in migrants moving from high-incidence to low-incidence countries : a population-based cohort study of 519 955 migrants screened before entry to England, Wales, and Northern Ireland. Lancet. 2016;388:2510–8. https://doi.org/10.1016/S0140-6736(16)31008-X.

32. Baral S, Beyrer C, Muessig K, Poteat T, Wirtz AL, Decker MR, et al. Burden of HIV among female sex workers in low-income and middle-income countries: a systematic review and meta-analysis. Lancet Infect Dis. 2012;12:538–49.

33. Scorgie F, Chersich MF, Ntaganira I, Gerbase A, Lule F, Lo Y-R. Socio-demographic characteristics and behavioral risk factors of female sex workers in sub-Saharan Africa: a systematic review. AIDS Behav. 2012;16:920–33.

34. Burgazli KM, Mericliler M, Sen C, Tuncay M, Nayir B, Sinterhauf K, et al. The prevalence of hepatitis B virus (HBV) among turkish immigrants in Germany. Eur Rev Med Pharmacol Sci. 2014;18(6):869–74. https://www.ncbi.nlm.nih.gov/pubmed/24706312. Accessed 25 July 2018.

35. Toy M, Önder FO, Wörmann T, Bozdayi AM, Schalm SW, Borsboom GJ, et al. Age- and region-specific hepatitis B prevalence in Turkey estimated using generalized linear mixed models: a systematic review. BMC Infect Dis. 2011;11:337.

36. Ay P, Torunoglu MA, Com S, Çipil Z, Mollahaliloğlu S, Erkoç Y, et al. Trends of hepatitis B notification rates in Turkey, 1990 to 2012. Euro Surveill. 2013;18(47)

37. Greenaway C, Ma AT, Kloda LA, Klein M, Cnossen S. The seroprevalence of hepatitis C antibodies in immigrants and refugees from intermediate and high endemic countries : a systematic review and meta-analysis 2015;1–19.

38. UK Visas and Immigration; The Rt Hon Mark Harper. UK Tuberculosis Technical Instructions. 2013. https://www.gov.uk/government/publications/uk-tuberculosis-technical-instructions. Accessed 25 July 2018.

39. Public Health England. Guidance: The Complete Routine Immunisation Schedule. Immunisation. 2017. https://www.gov.uk/government/publications/the-complete-routine-immunisation-schedule. Accessed 25 July 2018.

40. World Health Organization. Global hepatitis report 2017. World Health Organization. 2017. ISBN: 978-92-4-156545-5. http://www.who.int/hepatitis/publications/global-hepatitis-report2017/en/. Accessed 25 July 2018.

41. UNHCR. UNHCR Resettlement Handbook: Country chapter - United Kingdom. 2018. http://www.unhcr.org/40ee6fc04.html. Accessed 25 July 2018.

42. UNHCR. Procedural Standards for Refugee Status Determination under UNHCR' s Mandate Procedural Standards for RSD under UNHCR' s Mandate. 2005

9

Gender differences in tuberculosis treatment outcomes: a post hoc analysis of the REMoxTB study

M. E. Murphy[1][*][†], G. H. Wills[2][†], S. Murthy[1], C. Louw[3,4], A. L. C. Bateson[1], R. D. Hunt[1], T. D. McHugh[1], A. J. Nunn[2], S. K. Meredith[2], C. M. Mendel[5], M. Spigelman[5], A. M. Crook[2], S. H. Gillespie[6] and for the REMoxTB consortium

Abstract

Background: In the REMoxTB study of 4-month treatment-shortening regimens containing moxifloxacin compared to the standard 6-month regimen for tuberculosis, the proportion of unfavourable outcomes for women was similar in all study arms, but men had more frequent unfavourable outcomes (bacteriologically or clinically defined failure or relapse within 18 months after randomisation) on the shortened moxifloxacin-containing regimens. The reason for this gender disparity in treatment outcome is poorly understood.

Methods: The gender differences in baseline variables were calculated, as was time to smear and culture conversion and Kaplan-Meier plots were constructed. In post hoc exploratory analyses, multivariable logistic regression modelling and an observed case analysis were used to explore factors associated with both gender and unfavourable treatment outcome.

Results: The per-protocol population included 472/1548 (30%) women. Women were younger and had lower rates of cavitation, smoking and weight (all $p < 0.05$) and higher prevalence of HIV (10% vs 6%, $p = 0.001$). They received higher doses (mg/kg) than men of rifampicin, isoniazid, pyrazinamide and moxifloxacin ($p \leq 0.005$). There was no difference in baseline smear grading or mycobacterial growth indicator tube (MGIT) time to positivity. Women converted to negative cultures more quickly than men on Lowenstein-Jensen (HR 1.14, $p = 0.008$) and MGIT media (HR 1.19, $p < 0.001$). In men, the presence of cavitation, positive HIV status, higher age, lower BMI and 'ever smoked' were independently associated with unfavourable treatment outcome. In women, only 'ever smoked' was independently associated with unfavourable treatment outcome. Only for cavitation was there a gender difference in treatment outcomes by regimen; their outcome in the 4-month arms was significantly poorer compared to the 6-month treatment arm ($p < 0.001$). Women, with or without cavities, and men without cavities had a similar outcome on all treatment arms ($p = 0.218$, 0.224 and 0.689 respectively). For all other covariate subgroups, there were no differences in treatment effects for men or women.

Conclusions: Gender differences in TB treatment responses for the shorter regimens in the REMoxTB study may be explained by poor outcomes in men with cavitation on the moxifloxacin-containing regimens. We observed that women with cavities, or without, on the 4-month moxifloxacin regimens had similar outcomes to all patients on the standard 6-month treatment. The biological reasons for this difference are poorly understood and require further exploration.

Keywords: Gender, Tuberculosis, Treatment outcome, Cavitation, Clinical trials, REMoxTB

* Correspondence: michael.murphy@ucl.ac.uk
[†]M. E. Murphy and G. H. Wills contributed equally to this work.
[1]UCL Centre for Clinical Microbiology, Division of Infection and Immunity, University College London, Royal Free Campus, Rowland Hill Street, London NW3 2PF, England, UK
Full list of author information is available at the end of the article

Background

Tuberculosis (TB) is amongst the leading causes of death in reproductive-age women. In 2014, there were 3.2 million incident TB cases in women and almost half a million deaths [1]. In pregnant women, TB is associated with significant increases in premature birth, low birth weight and death. In those co-infected with HIV, the risk of active TB is high, and there is a threefold risk of mother and child death [2].

While men are notified as having higher incident TB (5.4 million in 2015), and have higher mortality (16.5% vs 15%), there is a wide-ranging variation in gender differences geographically, and mortality is roughly equal in areas of highest HIV co-infection in Africa [1]. It is uncertain whether, in settings where there are low levels of HIV, women are biologically less susceptible to TB infection and reactivation or whether gender differences in TB incidence may reflect gender-specific sociocultural factors influencing TB exposure and/or access to healthcare [3, 4].

Most gender-specific TB research has focussed on differences in women's access to healthcare and subsequent delays in seeking health services, with one study finding the status of being a married woman, a housewife or being a woman as being significantly associated with diagnostic delays [5]. There is evidence that women, once enrolled in healthcare, are more likely than men to adhere to the full course of treatment resulting in better treatment outcomes [6]. However, there are limited and sometimes conflicting data on gender differences in TB treatment responses and there may be specific factors, affecting either gender, influencing responses to treatment [7–9].

In the REMoxTB study of 4-month-treatment shortening regimens containing moxifloxacin, the proportion of favourable outcomes for women on the moxifloxacin-containing arms was similar to those on the standard 6-month treatment arm and would be considered non-inferior [10]. However, male patients, who comprised 70% of the study population, had significantly more unfavourable outcomes on the moxifloxacin-containing regimens. Specifically, while 8% of both males and females had unfavourable outcomes on the control regimen, male vs female breakdown of unfavourable rates for the isoniazid-moxifloxacin arm was 19% vs 7% and for the ethambutol-moxifloxacin regimen was 23% vs 13%. Although the study was not designed or powered to detect differences in treatment outcome by gender, the biological reasons for the observed gender disparity remain unclear and warrant further exploration.

The aim of this analysis was to better understand the biological and epidemiological factors associated with gender differences in TB treatment responses to inform future TB treatment and targeted public health interventions.

Methods

We undertook an analysis of the REMoxTB study database [11]. Patients included in this secondary analysis were those in the pre-specified per-protocol population in whom the gender-by-treatment interaction was detected in the main REMoxTB study [10]. This was the primary analysis population for the trial including patients who had adhered to at least 80% of study drug.

Patient treatment

Adult patients with sputum smear positive for acid-fast bacilli (AFB) were invited to be screened for enrolment to the REMoxTB study; a placebo-controlled, randomised, double-blind, phase 3 trial to test the non-inferiority of two experimental 4-month treatment arms containing moxifloxacin compared to standard 6-month treatment (see below). AFB-positive smears were confirmed on a new sputum sample in the study laboratory and additional blood and medical history were collected at the screening to determine patients' eligibility, which are described elsewhere [10]. Patients with HIV infection could enrol with a CD4 > 250 cells/μL. Study sites were in Africa, Asia and Central America. Those eligible and consenting to enrolment in the study were randomised to receive the control regimen—2 months of rifampicin (R), isoniazid (H), ethambutol (E) and pyrazinamide (Z), followed by 4 months of rifampicin and isoniazid 2EHRZ/4HR —or one of the two experimental arms in which moxifloxacin (M) replaced either ethambutol (2MHRZ/2MHR; the isoniazid-arm) or isoniazid (2EMRZ/2MR; the ethambutol arm). Drug dosing was stratified by patient weight for rifampicin (< 45 kg, 450 mg; ≥ 45 kg, 600 mg), pyrazinamide (< 55 kg, 1000 mg; ≥ 55–75 kg, 1500 mg; > 75 kg, 2000 mg), and ethambutol (< 40 kg, 15 mg/kg rounded to nearest 100 mg; 40–55 kg, 800 mg; > 55–75 kg, 1200 mg; > 75 kg, 1600 mg), while patients received moxifloxacin 400 mg and isoniazid 300 mg, all according to their randomised allocated regimen.

Microbiology

Patients enrolled in the REMoxTB study provided two sputum samples prior to commencing study drug. Further sputum samples were collected at regular study visits: weekly during the first 8 weeks of intensive phase treatment, at monthly visits until completion of study treatment at 6 months and three monthly for a further 12 months, with two samples being collected at each visit in the post-treatment phase. Each sputum sample was processed for smear microscopy and culture both on solid and in liquid media as per the REMoxTB-specific laboratory manual [12]. In brief, sputum samples were decontaminated and stained using Ziehl-Neelsen method and graded according to ATS guidelines as a semi-quantitative measure of mycobacterial burden [13]. Sputum samples were processed for culture on solid Lowenstein-Jensen (LJ) medium and in the fully automated BACTEC Mycobacterial Growth Indicator Tube system (MGIT; BBL™ MGIT™ 960, Becton Dickinson (BD) Microbiology Systems, Sparks, MD, USA). Time to detection (TTD) was recorded as a measure of mycobacterial burden. Drug susceptibility was performed on all isolates, and patients with multi-drug resistant TB, i.e. resistance to rifampicin ± isoniazid, were excluded.

Statistical analyses

Clinical trial data were recorded in the study database along with patient demographics: gender, age, weight and individual drug dose per kilogramme, HIV status and smoking history. The extent of lung disease was quantified using a binary variable for cavitation (yes/no). In addition, Ralph et al. scoring was performed which provides a score out of 140 comprising percentage of lung involvement evident on chest radiograph with an additional 40 points for those with cavitation [14]. Treatment outcomes were as defined by the REMoxTB study in which the primary efficacy outcome was the proportion of patients who had bacteriologically or clinically defined failure or relapse within 18 months after randomisation (a composite unfavourable outcome). Differences in baseline characteristics, including mycobacterial burden, between males and females were compared using chi-squared (χ^2) and Mann-Whitney U test. Kaplan-Meier plots were constructed to compare male and female time to smear and culture conversion, from randomisation to the study visit of the first negative result, summarised by a hazard ratio (HR) and compared using the logrank test. Factors found to be associated with gender ($p < 0.1$) were then included in a multivariable logistic regression model for unfavourable outcome, separately for men and women. Treatment effects within subgroups defined by covariates independently associated with outcome were explored, and an observed case analysis was conducted. All these analyses are post hoc and considered exploratory with no adjustments made for multiple testing. All analyses were conducted in Stata Version 14.0.

Results

The per-protocol population of the REMoxTB study comprised 1548 patients, 472 (30%) of whom were female. Female patients were younger and had a higher BMI. They had lower rates of cavitation and smoking. Females received higher doses of rifampicin (11.28 mg/kg vs 10.99 mg/kg; $p = 0.005$), isoniazid (6.36 mg/kg vs 5.76 mg/kg; $p = < 0.001$), pyrazinamide (23.26 mg/kg vs 22.42 mg/kg; $p < 0.001$) and moxifloxacin (8.48 mg/kg vs 7.68 mg/kg; < 0.001), but not for ethambutol which had a higher dose in men (17.39 mg/kg vs 17.58 mg/kg; $p = 0.018$). Compared to males, females had higher prevalence of HIV (10% vs 6%; $p = 0.001$); but CD4 cell counts were comparable (437 and 405 cells/μL, $p = 0.32$) (see Table 1).

There was no difference in pre-treatment smear gradings and MGIT time to positivity (TTP) (Table 1). The median LJ TTD was 14 days, with an interquartile range of 14–21 days, for both women and men, but there was a significant difference in their rankings with a lower LJ time to detection (TTD) suggesting higher mycobacterial burden in women ($p = 0.04$). Women were faster to convert to culture negative than men on both LJ (HR 1.14; 0.008) and in MGIT media (HR 1.19; $p < 0.001$). There was no difference in time to smear conversion (HR 1.07; $p = 0.14$). Kaplan-Meier plots are shown in Fig. 1.

Significant univariable baseline factors associated with an unfavourable outcome included cavitation (OR 2.19, $p < 0.001$), a current/ex-smoker (OR 2.07, $p < 0.001$), a low BMI (under 18.5 vs 18.5 and above) (OR 1.53, $p = 0.004$), being older (30 years and under vs over 30 years) (OR 1.6, $p = 0.003$) and HIV (OR 2.26, $p < 0.001$) and were included in the final adjusted logistic regression models for unfavourable outcome including treatment arm, for men and women separately. Drug dosing and baseline smear and culture results were not significantly associated with unfavourable outcome and were not included in the model. Ralph scoring, which includes a measure of the percentage of lung involvement in addition to the binary cavity variable, showed borderline evidence that men had a higher overall percentage of lung involvement than women (21.1% vs 19.7%; $p = 0.05$), but inclusion of this variable in the model did not improve the overall fit of the models when considered in place of the binary cavitation variable. Results are shown in Tables 2 and 3. For men, all factors included remained significantly associated with unfavourable outcome in multivariable analysis, except for race. For women, only current/ex-smoking status was significantly associated with the unfavourable response. No significant treatment-by-covariate interactions were observed in the multivariable models, which might have been expected given the small numbers in each subgroup.

In exploring the treatment effects within subgroups descriptively, cavitation emerged as the only covariate whose statistical significance differed substantially between genders in terms of treatment outcomes by regimen. Men with cavities had significantly poorer outcomes compared to women with cavities (19% vs 9%, $p < 0.001$; Table 4). In contrast, men and women without cavitation had similar treatment outcomes (both 9%, $p = 0.975$). Men with cavities had worse treatment outcomes than men without cavities and had significantly poorer outcomes on the experimental arms compared to control ($p < 0.001$;

Table 1 Baseline characteristics stratified by gender and treatment group. Baseline characteristics of patients in the per-protocol population. Numbers are N (%) unless otherwise stated

Characteristics	Control group (N = 510)		Isoniazid group (N = 514)		Ethambutol group (N = 524)		All patients (N = 1548)	
Sex	Male (N = 356)	Female (N = 154)	Male (N = 351)	Female (N = 163)	Male (N = 369)	Female (N = 155)	Male (N = 1076)	Female (N = 472)
Age group*								
≤ 30 years	155 (44)	89 (58)	170 (48)	84 (52)	161 (44)	80 (52)	486 (45)	253 (54)
> 30 years	201 (56)	65 (42)	181 (52)	79 (48)	208 (56)	75 (48)	590 (55)	219 (46)
Weight group*								
< 40 kg	14 (4)	36 (23)	14 (4)	30 (18)	29 (8)	29 (19)	57 (5)	95 (20)
40–45 kg	45 (13)	35 (23)	54 (15)	36 (22)	54 (15)	28 (18)	153 (14)	99 (21)
>45–55 kg	163 (46)	43 (28)	159 (45)	51 (31)	149 (40)	55 (35)	471 (44)	149 (32)
> 55 kg	134 (38)	40 (26)	124 (35)	46 (28)	137 (37)	43 (28)	395 (37)	129 (27)
BMI								
< 18.5	196 (55)	71 (46)	199 (57)	73 (45)	211 (57)	64 (41)	606 (56)	208 (44)
≥ 18.5	160 (45)	83 (54)	152 (43)	90 (55)	158 (43)	91 (59)	470 (44)	264 (56)
Race or ethnic group*‡								
Black	171 (48)	67 (44)	150 (43)	60 (37)	173 (47)	64 (41)	494 (46)	191 (40)
Asian	109 (31)	51 (33)	107 (30)	47 (29)	119 (32)	42 (27)	335 (31)	140 (30)
Mixed race or other	76 (21)	36 (23)	94 (27)	56 (34)	77 (21)	49 (32)	247 (23)	141 (30)
Smoking status*								
Never	133 (37)	113 (73)	121 (34)	110 (67)	127 (34)	103 (66)	381 (35)	326 (69)
Past	105 (29)	14 (9)	100 (28)	11 (7)	117 (32)	17 (11)	322 (30)	42 (9)
Current	118 (33)	27 (18)	130 (37)	42 (26)	125 (34)	35 (23)	373 (35)	104 (22)
HIV positivity*	21 (6)	17 (11)	23 (7)	14 (9)	17 (5)	18 (12)	61 (6)	49 (10)
Cavitation*||	268 (75)	100 (65)	244 (70)	113 (69)	264 (72)	103 (66)	776 (72)	316 (67)
Area of lung involvement (%, (SD))	21.5 (12.5)	20.1 (12.4)	20.9 (13.1)	19.2 (12.1)	20.9 (12.2)	19.7 (11.0)	21.1 (12.6)	19.7 (11.9)
Smear grading								
Neg	14 (4)	7 (5)	14 (4)	5 (3)	17 (5)	7 (5)	45 (4)	19 (4)
1+	32 (9)	15 (10)	24 (7)	17 (10)	25 (7)	14 (9)	81 (8)	46 (10)
2+	43 (12)	19 (12)	52 (15)	26 (16)	62 (17)	22 (14)	157 (15)	67 (14)
3+	86 (24)	42 (27)	79 (23)	37 (23)	82 (22)	32 (21)	247 (23)	111 (24)
4+	181 (51)	71 (46)	182 (52)	78 (48)	183 (50)	80 (52)	546 (51)	229 (49)
LJ								
Positive	283 (79)	117 (76)	277 (79)	137 (84)	294 (80)	132 (85)	854 (81)	386 (82)
Negative	33 (9)	14 (9)	25 (7)	12 (7)	31 (8)	4 (3)	89 (8)	30 (6)

Table 1 Baseline characteristics stratified by gender and treatment group. Baseline characteristics of patients in the per-protocol population. Numbers are N (%) unless otherwise stated (Continued)

Characteristics	Control group (N = 510)		Isoniazid group (N = 514)		Ethambutol group (N = 524)		All patients (N = 1548)	
Contaminated	29 (8)	16 (10)	38 (11)	14 (9)	33 (9)	16 (10)	100 (9)	46 (10)
Indeterminate	11 (3)	7 (5)	11 (3)	0 (0)	11 (3)	3 (2)	33 (3)	10 (2)
TTD (median [IQR])	14 [14–21]	14 [14–21]	14 [14–25]	14 [14–21]	21 [14–28]	14 [14–21]	14 [14–21]	14 [14–21]
MGIT								
Positive	329 (92)	141 (92)	319 (93)	157 (96)	332 (90)	147 (95)	980 (93)	445 (94)
Negative	5 (1)	2 (1)	4 (1)	0 (0)	7 (2)	2 (1)	16 (2)	4 (1)
Contaminated	11 (3)	4 (3)	10 (3)	6 (4)	15 (4)	3 (2)	36 (3)	13 (3)
False positive	2 (1)	0 (0)	5 (1)	0 (0)	4 (1)	0 (0)	11 (1)	0 (0)
Indeterminate	9 (3)	7 (5)	13 (4)	0 (0)	11 (3)	3 (2)	13 (1)	10 (2)
TTP (median [IQR])	4.81 [3.71–6.66]	5.13 [3.79–6.79]	4.92 [3.70–6.39]	5.04 [4.03–6.43]	4.83 [3.67–6.58]	4.73 [3.70–6.50]	4.83 [3.71–6.50]	5.04 [3.88–6.46]

p values for categorical variables are calculated using chi-squared test and for the continuous variable using Mann-Whitney U test

HIV human immunodeficiency virus, TTD time to detect a positive culture in days on LJ media, TTP time to detect a positive culture in days in MGIT, IQR interquartile range

*Males and females were significantly different at baseline for weight, age, race, smoking, HIV, cavitation, area of lung involvement and LJ TTD; p values were ≤0.001, 0.002, 0.013, ≤0.001, 0.001, 0.022, 0.05 and 0.04 respectively

‡Race or ethnic group was reported by the investigator. Asian category included both South Asians and East Asians. Mixed race or other included mixed race, coloured and Caucasian

∥Cavitation status was missing for 148 patients

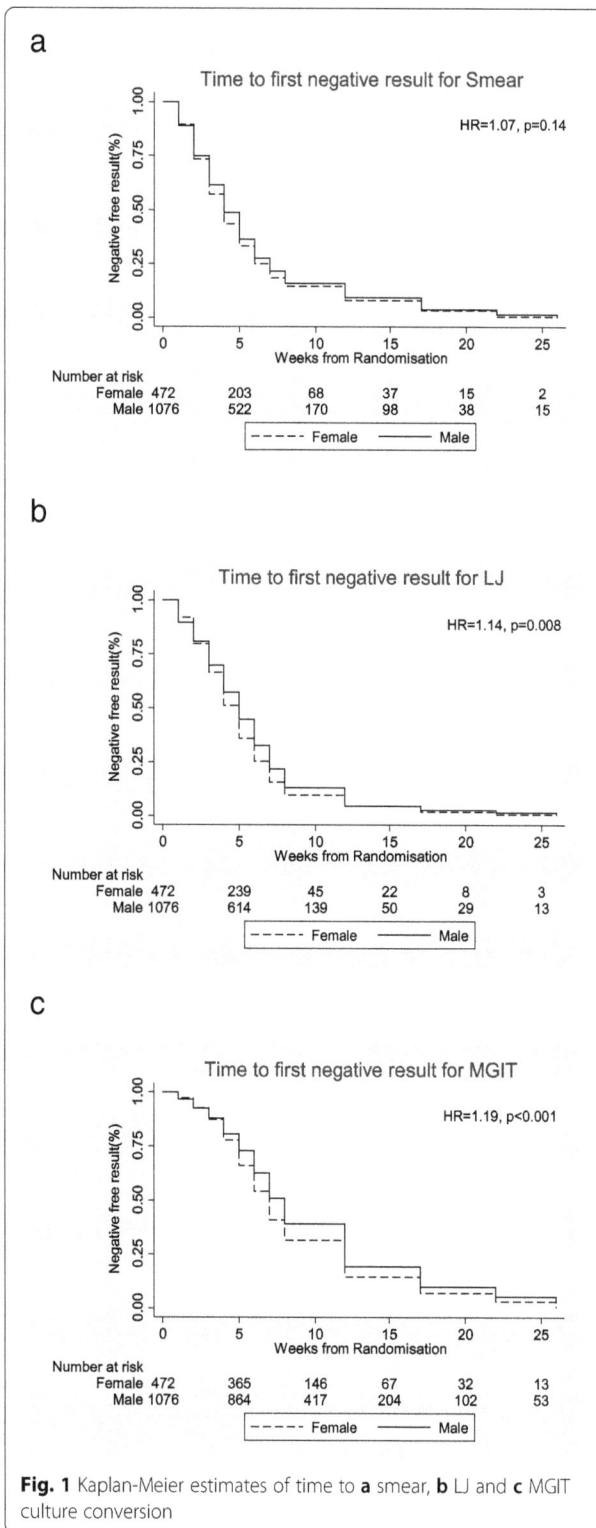

Fig. 1 Kaplan-Meier estimates of time to **a** smear, **b** LJ and **c** MGIT culture conversion

regardless of the treatment regimen ($p = 0.218$, 0.224 and 0.689 respectively).

To ensure that this result is not impacted by missing cavitation results, we repeated these analyses using imputed values ($N = 148$) employing a multiple imputation approach, and this produced similar results (data not shown). No other treatment effect differences across covariate subgroups within gender including HIV status, smoking and BMI were observed to explain the gender-by-treatment interaction found in the REMoxTB study (see Additional file 1: Tables S1).

Discussion

Women receiving 4-month moxifloxacin-containing regimens in the REMoxTB study had similar outcomes to those on 6-month control regimens. This held true for all covariate subgroups of women including HIV, smoking and low BMI and seems biologically plausible as women responded faster to TB treatment than men, despite comparable pre-treatment mycobacterial burdens. In contrast, the 4-month regimens, men had a significantly worse outcome compared to standard 6-month therapy, particularly the ethambutol-containing regimen. Cavitation was the only baseline characteristic measured which could potentially explain the observed difference in treatment outcomes between men and women.

Our analyses show that failure in the REMoxTB study was driven by poorer outcomes in men with cavitation in the moxifloxacin-containing arms. Importantly, men without cavities and women, with or without cavities, had similar outcomes in the moxifloxacin-containing and standard regimens. In addition to cavitation, men had poorer treatment outcomes on the experimental arms compared to control in all other covariate subgroups. While age, BMI, smoking status and HIV status were associated with an unfavourable outcome in males, they could not explain the different outcome in the individual treatment regimens. Similarly, for women, a history of smoking increased the hazard of a poor outcome, but there was no difference in outcomes across treatment regimens.

It is already established in a previous paper from our group that cavities visible on posterior-anterior chest radiograph are associated with the mycobacterial load as measured by time to positivity (TTP) and directly related to the size of the cavity [15]. The rate of decline of mycobacterial burden in that paper was unrelated to baseline load suggesting that patients with higher mycobacterial burdens at baseline would take longer to culture convert. However, in the current study, while the poor outcomes of men with cavitation were the only factor which may in part possibly explain the gender-by-treatment interaction, males and females had comparable mycobacterial burdens as measured by MGIT TTP prior to starting the

Table 5). However, women with cavities had no difference in treatment outcome compared to women without cavities (Table 4), and women, with or without cavities, and men without cavities had similar treatment outcomes

Table 2 Treatment and covariate effects on unfavourable outcome for men (N = 974)

	r/n	OR (unadjusted), 95% CI	p	aOR (adjusted), 95% CI	p
Treatment					
HRZE	30/326 (33)			1.0	
2MHRZ/2MHR	55/312 (32)	2.22 (1.36–3.62)	0.001	2.24 (1.37–3.65)	0.001
2EMRZ/2MR	78/336 (35)	3.31 (2.07–5.29)	< 0.001	3.31 (2.07–5.28)	< 0.001
Age					
≤ 30 years	58/435	1.0		1.0	
> 30 years	105/539	1.46 (1.00–2.12)	0.045	1.48 (1.02–2.14)	0.037
BMI					
< 18.5	105/547	1.0		1.0	
≥ 18.5	58/427	0.65 (0.45–0.93)	0.020	0.64 (0.44–0.92)	0.017
Race					
Asian	50/311	1.0			
Black	70/430	0.85 (0.55–1.32)	0.469	–	–
Mixed race and Caucasian	43/233	0.97 (0.58–1.61)	0.902		
Smoking					
Never smoked	39/334	1.0		1.0	
Ever smoked	124/640	1.61 (1.04–2.49)	0.034	1.60 (1.07–2.40)	0.023
HIV					
Negative	143/922 (95)	1.0		1.0	
Positive	20/52	4.26 (2.22–8.18)	< 0.001	3.97 (2.12–7.42)	< 0.001
Cavities					
No cavities	16/198	1.0		1.0	
Cavities	147/776	2.78 (1.59–4.85)	< 0.001	2.78 (1.59–4.84)	< 0.001

r number with unfavourable outcome
n total in category

treatment, yet women were faster to culture convert. The significant difference in the mycobacterial burden on LJ was more likely related to the ranking of categorical TTD data, recorded weekly than any real difference. In any case, this suggested a higher mycobacterial burden in women and would therefore have been expected to favour males. Furthermore, although we did not measure cavity volume specifically, and while there was borderline evidence of a higher percentage of lung involvement for men compared to women, this additional information did not improve the fit of our statistical model.

Cavitation has previously been identified as a risk factor for poor outcomes in TB treatment regimens, but these have not been stratified by gender [16]. The poor outcome of males with cavities on the experimental regimens compared to females with cavities cannot easily be explained. It may be that males had a higher volume of cavities, which is a factor that is not measured by the Ralph score, as this measure includes a single binary 'penalty' for cavities that is added to the score for percentage lung involvement. Studies of TB immunopathology have identified matrix-metalloproteinases as crucial

factors controlling the pulmonary extracellular matrix involved in cavity formation [17]. A recent study of the collagenase MMP-8 in plasma has shown this to be higher in males than in females which may support greater cavitation in male patients and deserves further consideration, along with other potential gender-specific immunological factors which might explain the findings of this study [18].

An earlier randomised control trial comparing 4-month and 6-month standard regimens in 394 patients, including 154 women, with non-cavitary disease, and who culture converted after 2 months standard treatment, was halted due to an unacceptable failure rate in the 4-month arms (7.0% vs 1.6%). This suggests that cavitation may not entirely explain the gender difference in treatment outcome observed in the REMoxTB study, however, again, the results of this study were not reported by gender [19]. A re-analysis of previous trial data from the UK MRC comparing 4- and 6-month regimens also identified higher rates of failure in the shorter regimens (5.9% vs 0%) [20]. However, unpublished data from two previous MRC trials involving unsuccessful

Table 3 Treatment and covariate effects on unfavourable outcome for women ($N = 426$)

	r/n	OR (unadjusted), 95% CI	p	aOR (adjusted), 95% CI	p
Treatment					
HRZE	10/138				
2MHRZ/2MHR	11/149	0.98 (0.40–2.43)	0.973	–	–
2EMRZ/2MR	18/139	1.93 (0.84–4.39)	0.119		
Age					
≤ 30 years	20/223	1.0		–	–
> 30 years	19/203	0.95 (0.48–1.88)	0.881		
BMI					
< 18.5	19/189	1.0		–	–
≥ 18.5	20/237	1.03 (0.51–2.12)	0.926		
Race					
Asian	15/135	1.0			
Black	9/163	0.39 (0.14–1.08)	0.070	–	–
Mixed race and Caucasian	15/128	0.45 (0.14–1.45)	0.182		
Smoking					
Never smoked	21/292	1.0		1.0	
Ever smoked	18/134	2.69 (0.92–7.90)	0.071	2.00 (1.03–3.90)	0.041
HIV					
Negative	36/385	1.0		–	–
Positive	3/41	1.16 (0.28–4.84)	0.835		
Cavities					
No cavities	9/110	1.0		–	–
Cavities	30/316	1.16 (0.51–2.63)	0.715		

4-month regimens, including one containing moxifloxacin, indicated that women had significantly better outcomes than men in an analysis stratified by cavitation, as in our study (Personal communication: Professor Andrew Nunn, MRC Clinical Trials Unit at UCL).

Gender-specific pharmacodynamics might potentially explain the observed differences in the treatment outcome. In the REMoxTB study, women, on average, received small increased doses of four of five study drugs, including moxifloxacin, known to be essential for bacterial sterilisation and cure. Increased dosing may therefore go some way to explaining the faster bacteriological response to treatment, but these were not found to be significantly associated with treatment outcome on univariable analyses. No gender difference in the pharmacokinetics of moxifloxacin has been described to explain the differences in unfavourable outcome between men and women with and without cavitation on the moxifloxacin-containing regimens. Poor outcomes on the ethambutol arms may be due to the superior bactericidal effect of isoniazid or the presence of three drugs over a 4-month period. Compliance with study regimens may also be a factor. To be included in the per-protocol analysis in which the gender-by-treatment interaction was identified, all patients had to have taken more than 80% of their medication. However, as data collection was not sufficiently detailed to address adherence further by gender, we do not know whether, within the per-protocol population of the REMoxTB study taking >80% of study medication, females may have had

Table 4 Unfavourable outcome within gender and subgroups defined by cavities

Cavities ($N = 1092$)				No cavities ($N = 308$)			
Male N (%)		Female N (%)		Male N (%)		Female N (%)	
776 (71)		316 (29)		198 (64)		110 (36)	
Favourable	Un-fav	Favourable	Un-fav	Favourable	Un-fav	Favourable	Un-fav
629 (81)	147 (19)	286 (91)	30 (9)	182 (92)	16 (8)	101 (92)	9 (8)
p < 0.001				p = 0.975			

Table 5 Unfavourable outcome by treatment group within gender and subgroups defined by cavities

	2EHRZ/4HR	2MHRZ/2MHR	2EMRZ/2MR
Men with cavities	268	244	264
Favourable	241 (90)	193 (79)	195 (74)
Unfavourable	27 (10)	51 (21)	69 (26)
$p < 0.001$			
Men without cavities	58	68	72
Favourable	55 (95)	64 (94)	63 (88)
Unfavourable	3 (5)	4 (6)	9 (13)
$p = 0.224$			
Women with cavities	100	113	103
Favourable	93 (93)	104 (92)	89 (86)
Unfavourable	7 (7)	9 (8)	14 (14)
$p = 0.218$			
Women without cavities	38	36	36
Favourable	35 (92)	34 (94)	32 (89)
Unfavourable	3 (8)	2 (6)	4 (11)
$p = 0.689$			

significantly greater compliance, nearer 100%, compared to men, or, indeed, vice versa. A previous systematic review of previous studies found a higher likelihood of compliance amongst females, so it would be important to consider the potential impact in future studies [6]. Furthermore, we were unable to further stratify compliance by gender and cavitation, and we cannot comment on whether there were differences in treatment compliance in men and women with cavitation which might explain the differences observed in the REMoxTB study.

To date, reports of gender differences in outcome have often been excluded from published clinical trials of moxifloxacin, and thus, there is limited data on the outcomes by gender for the many indications of moxifloxacin [21]. Two other clinical trials of fluoroquinolones for tuberculosis were published at the same time as the REMoxTB study but neither included analysis by gender [22, 23]. The US Food and Drug Administration, guidelines support reporting of gender differences in the clinical evaluation of drugs and journals are increasingly introducing editorial policies requiring the reporting of result by gender [24, 25]. Our observation emphasises the importance of such policies and supports the reporting of outcomes by gender so that we can better understand the factors bearing on these differences. This is particularly true for studies of moxifloxacin given that it is commonly used to treat with complicated and/or severe disease including patients intolerant of other first-line drugs and in patients with TB meningitis.

Although we should bear in mind that these analyses were all post hoc, considered exploratory and based on

relatively small numbers not powered to detect a gender-treatment interaction, the findings suggest that possibly the shorter regimens may be appropriate in females. Yet, how gender-specific therapy, if indicated, could be implemented within current standard National TB Programmes requires operational consideration. Research on gender difference in tuberculosis has thus far focussed on improving access to healthcare for women, presuming that, once engaged, women will have greater adherence to therapy. It is axiomatic that we need to improve patient engagement and adherence to approved regimens, but our study suggests a greater focus on men may be required to improve their treatment outcomes. This is supported by the findings of a recent meta-analysis that reported men as disadvantaged in seeking or accessing TB services and suggested that men were a high-risk group requiring improved access to TB [4]. Other factors associated with poor outcomes in men and/or women, including smoking and HIV, should further assist in directing public health responses.

Conclusions

Gender differences in TB treatment responses for the shorter regimens in the REMoxTB study may be explained by poor outcomes in men with cavitation on the moxifloxacin-containing regimens. We observed that women with cavities, or without, on the 4-month moxifloxacin regimens had similar outcomes to all patients on the standard 6-month treatment. The biological reasons for this difference are poorly understood and require further exploration.

Abbreviations

AFB: Acid-fast bacilli; ATS: American Thoracic Society; BMI: Body mass index; E: Ethambutol; H: Isoniazid; HIV: Human immunodeficiency virus; HR: Hazard ratio; IQR: Interquartile range; LJ: Lowenstein-Jensen; M: Moxifloxacin; MGIT: Mycobacterial growth indicator tube; MMP: Matrix metalloproteinase; MRC: Medical Research Council; Neg: Negative; OR: Odds ratio; R: Rifampicin; REMoXTB: Rapid regulatory evaluation of moxifloxacin for TB; TB: Tuberculosis; TTD: Time to detection; TTP: Time to positivity; UCL: University College London; UK: United Kingdom; Un-fav: Unfavourable (outcome); US: United States; WHO: World Health Organization; Z: Pyrazinamide; ZN: Ziehl-Neelsen

Acknowledgements

We thank all the participants in the REMoxTB clinical trial, without whom, this study would not have been possible; the study clinicians and nursing staff; and all the staff involved in the REMoxTB study at all of our study sites. The REMoxTB Consortium: Task Applied Sciences and Stellenbosch University, South Africa—Andreas Diacon, Madeleine Hanekom, Amour Venter; University of Cape Town, South Africa—Rodney Dawson, Kimberley Narunsky; Mbeya Medical Research Programme, Tanzania—B. Mtafya, N. Elias Ntinginya, Andrea Rachow; Centre for Respiratory Disease Research at KEMRI, Kenya—Evans

Amukoye, B. Miheso, M. Njoroje; Kilimanjaro Christian Medical Centre, Tanzania—Noel Sam, D. Damas, Alphonce Liyoyo; Institute of Respiratory Medicine, Jalan Pahang, Malaysia—A. Ahmad Mahayiddin; Chest Disease Institute, Thailand—C. Chuchottaworn, J. Boonyasopun, B. Saipan; University of Zambia and University Teaching Hospital, Zambia—Shabir Lakhi, D. Chanda, J. Mcyeze; Medical Research Council, South Africa—Alexander Pym, N. Ngcobo; Madibeng Centre for Research, South Africa—Cheryl Louw, H. Veldsman; Hospital General de Occidente de la Secretaría de Salud del Estado de Jalisco, Mexico—Gerardo Amaya-Tapia, T. Vejar Aguirre; Dr. D. K. Chauhan Clinic, India—D. K. Chauhan; Dr. R. K. Garg's Clinic, India—R. K. Garg; Dr.Nirmal Kumar Jain Clinic, India—N.K Jain; Indra Nursing Home and Maternity Centre, India—A. Aggarwal; Mahatma Gandhi Medical College & Hospital, India 302022—M. Mishra; Dr. Sanjay Teotia Clinic, India—S. Teotia; Aurum, Tembisa Hospital, South Africa—S. Charalambous, N. Hattidge, L. Pretorious; University of KwaZulu Natal, South Africa (ACTG Site)—N. Padayachi; Perinatal HIV Research Unit, Chris Hani Baragwanath Hospital, South Africa (ACTG Site)—L. Mohapi; Beijing Tuberculosis and Thoracic Tumor Research Institute, China—M. Gao, X. Li, L. Zhang; Shanghai Pulmonary Hospital, China—Q. Zhang; Siddharth Nursing Home, India—S. Aggarwal; TB Alliance—Ketty Belizaire, Majda Benhayoun, D. Everitt, Ann Ginsberg, Martino Laurenzi, Bridget Rawls, Christopher Ridali, Mel Spigelman, Almarie Uys, Christo van Niekerk; University College London—Anna LC Bateson, Matthew Betteridge, S. Birkby, Emily Bongard, Michael Brown, Holly Ciesielczuk, C. Cook, E Cunningham, James Huggett, Robert Hunt, Clare Ling, Marc Lipman, Paul Mee, Michael E Murphy, Saraswathi E Murthy, Felicity MR Perrin, Robert Shorten, Kasha P Singh, K. Smith, Victoria Yorke-Edwards, Alimuddin Zumla

Funding

This study was supported by the Global Alliance for TB Drug Development with support from the Bill and Melinda Gates Foundation, the European and Developing Countries Clinical Trials Partnership (grant IP.2007.32011.011), US Agency for International Development, UK Department for International Development, Directorate General for International Cooperation of the Netherlands, Irish Aid, Australia Department of Foreign Affairs and Trade and National Institutes of Health, AIDS Clinical Trials Group and by grants from the National Institute of Allergy and Infectious Diseases (NIAID) (UM1AI068634, UM1 AI068636 and UM1AI106701) and by NIAID grants to the University of KwaZulu Natal, South Africa, AIDS Clinical Trials Group (ACTG) site 31422 (1U01AI069469); to the Perinatal HIV Research Unit, Chris Hani Baragwanath Hospital, South Africa, ACTG site 12301 (1U01AI069453); and to the Durban International Clinical Trials Unit, South Africa, ACTG site 11201 (1U01AI069426); Bayer Healthcare for the donation of moxifloxacin and Sanofi for the donation of rifampin. Role of the funding source

Senior staff at the Global Alliance for TB Drug Development, including CM, were members of the REMoxTB senior team who reviewed the data from this study, contributed to the data interpretation, commented on the manuscript and provided approval for publication. No other funders had any role in this study or the decision to publish.

Authors' contributions

MM, GW designed the study, performed data analysis and data interpretation, and wrote the manuscript. SM and SHG performed Ralph scoring. SM, CL, AB, RH, AJN, SKM, CM, MS contributed to interpretation of data. SHG, AC, TDM contributed to study design and analyses and supervised this study. All authors reviewed and commented on the manuscript.

Authors' information

MM—UCL Clinician and Research Associate; GW—Statistician, MRC Clinical Trials Unit at UCL; SM—Clinician and Research Associate, UCL; CL—Clinician and Principal Investigator, Madibeng Centre for Research, South Africa; AB—Post-doctoral Scientist, UCL; RH—Senior Research Associate, UCL; TDM—Professor of Clinical Microbiology, UCL, and Director, UCL Centre for Clinical Microbiology; AJN—Senior scientist at MRC Clinical Trials Unit at UCL;

SKM—Professor of Clinical Trials, MRC Clinical Trials Unit at UCL; CM—Senior VP Research and Development, TB Alliance; MS—President and CEO, TB Alliance; AC—Senior Statistician, MRC Clinical Trials Unit at UCL; SHG—Sir James Black Professor of Medicine, University of St Andrews.

Competing interests

The authors declare that they have no competing interests.

Author details

[1]UCL Centre for Clinical Microbiology, Division of Infection and Immunity, University College London, Royal Free Campus, Rowland Hill Street, London NW3 2PF, England, UK. [2]MRC Clinical Trials Unit at UCL, Institute for Clinical Trials and Methodology, Aviation House, 125 Kingsway, London WC2B 6NH, England, UK. [3]Madibeng Centre for Research, Brits, South Africa. [4]Department of Family Medicine, School of medicine, University of Pretoria, Pretoria, South Africa. [5]Global Alliance for Tuberculosis Drug Development, New York, NY 10005, USA. [6]School of Medicine, Medical and Biological Sciences Building, University of St Andrews, North Haugh, St Andrews KY16 9TF, Scotland, UK.

References

1. WHO: Global tuberculosis report. 2015.
2. WHO: Tuberculosis in women. 2014.
3. Weiss MG, Sommerfeld J, Uplekar MW. Social and cultural dimensions of gender and tuberculosis. Int J Tuberc Lung Dis. 2008;12(7):829–30.
4. Horton KC, MacPherson P, Houben RM, White RG. Sex differences in tuberculosis burden and notifications in low- and middle-income countries: a systematic review and meta-analysis. PLoS Med. 2016;13(9):e1002119.
5. Gosoniu GD, Ganapathy S, Kemp J, Auer C, Somma D, Karim F, Weiss MG. Gender and socio-cultural determinants of delay to diagnosis of TB in Bangladesh, India and Malawi. Int J Tuberc Lung Dis. 2008;12(7):848–55.
6. Susan van den Hof CAN, E Bloss, M Straetemans: A systematic review on the role of gender in tuberculosis control; 2010.
7. Kosgei RJ, Sitienei JK, Kipruto H, Kimenye K, Gathara D, Odawa FX, Gichangi P, Callens S, Temmerman M, Sitienei JC, et al. Gender differences in treatment outcomes among 15–49 year olds with smear-positive pulmonary tuberculosis in Kenya. Int J Tuberc Lung Dis. 2015; 19(10):1176–81.
8. Feng JY, Huang SF, Ting WY, Chen YC, Lin YY, Huang RM, Lin CH, Hwang JJ, Lee JJ, Yu MC, et al. Gender differences in treatment outcomes of tuberculosis patients in Taiwan: a prospective observational study. Clin Microbiol Infect. 2012;18(9):E331–7.
9. Allotey P, Gyapong M. Gender in tuberculosis research. Int J Tuberc Lung Dis. 2008;12(7):831–6.
10. Gillespie SH, Crook AM, McHugh TD, Mendel CM, Meredith SK, Murray SR, Pappas F, Phillips PP, Nunn AJ. Four-month moxifloxacin-based regimens for drug-sensitive tuberculosis. N Engl J Med. 2014;371(17):1577–87.
11. Corbett EL, Watt CJ, Walker N, Maher D, Williams BG, Raviglione MC, Dye C. The growing burden of tuberculosis: global trends and interactions with the HIV epidemic. Arch Intern Med. 2003;163(9):1009–21.
12. REMox Laboratory Manual. 2012. https://www.ucl.ac.uk/infection-immunity/ sites/infection-immunity/files/remox-laboratory-manual.pdf. Accessed 17 Sept 2018.

13. ATS: Diagnostic standards and classification of tuberculosis in adults and children. This official statement of the American Thoracic Society and the Centers for Disease Control and Prevention was adopted by the ATS Board of Directors, July 1999. This statement was endorsed by the Council of the Infectious Disease Society of America, September 1999. *Am J Respir Crit Care Med* 2000, 161(4 Pt 1):1376–1395.

14. Ralph AP, Ardian M, Wiguna A, Maguire GP, Becker NG, Drogumuller G, Wilks MJ, Waramori G, Tjitra E, Sandjaja, et al. A simple, valid, numerical score for grading chest X-ray severity in adult smear-positive pulmonary tuberculosis. Thorax. 2010;65(10):863–9.

15. Perrin FM, Woodward N, Phillips PP, McHugh TD, Nunn AJ, Lipman MC, Gillespie SH. Radiological cavitation, sputum mycobacterial load and treatment response in pulmonary tuberculosis. Int J Tuberc Lung Dis. 2010; 14(12):1596–602.

16. Benator D, Bhattacharya M, Bozeman L, Burman W, Cantazaro A, Chaisson R, Gordin F, Horsburgh CR, Horton J, Khan A, et al. Rifapentine and isoniazid once a week versus rifampicin and isoniazid twice a week for treatment of drug-susceptible pulmonary tuberculosis in HIV-negative patients: a randomised clinical trial. Lancet. 2002;360(9332):528–34.

17. Elkington PT, D'Armiento JM, Friedland JS. Tuberculosis immunopathology: the neglected role of extracellular matrix destruction. Sci Transl Med. 2011; 3(71):71ps76.

18. Sathyamoorthy T, Sandhu G, Tezera LB, Thomas R, Singhania A, Woelk CH, Dimitrov BD, Agranoff D, Evans CA, Friedland JS, et al. Gender-dependent differences in plasma matrix metalloproteinase-8 elevated in pulmonary tuberculosis. PLoS One. 2015;10(1):e0117605.

19. Johnson JL, Hadad DJ, Dietze R, Maciel EL, Sewali B, Gitta P, Okwera A, Mugerwa RD, Alcaneses MR, Quelapio MI, et al. Shortening treatment in adults with noncavitary tuberculosis and 2-month culture conversion. Am J Respir Crit Care Med. 2009;180(6):558–63.

20. Phillips PP, Nunn AJ, Paton NI. Is a 4-month regimen adequate to cure patients with non-cavitary tuberculosis and negative cultures at 2 months? Int J Tuberc Lung Dis. 2013;17(6):807–9.

21. Chilet-Rosell E, Ruiz-Cantero MT, Pardo MA. Gender analysis of moxifloxacin clinical trials. J Womens Health. 2014;23(1):77–104.

22. Jindani A, Harrison TS, Nunn AJ, Phillips PP, Churchyard GJ, Charalambous S, Hatherill M, Geldenhuys H, McIlleron HM, Zvada SP, et al. High-dose rifapentine with moxifloxacin for pulmonary tuberculosis. N Engl J Med. 2014;371(17):1599–608.

23. Merle CS, Fielding K, Sow OB, Gninafon M, Lo MB, Mthiyane T, Odhiambo J, Amukoye E, Bah B, Kassa F, et al. A four-month gatifloxacin-containing regimen for treating tuberculosis. N Engl J Med. 2014;371(17):1588–98.

24. Wright CA, Hesseling AC, Bamford C, Burgess SM, Warren R, Marais BJ. Fine-needle aspiration biopsy: a first-line diagnostic procedure in paediatric tuberculosis suspects with peripheral lymphadenopathy? Int J Tuberc Lung Dis. 2009;13(11):1373–9.

25. Schiebinger L, Leopold SS, Miller VM. Editorial policies for sex and gender analysis. Lancet. 2016;388(10062):2841–2.

The association of depression and all-cause and cause-specific mortality

Myrela O. Machado[1†], Nicola Veronese[2,3†], Marcos Sanches[4], Brendon Stubbs[2,5,6,7], Ai Koyanagi[8], Trevor Thompson[9], Ioanna Tzoulaki[10,11,12], Marco Solmi[2,13], Davy Vancampfort[14,15], Felipe B. Schuch[16,17], Michael Maes[18,19], Giovanni A. Fava[20,21], John P. A. Ioannidis[22,23,24,25] and André F. Carvalho[26,27*]

Abstract

Background: Depression is a prevalent and disabling mental disorder that frequently co-occurs with a wide range of chronic conditions. Evidence has suggested that depression could be associated with excess all-cause mortality across different settings and populations, although the causality of these associations remains unclear.

Methods: We conducted an umbrella review of systematic reviews and meta-analyses of observational studies. PubMed, PsycINFO, and Embase electronic databases were searched through January 20, 2018. Systematic reviews and meta-analyses that investigated associations of depression and all-cause and cause-specific mortality were selected for the review. The evidence was graded as convincing, highly suggestive, suggestive, or weak based on quantitative criteria that included an assessment of heterogeneity, 95% prediction intervals, small-study effects, and excess significance bias.

Results: A total of 26 references providing 2 systematic reviews and data for 17 meta-analytic estimates met inclusion criteria (19 of them on all-cause mortality); data from 246 unique studies ($N = 3,825,380$) were synthesized. All 17 associations had $P < 0.05$ per random effects summary effects, but none of them met criteria for convincing evidence. Associations of depression and all-cause mortality in patients after acute myocardial infarction, in individuals with heart failure, in cancer patients as well as in samples from mixed settings met criteria for highly suggestive evidence. However, none of the associations remained supported by highly suggestive evidence in sensitivity analyses that considered studies employing structured diagnostic interviews. In addition, associations of depression and all-cause mortality in cancer and post-acute myocardial infarction samples were supported only by suggestive evidence when studies that tried to adjust for potential confounders were considered.

Conclusions: Even though associations between depression and mortality have nominally significant results in all assessed settings and populations, the evidence becomes weaker when focusing on studies that used structured interviews and those that tried to adjust for potential confounders. A causal effect of depression on all-cause and cause-specific mortality remains unproven, and thus interventions targeting depression are not expected to result in lower mortality rates at least based on current evidence from observational studies.

Keywords: Depression, Mortality, All-cause, Cause-specific, Systematic reviews, Meta-analyses, Survival, Umbrella review, Psychiatry

* Correspondence: andre.carvalho@camh.ca; andrefc7@hotmail.com
†Myrela O. Machado and Nicola Veronese contributed equally to this work.
[26]Department of Psychiatry, University of Toronto, Toronto, ON, Canada
[27]Centre for Addiction & Mental Health (CAMH), 33 Russel Street, room RS1050S, Toronto, ON M5S 2S1, Canada
Full list of author information is available at the end of the article

Background

Major depressive disorder is a chronic and recurring condition with an estimated lifetime prevalence of 14.6% and 11.1% in high- and lower- and middle-income countries, respectively [1, 2]. In addition, major depressive disorder is a leading source of disability worldwide [3, 4], and is associated with diminished quality of life and medical morbidity [2, 4, 5]. An accumulating body of evidence also indicates that major depressive disorder may confer a higher risk for several non-communicable diseases (for example, diabetes [6], obesity [7], stroke [8], acute myocardial infarction [9], dementia [10], and physical health multimorbidity [11]), while these chronic health conditions appear to increase the likelihood of developing depression [7, 12–15].

It has long been suggested that depression is associated with elevated all-cause mortality [16, 17], and is an established risk factor for completed suicide [18]. In addition, depression has been associated with higher mortality rates across several settings and populations, including community samples, inpatients/outpatients, and patients with specific medical conditions (for example, stroke, diabetes, and coronary heart disease) [9, 16, 19, 20]. However, consistent evidence has not shown that specific interventions targeting depression may increase survival in both community and clinical samples. Furthermore, several confounding variables may account for the observed associations between depression and survival, namely sociodemographic variables [21], physical inactivity [22, 23], higher smoking rates [24], follow-up duration of studies [16], and co-occurring medical and psychiatric conditions [5, 25].

Several individual systematic reviews and meta-analyses have investigated the association between depression and mortality across distinct populations (for example, in community samples as well as in samples with specific chronic diseases) [16, 20, 26–28]. To synthesize and evaluate the available evidence we conducted an umbrella review of systematic reviews and meta-analyses that assessed the association of depression and all-cause and cause-specific mortality. The strength of the evidence supporting these associations and hints of bias were evaluated using standardized approaches [8, 29–31].

Methods

Literature search

We conducted an umbrella review, which is the systematic collection and assessment of multiple systematic reviews and meta-analyses done in a specific research topic [29]. The PubMed/MEDLINE, EMBASE, and PsycINFO databases were searched from inception up to January 20, 2018, for systematic reviews and meta-analyses of observational studies which examined the association of depression and all-cause or cause-specific mortality. A pre-defined search strategy was used (Additional file 1).

Eligibility criteria

We included systematic reviews and meta-analyses of observational epidemiological studies performed in humans that assessed the impact of depression on all-cause or cause-specific mortality in any specific population (for example, community samples, samples with a specific medical condition, inpatients, etc.). In addition, systematic reviews and meta-analyses that solely investigated the association of depression and suicide-related deaths were not considered; this was not an aim of the current effort as depression is an established risk factor for completed suicide [18]. However, suicide-related deaths were considered in meta-analyses that estimated the association of depression and all-cause mortality across different populations. No language restrictions were considered for the selection of systematic reviews and meta-analyses for this umbrella review. We included unique observational studies derived from all available systematic reviews and meta-analyses on a specific topic. Whenever a meta-analysis included a lower number of component studies compared to another meta-analysis on the same topic, the former was excluded only if all its individual datasets were included in the larger meta-analysis. Otherwise, we also extracted data from non-overlapping datasets included only in the meta-analysis with fewer studies. This approach aimed to synthesize the largest evidence possible derived from available systematic reviews and meta-analyses. Across each eligible systematic review and/ or meta-analysis we considered studies in which the case definition of depression was based on either *International Classification of Disease* [32] (ICD), *Diagnostic and Statistical Manual of Mental Disorders* [33] (DSM), or other consensus-based acceptable criteria (e.g., the Research Diagnostic Criteria [34]). We also included studies where depression was assessed by means of a screening instrument with a specific cutoff score (e.g., the Patient Health Questionnaire-9 and the Beck Depression Inventory). We excluded individual studies from eligible systematic reviews and meta-analyses according to the following criteria: (1) reported an association only for depressive symptoms (i.e., the association was reported for an increase in scores of a depression rating scale instead of a possible diagnosis of depression based on a screening tool with a cutoff point); (2) considered other mental disorders (e.g., dysthymia) in the mortality outcome assessment unless data for depression, as defined above, was provided separately; (3) a diagnosis of depression was based only on clinical evaluation without any specification of the diagnostic criteria; (4) a diagnosis of depression was based only on the use of antidepressants or otherwise on a self-reported (or record-based) history of depression; (5) the association was reported considering other outcomes in addition to mortality (e.g., recurrence); and (6) studies that provided results based on controls that were not included in the original sample (for example, studies that estimated the associations of depression and mortality through standardized mortality ratios compared with general population data external to the study sample).

Two authors (MOM and NV) independently screened the titles and abstracts of retrieved references for eligibility. The full-text articles of potentially eligible articles were then independently scrutinized in detail by two investigators (MOM and NV). Disagreements were resolved through consensus or discussion with a third investigator (CAK or AFC).

Data extraction

Data extraction was done independently by two investigators (MOM and NV) and, in case of discrepancies, a third investigator made the final decision (CAK and AFC). For each eligible reference, we recorded the first author, year, journal of publication, specific populations evaluated and the number of included studies. If a quantitative synthesis was performed, we also extracted the most fully adjusted study-specific risk estimates (relative risk, odds ratio, hazard ratio, or incident risk ratio) and corresponding 95% confidence intervals (CIs). When available, we also extracted the following variables from each study: number of cases (number of death events in participants with depression), sample size, follow-up time, covariates included in multivariable models, method used to define depression (i.e., structured diagnostic interview or screening instrument), study design (case-control, prospective cohort, or retrospective cohort), specific population, as well as the setting and country where the study was conducted. Whenever studies used several control groups, we considered data from healthy controls as the control group. For studies with no quantitative synthesis, the authors' main interpretations about their findings and reasons why a meta-analysis was not conducted were recorded.

Statistical analysis and methodological quality appraisal

We based our analysis on the largest meta-analysis that evaluated the association of depression and all-cause or cause-specific mortality. Furthermore, all datasets from similar meta-analyses that were not included in the largest available one were also considered (i.e., we included all datasets from the smaller meta-analysis that did not overlap with the larger one). We then estimated effect sizes (ES) and 95% CIs through both fixed and random effects models [35]. We also estimated the 95% prediction interval, which further accounts for between-study heterogeneity, and evaluates the uncertainty of the effect that would be expected in a new study addressing the same association [36, 37]. For the largest dataset of each meta-analysis, we calculated the standard error of the ES. If the standard error is < 0.1, then the 95% CI will be < 0.20 (i.e., less than the magnitude of a small ES). We calculated the I^2 metric to quantify between-study heterogeneity. Values ≥ 50% indicate large heterogeneity,

and values ≥ 75% are indicative of very large heterogeneity [38, 39]. To assess evidence for small-study effects we used the asymmetry test developed by Egger et al. [40]. A P value < 0.10 in the Egger's test and the ES of the largest study being more conservative than the summary random effects ES of the meta-analysis were considered indicative of small-study effects [41]. Finally, evidence of an excess of significance was assessed by the Ioannidis test [42]. Briefly, this test estimates whether the number of studies with nominally significant results (i.e., $P < 0.05$) among those included in a meta-analysis is too large considering their power to detect significant effects at an alpha level of 0.05. First, the power of each study is estimated with a non-central t distribution. The sum of all power estimates provides the expected (E) number of datasets with nominal statistical significance. The actual observed (O) number of statistically significant datasets is then compared to the E number using a χ^2-based test [42]. Since the true ES of a meta-analysis cannot be precisely determined, we considered the ES of the largest dataset as the plausible true ES. This decision was based on the fact that simulations indicate that the most appropriate assumption is the ES of the largest dataset included in the meta-analysis [43]. Excess significance for a single meta-analysis was considered if $P < 0.10$ in Ioannidis's test and O > E. We graded the credibility of each association with standard approaches on the following categories [31, 44]: convincing (class I), highly suggestive (class II), suggestive (class III), weak evidence, and non-significant associations (Table 1).

For associations supported by either class I or II evidence, we conducted additional analyses. First, grading of the evidence was re-assessed through sensitivity analyses (when at least three independent datasets were available for each subgroup). The following analyses were considered: (1) prospective cohort studies; (2) studies in which the ascertainment of depression was performed by means of a structured diagnostic interview; (3) studies that provided estimates adjusted for potential confounding variables through multivariable models; (5) studies from which estimates were adjusted at least for sex and age; (6) studies that adjusted for characteristics of the underlying somatic disease (i.e., whenever the association of depression and mortality was assessed in a population with a specific somatic condition); (7) studies that adjusted estimates for the presence of co-morbid diseases (including mental and/or somatic conditions); (8) settings where samples were derived from (community, primary care, outpatient samples, or inpatient samples); and (9) studies in which the follow-up time was longer than 5 years. Finally, we used credibility ceilings, which is a method of sensitivity analyses to account for potential methodological limitations of observational studies that might lead to spurious precision of combined effect estimates. In

Table 1 Criteria for classification of the credibility of the evidence (adapted from reference [31])

Classification	Criteria
Convincing evidence (Class I)	More than 1000 death events
	Significant summary associations ($P < 10^{-6}$) per random effects calculations
	No evidence of small-study effects
	No evidence of excess of significance
	Prediction intervals not including the null
	Not large heterogeneity (i.e., $I^2 < 50\%$)
Highly-suggestive evidence (Class II)	Significant summary associations ($P < 10^{-6}$) per random effects calculation
	More than 1000 death events
	The largest study with 95% confidence intervals excluding the null
Suggestive evidence (Class III)	More than 1000 death events
	Significant summary associations ($P < 10^{-3}$) per random effects calculations
Weak evidence	All other associations with $P < 0.05$
Non-significant associations	All associations with $P > 0.05$

brief, this method assumes that every observational study has a probability c (credibility ceiling) that the true effect size is in a different direction from the one suggested by the point estimate [45, 46]. The pooled effect sizes were re-estimated considering a wide range of credibility ceiling values [30, 45]. All analyses were conducted in STATA/MP 14.0 (StataCorp, USA) with the metan package.

Two investigators (MOM and NV) independently rated the methodological quality of included systematic reviews and meta-analyses with the Assessment of Multiple Systematic Reviews (AMSTAR) instrument, which has been validated for this purpose [47–49]. Scores range from 0 to 11 with higher scores indicating greater quality. The AMSTAR tool involves dichotomous scoring (i.e., 0 or 1) of 11 related items to assess methodological rigor of systematic reviews and meta-analyses (e.g., comprehensive search strategy, publication bias assessment). AMSTAR scores are graded as high (8–11), medium (4–7), and low quality (0–3) [47].

Results

Overall, the title and abstract of 4983 references were screened for eligibility. The full-text of 52 references were then scrutinized in detail, of which 19 were excluded with reasons (Additional file 1: Table S1), while 26 references met inclusion criteria (Fig. 1). Overall, 24 references provided quantitative synthesis of evidence [16, 19, 20, 26–28, 50–67], and 2 references were qualitative systematic reviews [68, 69]. This umbrella review included 238 prospective studies and 8 retrospective cohort studies and comprised data from 3,825,380

participants, including 293,073 participants with depression and 282,732 death events, which were grouped in 17 meta-analytic estimates (Additional file 1: Table S2). Overall, 246 eligible studies were derived from included meta-analyses, while 667 component studies were excluded from eligible meta-analyses due to the following reasons: datasets were included in more than one meta-analysis ($k = 375$); other mental disorders (e.g., dysthymia) were considered in the association between depression and mortality ($k = 14$); a diagnosis of depression was based only on clinical evaluation without any specification of the diagnostic criteria ($k = 7$); a diagnosis of depression was based only on the use of antidepressants ($k = 5$); the association included other outcomes besides mortality (e.g., recurrence) ($k = 5$); overlapping samples ($k = 20$); did not provide data for ES estimation ($k = 12$); a diagnosis of depression was not established according to inclusion criteria ($k = 223$); and assessed the impact of depression on mortality considering standardized mortality ratios against general population data external to the study ($k = 6$). Overall, 165 studies (67.1%) provided adjusted association metrics, with a median number of 5 (IQR 3–8) covariates controlled for in multivariable models (see Additional file 1: Table S3 for the list of factors that were considered in multivariable models in studies derived from eligible meta-analyses). The median follow-up time of included studies was 4.5 years (IQR 2–7.5). The median AMSTAR score of eligible systematic reviews and meta-analyses was 6 (IQR 5–7.5). Scores of each domain of the AMSTAR instrument are provided in Additional file 1: Table S4.

Evidence from qualitative systematic reviews

A systematic review that included 3 studies suggested that depression could be associated with reduced long-term survival in patients with head and neck cancers [68]. In addition, a systematic review that included 11 studies that assessed the association of depression and mortality in chronic pulmonary obstructive pulmonary disease (COPD) met inclusion criteria. The authors concluded that depression could be associated with an increase in early mortality in patients with COPD [69].

Summary effect sizes

At a threshold of $P < 0.05$, summary ESs were significant for all 17 (100%) meta-analytic estimates in both fixed and random effects models (Additional file 1: Table S2). At a more conservative threshold of $P < 0.001$, 16 (94.1%) and 9 (52.9%) estimates were significant in fixed and random effects models, respectively. At a threshold of $P < 10^{-6}$, 12 (70.6%) and 5 (29.4%) meta-analyses were statistically significant in fixed and random effects models, respectively.

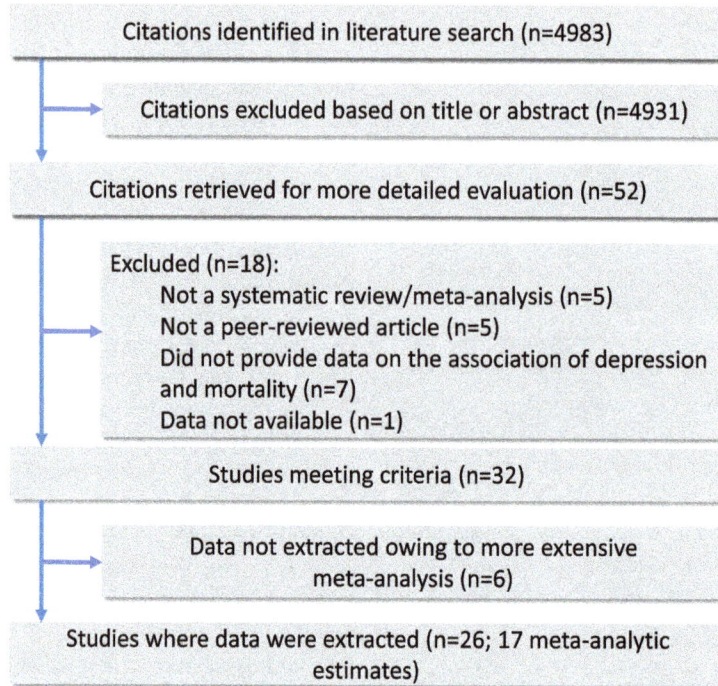

```
┌─────────────────────────────────────────────────────────────────┐
│        Citations identified in literature search (n=4983)         │
└─────────────────────────────────────────────────────────────────┘
                 │
                 │   ┌─────────────────────────────────────────────────┐
                 ├──▶│ Citations excluded based on title or abstract (n=4931) │
                 │   └─────────────────────────────────────────────────┘
                 ▼
┌─────────────────────────────────────────────────────────────────┐
│      Citations retrieved for more detailed evaluation (n=52)      │
└─────────────────────────────────────────────────────────────────┘
                 │
                 │   ┌─────────────────────────────────────────────────┐
                 ├──▶│ Excluded (n=18):                                 │
                 │   │    Not a systematic review/meta-analysis (n=5)   │
                 │   │    Not a peer-reviewed article (n=5)             │
                 │   │    Did not provide data on the association of depression │
                 │   │    and mortality (n=7)                           │
                 │   │    Data not available (n=1)                      │
                 │   └─────────────────────────────────────────────────┘
                 ▼
┌─────────────────────────────────────────────────────────────────┐
│                Studies meeting criteria (n=32)                     │
└─────────────────────────────────────────────────────────────────┘
                 │
                 │   ┌─────────────────────────────────────────────────┐
                 ├──▶│ Data not extracted owing to more extensive       │
                 │   │ meta-analysis (n=6)                              │
                 │   └─────────────────────────────────────────────────┘
                 ▼
┌─────────────────────────────────────────────────────────────────┐
│ Studies where data were extracted (n=26; 17 meta-analytic         │
│ estimates)                                                         │
└─────────────────────────────────────────────────────────────────┘
```

Fig. 1 Study flowchart

Heterogeneity between studies

Six meta-analyses (35.6%) showed large heterogeneity ($I^2 = 50$–75%) and 5 (29.4%) exhibited very large heterogeneity ($I^2 > 75\%$) (Additional file 1: Table S5). We further assessed the uncertainty of the summary effects by calculating their 95% prediction intervals; the null value was excluded in only 3 associations, namely in all-cause mortality in coronary artery bypass graft patients, coronary heart disease patients, and COPD patients.

Small-study effects

Evidence of small-study effects was verified in 13 meta-analyses, including associations of depression and all-cause mortality in patients after coronary artery bypass grafting, with acute coronary syndrome or coronary heart disease, after stroke, post-transplant patients, and people with HIV, chronic kidney disease, heart failure, COPD, diabetes mellitus, and mixed settings, as well as associations with depression and fatal stroke and cardiovascular mortality after acute myocardial infarction (Additional file 1: Table S5) [51].

Excess significance

We assessed excess of significance bias (i.e., the likelihood that the observed number of nominally significant studies could exceed the expected number of 'positive' studies for a given estimate). Eleven (64.7%) meta-analyses had evidence of excess significance bias, namely those investigating the associations of all-cause mortality and cancer,

heart failure, mixed settings, coronary heart disease, acute coronary syndrome, stroke, post-transplant patients, chronic kidney disease, as well as associations of depression and fatal stroke, cardiovascular mortality in patients with diabetes mellitus, and cardiovascular mortality in mixed settings (Additional file 1: Table S5).

Grading of the evidence

We explored whether the nominally significant associations between mortality and depression were supported by convincing, highly suggestive, suggestive, or weak evidence (Table 2). Overall, no association was supported by convincing evidence, while associations of depression and all-cause mortality among patients with cancer, patients after acute myocardial infarction, patients with heart failure, and mixed settings (including inpatients, outpatients, and community as well as primary care samples) were supported by highly suggestive evidence. Furthermore, associations between depression and all-cause mortality in patients with coronary heart disease and diabetes mellitus were supported by suggestive evidence. Finally, the remaining 11 (64.7%) associations were supported by weak evidence (Table 2).

Sensitivity analyses

Sensitivity analyses were performed for the four associations supported by highly suggestive evidence as per our protocol (Table 3). It is worth noting that, when studies that employed structured/semi-structured diagnostic

Table 2 Details of evidence grading for meta-analyses investigating associations of depression and mortality

Author, year	Population	Mortality type	Sample size MDD/Deaths	k	Largest study ES (95% CI)[a]	Random effects summary RR[b] (95% CI)	Random effects P value[c]	95% prediction interval	I² (%)	Excess significance O/E[d]	Excess significance P-value
Associations supported by highly suggestive evidence											
Cuijpers, 2014 [51] Satin, 2009 [62]	Cancer	All-cause	4034/4817	23	1.37 (1.26–1.50)	1.55 (1.32–1.81)	$<10^{-6}$	0.80–2.50	69.6	11/4.53	< 0.001
Cuijpers, 2014 [51] Sorensen, 2005 [64] Meijer, 2013 [67] van Melle, 2004 [58]	Post-AMI	All-cause	4183/2358	20	1.48 (1.12–1.96)	2.09 (1.66–2.63)	$<10^{-6}$	0.89–3.54	66.6	12/11.0	0.64
Cuijpers, 2014 [51] Fan, 2014 [28] Gathright 2017 [54] Sokoreli, 2016 [63]	HF	All-cause	3418/4345	22	1.33 (1.19–1.42)	1.46 (1.30–1.65)	$<10^{-6}$	0.89–1.92	81.0	14/6.5	< 0.001
Baxter, 2011 [50] Cuijpers, 2002 [19] Cuijpers, 2014 [51] Walker, 2015 [16]	Mixed-sample[e]	All-cause	87,633/242577	111	1.77 (1.41–2.17)	1.48 (1.39–1.58)	$<10^{-6}$	0.84–2.23	89.3	55/17.8	0.00
Associations supported by suggestive evidence											
Barth, 2004 [26] Cuijpers, 2014 [51] Leung, 2012 [56] Meijer, 2013 [67]	CHD	All-cause	2284/1533	10	1.21 (1.04–1.42)	1.57 (1.27–1.94)	$<10^{-4}$	1.16–1.47	62.6	5/1.18	< 0.001
Cuijpers, 2014 [51] Hofmann, 2013 [55] Park, 2013 [60]	DM	All-cause	4373/7452	12	1.06 (0.96–1.18)	1.60 (1.30–1.80)	$<10^{-6}$	0.90–3.21	83.6	8/5.72	0.18
Associations supported by weak evidence											
Cuijpers, 2014 [51] Stenman, 2016 [65]	CABG	All-cause	503/347	4	2.40 (1.40–4.00)	1.93 (1.43–2.60)	$<10^{-4}$	1.09–3.18	0	2/2.32	0.74
Cuijpers, 2014 [51] Meijer, 2013 [67]	ACS	All-cause	324/163	3	2.80 (1.40–5.07)	1.82 (1.02–3.26)	0.04	0.06–48.2	86.4	2/0.54	0.02

Table 2 Details of evidence grading for meta-analyses investigating associations of depression and mortality (Continued)

Author, year	Population	Mortality type	Sample size MDD/Deaths	k	Largest study ES (95% CI)[a]	Random effects summary RR[b] (95% CI)	Random effects P value[c]	95% prediction interval	I^2 (%)	Excess significance O/E[d]	Excess significance P- value
Bartoli, 2013 [20] Cuijpers, 2014 [51] Pan, 2011 [59]	Stroke	All-cause	3103/414	7	1.13 (1.06–1.21)	1.46 (1.15–1.85)	0.002	0.80–2.13	62.1	4/0.04	0.00
Pan, 2011 [59]	Stroke	Fatal Stroke	1600/377	4	1.66 (1.16–2.39)	1.58 (1.00–2.50)	0.049	0.21–8.07	46.7	2/0.02	0.00
Cuijpers, 2014 [51] Dew, 2015 [52]	Post-transplant patients[f]	All-cause	405/433	6	1.66 (1.12–2.47)	1.64 (1.37–1.95)	$< 10^{-2}$	0.71–2.65	36.5	4/0.86	$< 10^{-3}$
Cuijpers, 2014 [51]	HIV	All-cause	1977/1580	4	1.60 (1.32–1.92)	1.30 (1.05–1.61)	0.017	0.61–2.70	55.1	1/1.79	0.42
Meijer, 2011 [57]	AMI	Cardiovascular Mortality	995/114	5	5.51 (0.61–49.18)	2.98 (1.65–5.38)	$< 10^{-3}$	0.26–15.80	42.3	3/2.37	0.57
Cuijpers, 2014 [51] Palmer, 2013 [27]	CKD	All-cause	922/930	12	0.98 (0.72–1.34)	1.66 (1.20–2.30)	$< 10^{-2}$	0.84–1.40	44.4	4/0.17	0.00
Cuijpers, 2014 [51]	COPD	All-cause	338/261	5	1.93 (1.04–3.58)	2.34 (1.69–3.24)	$< 10^{-6}$	1.23–3.63	0.00	4/3.01	0.25
van Dooren, 2013 [53]	DM	Cardiovascular	1255/536	4	1.25 (0.83–1.86)	1.48 (1.08–2.03)	0.014	0.61–3.00	52.5	2/0.38	$< 10^{-2}$
Correll, 2017 [66]	Mixed samples[g]	Cardiovascular mortality	175,726/14495	4	1.00 (0.85–1.17)	1.56 (1.08–2.24)	0.018	0.34–6.82	87.8	3/1.00	0.02

ACS acute coronary syndrome, AMI acute myocardial infarction, CA cancer, CABG coronary artery bypass grafting, CHD coronary heart disease, CI confidence interval, CKD chronic kidney disease, COPD chronic pulmonary obstructive disease, DM diabetes mellitus, E expected, ES effect size, HF heart failure, MDD major depressive disorder, O observed, RR risk ratio

[a]Relative risk and 95% confidence interval of largest study (smallest standard error) in each meta-analysis

[b]Random effects refer to summary effect size (95% confidence interval) using the random effects model

[c]P value of summary random effects estimate

[d]Expected number of statistically significant studies using the point estimate of the largest study (smallest standard error) as the plausible effect size

[e]Kidney, liver, heart, and lung transplantation

[f]Includes community samples, inpatients, outpatients, and primary care samples

[g]Includes community, outpatient, and inpatient samples

Table 3 Sensitivity analyses for associations of depression and all-cause mortality supported by highly suggestive (class II) evidence

Subgroup	Sample size MDD/Deaths	k	Largest study ES (95% CI)[a]	Random effects summary ES[b] (95% CI)	Random effects P value[c]	95% prediction interval	I² (%)	Excess significance O/E[d]	P value	Classification
All-cause in cancer										
Structured interview	145/462	5	2.85 (2.29–3.54)	1.56 (0.87–2.8)	0.133	0.28–8.56	71.9	1/1.02	0.979	Weak
Adjusted estimates only	1066/2273	13	1.2 (0.9–1.4)	1.6 (1.35–1.9)	$< 10^{-6}$	1.02–2.51	42.3	8/5.16	0.097	Class III
Adjusted at least for age and sex	691/1030	6	1.2 (0.9–1.4)	1.69 (1.23–2.31)	0.001	0.77–3.68	51.6	4/3.3	0.563	Class III
Adjusted comorbidities	910/1951	9	1.2 (0.9–1.4)	1.52 (1.27–1.83)	< 0.001	0.97–2.4	43.3	5/3.54	0.3	Class III
Inpatients	764/618	10	1.66 (1.16–2.37)	1.7 (1.35–2.13)	< 0.001	0.96–3	40.9	6/3.55	0.106	Weak
Outpatients	453/1418	10	1.3 (0.98–1.73)	1.56 (1.11–2.17)	0.009	0.57–4.28	75.3	4/2.57	0.291	Class III
Prospective studies	4034/4817	23	1.37 (1.26–1.5)	1.55 (1.32–1.81)	$< 10^{-6}$	0.86–2.78	69.6	11/6.21	0.023	Class II
Follow-up ≤ 5 years	946/1580	15	1.2 (0.9–1.4)	1.8 (1.42–2.28)	< 0.001	0.83–3.9	68.1	9/6.64	0.22	Class III
Follow-up > 5 years	3088/3237	8	1.37 (1.26–1.5)	1.29 (1.14–1.47)	< 0.001	1–1.68	22.5	2/1.52	0.658	Class III
All-cause in heart failure patients[e]										
Adjusted estimates only	3383/4275	21	1.33 (1.19–1.42)	1.46 (1.29–1.64)	$< 10^{-6}$	0.93–2.27	79.1	14/9.83	0.068	Class II
Adjusted at least for age and sex	2526/2935	13	1.33 (1.19–1.42)	1.36 (1.22–1.52)	$< 10^{-6}$	0.99–1.86	54.3	9/5.39	0.042	Class II
Adjusted for comorbidities	2395/3371	12	1.33 (1.19–1.42)	1.43 (1.26–1.62)	$< 10^{-6}$	1–2.04	60.5	8/6.58	0.41	Class II
Inpatients	1245/1500	7	2.02 (1.48–2.76)	1.82 (1.28–2.6)	< 0.001	0.64–5.19	77.7	4/5.12	0.339	Class III
Outpatients	639/583	6	1.31 (1.07–1.6)	1.46 (1.08–1.96)	0.013	0.67–3.16	75.2	4/1.8	0.049	Weak
Prospective studies	3418/4345	22	1.33 (1.19–1.42)	1.46 (1.3–1.65)	$< 10^{-6}$	0.94–2.28	78.4	14/10.02	0.088	Class II
Follow-up ≤ 5 years	2417/2358	16	1.33 (1.19–1.42)	1.52 (1.3–1.77)	$< 10^{-6}$	0.93–2.47	80.0	10/6.55	0.079	Class II
Follow-up > 5 years	1001/1987	6	1.31 (1.07–1.6)	1.4 (1.14–1.72)	0.001	0.76–2.57	72.5	4/3.41	0.627	Class III
All-cause in mixed sample[e]										
Structured interview	4746/29667	19	2.3 (2.1–2.5)	1.64 (1.3–2.08)	< 0.001	0.62–4.38	88.7	11/13.06	0.277	Class III
Adjusted estimates only	83,470/212385	81	1.77 (1.41–2.17)	1.42 (1.33–1.5)	$< 10^{-6}$	0.93–2.15	86.5	44/16.69	0	Class II
Adjusted at least for age and sex	51,332/161660	42	1.1 (1.07–1.13)	1.34 (1.25–1.43)	$< 10^{-6}$	0.96–1.85	82.4	23/15.72	0.017	Class II
Adjusted for comorbidities	34,122/41488	53	1.77 (1.41–2.17)	1.38 (1.29–1.47)	$< 10^{-6}$	0.97–1.96	71.6	31/3.66	0	Class II
Community	32,269/69181	62	1.77 (1.41–2.17)	1.48 (1.36–1.61)	$< 10^{-6}$	0.83–2.63	88.2	31/8.76	0	Class II
Inpatients	2209/2334	16	1.44 (1.1–1.88)	1.58 (1.33–1.87)	$< 10^{-6}$	0.93–2.68	56.0	10/5.69	0.019	Class II
Outpatients	811/497	6	1.55 (1.06–2.26)	1.47 (1.13–1.91)	0.004	0.8–2.68	34.5	4/0.58	0	Weak
Primary care	8730/4558	6	1.04 (0.93–1.15)	1.44 (1.11–1.86)	0.006	0.67–3.1	82.0	4/2.13	0.11	Class III
Prospective studies	46,951/96860	95	1.77 (1.41–2.17)	1.51 (1.4–1.62)	$< 10^{-6}$	0.86–2.63	87.1	51/11.97	0	Class II
Follow-up ≤ 5 years	24,944/26135	61	1.37 (1.19–1.48)	1.62 (1.48–1.77)	$< 10^{-6}$	0.96–2.71	75.7	34/17.79	0	Class II
Follow-up > 5 years	62,689/216442	40	1.77 (1.41–2.17)	1.36 (1.24–1.48)	$< 10^{-6}$	0.81–2.26	93.8	21/8.41	0	Class II
All-cause in post-AMI										
Structured interview	1688/638	5	1.48 (1.12–1.96)	2.37 (1.36–4.14)	0.002	0.41–13.76	86.3	4/4.12	0.886	Weak
Adjusted estimates only	2381/1771	9	1.48 (1.12–1.96)	2.2 (1.51–3.2)	< 0.001	0.71–6.81	80.7	7/7.88	0.374	Class III
Adjusted for comorbidities	1507/579	3	1.48 (1.12–1.96)	1.56 (1.18–2.06)	0.001	0.79–3.1	5.1	2/2.15	0.843	Weak
Inpatients	3998/2196	17	1.48 (1.12–1.96)	2.09 (1.63–2.69)	$< 10^{-6}$	0.9–4.85	70.3	10/12.89	0.102	Class II
Prospective studies	4183/2358	20	1.48 (1.12–1.96)	2.09 (1.66–2.63)	$< 10^{-6}$	0.95–4.62	66.6	12/14.72	0.168	Class II
Follow-up ≤ 5 years	3602/1789	16	1.67 (1.31–2.12)	2.18 (1.66–2.86)	$< 10^{-6}$	0.89–5.32	69.4	9/12.4	0.042	Class II
Follow-up > 5 years	533/560	3	1.48 (1.12–1.96)	1.57 (1.25–1.99)	< 0.001	0.94–2.63	0.0	2/1.31	0.42	Weak

AMI acute myocardial infarction, *CI* confidence interval, *E* expected, *ES* effect size, *MDD* major depressive disorder, *NA* not available, *NE* not evaluated, *NS* not significant, *O* observed

[a]ES and 95% confidence interval of largest study (smallest standard error) in each meta-analysis

[b]Random effects refer to summary effect size (95% CI) using the random effects model

[c]P value of summary random effects estimate

[d]Expected number of statistically significant studies using the point estimate of the largest study (smallest standard error) as the plausible effect size

[e]Include community samples, inpatients, outpatients and primary care

interviews were considered, associations of depression and all cause-mortality in cancer as well as post-acute myocardial infarction became supported by weak evidence, while the association of depression and all-cause mortality in mixed settings dropped to suggestive evidence. Furthermore, when only studies that provided adjusted estimates were considered, associations of depression and all-cause mortality in cancer and post-acute myocardial infarction dropped to suggestive evidence. Moreover, the association of depression and all-cause mortality in cancer was supported by suggestive evidence only when studies that adjusted at least for age and sex were assessed in analysis.

Sensitivity analyses through credibility ceilings were also conducted for the four associations supported by highly suggestive evidence (Additional file 1: Table S6). All associations remained significant when 10% credibility ceilings were considered, while no associations were nominally significant when 20% credibility ceilings were considered.

Discussion

The associations between mental disorders and mortality have been investigated for more than 150 years [70, 71]. The associations between depression and all-cause and cause-specific mortality has been particularly investigated across different types of settings and populations. All meta-analyses have obtained nominally statistically significant results for a higher risk of mortality in almost all the tested populations. However, no associations met criteria for convincing evidence, while only four associations, namely those of depression and all-cause mortality in cancer, heart failure, mixed settings as well as among patients after acute myocardial infarction, were supported by highly suggestive evidence. Nevertheless, our sensitivity analyses indicate that differences in case ascertainment of depression as well as the lack of proper adjustment for confounding variables and other major risk factors could render several associations supported by lower levels of evidence. Therefore, the current work suggests that causal inferences between depression and all-cause mortality across distinct populations do not appear to be as conclusive as once thought [16, 21, 72].

Several variables and mechanisms may contribute to the observed associations of depression and all-cause mortality. Some effects may be direct. For example, it has been suggested that depression activates several pathophysiological mechanisms that could contribute to the emergence of chronic somatic diseases that are consistently related to lowered survival. For instance, it has been claimed that depression is associated with peripheral inflammation [73] and oxidative stress [74], mechanisms which may contribute to the association of depression and obesity and cardio-metabolic conditions [66, 75–77]. However, depression may also exert indirect

effects on survival. For example, a large body of evidence suggests that depression alters illness behavior [78], leading to a meaningful decrease in treatment adherence across several conditions [79, 80] as well as unhealthy lifestyles (e.g., sedentary behavior, higher prevalence of smoking, and non-salutary diet) [23, 73, 81, 82]. Depression also often co-exists with other mental health conditions that may also be associated with elevated mortality rates [25, 72]. Multivariable adjustment has varied across included studies, and only approximately 40% of included studies controlled their results at least for age and sex. Mortality analyses that do not account for at least these two major determinants of death risk are problematic. We observed that, when only studies that controlled for age and sex were considered, the association of depression and all-cause mortality in cancer was no longer supported by highly suggestive evidence. Furthermore, no association was supported by highly suggestive evidence when only studies that employed structured/semi-structured diagnostic interviews were considered. This is a relevant finding since recent evidence suggests that the selective use of different cutoff points may bias accuracy estimates of screening instruments for depression, even if these instruments are considered to be validated, whilst this type of bias does not apparently occur in gold-standard structured diagnostic interviews [83]. It is worthy to note, however, that the association between depression and all-cause mortality among patients with heart failure remained supported by highly suggestive evidence when only studies that provided either adjusted estimates or, otherwise, that adjusted for age and sex were considered, while due to the lack of available datasets sensitivity analyses considering studies that used structured/semi-structured diagnostic interviews could not be performed. Therefore, further studies should be conducted to evaluate this association.

Comparison with other studies

Cuijpers et al. [51] performed the largest meta-analysis to date assessing the impact of depression on mortality. Although this previous meta-analysis concluded that depression is associated with all-cause mortality, fewer studies were available when that study was conducted. In addition, the inclusion criteria differed from ours. For example, Cuijpers et al. [51] included studies in which a diagnosis of depression was based on previous exposure to antidepressants, which are drugs used for several other medical and psychiatric indications, whilst we limited our inclusion criteria to investigations in which depression was assessed by either a structured/unstructured diagnostic interview or a screening instrument with a cut-off score, and also large-scale studies that used a coded diagnosis of depression based on well-established criteria. In addition, we estimated the credibility of the evidence in different settings and populations with state-of-the art statistical methods used in previous umbrella reviews [8, 30].

A previous meta-review investigated the associations between severe mental disorders (including depression) and all-cause and suicide-related mortality [72]. Although the authors concluded that depression was associated with an excess of all-cause mortality, only three references were included and the credibility of the evidence was not quantitatively assessed. Finally, a recent study pooled evidence from 15 systematic reviews and meta-analyses and observed that evidence that depression is associated with all-cause mortality remains inconclusive [84]. This previous effort is the most comprehensive assessment of the impact of depression on mortality conducted to date. The inclusion criteria differed from ours. Furthermore, in the current effort, an attempt to demarcate the putative impact of depression on survival in different populations was performed. In addition, we assessed several hints of biases in this literature. Our findings provide further quantitative evidence that the causality of associations between depression and elevated all-cause mortality across different populations and settings remains to be proven.

Strengths and limitations

Our umbrella review might have missed some available evidence, e.g., recently published studies that had not been included in the prior meta-analyses [29]. However, in this effort, we assessed all available systematic reviews and meta-analyses, and all unique datasets which met inclusion criteria were synthesized for each estimate from all available meta-analyses and most considered meta-analyses were very recent. Although several hints of bias were found to be prevalent in this literature, it is relevant to mention that this finding does not exclude the presence of genuine (i.e., true) heterogeneity in this field. Moreover, the Ioannidis test has relatively low power in a context of high heterogeneity [42], while the assumption that the largest study could approximate the underlying 'true' effect size of a meta-analysis may be less straightforward for observational studies than for randomized controlled trials. Depression is a heterogeneous phenotype with different symptomatic dimensions and subtypes [85]. For example, a model has proposed that the duration and specific dimensions of depression (i.e., 'cognitive/affective' versus 'somatic/affective') may have a differential impact on the progression of coronary artery disease after acute coronary syndrome [86]. This framework was supported by a previous meta-analysis that has shown that somatic/affective symptoms of depression may exert a stronger deleterious effect upon mortality compared to cognitive/affective symptoms in patients with heart disease [87]. In addition, a recent individual-patient meta-analysis suggested that, following proper adjustment for cardiovascular factors, the

association between depression and all-cause mortality is notably attenuated in patients after an acute myocardial infarction [67]. This finding underscores that the extent of proper or suboptimal adjustment of clinical and sociodemographic variables may render the association between depression and mortality less consistent across populations with chronic diseases. Although we conducted several sensitivity analyses, the reporting and multivariable adjustment to potential confounders was not consistent across included studies, thus limiting the quality of available evidence. It is possible that more studies adjusted their results at least to age and sex but considered it so trivial that they did not even report on this. Therefore, more thorough reporting of model specification and adjustment is needed in future studies.

Finally, depression may manifest in samples with chronic somatic conditions differently. For example, the diagnosis of depression in cancer patients has been a matter of debate, and may also be ascribed as a spectrum of syndromes [88, 89], some of which may not be properly captured by conventional diagnostic criteria (e.g., DSM-5 or ICD-10) [88]. Furthermore, there is a spectrum related to the timing of appearance with symptoms. In some circumstances, depression may either antedate or be considered an initial manifestation of chronic somatic diseases [78, 90], whilst in other circumstances depression may occur after the onset of the medical condition [78], and also as a result of treatment and its complications. The current effort could not elucidate how the temporal relationship between depression and the respective chronic medical condition could potentially influence mortality rates.

Implications

Our findings suggest that available evidence does not consistently allow the establishment of causal inferences linking depression to all-cause and cause-specific mortality across different settings and populations. Yet, the association of depression and all-cause mortality appears to be complex, and may be influenced by several sociodemographic and clinical variables. Moreover, we do not question the association between depression and suicide where the evidence is unquestionable [18, 91, 92]. However, suicides appear to account for a relatively smaller fraction of deaths compared to natural causes of death among people with depression [93–95].

The current data may also reconcile some controversies in existing literature. For example, although previous evidence has suggested that post-acute myocardial infarction depression might be associated with diminished survival, no conclusive evidence indicated that the treatment of depression translates to an increased survival in this specific population [96, 97]. Therefore, findings from this umbrella review of observational studies and data from intervention studies conducted to date appear to concur in that associations between depression and all-cause and cause-specific mortality are unlikely to be causal.

For other conditions, such as cancer, it remains unclear if prevention and treatment of depression may increase overall survival. Management of depression is worthwhile for various other reasons, e.g., improvement of quality of life, but not with the expectation that death risk will decrease. Furthermore, interventions aiming to promote a healthy lifestyle as well as the proper care of co-occurring somatic conditions in those with depression may also lead to a decrease in all-cause mortality [25]. However, the impact of those interventions at an individual, societal, and health system levels upon all-cause survival warrant further investigation.

Conclusions

The associations between depression and all-cause and specific natural cause mortality has been extensively investigated in a wide range of populations and settings. However, this umbrella review of observational studies indicates that the evidence for causal associations of depression and all-cause mortality remains inconclusive. To draw firmer conclusions, further prospective and collaborative studies with transparent a priori-defined protocols and a proper multivariable adjustment to confounders and other important risk determinants for mortality are warranted.

Abbreviations
AMSTAR: Assessment of Multiple Systematic Reviews; CI: confidence interval; COPD: chronic pulmonary obstructive disease; E: expected; ES: effect size; O: observed

Acknowledgements
CAK is supported by a postdoctoral research fellowship from the Coordenação de Aperfeiçoamento de Pessoal de Nível Superior (CAPES, Brazil). AK's work was supported by the Miguel Servet contract financed by the CP13/00150 and PI15/00862 projects, integrated into the National R + D + I and funded by the ISCIII - General Branch Evaluation and Promotion of Research - and the European Regional Development Fund (ERDF-FEDER).

Authors' contributions
All authors designed this research. MOM, NV, and CAK extracted data. CAK, IT, JPAI, and AFC analyzed the data. MOM, NV, CAK, JPAI, and AFC wrote the first draft of the manuscript. All authors contributed to the interpretation of findings and wrote the final version of the manuscript. The final version was read and approved by all authors.

Competing interests
The authors declare that they have no competing interests.

Author details
[1]Department of Clinical Medicine and Translational Psychiatry Research Group, Faculty of Medicine, Federal University of Ceará, Fortaleza, CE 60430-140, Brazil. [2]Institute for Clinical Research and Education in Medicine (IREM), 35128 Padova, Italy. [3]National Research Council, Neuroscience Institute, Aging Branch, 35128 Padova, Italy. [4]Biostatistical Consulting Unit, Centre for Addiction and Mental Health (CAMH), Toronto, ON, Canada. [5]South London and Maudsley NHS Foundation Trust, Denmark Hill, London SE5 8AZ, UK. [6]Institute of Psychiatry, Psychology and Neuroscience (IoPPN), King's College London, De Crespigny Park, London, AF SE5 8, UK. [7]Faculty of Health, Social Care and Education, Anglia Ruskin University, Chelmsford CM1 1SQ, UK. [8]Parc Sanitari Sant Joan de Déu, Universitat de Barcelona, Fundació Sant Joan de Déu/CIBERSAM, 08950 Barcelona, Spain. [9]Faculty of Education and Health, University of Greenwich, London SE10 9LS, UK. [10]Department of Epidemiology and Biostatistics, School of Public Health, Imperial College London, W2 1PG, London, UK. [11]MRC-PHE Centre for Environment, School of Public Health, Imperial College London, London W2 1PG, UK. [12]Department of Hygiene and Epidemiology, University of Ioannina Medical School, Ioannina, Greece. [13]Department of Neuroscience, University of Padova, 35100 Padova, Italy. [14]Department of Rehabilitation Sciences, KU Leuven - University of Leuven, 3001 Leuven, Belgium. [15]KU Leuven - University of Leuven, University Psychiatric Center KU Leuven, 3070 Leuven, Kortenberg, Belgium. [16]Centro Universitário La Salle, Canoas, Brazil. [17]Hospital de Clínicas de Porto Alegre, Porto Alegre, Brazil. [18]Department of Psychiatry, Faculty of Medicine, Chulalongkorn University, Bangkok 10330, Thailand. [19]IMPACT Strategic Research Center, Barwon Health, Deakin University, Geelong, VIC, Australia. [20]Department of Psychology, University of Bologna, viale Berti Pichat 5, 40127 Bologna, Italy. [21]Department of Psychiatry, Erie County Medical Center, 462 Grider Street, Buffalo, NY 14215, USA. [22]Department of Medicine, Stanford University, Palo Alto, CA 94305, USA. [23]Department of Health Research and Policy, Stanford University, Palo Alto, CA 94305, USA. [24]Department of Statistics, Stanford University, Palo Alto, CA 94305, USA. [25]Department of Meta-Research Innovation Center at Stanford (METRICS), Stanford University, Palo Alto, CA 94305, USA. [26]Department of Psychiatry, University of Toronto, Toronto, ON, Canada. [27]Centre for Addiction & Mental Health (CAMH), 33 Russel Street, room RS1050S, Toronto, ON M5S 2S1, Canada.

References
1. Bromet E, Andrade LH, Hwang I, Sampson NA, Alonso J, de Girolamo G, de Graaf R, Demyttenaere K, Hu C, Iwata N, et al. Cross-national epidemiology of DSM-IV major depressive episode. BMC Med. 2011;9:90.
2. Kessler RC, Bromet EJ. The epidemiology of depression across cultures. Annu Rev Public Health. 2013;34:119–38.
3. Global Burden of Disease Study 2013 Collaborators. Global, regional, and national incidence, prevalence, and years lived with disability for 301 acute and chronic diseases and injuries in 188 countries, 1990–2013: a systematic analysis for the Global Burden of Disease Study 2013. Lancet. 2015; 386(9995):743–800.
4. Ferrari AJ, Charlson FJ, Norman RE, Patten SB, Freedman G, Murray CJ, Vos T, Whiteford HA. Burden of depressive disorders by country, sex, age, and year: findings from the global burden of disease study 2010. PLoS Med. 2013; 10(11):e1001547.
5. Rackley S, Bostwick JM. Depression in medically ill patients. Psychiatr Clin North Am. 2012;35(1):231–47.
6. Rotella F, Mannucci E. Depression as a risk factor for diabetes: a meta-analysis of longitudinal studies. J Clin Psychiatry. 2013;74(1):31–7.

7. Luppino FS, de Wit LM, Bouvy PF, Stijnen T, Cuijpers P, Penninx BW, Zitman FG. Overweight, obesity, and depression: a systematic review and meta-analysis of longitudinal studies. Arch Gen Psychiatry. 2010;67(3):220–9.

8. Tsilidis KK, Kasimis JC, Lopez DS, Ntzani EE, Ioannidis JP. Type 2 diabetes and cancer: umbrella review of meta-analyses of observational studies. BMJ. 2015;350:g7607.

9. Wu Q, Kling JM. Depression and the risk of myocardial infarction and coronary death: a meta-analysis of prospective cohort studies. Medicine (Baltimore). 2016;95(6):e2815.

10. Cherbuin N, Kim S. Dementia risk estimates associated with measures of depression: a systematic review and meta-analysis. BMJ Open. 2015; 5(12):e008853.

11. Read JR, Sharpe L, Modini M, Dear BF. Multimorbidity and depression: a systematic review and meta-analysis. J Affect Disord. 2017;221:36–46.

12. Rotella F, Mannucci E. Diabetes mellitus as a risk factor for depression. A meta-analysis of longitudinal studies. Diabetes Res Clin Pract. 2013; 99(2):98–104.

13. Hackett ML, Pickles K. Part I: frequency of depression after stroke: an updated systematic review and meta-analysis of observational studies. Int J Stroke. 2014;9(8):1017–25.

14. Lichtman JH, Froelicher ES, Blumenthal JA, Carney RM, Doering LV, Frasure-Smith N, Freedland KE, Jaffe AS, Leifheit-Limson EC, Sheps DS, et al. Depression as a risk factor for poor prognosis among patients with acute coronary syndrome: systematic review and recommendations: a scientific statement from the American Heart Association. Circulation. 2014;129(12):1350–69.

15. Bennett S, Thomas AJ. Depression and dementia: cause, consequence or coincidence? Maturitas. 2014;79(2):184–90.

16. Walker ER, McGee RE, Druss BG. Mortality in mental disorders and global disease burden implications: a systematic review and meta-analysis. JAMA Psychiatry. 2015;72(4):334–41.

17. Pratt LA, Druss BG, Manderscheid RW, Walker ER. Excess mortality due to depression and anxiety in the United States: results from a nationally representative survey. Gen Hosp Psychiatry. 2016;39:39–45.

18. Bolton JM, Gunnell D, Turecki G. Suicide risk assessment and intervention in people with mental illness. BMJ. 2015;351:h4978.

19. Cuijpers P, Smit F. Excess mortality in depression: a meta-analysis of community studies. J Affect Disord. 2002;72(3):227–36.

20. Bartoli F, Lillia N, Lax A, Crocamo C, Mantero V, Carra G, Agostoni E, Clerici M. Depression after stroke and risk of mortality: a systematic review and meta-analysis. Stroke Res Treat. 2013;2013:862978.

21. Cuijpers P, Vogelzangs N, Twisk J, Kleiboer A, Li J, Penninx BW. Is excess mortality higher in depressed men than in depressed women? A meta-analytic comparison. J Affect Disord. 2014;161:47–54.

22. Rethorst CD, Leonard D, Barlow CE, Willis BL, Trivedi MH, DeFina LF. Effects of depression, metabolic syndrome, and cardiorespiratory fitness on mortality: results from the Cooper Center longitudinal study. Psychol Med. 2017;47(14):1–7.

23. Schuch F, Vancampfort D, Firth J, Rosenbaum S, Ward P, Reichert T, Bagatini NC, Bgeginski R, Stubbs B. Physical activity and sedentary behavior in people with major depressive disorder: a systematic review and meta-analysis. J Affect Disord. 2017;210:139–50.

24. Prochaska JJ, Das S, Young-Wolff KC. Smoking, mental illness, and public health. Annu Rev Public Health. 2017;38:165–85.

25. Liu NH, Daumit GL, Dua T, Aquila R, Charlson F, Cuijpers P, Druss B, Dudek K, Freeman M, Fujii C, et al. Excess mortality in persons with severe mental disorders: a multilevel intervention framework and priorities for clinical practice, policy and research agendas. World Psychiatry. 2017;16(1):30–40.

26. Barth J, Schumacher M, Herrmann-Lingen C. Depression as a risk factor for mortality in patients with coronary heart disease: a meta-analysis. Psychosom Med. 2004;66(6):802–13.

27. Palmer SC, Vecchio M, Craig JC, Tonelli M, Johnson DW, Nicolucci A, Pellegrini F, Saglimbene V, Logroscino G, Hedayati SS, et al. Association between depression and death in people with CKD: a meta-analysis of cohort studies. Am J Kidney Dis. 2013;62(3):493–505.

28. Fan H, Yu W, Zhang Q, Cao H, Li J, Wang J, Shao Y, Hu X. Depression after heart failure and risk of cardiovascular and all-cause mortality: a meta-analysis. Prev Med. 2014;63:36–42.

29. Ioannidis JP. Integration of evidence from multiple meta-analyses: a primer on umbrella reviews, treatment networks and multiple treatments meta-analyses. CMAJ. 2009;181(8):488–93.

30. Kyrgiou M, Kalliala I, Markozannes G, Gunter MJ, Paraskevaidis E, Gabra H, Martin-Hirsch P, Tsilidis KK. Adiposity and cancer at major anatomical sites: umbrella review of the literature. BMJ. 2017;356:j477.

31. Belbasis L, Bellou V, Evangelou E, Ioannidis JP, Tzoulaki I. Environmental risk factors and multiple sclerosis: an umbrella review of systematic reviews and meta-analyses. Lancet Neurol. 2015;14(3):263–73.

32. World Health Organization. The ICD-10 Classification of Mental and Behavioural Disorders: Diagnostic Criteria for Research. Geneva: World Health Organization; 1993.

33. American Psychiatric Association. Diagnostic and Statistical Manual of Mental Disorders (DSM-5®). Arlington: American Psychiatric Pub; 2013.

34. Spitzer RL, Endicott J, Robins E. Research diagnostic criteria: rationale and reliability. Arch Gen Psychiatry. 1978;35(6):773–82.

35. Lau J, Ioannidis JP, Schmid CH. Quantitative synthesis in systematic reviews. Ann Intern Med. 1997;127(9):820–6.

36. Higgins JP, Thompson SG, Spiegelhalter DJ. A re-evaluation of random-effects meta-analysis. J R Stat Soc Ser A Stat Soc. 2009;172(1):137–59.

37. IntHout J, Ioannidis JP, Rovers MM, Goeman JJ. Plea for routinely presenting prediction intervals in meta-analysis. BMJ Open. 2016;6(7):e010247.

38. Higgins JP, Thompson SG. Quantifying heterogeneity in a meta-analysis. Stat Med. 2002;21(11):1539–58.

39. Ioannidis JP, Patsopoulos NA, Evangelou E. Uncertainty in heterogeneity estimates in meta-analyses. BMJ. 2007;335(7626):914–6.

40. Egger M, Davey Smith G, Schneider M, Minder C. Bias in meta-analysis detected by a simple, graphical test. BMJ. 1997;315(7109):629–34.

41. Carvalho AF, Kohler CA, Brunoni AR, Miskowiak KW, Herrmann N, Lanctot KL, Hyphantis TN, Quevedo J, Fernandes BS, Berk M. Bias in peripheral depression biomarkers. Psychother Psychosom. 2016;85(2):81–90.

42. Ioannidis JP, Trikalinos TA. An exploratory test for an excess of significant findings. Clin Trials. 2007;4(3):245–53.

43. Ioannidis JP. Clarifications on the application and interpretation of the test for excess significance and its extensions. J Math Psychol. 2013; 57(5):184–7.

44. Bortolato B, Kohler CA, Evangelou E, Leon-Caballero J, Solmi M, Stubbs B, Belbasis L, Pacchiarotti I, Kessing LV. Systematic assessment of environmental risk factors for bipolar disorder: an umbrella review of systematic reviews and meta-analyses. Bipolar Disord. 2017;19(2):84–96.

45. Salanti G, Ioannidis JP. Synthesis of observational studies should consider credibility ceilings. J Clin Epidemiol. 2009;62(2):115–22.

46. Papatheodorou SI, Tsilidis KK, Evangelou E, Ioannidis JP. Application of credibility ceilings probes the robustness of meta-analyses of biomarkers and cancer risk. J Clin Epidemiol. 2015;68(2):163–74.

47. Shea BJ, Grimshaw JM, Wells GA, Boers M, Andersson N, Hamel C, Porter AC, Tugwell P, Moher D, Bouter LM. Development of AMSTAR: a measurement tool to assess the methodological quality of systematic reviews. BMC Med Res Methodol. 2007;7:10.

48. Shea BJ, Hamel C, Wells GA, Bouter LM, Kristjansson E, Grimshaw J, Henry DA, Boers M. AMSTAR is a reliable and valid measurement tool to assess the methodological quality of systematic reviews. J Clin Epidemiol. 2009;62(10): 1013–20.

49. Pieper D, Buechter RB, Li L, Prediger B, Eikermann M. Systematic review found AMSTAR, but not R(evised)-AMSTAR, to have good measurement properties. J Clin Epidemiol. 2015;68(5):574–83.

50. Baxter AJ, Page A, Whiteford HA: Factors influencing risk of premature mortality in community cases of depression: a meta-analytic review. Epidemiol Res Int 2011, 2011:832945.

51. Cuijpers P, Vogelzangs N, Twisk J, Kleiboer A, Li J, Penninx BW. Comprehensive meta-analysis of excess mortality in depression in the general community versus patients with specific illnesses. Am J Psychiatry. 2014;171(4):453–62.

52. Dew MA, Rosenberger EM, Myaskovsky L, DiMartini AF, DeVito Dabbs AJ, Posluszny DM, Steel J, Switzer GE, Shellmer DA, Greenhouse JB. Depression and anxiety as risk factors for morbidity and mortality after organ transplantation: a systematic review and meta-analysis. Transplantation. 2015;100(5):988–1003.

53. van Dooren FE, Nefs G, Schram MT, Verhey FR, Denollet J, Pouwer F. Depression and risk of mortality in people with diabetes mellitus: a systematic review and meta-analysis. PLoS One. 2013;8(3):e57058.

54. Gathright EC, Goldstein CM, Josephson RA, Hughes JW. Depression increases the risk of mortality in patients with heart failure: a meta-analysis. J Psychosom Res. 2017;94:82–9.

55. Hofmann M, Kohler B, Leichsenring F, Kruse J. Depression as a risk factor for mortality in individuals with diabetes: a meta-analysis of prospective studies. PLoS One. 2013;8(11):e79809.

56. Leung YW, Flora DB, Gravely S, Irvine J, Carney RM, Grace SL. The impact of premorbid and postmorbid depression onset on mortality and cardiac morbidity among patients with coronary heart disease: meta-analysis. Psychosom Med. 2012;74(8):786–801.

57. Meijer A, Conradi HJ, Bos EH, Thombs BD, van Melle JP, de Jonge P. Prognostic association of depression following myocardial infarction with mortality and cardiovascular events: a meta-analysis of 25 years of research. Gen Hosp Psychiatry. 2011;33(3):203–16.

58. Van Melle JP, De Jonge P, Spijkerman TA, Tijssen JGP, Ormel J, Van Veldhuisen DJ, Van Den Brink RHS, Van Den Berg MP. Prognostic association of depression following myocardial infarction with mortality and cardiovascular events: a meta-analysis. Psychosom Med. 2004;66(6):814–22.

59. Pan A. Depression and risk of stroke morbidity and mortality: A meta-analysis and systematic review. JAMA. 2011;306(11):1241–9.

60. Park M, Katon WJ, Wolf FM. Depression and risk of mortality in individuals with diabetes: a meta-analysis and systematic review. Gen Hosp Psychiatry. 2013;35(3):217–25.

61. Pederson JL, Warkentin LM, Majumdar SR, McAlister FA. Depressive symptoms are associated with higher rates of readmission or mortality after medical hospitalization: a systematic review and meta-analysis. J Hosp Med. 2016;11(5):373–80.

62. Satin JR, Linden W, Phillips MJ. Depression as a predictor of disease progression and mortality in cancer patients: a meta-analysis. Cancer. 2009; 115(22):5349–61.

63. Sokoreli I, de Vries JJG, Pauws SC, Steyerberg EW. Depression and anxiety as predictors of mortality among heart failure patients: systematic review and meta-analysis. Heart Fail Rev. 2016;21(1):49–63.

64. Sorensen C, Friis-Hasche E, Haghfelt T, Bech P. Postmyocardial infarction mortality in relation to depression: a systematic critical review. Psychother Psychosom. 2005;74(2):69–80.

65. Stenman M, Holzmann MJ, Sartipy U. Association between preoperative depression and long-term survival following coronary artery bypass surgery - a systematic review and meta-analysis. Int J Cardiol. 2016;222:462–6.

66. Correll CU, Solmi M, Veronese N, Bortolato B, Rosson S, Santonastaso P, Thapa-Chhetri N, Fornaro M, Gallicchio D, Collantoni E, et al. Prevalence, incidence and mortality from cardiovascular disease in patients with pooled and specific severe mental illness: a large-scale meta-analysis of 3,211,768 patients and 113,383,368 controls. World Psychiatry. 2017;16(2):163–80.

67. Meijer A, Conradi HJ, Bos EH, Anselmino M, Carney RM, Denollet J, Doyle F, Freedland KE, Grace SL, Hosseini SH, et al. Adjusted prognostic association of depression following myocardial infarction with mortality and cardiovascular events: individual patient data meta-analysis. Br J Psychiatry. 2013;203(2):90–102.

68. Barber B, Dergousoff J, Slater L, Harris J, O'Connell D, El-Hakim H, Biron VL, Mitchell N, Seikaly H. Depression and survival in patients with head and neck Cancer: a systematic review. JAMA Otolaryngol Head Neck Surg. 2016; 142(3):284–8.

69. Salte K, Titlestad I, Halling A. Depression is associated with poor prognosis in patients with chronic obstructive pulmonary disease - a systematic review. Dan Med J. 2015;62(10):A5137.

70. Ødegård Ø. The excess mortality of the insane. Acta Psychiatr Scand. 1952; 27(3–4):353–67.

71. Jarvis E. On the comparative liability of males and females to insanity, and their comparative curability and mortality when insane. Am J Psychiatr. 1850;7(2):142–71.

72. Chesney E, Goodwin GM, Fazel S. Risks of all-cause and suicide mortality in mental disorders: a meta-review. World Psychiatry. 2014;13(2):153–60.

73. Slyepchenko A, Maes M, Jacka FN, Kohler CA, Barichello T, McIntyre RS, Berk M, Grande I, Foster JA, Vieta E, et al. Gut microbiota, bacterial translocation, and interactions with diet: pathophysiological links between major depressive disorder and non-communicable medical comorbidities. Psychother Psychosom. 2017;86(1):31–46.

74. Black CN, Bot M, Scheffer PG, Cuijpers P, Penninx BW. Is depression associated with increased oxidative stress? A systematic review and meta-analysis. Psychoneuroendocrinology. 2015;51:164–75.

75. de Melo LGP, Nunes SOV, Anderson G, Vargas HO, Barbosa DS, Galecki P, Carvalho AF, Maes M. Shared metabolic and immune-inflammatory, oxidative and nitrosative stress pathways in the metabolic syndrome and mood disorders. Prog Neuro-Psychopharmacol Biol Psychiatry. 2017;78:34–50.

76. Penninx BW. Depression and cardiovascular disease: epidemiological evidence on their linking mechanisms. Neurosci Biobehav Rev. 2017;74(Pt B):277–86.

77. Vancampfort D, Stubbs B, Mitchell AJ, De Hert M, Wampers M, Ward PB, Rosenbaum S, Correll CU. Risk of metabolic syndrome and its components in people with schizophrenia and related psychotic disorders, bipolar disorder and major depressive disorder: a systematic review and meta-analysis. World Psychiatry. 2015;14(3):339–47.

78. Fava GA, Cosci F, Sonino N. Current psychosomatic practice. Psychother Psychosom. 2017;86(1):13–30.

79. Crawshaw J, Auyeung V, Norton S, Weinman J. Identifying psychosocial predictors of medication non-adherence following acute coronary syndrome: a systematic review and meta-analysis. J Psychosom Res. 2016;90:10–32.

80. Smith SG, Sestak I, Forster A, Partridge A, Side L, Wolf MS, Horne R, Wardle J, Cuzick J. Factors affecting uptake and adherence to breast cancer chemoprevention: a systematic review and meta-analysis. Ann Oncol. 2016; 27(4):575–90.

81. Prince M, Patel V, Saxena S, Maj M, Maselko J, Phillips MR, Rahman A. No health without mental health. Lancet. 2007;370(9590):859–77.

82. Jacka FN, Pasco JA, Mykletun A, Williams LJ, Hodge AM, O'Reilly SL, Nicholson GC, Kotowicz MA, Berk M. Association of Western and traditional diets with depression and anxiety in women. Am J Psychiatry. 2010;167(3):305–11.

83. Levis B, Benedetti A, Levis AW, Ioannidis JPA, Shrier I, Cuijpers P, Gilbody S, Kloda LA, McMillan D, Patten SB, et al. Selective cutoff reporting in studies of diagnostic test accuracy: a comparison of conventional and individual-patient-data meta-analyses of the patient health Questionnaire-9 depression screening tool. Am J Epidemiol. 2017;185(10):954–64.

84. Miloyan B, Fried E. A reassessment of the relationship between depression and all-cause mortality in 3,604,005 participants from 293 studies. World Psychiatry. 2017;16(2):219–20.

85. Lichtenberg P, Belmaker RH. Subtyping major depressive disorder. Psychother Psychosom. 2010;79(3):131–5.

86. Ormel J, de Jonge P. Unipolar depression and the progression of coronary artery disease: toward an integrative model. Psychother Psychosom. 2011; 80(5):264–74.

87. de Miranda Azevedo R, Roest AM, Hoen PW, de Jonge P. Cognitive/affective and somatic/affective symptoms of depression in patients with heart disease and their association with cardiovascular prognosis: a meta-analysis. Psychol Med. 2014;44(13):2689–703.

88. Caruso R, GiuliaNanni M, Riba MB, Sabato S, Grassi L. Depressive spectrum disorders in cancer: diagnostic issues and intervention. A Critical Review. Curr Psychiatry Rep. 2017;19(6):33.

89. Lambert SD, Clover K, Pallant JF, Britton B, King MT, Mitchell AJ, Carter G. Making sense of variations in prevalence estimates of depression in Cancer: a co-calibration of commonly used depression scales using Rasch analysis. J Natl Compr Cancer Netw. 2015;13(10):1203–11.

90. Cosci F, Fava GA, Sonino N. Mood and anxiety disorders as early manifestations of medical illness: a systematic review. Psychother Psychosom. 2015;84(1):22–9.

91. Harris EC, Barraclough B. Excess mortality of mental disorder. Br J Psychiatry. 1998;173:11–53.

92. Laursen TM, Munk-Olsen T, Nordentoft M, Mortensen PB. Increased mortality among patients admitted with major psychiatric disorders: a register-based study comparing mortality in unipolar depressive disorder, bipolar affective disorder, schizoaffective disorder, and schizophrenia. J Clin Psychiatry. 2007; 68(6):899–907.

93. Laursen TM, Musliner KL, Benros ME, Vestergaard M, Munk-Olsen T. Mortality and life expectancy in persons with severe unipolar depression. J Affect Disord. 2016;193:203–7.

94. Fekadu A, Medhin G, Kebede D, Alem A, Cleare AJ, Prince M, Hanlon C, Shibre T. Excess mortality in severe mental illness: 10-year population-based cohort study in rural Ethiopia. Br J Psychiatry. 2015;206(4):289–96.

95. Markkula N, Harkanen T, Perala J, Partti K, Pena S, Koskinen S, Lonnqvist J, Suvisaari J, Saarni SI. Mortality in people with depressive, anxiety and alcohol use disorders in Finland. Br J Psychiatry. 2012;200(2):143–9.

96. Pizzi C, Rutjes AW, Costa GM, Fontana F, Mezzetti A, Manzoli L. Meta-analysis of selective serotonin reuptake inhibitors in patients with depression and coronary heart disease. Am J Cardiol. 2011;107(7):972–9.

97. Whalley B, Thompson DR, Taylor RS. Psychological interventions for coronary heart disease: Cochrane systematic review and meta-analysis. Int J Behav Med. 2014;21(1):109–21.

11

Human antibodies activate complement against *Plasmodium falciparum* sporozoites, and are associated with protection against malaria in children

Liriye Kurtovic[1,2], Marije C. Behet[3], Gaoqian Feng[1], Linda Reiling[1], Kiprotich Chelimo[4], Arlene E. Dent[5], Ivo Mueller[6,7], James W. Kazura[5], Robert W. Sauerwein[3], Freya J. I. Fowkes[1,8,9] and James G. Beeson[1,2,10,11]*

Abstract

Background: Antibodies targeting *Plasmodium falciparum* sporozoites play a key role in human immunity to malaria. However, antibody mechanisms that neutralize sporozoites are poorly understood. This has been a major constraint in developing highly efficacious vaccines, as we lack strong correlates of protective immunity.

Methods: We quantified the ability of human antibodies from malaria-exposed populations to interact with human complement, examined the functional effects of complement activity against *P. falciparum* sporozoites *in vitro*, and identified targets of functional antibodies. In children and adults from malaria-endemic regions, we determined the acquisition of complement-fixing antibodies to sporozoites and their relationship with antibody isotypes and subclasses. We also investigated associations with protective immunity in a longitudinal cohort of children (*n* = 206) residing in a malaria-endemic region.

Results: We found that antibodies to the major sporozoite surface antigen, circumsporozoite protein (CSP), were predominately IgG1, IgG3, and IgM, and could interact with complement through recruitment of C1q and activation of the classical pathway. The central repeat region of CSP, included in leading vaccines, was a key target of complement-fixing antibodies. We show that antibodies activate human complement on *P. falciparum* sporozoites, which consequently inhibited hepatocyte cell traversal that is essential for establishing liver-stage infection, and led to sporozoite death *in vitro*. The natural acquisition of complement-fixing antibodies in malaria-exposed populations was age-dependent, and was acquired more slowly to sporozoite antigens than to merozoite antigens. In a longitudinal cohort of children, high levels of complement-fixing antibodies were significantly associated with protection against clinical malaria.

Conclusions: These novel findings point to complement activation by antibodies as an important mechanism of anti-sporozoite human immunity, thereby enabling new strategies for developing highly efficacious malaria vaccines. We also present evidence that complement-fixing antibodies may be a valuable correlate of protective immunity in humans.

Keywords: Antibodies, Circumsporozoite protein, Sporozoite, Complement, Malaria, *Plasmodium falciparum*, Vaccines

* Correspondence: beeson@burnet.edu.au
[1]Burnet Institute, Melbourne, Australia
[2]Department of Immunology and Pathology, Monash University, Melbourne, Australia
Full list of author information is available at the end of the article

Background

Malaria is a substantial cause of global morbidity and mortality, and the effectiveness of current interventions is under threat due to increasing reports of drug and insecticide resistance. To achieve malaria control and elimination, there is a pressing need to develop and license highly efficacious malaria vaccines. This is a global priority, and the World Health Organization has set the ambitious goal to license a malaria vaccine that is at least 75% efficacious against clinical malaria by 2030 [1]. Currently, there is no licensed vaccine against *Plasmodium falciparum*, the main cause of malaria morbidity and mortality [2]. Vaccine development is significantly challenged by the lack of knowledge on the targets and mechanisms of functional immunity that confer protection against malaria, and a lack of correlates of protection. Defining these mechanisms is crucial for identifying strong correlates of protection, which will aid vaccine evaluation and enhance current vaccine candidates by inducing potent functional immune responses [3].

Plasmodium sporozoites are transmitted to humans when an infected female *Anopheles* mosquito probes the skin in search of a blood vessel [4]. Sporozoites are passively carried in the blood circulation to the liver, where they develop within hepatic cells, generating thousands of merozoites [5], which initiate blood-stage replication and subsequently cause symptomatic and severe malaria. Vaccines targeting sporozoites are attractive because fewer than 100 sporozoites are transmitted to humans [6] and blocking sporozoites will prevent infection and subsequent disease. Even partial immunity to sporozoites could reduce the number of successful hepatocyte infections and subsequent blood-stage parasitemia, which may confer protection against clinical malaria or reduce disease severity.

The predominant sporozoite surface antigen is circumsporozoite protein (CSP). Antibodies to CSP have been directly shown to confer protection against infection in animal malaria models [7, 8], have had some association with protection in human vaccine trials [9], and can be acquired through natural exposure to malaria [10, 11]. However, an enduring question that remains unanswered is how antibodies to sporozoites and CSP function to protect against infection. The most advanced malaria vaccine candidate, RTS,S/AS01 (RTS,S), is based on the central-repeat and C-terminal regions of CSP [12], and induces antibody and CD4+ T cell responses [13]. RTS,S was only partially efficacious against clinical malaria in phase III clinical trials (vaccine efficacy 29–36% in children aged 5–17 months after 48 months of follow-up) [14], and the functional mechanisms of vaccine-induced immunity remain unknown. These knowledge gaps severely impair our ability to enhance current vaccines and to design new vaccines that induce potent functional immunity for greater efficacy.

Sporozoites can take several hours to reach the liver [4], leaving them highly susceptible to immune attack at the inoculation site in the skin and in the circulation. The success of invasion and development in the liver is dependent on sporozoite motility, which includes: (i) gliding to migrate out of the skin [15], (ii) traversal to pass through cells, and (iii) hepatocyte invasion and maturation [16]. Anti-CSP antibodies can neutralize motility *in vitro*, although the relationship between function and protective immunity has not been demonstrated [17–19], and direct inhibitory activity of antibodies generally requires relatively high antibody concentrations [18, 20]. Furthermore, there are few data on whether the immunoglobulin G (IgG) subclass influences antibody function and what epitopes are primarily targeted.

We hypothesized that antibodies of the right type and specificity may fix and activate complement to neutralize *P. falciparum* sporozoites. Harnessing complement activity using antibodies is an attractive mechanism of functional immunity because complement could act early following inoculation to combat sporozoites (Additional file 1: Figure S1). Complement activation can occur via the classical pathway whereby C1q interacts with immune complexes, referred to as C1q-fixation [21]. This leads to sequential activation of downstream complement proteins such as C3, and formation of the membrane attack complex (MAC), which mediates cell death. Activation can also occur via the alternative pathway involving direct C3 activation against pathogens [21]. Currently it is unknown if *P. falciparum* sporozoites are susceptible to complement deposition and attack, and whether antibodies function to promote complement activation and consequently neutralize sporozoite function or lead to sporozoite death.

We investigated the ability of antibodies to CSP and *P. falciparum* sporozoites to recruit human complement proteins, and demonstrated the functional effects of complement activation against sporozoites *in vitro*. We also explored the natural acquisition of complement-fixing antibodies, and then assessed whether functional antibodies were associated with protection in a prospective longitudinal cohort of children.

Methods
Aims and study participants

There were several aims to this study: (i) to determine whether human antibodies fix complement, (ii) to explore the relationship between functional antibodies and isotype, subclass, and specificity, (iii) to examine the natural acquisition of functional antibodies in young children, and (iv) to assess the association between functional antibodies and protection against malaria in children. To meet these aims, we tested antibody samples from previously described cohort studies as summarized below. Note that all three study sites were considered to be malaria holo- or hyper-endemic, and no bed nets of any type were in place at this time.

(i) To maximize the likelihood of detecting functional anti-CSP antibodies, we tested two cohorts of malaria-exposed adults from distinct areas, as anti-CSP antibodies have been previously reported to be acquired with age as a result of repeated malaria exposure. Sera from adults living in Madang District (Papua New Guinea, PNG, $N = 116$) were collected in 2001 and 2002 [22], and plasma from adults living in the Kanyawegi subdistrict, Kisumu county (Kenya, $N = 104$) were collected in August 2007 [23].

(ii) We then preferentially selected 30 samples from each adult cohort (PNG and Kenyan) to characterize the antibody response further, based on IgG/C1q-fixation reactivity to CSP and sample availability.

(iii) The majority of malaria morbidity occurs in children under 5 years, and so we tested a cohort of young children (0.3–5.9 years) to examine the acquisition of functional antibodies, and compared this cohort to adults from the same area. Plasma from children/adults living in the Chulaimbo subdistrict, Kisumu county (Kenya, $N = 75$) were collected in February and March 2007 [24]. Samples were categorized into groups based on the median ages of 0.5, 1, 2, 5 and 35 years (age ranges were 0.3–0.7, 1–1.5, 1.8–3.0, 4.7–5.9, and 19.6–69.2 with $n = 11$, $n = 14$, $n = 18$, $n = 16$, and $n = 16$, respectively).

(iv) To assess the relationship between functional antibodies and protection against malaria, we tested samples from a longitudinal prospective treatment-to-reinfection study. Plasma samples from children living in Madang Province (PNG, $N = 206$) aged 5–14 years (median = 9.3 years) were collected at enrolment in 2004 and 2005 [25]. Children were treated to clear parasitemia present at baseline, and then actively followed every 2 weeks for symptomatic illness and parasitemia, and by passive case detection over a period of 6 months. A clinical episode of *P. falciparum* malaria was defined as fever and *P. falciparum* parasitemia >5000 parasites/µl.

We also generated two pools of Kenyan donors with high C1q-fixation reactivity from the adult Kenyan cohort. Pool 1 ($n = 10$) was used in IgG-purification experiments, using the Melon gel purification kit as described by the manufacturer (Thermo Fisher Scientific, Waltham, USA). Pool 2 ($n = 19$) was used in the *in vitro* hepatocyte traversal experiments. To minimize potential background reactivity from any residual complement that may remain after heat inactivation, antibodies from pool 2 (and a control pool from residents of Melbourne, Australia) were purified by ammonium sulfate precipitation [26]. Sterile saturated ammonium sulfate was slowly added with continuous agitation to plasma (diluted 1/5 in sterile saline) to a final concentration of 50%.

Following 30 min incubation on ice, the precipitate was pelleted (20,000 relative centrifugal force (RCF) × 10 min), then washed in 50% sterile saturated ammonium sulfate. The precipitate was repeatedly washed in excess phosphate-buffered saline (PBS) using a centrifugation concentration device, as described by the manufacturer (100 kDa cut-off, Millipore, Burlington, USA), and resuspended to the same starting volume of plasma.

Parasites

Aseptic, purified, non-attenuated cryopreserved *P. falciparum* 3D7 sporozoites (Sanaria, Rockville, USA) were provided by PATH's Malaria Vaccine Initiative or purchased from Sanaria. Freshly dissected *P. falciparum* NF54 and NF166.C8 sporozoites were generated at Radboud University Medical Center (Radboudumc, Nijmegen, The Netherlands), as described previously [20, 27].

Antigens and antibodies

Recombinant *P. falciparum* CSP was expressed in *Pichia pastoris* and purified using high-performance liquid chromatography (Sanaria) [28]. The protein was based on the 3D7 sequence beginning at amino acid residue 50 and contained 22 NANP repeats and four NVDP repeats. A peptide representative of the *P. falciparum* CSP central repeat B-cell epitope $(NANP)_{15}$ was synthesized and purified using high-performance liquid chromatography (Life Tein, Hillsborough, USA). Full-length recombinant merozoite surface protein 2 (MSP2) was expressed in *Escherichia coli* as previously described [29].

Rabbits were immunized with three doses of 200 µg CSP 4 weeks apart (the first immunization was administered in complete Freud's adjuvant and the last two in incomplete Freud's adjuvant). The terminal bleed was obtained 12 days after the final immunization, and anti-CSP IgG was purified at the Walter and Eliza Hall Institute. Pre-immune IgG was purified in-house using the Melon gel purification kit, as described by the manufacturer (Thermo Fisher Scientific). Animal immunizations were approved by the Animal Ethics Committee of the Walter and Eliza Hall Institute. We were provided with subclass switched mouse anti-NANP monoclonal antibodies (MAbs) 2H8-IgG1/IgG2a and 3C1-IgG1/IgG3 (LakePharma, Belmont, USA) by PATH's MVI [30].

Antibody isotypes and subclasses by enzyme-linked immunosorbent assay

The procedure for the enzyme-linked immunosorbent assay (ELISA) was as follows. Flat bottom 96-well MaxiSorp plates (Thermo Fisher Scientific) were coated with 0.5 µg/ml antigen in PBS overnight at 4 °C. Plates were washed thrice in PBS-Tween20 0.05% (v/v), blocked using 1% (w/v) casein in PBS for 2 h at 37 °C, and then washed again. Human antibody samples were applied in duplicate at 1/2000 (IgG/M) or 1/500 (IgG subclasses) dilutions in 0.1% (w/v) casein in PBS (diluting buffer) for 2 h at room temperature (RT), and then washed. Antibody isotypes were detected using goat anti-human IgG/IgM horse radish peroxidase (HRP) conjugated antibodies (Millipore) at 1/2500 dilution for 1 h at RT, followed by washing and incubation with 2,2′-azino-bis(3-ethylbenzothiazoline-6-sulfonic acid) (ABTS) substrate (Sigma-Aldrich, St. Louis, USA) for 1 h at RT in the dark. The reaction was stopped using 1% (w/v) sodium dodecyl sulfate in PBS. The optical density (OD) was measured at 405 nm. IgG subclasses were detected using mouse anti-human IgG1/IgG2/IgG3/IgG4 antibodies (Invitrogen) at 1/1000 dilution for 1 h at RT, followed by washing and incubation with goat anti-mouse IgG HRP conjugated antibodies (Millipore) at 1/1000 dilution for 1 h at RT. Plates were washed and incubated with a tetramethylbenzidine substrate (Sigma-Aldrich) for 1 h at RT in the dark, and the reaction was stopped using 1 M sulfuric acid (OD measured at 450 nm). Rabbit and murine antibodies were detected using goat anti-rabbit/mouse HRP conjugated antibodies (Millipore, Abcam) at 1/2000 and ABTS substrate.

Complement-fixation by ELISA and Western blot

Again, 96-well flat bottom MaxiSorp plates were coated with antigen, blocked and washed as described above. Human antibody samples were applied in duplicate at 1/100–1/250 dilution for 2 h at RT, and then washed. Plates were incubated with 10 µg/ml human C1q, C1q-depleted serum (Millipore), C5-depleted serum (for C2/C3/C4 fixation, Millipore) or fresh pooled non-immune serum (for C5b-C9 fixation) at 1/10 dilution for 30 min at RT, washed, and detected using anti-C1q/C2/C3/C4/C5b-C9 antibodies at 1/1000–1/2000 dilution (Dako, Santa Clara, USA; Abcam, Cambridge, UK; Millipore) for 1 h at RT. Plates were washed and incubated with the appropriate HRP conjugated antibodies (Abcam, Sigma-Aldrich, Millipore) at 1/2000 dilution for 1 h at RT followed by washing. Complement-fixation was detected using a tetramethylbenzidine substrate as described above (MSP2 experiments utilized ABTS). Complement-fixation using murine and rabbit antibodies were conducted using the same methods.

Complement-fixation to 3D7 *P. falciparum* sporozoites by ELISA was conducted using the same method as above (coating of 10,000 cells per well); however, all incubation times did not exceed 1 h, were conducted at RT, and the washing buffer contained PBS only. To measure complement-fixation by Western blot, 10,000 sporozoites were incubated with human antibody samples at 1/10 dilution and fresh normal human serum at 25% in PBS for 15 min at 37 °C with agitation. Sporozoites were washed twice in cold protease inhibitor (1600 x

RCF, 4 min), processed for SDS-PAGE and then blotted into nitrocellulose membrane (under reducing conditions). The membrane was blocked in 10% (w/v) skimmed milk in PBS-Tween20 0.5% (v/v) and probed using anti-C1q/iC3b antibodies (Serotec, Kidlington, UK) followed by HRP conjugated antibodies, with membrane stripping (Sigma-Aldrich), washing and blocking in between. Protein bands were detected using chemiluminescent substrate and autoradiography film (GE Life Sciences, Chicago, USA). Membranes were also probed with anti-CSP antibodies as a loading control.

Experimental controls and standardization

Human antibody samples (serum/plasma) tested by ELISA were excluded if duplicates varied by greater than 25% (unless duplicates differed by OD < 0.1). OD values were corrected by subtracting the background reactivity of control wells containing no serum or plasma. Cohort experiments that spread across multiple ELISA plates were standardized for plate-to-plate variation using positive control wells containing highly reactive samples from malaria-exposed individuals. Malaria-naïve sera from Melbourne donors were tested as negative controls. Test samples giving ODs greater than the mean + 3 standard deviations of malaria naïve controls were considered positive. This positive cut-off value was used to convert OD into arbitrary units (AU) as follows: AU = sample corrected OD / positive cut-off OD, so that samples with AU > 1 were considered positive. All plasma/serum samples were heat inactivated at 56 °C for 45 min prior to use.

Sporozoite cell traversal

Traversal was conducted as previously described [20] using freshly dissected *P. falciparum* NF54 and NF166. C8 sporozoites. Briefly, sporozoites were pre-incubated with pooled human antibody samples (malaria-exposed Kenyan and malaria-naïve Melbourne pools purified by ammonium sulfate precipitation) at 1/10 dilution, or vaccine-induced rabbit anti-CSP IgG and pre-immune IgG at 1 and 10 µg/ml, for 30 min on ice. Sporozoite/antibody samples were added to HC-04 cells seeded on 96-well plates, along with 10% normal human serum (NHS; active complement) or heat-inactivated serum (HIS; inactive complement), and tetramethylrhodamine (Rh) labelled dextran (50,000 sporozoites and 50,000 HC-04 cells per well). Sporozoites were allowed to traverse HC-04 cells under these conditions (in the presence of immune/non-immune antibodies and active/inactive complement) for 2 h at 37 °C in 5% CO_2, and were then washed in PBS. HC-04 cells were then trypsinized, washed in 10% fetal bovine serum in PBS, and resuspended in 1% paraformaldehyde. Traversed HC-04 cells were measured as Rh positive, and quantified by flow cytometry using the Cyan (Beckman Coulter) and FlowJo software (gating strategy shown in Additional file 1: Figure S2A). The percentage of Rh positive cells was corrected for background reactivity using HC-04 cells treated with dextran only. Traversal inhibition by immune antibodies (Kenyan pool and rabbit anti-CSP IgG) compared to non-immune antibodies (Melbourne pool and rabbit pre-immune IgG) in the presence of NHS and HIS was calculated as

$$\left(1 - \frac{\%\text{traversed cells in the presence of immune antibodies}}{\%\text{traversed cells in the presence of non-immune antibodies}}\right) \times 100$$

Sporozoites were also pre-incubated with anti-CSP MAb 3SP2 as a positive control.

Sporozoite cell death by flow cytometry

Altogether, 50,000 3D7 *P. falciparum* sporozoites were incubated with rabbit anti-CSP antibodies at 1/10 dilution and 20% human serum (normal or C5-depleted) for 10 min at 37 °C. Sporozoites were placed on ice and dead cells were stained using the DNA-binding dye, propidium iodide (PI). PI positive cells were quantified by flow cytometry using FACSVerse (BD Biosciences) and FlowJo software (gating strategy shown in Additional file 1: Figure S2B).

Statistical analysis

Data were analyzed using GraphPad Prism version 6. 05 and Stata 13.1. The following two-tailed non-parametric tests were performed where appropriate: Spearman's correlation coefficient (rho), Wilcoxon matched-pairs signed rank test, Man Whitney U test, and Kruskal–Wallis test. To investigate the association between anti-CSP IgG and IgM with C1q fixation in PNG adults, we performed a multiple linear regression with robust standard errors. To evaluate associations between specific antibodies (C1q fixation activity or IgG reactivity to CSP) and malaria risk in the longitudinal study, Kaplan–Meier survival curves were plotted to show the cumulative proportion of children who had experienced an episode of malaria during follow-up, stratified by antibody response group defined as negative, low positive, and high positive (positive samples were defined as those with reactivity > 3 standard deviations above the mean of the malaria-naïve control samples, high-positive samples were those defined as being above the median of the positive samples, and low positive were those below the median of positive samples). Hazard ratios (HRs) of the risk of malaria during follow-up were calculated using the Cox proportional hazards model (using the first episodes of malaria only), and adjusted HRs were calculated by including age, location of residence, and parasitemia status at enrolment [25].

Results

Naturally acquired anti-CSP antibodies are predominately IgG1, IgG3, and IgM

Antibody isotype and subclass influence the ability to fix C1q and activate the classical pathway. Therefore, we characterized naturally acquired antibodies to the most abundant sporozoite surface protein, CSP, for possible interaction with complement. We measured antibody levels by ELISA and converted OD into AU. Among a selection of malaria-exposed adults from PNG and Kenya ($n = 30$ in each group), 40% and 75% were positive for anti-CSP IgM, respectively (Fig. 1a and b). IgM antibodies are potent complement activators whereas IgG complement activity is mediated primarily by the IgG1 and IgG3 subclasses, whereby IgG3 generally has greater activity [31]. The predominant subclasses in PNG and Kenyan adults were the complement-fixing subclasses IgG1 (seropositivity 67% and 100%, respectively) and IgG3 (seropositivity 76% and 97%, respectively). In contrast, the seroprevalence of IgG2 and IgG4 antibodies were lower (PNG seropositivity 15% and 7%; Kenyan seropositivity 48% and 16%, respectively).

Naturally acquired human antibodies and vaccine-induced antibodies promote complement-fixation to recombinant CSP

We next investigated whether naturally acquired antibodies in humans and vaccine-induced antibodies in animals were capable of promoting complement activation. Since the classical pathway is initiated by antibody-C1q interactions [31, 32], we tested whether antibodies to CSP could fix C1q using ELISA-based methods. Among a selection of PNG adults ($n = 30$), 77% of individuals were positive for this activity. Furthermore, human anti-CSP antibodies also fixed other complement components downstream of C1q, including C4, C2, C3, and C5b-C9 (reflecting MAC-formation) [21], all of which strongly positively correlated with C1q-fixation (Spearman's correlation coefficient rho = 0.794, 95% confidence interval (CI) 0.591 to 0.903; rho = 0.763, 95% CI 0. 548 to 0.884; rho = 0.784, 95% CI 0.584 to 0.895; and rho = 0.836, 95% CI 0.674 to 0.921; $p < 0.001$ for all tests, respectively) (Fig. 1c and d). We confirmed that C3-fixation was mediated by anti-CSP antibodies and the classical pathway and not by the alternative pathway using C1q-depleted serum as a source of complement, which significantly reduced reactivity by 61–88% ($p = 0.031$) (Fig. 1e). We next addressed whether complement-fixing antibodies could be elicited by CSP immunization of rabbits, as rabbit IgG is known to engage [33] and activate the human complement [34]. Vaccine-induced IgG demonstrated strong reactivity to recombinant CSP and to the central repeat region of CSP represented by the synthetic (NANP)$_{15}$ peptide, and promoted C1q and C3-

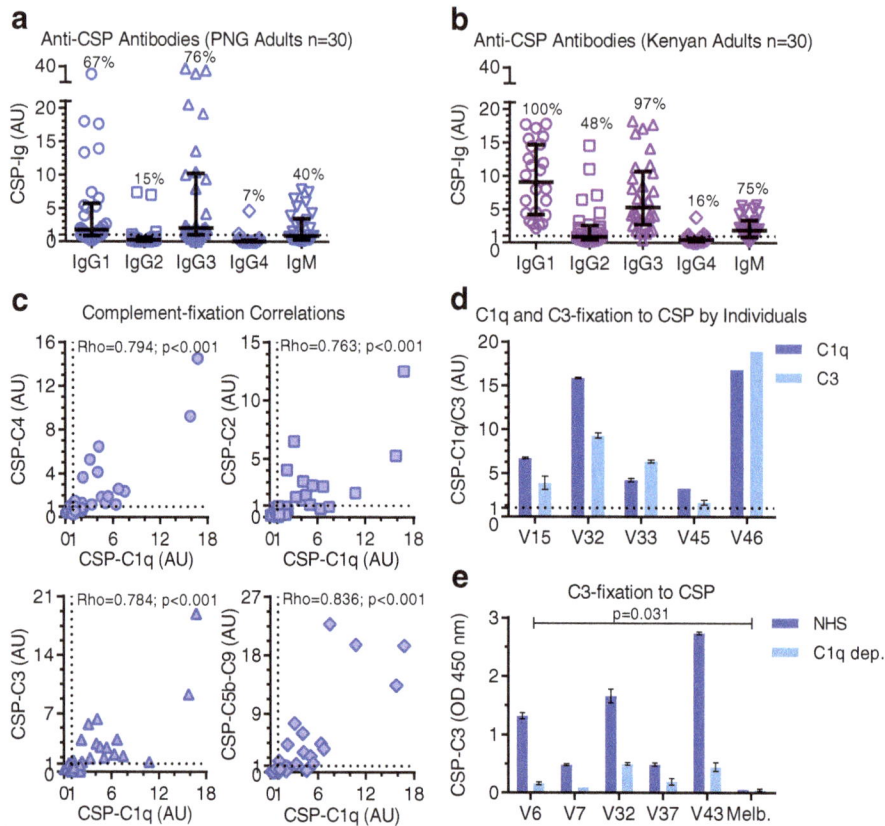

Fig. 1 Naturally acquired human anti-CSP antibodies are predominately IgG1, IgG3, and IgM, and can promote complement fixation to CSP. Antibodies from malaria-exposed adults (n = 30 in each group) living in PNG (**a**, **c-e**) and Kenyan (**b**) were tested for IgG/IgM and complement-fixation to CSP by ELISA. Results were standardized to arbitrary units (AU) based on malaria-naïve negative controls from Melbourne (seropositivity defined as AU > 1, shown as dotted lines), and mean and range of duplicates were graphed (mean only for scatter plots). **a,b** IgG subclasses and IgM reactivity to CSP. The median, interquartile range, and percentage of positive samples are shown. **c** Correlations between C1q-fixation and C4/C3/C5b-C9-fixation to CSP (Spearman's correlation coefficient, rho). **d** Examples of C1q and C3-fixation to CSP by individual serum samples (V15, V32, V33, V45, and V46 from PNG donors, n = 5). **e** C3-fixation to CSP by individual samples (V6, V7, V32, V37, and V43 from PNG donors, n = 5) in the presence of normal human serum (NHS) and serum depleted of C1q (C1q dep.) (Wilcoxon matched-pairs signed rank test). Non-standardized data are shown, as only one Melbourne control (Melb.) was tested. AU arbitrary units, CSP circumsporozoite protein, dep. depleted, ELISA enzyme-linked immunosorbent assay, Melb. Melbourne, NHS normal human serum, PNG Papua New Guinea

fixation to CSP (Fig. 2). Collectively these data demonstrate that antibodies can fix C1q and activate the classical pathway against CSP.

Anti-CSP antibody isotype and subclass are associated with complement-fixation

We examined the relationship between IgG and C1q-fixation to CSP in two different cohorts of malaria-exposed adults from PNG (n = 116) and Kenya (n = 104). Although there was a consistent positive trend between IgG and C1q-fixation in both populations, we observed marked differences in the ability to fix C1q among individuals with similar levels of anti-CSP IgG (Fig. 3). This suggests that additional factors or antibody properties influence this function.

To confirm that IgG alone is capable of promoting C1q-fixation, we compared purified IgG and whole

plasma from a pool of Kenyan adults with high levels of C1q-fixing antibodies (n = 10). Purified IgG could fix C1q, but less effectively than plasma, possibly due to the loss of IgM, which is known to activate complement potently (Additional file 1: Figure S3A). To explore in more detail the relative contributions of IgG and IgM in promoting C1q-fixation, we performed a linear regression with data from PNG adults (n = 116). For every unit increase in anti-CSP IgG, there was an increase in C1q-fixation of 0.785 AU (95% CI 0.585 to 0.985; $p < 0.001$), and this value was lower after adjusting for anti-CSP IgM (0.579, 95% CI 0.342 to 0.851; $p < 0.001$) (Additional file 1: Table S1). The inclusion of IgM only slightly improved the fit of the model (IgG R-squared = 0.67 and IgG/IgM R-squared = 0.71), suggesting that most variation in C1q-fixation responses could be explained by anti-CSP IgG for these samples.

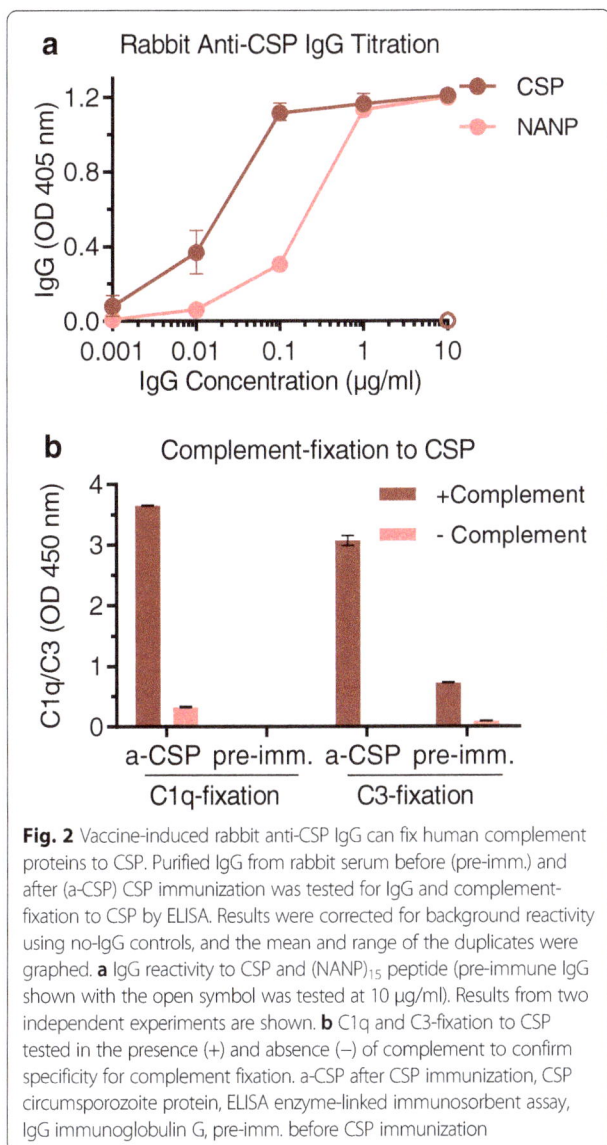

Fig. 2 Vaccine-induced rabbit anti-CSP IgG can fix human complement proteins to CSP. Purified IgG from rabbit serum before (pre-imm.) and after (a-CSP) CSP immunization was tested for IgG and complement-fixation to CSP by ELISA. Results were corrected for background reactivity using no-IgG controls, and the mean and range of the duplicates were graphed. **a** IgG reactivity to CSP and (NANP)$_{15}$ peptide (pre-immune IgG shown with the open symbol was tested at 10 μg/ml). Results from two independent experiments are shown. **b** C1q and C3-fixation to CSP tested in the presence (+) and absence (−) of complement to confirm specificity for complement fixation. a-CSP after CSP immunization, CSP circumsporozoite protein, ELISA enzyme-linked immunosorbent assay, IgG immunoglobulin G, pre-imm. before CSP immunization

Of the IgG subclasses, IgG1 and IgG3 are the most potent at activating the classical complement pathway. As expected, anti-CSP IgG1 and IgG3 both strongly correlated with C1q-fixation to CSP among a selection of PNG adults ($n = 30$, rho = 0.829, 95% CI 0.662 to 0.917 and rho = 0.792, 95% CI 0.592 to 0.900; $p < 0.001$ for both tests). These antibodies also strongly correlated with C4, C2, C3, and C5b-C9-fixation (Table 1), which further supported that complement activation was via the antibody-dependent classical pathway. To identify which subclass was prevalent in samples with high levels of C1q-fixing antibodies (above median AU = 2.2, $n = 14$), we compared the ratio of anti-CSP IgG1 to IgG3 (Additional file 1: Figure S3B). There tended to be an increased IgG3 response, whereas the ratio of anti-CSP IgG to IgM was highly variable, indicating that IgM may

be important in some individuals (Additional file 1: Figure S3C). Overall, characterizing the antibody response is an important consideration when assessing functional antibody responses.

P. falciparum sporozoites are susceptible to complement-fixation by human antibodies

Initially, we tested antibodies from a highly reactive PNG adult for the ability to promote complement-fixation on sporozoites by ELISA (Fig. 4a; reactivity to CSP shown in Additional file 1: Figure S4A). Consistent with complement-fixation to CSP, we observed greater C1q and C3-fixation in the presence of antibodies from the PNG individual than the malaria-naïve individual. It is noteworthy that some C3-fixation was observed in the presence of malaria-naïve antibodies, suggesting that C3 may bind directly to the sporozoite surface to some extent, although this was substantially lower than C3-fixation in the presence of malaria-exposed antibodies. To confirm these findings, we tested antibodies from a highly reactive Kenyan adult for complement-fixation on sporozoites by Western blot (Fig. 4a; reactivity to CSP shown in Additional file 1: Figure S4A). C1q and enhanced C3-fixation occurred in the presence of malaria-exposed antibodies, and some direct C3-fixation was also observed in the presence of malaria-naïve antibodies (repeat Western blots with reduced exposure time to observe the C3b band more clearly are shown in Additional file 1: Figure S4B). These data show that naturally acquired antibodies from malaria-exposed individuals promote complement fixation on sporozoites via the antibody-dependent classical pathway.

Sporozoite traversal inhibition by human and vaccine-induced rabbit antibodies is enhanced by complement

We examined whether antibodies inhibited sporozoite traversal, and whether this was enhanced in the presence of an active complement. Sporozoites rely on their traversal form of motility to pass through the sinusoidal cell layer and several hepatic cells before encountering a terminal hepatocyte for cellular invasion and development [16]. We tested rabbit anti-CSP IgG previously shown to fix the human complement to evaluate whether the functional effect of antibodies to CSP was enhanced by complement. Rabbit anti-CSP IgG inhibited sporozoite traversal of HC-04 cells (compared to rabbit pre-immune IgG), and inhibitory activity was substantially enhanced in the presence of NHS compared to HIS, whereby complement proteins were active and inactive, respectively (Fig. 4b). To establish whether complement also enhanced the function of human antibodies that contain antibodies to CSP and other *Plasmodium* antigens, we tested purified antibodies

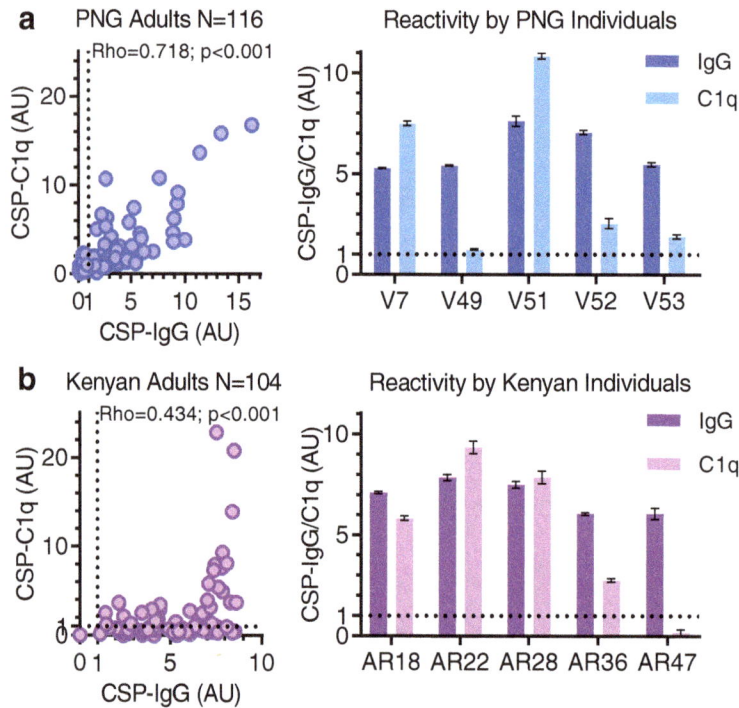

Fig. 3 Naturally acquired human anti-CSP IgG correlates with the ability to promote C1q-fixation to CSP, despite individual differences in reactivity. Antibodies from malaria-exposed adults living in PNG (**a**; $N = 116$) and Kenya (**b**; $N = 104$) were tested for IgG and C1q-fixation to CSP by ELISA. Results were standardized to arbitrary units (AU) based on malaria-naïve negative controls from Melbourne (seropositivity defined as AU > 1, shown as dotted lines), and the mean and range of duplicates were graphed (mean only for scatter plots). The left panels show correlations between IgG and C1q-fixation to CSP (Spearman's correlation coefficient, rho). The right panels show selected examples of IgG and C1q-fixation to CSP for individual serum samples from PNG donors (V7, V49, V51, V52, and V53) and Kenyan donors (AR18, AR22, AR28, AR36, and AR47). AU arbitrary units, CSP circumsporozoite protein, ELISA enzyme-linked immunosorbent assay, IgG immunoglobulin G, PNG Papua New Guinea

(including IgG and IgM) from a pool of malaria-exposed Kenyan adults ($n = 19$ samples, Additional file 1: Figure S5) and malaria-naïve Melbourne donors, and quantified *P. falciparum* sporozoite transversal (Fig. 4c). Kenyan antibodies inhibited NF54 sporozoite traversal (compared to Melbourne antibodies) twofold higher in the presence of an active complement compared to an inactive complement (mean and range of two independent experiments: 46% [45.7 to 46.2%] and 18.2% [11.8 to 24.6%],

respectively). We confirmed this effect using sporozoites from a second *P. falciparum* strain, NF166.C8, whereby inhibition of antibody-mediated traversal was observed only in the presence of active complement and was not detected when antibodies were tested with inactivated complement (30.7% [27.1 to 34.2%] and −4.7% [−14.6 to 5.2%], respectively). Therefore, the ability of antibodies to inhibit sporozoite traversal was enhanced in the presence of active human complement.

Table 1 Correlations between antibodies and complement fixation to CSP among malaria-exposed PNG adults ($n = 30$)

Antibody	Rho C1q	Rho C4	Rho C2	Rho C3	Rho C5b-C9
IgG	0.831 (0.666 to 0.919)	0.813 (0.625 to 0.912)	0.797 (0.606 to 0.901)	0.831 (0.666 to 0.919)	0.803 (0.616 to 0.904)
IgG1	0.829 (0.662 to 0.917)	0.839 (0.672 to 0.925)	0.830 (0.664 to 0.918)	0.895 (0.784 to 0.950)	0.745 (0.518 to 0.874)
IgG2	0.607 (0.276 to 0.809)	0.443 (0.046 to 0.720)	0.404 (0.008 to 0.691)	0.552 (0.198 to 0.779)	0.485 (0.108 to 0.740)
IgG3	0.792 (0.592 to 0.900)	0.795 (0.586 to 0.904)	0.788 (0.585 to 0.898)	0.801 (0.608 to 0.905)	0.754 (0.527 to 0.880)
IgG4	0.416 (0.039 to 0.689)	–	–	–	–
IgM	0.826 (0.656 to 0.916)	0.655 (0.363 to 0.830)	0.620 (0.325 to 0.805)	0.738 (0.506 to 0.870)	0.791 (0.596 to 0.898)

Spearman's correlation coefficient (rho) and 95% CI between anti-CSP antibodies and complement fixation to CSP. Values greater than 0.7 are underlined. Only significant correlations ($p < 0.05$) are shown
CI confidence interval, *CSP* circumsporozoite protein, *PNG* Papua New Guinea

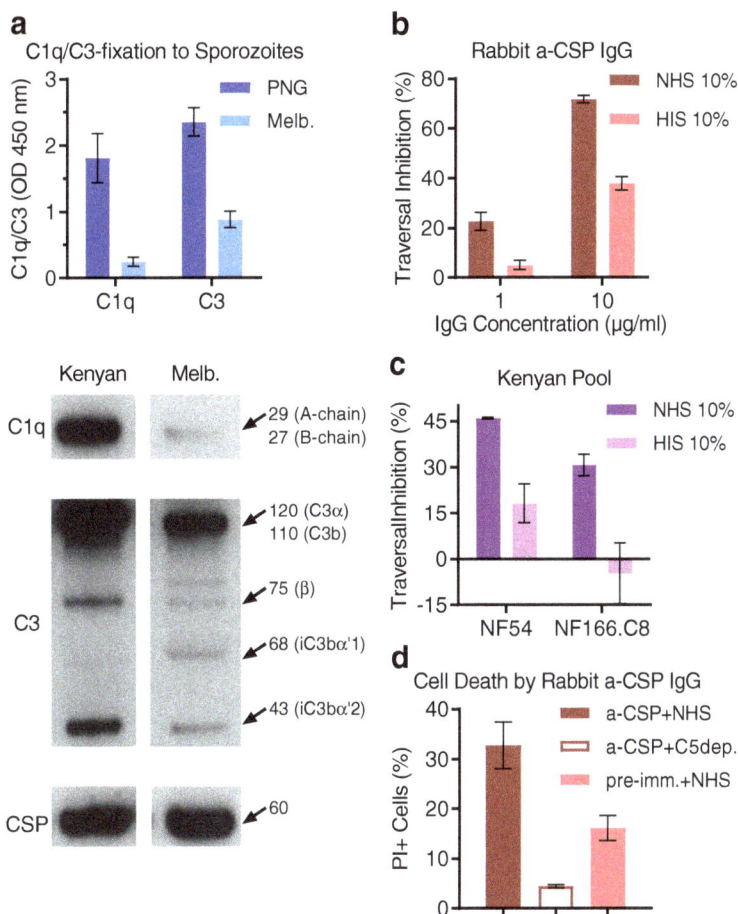

Fig. 4 Antibodies promote complement-fixation on *P. falciparum* sporozoites, which enhances antibody-mediated traversal inhibition and can lead to sporozoite death. **a** Antibody samples from malaria-exposed (PNG and Kenyan) and malaria-naïve (Melbourne) individuals were tested for the ability to fix human C1q and C3 to 3D7 *P. falciparum* sporozoites by ELISA and Western blot. ELISA samples (top panel) were tested in duplicate, and the mean and range were graphed (C1q-fixation data is from two independent experiments). Western blot sporozoites (bottom panel) were incubated with human antibody samples and normal human serum (NHS, active complement), and then washed and processed for Western blotting under reduced conditions. Any complement proteins that had deposited on the sporozoite surface were detected using C1q- and C3-specific antibodies, and the sporozoite surface antigen, CSP, was used as a loading control. **b,c** *In vitro* traversal inhibition of freshly dissected sporozoites incubated with HC-04 cells, in the presence of NHS and heat-inactivated human serum (HIS). Each condition was tested in duplicate, and the mean and range were graphed. **b** Traversal inhibition of NF54 sporozoites treated with rabbit anti-CSP IgG (compared to rabbit pre-immune IgG). **c** Traversal inhibition of NF54 and NF166.C8 sporozoites treated with malaria-exposed Kenyan pool (compared to malaria-naïve Melbourne pool). Results from two independent experiments are shown. **d** Percentage of dead 3D7 sporozoites (PI+ cells) treated with rabbit anti-CSP IgG and pre-immune IgG, in the presence of NHS or C5-depleted serum (C5dep.). The mean and range of two independent experiments are graphed. a-CSP after CSP immunization, C5dep. C5-depleted serum, CSP circumsporozoite protein, ELISA enzyme-linked immunosorbent assay, HIS heat-inactivated human serum, IgG immunoglobulin G, Melb. Melbourne, NHS normal human serum, OD optical density, PI propidium iodide, PNG Papua New Guinea, pre-imm. before CSP immunization

Antibody-mediated complement-fixation leads to sporozoite death

We examined whether sporozoites were susceptible to complement-mediated death since the formation of the MAC can lead to membrane damage and possible lysis of target cells. Cell death caused by complement might be a contributing mechanism in the inhibition of cell traversal. *P. falciparum* sporozoites were incubated with rabbit anti-CSP IgG and NHS containing an active complement, or C5-depleted serum as a negative control as MAC-formation is C5 dependent (Fig. 4d). We observed a twofold increase in the percentage of dead cells (PI positive) [35] when sporozoites were incubated with complement and anti-CSP IgG compared to pre-immune IgG (mean and range of two independent experiments: 32.8% [28.1 to 37.4%] and 16.1% [13.6 to 18.6%], respectively). Few PI-positive cells were detected following treatment with anti-CSP IgG and C5-depleted serum (4.4% [4.1 to 4.7%]). These data show that anti-CSP IgG and complement proteins interact to enhance complement-mediated sporozoite death.

The NANP-repeat epitope is a target of C1q-fixing antibodies

The NANP-repeat sequence is a major B-cell epitope of *P. falciparum* CSP and a key target of antibodies generated by the RTS,S vaccine [36]. Among PNG adults ($n = 30$), 55% were positive for C1q-fixation to $(NANP)_{15}$ peptide and 77% were positive for C1q-fixation to CSP. These variables were strongly correlated (rho = 0.841, 95% CI 0.679 to 0.925; $p < 0.001$), suggesting that NANP was a significant target of C1q-fixation to CSP (Fig. 5a). Among Kenyan adults ($n = 30$), a lower proportion of individuals were positive for C1q-fixation to $(NANP)_{15}$ and CSP (36% and 44%, respectively), and these variables only moderately correlated (rho = 0.489, 95% CI 0.094 to 0.751; $p = 0.015$) (Fig. 5b).

IgG and IgM isotype reactivity of PNG samples to $(NANP)_{15}$ positively correlated with C1q-fixation to CSP (rho = 0.525, 95% CI 0.185 to 0.752; $p = 0.004$ and rho = 0.812, 95% CI 0.622 to 0.911; $p < 0.001$, respectively) (Fig. 5a). To understand the role of antibody isotype further, we categorized samples into four groups based on low/high reactivity for NANP-specific IgG and IgM (defined by median AU) and compared C1q-fixation reactivity to CSP. Most samples were defined as either low or high for both antibody isotypes. Those with high NANP-IgG/IgM antibodies had significantly higher C1q-fixation levels to CSP (by AU = 4.9) than individuals with low NANP-IgG/IgM antibodies ($p < 0.001$) (Additional file 1: Figure S6A). Interestingly, two samples with high complement activity were classified as NANP-IgM high

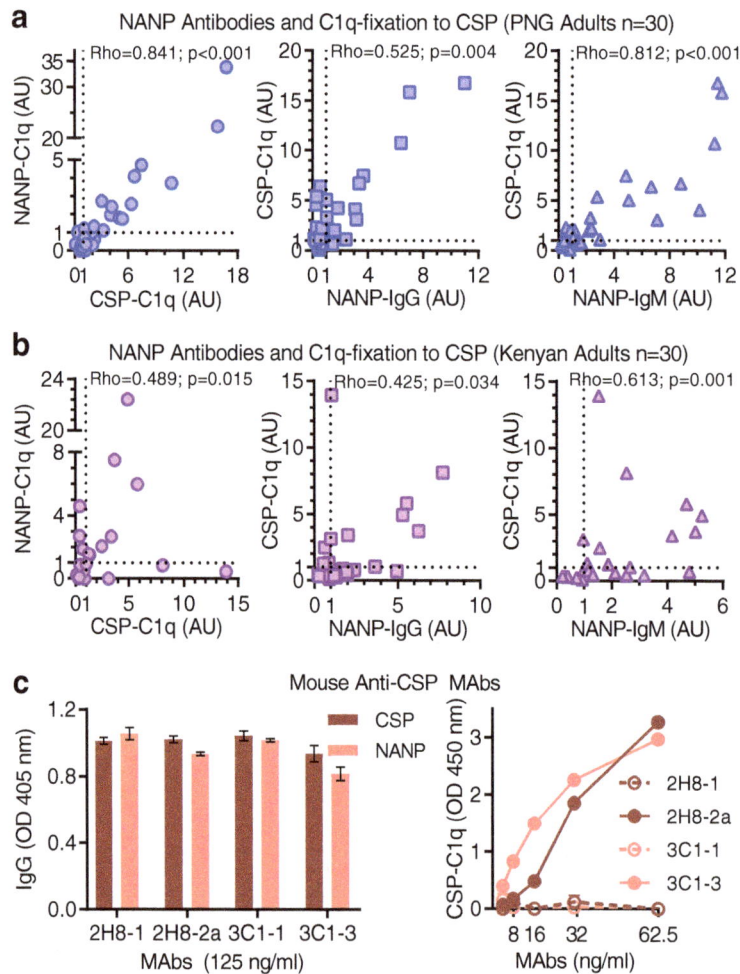

Fig. 5 Antibodies that target the NANP epitope of CSP can promote C1q-fixation. Antibodies from malaria-exposed adults living in PNG ($n = 30$) (**a**) and Kenya ($n = 30$) (**b**) were tested for IgG, IgM, and C1q-fixation to $(NANP)_{15}$ peptide by ELISA, and correlated with C1q fixation to CSP (Spearman's correlation coefficient, rho). Results were standardized to arbitrary units (AU) based on malaria-naïve negative controls from Melbourne (seropositivity defined as AU > 1, shown as dotted lines) and mean of duplicates were graphed. **c** Mouse anti-CSP MAbs 2H8-IgG1/IgG2a and 3C1-IgG1/IgG3 were tested for CSP-IgG, NANP-IgG, and C1q-fixation to CSP by ELISA. Results were corrected for background reactivity using no-IgG controls, and the mean and range of duplicates were graphed. AU arbitrary units, CSP circumsporozoite protein, ELISA enzyme-linked immunosorbent assay, IgG immunoglobulin G, IgM immunoglobulin M, MAb monoclonal antibody, OD optical density, PNG Papua New Guinea

and NANP-IgG low, suggesting the importance of IgM for complement-fixation in these individuals. The IgG and IgM isotype reactivity of Kenyan samples to $(NANP)_{15}$ moderately correlated with C1q-fixation to CSP (rho = 0.425, 95% CI 0.024 to 0.709; $p = 0.034$ and rho = 0.613, 95% CI 0.276 to 0.816; $p = 0.001$, respectively) (Fig. 5b) Furthermore, individuals with high NANP-IgG/IgM antibodies had only a minor increase in C1q-fixation to CSP (by AU = 1.86) than individuals with low NANP-IgG/IgM ($p = 0.043$) (Additional file 1: Figure S6B). Collectively, these data show that NANP-specific antibodies were variably associated with C1q-fixation to CSP among individuals, and between the two malaria-endemic populations.

To establish further that NANP-specific antibodies mediate C1q-fixation to CSP, we tested mouse anti-NANP MAbs (2H8 and 3C1) that had been subclass-switched so that there were 2H8-IgG1/IgG2a and 3C1-IgG1/IgG3 antibody pairs. All four MAbs demonstrated similar IgG-reactivity against CSP and $(NANP)_{15}$, but only 2H8-IgG2a and 3C1-IgG3 effectively fixed C1q compared to their IgG1 subclass counterparts, which is known not to fix human complement (Fig. 5c) [31].

Age-associated acquisition of naturally acquired complement-fixing antibodies to CSP

The bulk of malaria morbidity and mortality occurs in endemic areas where transmission is stable and relatively intense, particularly in children aged less than 5 years. We, therefore, investigated the acquisition of C1q-fixing antibodies to CSP among young children ($n = 59$) compared to adults ($n = 16$) living in a *P. falciparum* holoendemic area in western Kenya when transmission was high. We also compared complement-fixation responses to a major merozoite surface protein, MSP2, which is an established target of complement-fixing antibodies in blood-stage immunity [37]. In this setting, young children are known to be acquiring immunity to blood-stage infection and are susceptible to severe malaria, whereas adults have more established immunity due to extensive exposure to infections. Study participants were categorized into groups based on median ages of 0.5, 1, 2, 5, and 35 years (ages were in the ranges 0.3–0.7, 1–1.5, 1.8–3.0, 4.7–5.9, and 19.6–69.2 years, respectively). Reactivity for C1q-fixation and IgG to CSP was relatively low among children of all age groups and was significantly higher among adults ($p < 0.001$ for both tests) (Fig. 6a). In contrast, we observed higher reactivity for C1q-

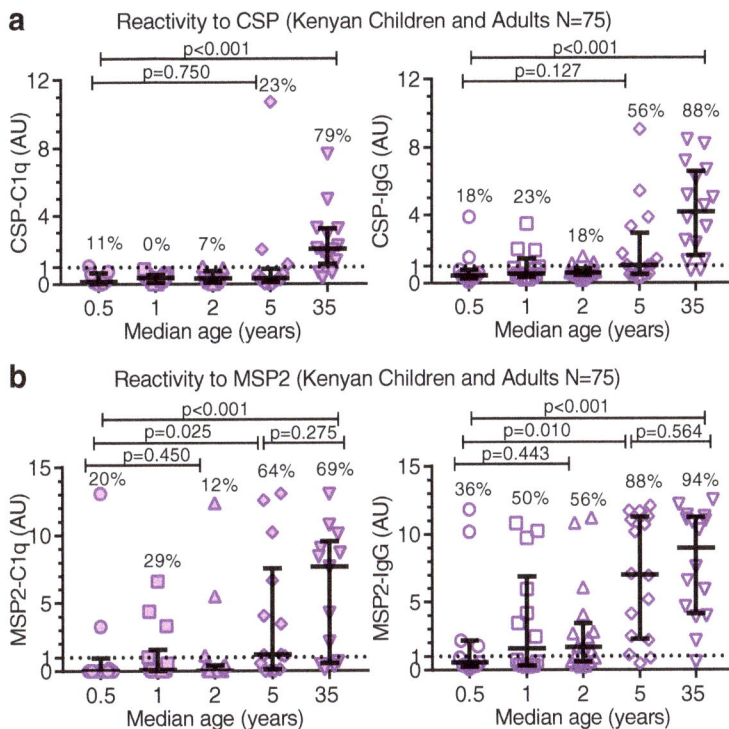

Fig. 6 Acquisition of C1q-fixing antibodies and total IgG to CSP and MSP2 antigens in malaria-exposed Kenyan children and adults. Kenyan children and adults ($N = 75$) were categorized into groups based on the median ages 0.5, 1, 2, 5, and 35 years ($n = 11$, $n = 14$, $n = 18$, $n = 16$, and $n = 16$, respectively). Samples were tested for C1q-fixation and total IgG to CSP (**a**) and MSP2 (**b**) by ELISA. Results were standardized to arbitrary units (AU) based on malaria-naive negative controls from Melbourne (seropositivity defined as AU > 1, shown as dotted lines), and the mean of duplicates were graphed along with the group median, interquartile range, and percentage of positive samples. Reactivity between two groups and more than two groups were compared using the Mann–Whitney U test and Kruskal–Wallis test, respectively. AU arbitrary units, CSP circumsporozoite protein, ELISA enzyme-linked immunosorbent assay, IgG immunoglobulin G, MSP2 Merozoite surface protein 2

fixation to MSP2, a known target of naturally acquired immunity [29]. Interestingly, children in the age group with a median of 5 years had C1q-fixing antibody levels similar to adults ($p = 0.275$), which were higher than those observed in younger children ($p < 0.001$). Taken together, these results suggest that complement-fixing antibodies to CSP are poorly acquired during early childhood compared to the merozoite antigen MSP2, and that C1q-fixing antibodies to CSP are overall acquired more slowly than those to blood-stage antigens.

High levels of C1q-fixing antibodies are associated with protection against clinical malaria in children

From a longitudinal cohort study of children ($N = 206$, 5–14 years) who were resident in a malaria-endemic region of PNG [25], only a minority had antibodies that promoted C1q-fixation to CSP (positivity 40%), weakly

correlating with anti-CSP IgG (rho = 0.280, 95% CI 0.140 to 0.409; $p < 0.001$). When stratified into four age groups (≤8, 8.1–9, 9.1–10, and ≥10 years), there was no significant association between age and C1q-fixing antibodies ($p = 0.211$) (Fig. 7a). However, children with concurrent parasitemia at the time of enrolment as determined by the polymerase chain reaction showed significantly higher C1q-fixation activity than uninfected children (positivity 45% and 31%, respectively; $p < 0.001$) (Fig. 7a), reflecting their recent exposure to sporozoites.

To obtain epidemiologic evidence supporting the importance of antibody-mediated complement-fixation to CSP in acquired immunity to malaria, we investigated whether the minority of PNG children with high levels of functional antibodies had a reduced risk of clinical malaria. Children were treated for malaria and then actively monitored for the duration of the study,

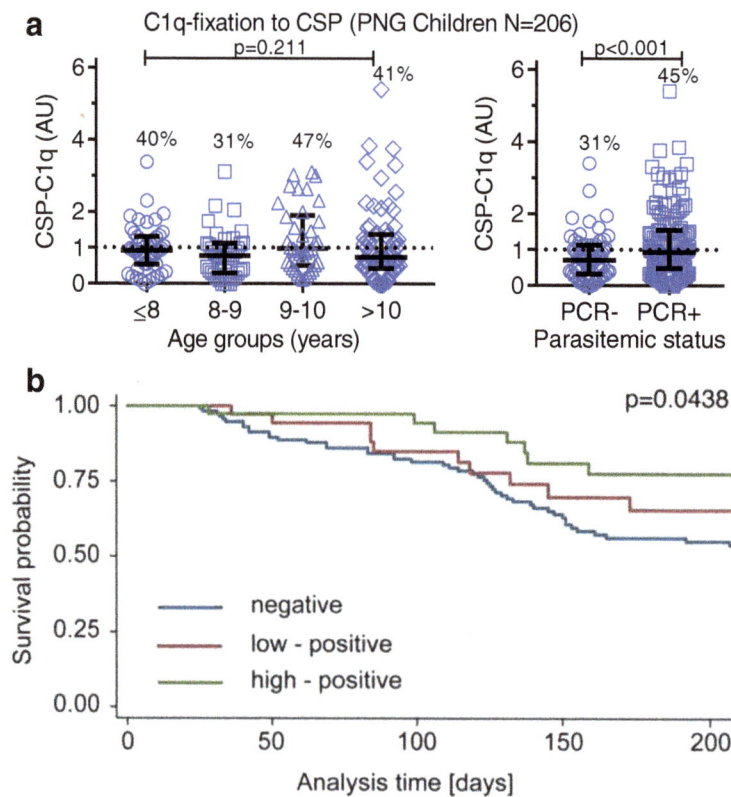

Fig. 7 High levels of C1q-fixing antibodies to CSP are associated with protection against clinical malaria in children. PNG children ($N = 206$) were tested for C1q-fixation to CSP by ELISA. Results were standardized to arbitrary units (AU) based on malaria-naïve negative controls from Melbourne (seropositivity defined as AU > 1, shown as dotted lines). **a** C1q-fixation to CSP was categorized by age (≤8, 8.1–9, 9.1–10, and ≥10 for $n = 47$, $n = 39$, $n = 38$, and $n = 71$, respectively), and parasitemic status at enrolment by PCR. Each sample was tested in duplicate, and the mean value was used to generate box plots. The top, center, and bottom horizontal lines represent the 75th percentile, median, and 25th percentile, respectively. The upper and lower whiskers represent the highest and lowest values within the 1.5×-interquartile range, respectively. Values that exceed this range are presented as symbols. Reactivity between two groups and more than two groups was compared using the Mann–Whitney U test and Kruskal–Wallis test, respectively. **b** Kaplan–Meier survival curve showing the cumulative proportion of children who had experienced an episode of malaria during the follow-up (time in days), stratified into three groups based on C1q-fixation reactivity: negative (AU < 1), low positive (bottom 50% of positive samples, 1 < AU ≤ 1.525), and high positive (top 50% of positive samples, AU > 1.525), as shown in blue, red, and green, respectively ($n = 116$, $n = 39$, and $n = 39$, respectively; $p = 0.0438$, Wilcoxon Breslow test, unadjusted for confounders). AU arbitrary units, CSP circumsporozoite protein, ELISA enzyme-linked immunosorbent assay, PCR polymerase chain reaction, PNG Papua New Guinea

enabling us to establish any association between C1q-fixing antibody levels at enrolment and the subsequent risk of developing clinical malaria. Children were divided into three response groups based on C1q-fixation reactivity: (i) negative (AU < 1), (ii) low positive (bottom 50% positive samples, $1 < AU \leq 1.525$), and (iii) high positive (top 50% of positive samples, AU > 1.525) (Additional file 1: Figure S7). In a Kaplan–Meier survival analysis, children with high levels of C1q-fixation had a lower rate of malaria during the follow-up (Fig. 7b). Importantly, we found that children with high levels of C1q-fixing antibodies at enrolment had a significantly reduced risk of clinical malaria compared to children who were negative for C1q-fixing antibodies (Cox proportional hazards model; HR = 0.39 [0.18–0.87], $p = 0.020$), which remained significant after adjusting for potential confounders of age, location of residence, and parasitemia at baseline (adjusted HR = 0.42 [0.19–0.94], $p = 0.034$). A significant association was not observed for children with low C1q-antibodies compared to those who were negative (HR = 0.70 [0.38–1.38], p was not significant and adjusted HR = 0.69 [0.35–1.37], $p = 0.2$). Furthermore, there was no significant association between IgG to CSP and risk of malaria (adjusted HR 0.50 [0.19–1.32] comparing children with high IgG responses compared to IgG-negative individuals). Although the prevalence of naturally acquired functional anti-CSP antibodies was generally low, these data suggest that high levels of C1q-fixing antibodies are associated with naturally acquired anti-malarial immunity and protection against disease.

Discussion

Developing highly efficacious vaccines requires knowledge of the functional mechanisms that contribute to protection against malaria, and the identification of correlates of protective immunity. Here we show that naturally acquired human anti-CSP antibodies can function by fixing C1q and activating the classical complement pathway, and this activity significantly correlated with IgG1, IgG3, and IgM antibodies. C1q-fixing antibodies were also shown to target the central NANP-repeat region of CSP. Importantly, we provide the first direct evidence that P. falciparum sporozoites are susceptible to human complement via the antibody-dependent classical pathway, resulting in enhanced traversal inhibition and sporozoite death in vitro. Furthermore, we found that the natural acquisition of C1q-fixing antibodies to CSP in children occurs more slowly than observed for blood-stage antigens. Although poorly acquired in general, the minority of children who acquired high levels of C1q-fixing antibodies to CSP had a significantly reduced risk of developing clinical malaria, which identified the first functional correlate of immunity to sporozoites in human studies. Together, these findings reveal that antibodies to CSP and P. falciparum sporozoites can function by activating human complement, and provide initial epidemiological evidence linking antibody function and protective immunity.

To detect functional anti-CSP antibodies, we measured their ability to fix C1q, which is unique to the antibody-dependent classical complement pathway, as well as downstream complement proteins. There were strong correlations between C1q fixation and C4/C2/C3/C5b-C9 fixation demonstrating that C1q-fixation alone was a sufficient measure of complement activity, which we used in subsequent cohort experiments.

We demonstrated that immune antibodies promote the deposition and activation of human complement against whole P. falciparum sporozoites and had functional effects. While anti-CSP antibodies can directly inhibit sporozoite traversal and invasion in vitro [17–19], high antibody concentrations have generally been required and the relationship between function and protection has not been established. Furthermore, the presence of anti-CSP IgG alone is an insufficient correlate of protection in humans. We found that naturally acquired human antibodies had only weak activity in the direct inhibition of P. falciparum sporozoite traversal, but activity was substantially enhanced by an active human complement. When using sporozoites from the NF54 line, there was a more than twofold increase in inhibitory activity when antibodies were tested in the presence of an active complement (compared to an inactivated complement), whereas substantial traversal inhibition of NF166.C8 sporozoites was seen only when antibodies were tested with active complement present. Inhibiting sporozoite traversal may be important, as it is essential for establishing liver-stage infection in animals [16, 38]. Mouse studies of the rodent species, P. berghei, reported that glycan-specific antibodies activated the mouse complement and inhibited the traversal and invasion of sporozoites [39]. Interestingly, this was not mediated by murine IgG2a, which we have shown is capable of fixing human C1q. There are important differences between human malaria immunity and murine models. Murine models typically use the rodent malaria P. berghei, which has substantial biological and functional differences from P. falciparum, including in the major target antigen CSP, as P. berghei does not have the major NANP epitope of P. falciparum CSP. Furthermore, complement activity in laboratory mice is much lower than for human complement, which plays an important role in immunity [40]. Murine immune responses to Plasmodium infection are typically dominated by murine IgG1, which does not fix complement, whereas human IgG1 and IgG3 dominate human responses and both subclasses potently activate complement. The future development of new animal models of malaria that better represent antibody–complement interactions may be valuable for vaccine development. Future research to define further the antibody titers, types, and specificity required for optimal complement fixation and functional effects would be valuable to help inform vaccine development.

Antibodies alone cannot kill target cells, but our findings suggest that they can mediate this effect by recruitment and activation of complement. We directly showed that incubation with antibodies and complement can lead to sporozoite death. It has previously been proposed that murine antibody–complement interactions lead to morphological changes and bleb formation in *P. falciparum* sporozoites [41]. However, in that prior study, complement-fixation and activation were not directly shown and the potential effect of the complement was not quantified (only qualitative data were presented), and antibodies were predominantly murine IgG1, which cannot interact with complement, as we have also shown [31]. Interestingly we found that sporozoites were partially susceptible to direct complement attack, as indicated by some direct C3 deposition and cell death. However, complement susceptibility was enhanced two-fold in the presence of immune antibodies.

The NANP-repeat sequence is a known B-cell epitope of CSP, and an important target of RTS,S-induced antibodies [36]. We found this epitope also to be a target C1q-fixation using synthetic NANP peptide and NANP-specific MAbs. This supports future investigation of whether RTS,S-induced antibodies mediate complement-fixation, as they are known to predominately target this epitope. NANP-specific antibodies can neutralize sporozoite function *in vitro* [42], and can reduce liver-stage burden in humanized mice that are susceptible to *P. falciparum* [8] or mice challenged with transgenic *P. falciparum/P. berghei* sporozoites [43], although high antibody concentrations appear to be required for function. Our data suggest that complement may substantially enhance the function of these antibodies, reducing the critical concentrations needed to mediate functional effects. There were significant correlations between C1q-fixation to NANP and CSP, and between NANP-specific IgG/IgM and C1q-fixation to CSP, but the strength of correlations varied between the PNG and Kenyan populations. It is possible that antibodies to other regions of CSP mediate complement-fixation, such as epitopes in the C-terminal and N-terminal regions, which warrants further investigation.

We identified a subset of individuals from PNG and Kenya with high anti-CSP IgG reactivity that demonstrated a weak ability to fix C1q. This highlights that total IgG reactivity is not wholly reflective of functional activity, and may explain why measuring anti-CSP IgG alone is a poor correlate of protective immunity. Anti-CSP IgG can directly fix C1q, and IgM is also likely to play some role, as we observed high levels of anti-CSP IgM in selected individuals that strongly fixed C1q. Anti-CSP IgG was predominately the IgG1 and IgG3 subclasses, which are known to active complement. However, IgG2 and IgG4 were also detected in some individuals, which may negatively impact C1q-fixation by outcompeting the complement-fixing subclasses; therefore, the overall isotype and subclass profile is important for functional activity. Other antibody factors, such as epitope specificity, affinity, and glycosylation, are also important in determining function.

A striking new finding is that children with high levels of C1q-fixing antibodies to CSP had a significantly reduced risk of clinical malaria compared to children who had no detectable functional antibodies. Previously, no association between anti-CSP antibodies and protection in malaria-exposed populations has been found [44, 45]. In contrast, we show important initial epidemiologic evidence of the potential role of anti-CSP antibodies that fix complement in malaria immunity, supported by findings on the functional outcomes of antibody–complement interactions. This is the first identification of a functional antibody response to sporozoite antigens that is associated with protective immunity in malaria-exposed children, suggesting that this is a significant new correlate of immunity. Our findings suggest that although the natural development of strong complement-fixing antibodies occurs only in a minority of children, when such antibodies do develop, they contribute to protective immunity. These findings support future investigation of whether C1q-fixing antibodies are induced by vaccines such as RTS,S, and whether functional antibodies are associated with vaccine efficacy and could be used a correlate of protection.

The cell-free high-throughput assay to detect and quantify functional, complement-fixing antibodies to CSP, which we developed in this study, could be applied in large-scale clinical trials for vaccine evaluation. Although this may not wholly represent all interactions that occur on the sporozoite surface, CSP is a well-validated antigen that is known to be the major target of naturally acquired immunity to sporozoites [11, 46, 47] and is the basis of the leading vaccine candidate, RTS,S [12]. Future studies should investigate other potentially important sporozoite antigens as targets of complement-fixing antibodies and the importance of non-repeat CSP epitopes, which may have important implications in vaccine development, and whether complement activation leads to additional effects or outcomes.

Conclusions

In summary, this study demonstrates for the first time that immune antibodies fix and activate human complement against CSP and *P. falciparum* sporozoites, which inhibited sporozoite traversal and lead to sporozoite death. These data provide key knowledge on antibody functional mechanisms against sporozoites, and help us to identify which antibody types and epitopes are important in mediating anti-malarial immunity. We also obtained promising evidence that a strong level of C1q-fixing antibodies to CSP is associated with protection against clinical malaria, and may be a valuable correlate of protective immunity. This is the first evidence of a functional antibody response to sporozoites associated with protection against malaria in children. The future application of these approaches to quantify functional immunity in vaccine trials may greatly aid our understanding of how vaccines work and why efficacy has been suboptimal in trials to date. The antibody C1q-fixation assay may be a suitable correlate of protective immunity in vaccine development and trial evaluation, and studies of acquired human immunity. Defining the functional mechanisms that confer protective immunity against malaria is essential for developing and evaluating much-needed highly efficacious malaria vaccines. These findings have strong translational significance by revealing a mechanism of anti-sporozoite immunity, and thereby enabling the development of strategies to maximize this effector mechanism in the development of highly efficacious malaria vaccines.

Abbreviations
ABTS: 2,2'-azino-bis(3-ethylbenzothiazoline-6-sulfonic acid); AU: Arbitrary units; CI: Confidence interval; CSP: Circumsporozoite protein; ELISA: Enzyme-linked immunosorbent assay; HIS: Heat-inactivated serum; HR: Hazard ratio; HRP: Horse radish peroxidase; IgG: Immunoglobulin G; IgM: Immunoglobulin M; MAb: Monoclonal antibody; MAC: Membrane attack complex; MSP2: Merozoite surface protein 2; NHS: Normal human serum; OD: Optical density; PBS: Phosphate-buffered saline; PI: Propidium iodide; PNG: Papua New Guinea; Rh: Tetramethylrhodamine; RT: Room temperature; RTS,S: RTS,S/AS01; SDS-PAGE: Sodium dodecyl sulphate-polyacrylamide gel electrophoresis

Acknowledgements
We thank all study participants, the staff of the Kenya Medical Research Institute, and the Institute of Medical Research in PNG for their assistance with clinical studies. We thank Emily Locke of PATH's Malaria Vaccine Initiative for helpful comments and providing reagents, Robin Anders for providing recombinant MSP2 antigen, Moriya Tsuji of Rockefeller University and Gennova, India, for providing CSP monoclonal antibodies, and the teams of Marga van de Vegte-Bolmer (Rianne Siebelink-Stoter and Wouter Graumans) and Geert-Jan van Gemert (Jolanda Klaasssen, Laura Pelser-Posthumus, Jacqueline Kuhnen, and Astrid Pouwelsen) from Radboud University Medical Center for technical assistance with the generation of infected mosquitoes and salivary gland dissections.

Funding
Funding was provided by PATH's Malaria Vaccine Initiative; the National Health and Medical Research Council (NHMRC) of Australia (program grant to JGB; research fellowships to JGB and IM); the National Institutes of Health; the Australian government's Research Training Program Scholarship; and the Nijmegen Institute for Infection, Inflammation and Immunity (N4i) for a PhD scholarship. The funders had no role in the study design, data collection and analysis, decision to publish, or preparation of the manuscript. The Burnet Institute is supported by an operational infrastructure support grant from Victoria's state government, and the infrastructure support scheme of the NHMRC Independent Research Institutes. This paper is published with permission from the director of the Kenya Medical Research Institute.

Authors' contributions
LK performed ELISAs. MCB and LK performed the sporozoite traversal experiment. GF and LK performed the sporozoite cell death experiment. LR and LK designed and optimized the complement-fixation assay and MCB optimized the sporozoite traversal assay. LR, FJIF, and LK analyzed the data. JGB, JWK, IM, KC, and AED were involved in cohort studies. LK, JGB, FJIF, MCB, and RS designed the study. LK and JGB wrote the manuscript, which was critically reviewed by all authors. All authors approved the final manuscript.

Competing interests
The authors declare they have no competing interests.

Author details
[1]Burnet Institute, Melbourne, Australia. [2]Department of Immunology and Pathology, Monash University, Melbourne, Australia. [3]Department of Medical Microbiology, Radboud University Medical Center, Nijmegen, The Netherlands. [4]Kenya Medical Research Institute, Kisumu, Kenya. [5]Center for Global Health and Diseases, Case Western University, Cleveland, USA. [6]Division of Population Health and Immunity, Walter and Eliza Hall Institute, Melbourne, Australia. [7]Department of Parasites and Insect Vectors, Institut Pasteur, Paris, France. [8]Department of Epidemiology and Preventative Medicine and Department of Infectious Diseases, Monash University, Melbourne, Australia. [9]Centre for Epidemiology and Biostatistics, Melbourne School of Population and Global Health, The University of Melbourne, Melbourne, Australia. [10]Department of Microbiology, Monash University, Clayton, Australia. [11]Department of Medicine, The University of Melbourne, 185 Commercial Road, Parkville, Australia.

References
1. World Health Organization: Malaria vaccine technology roadmap. 2013.
2. World Health Organization: World Malaria Report 2016 2016.
3. malERA Consultative Group on Vaccines. A research agenda for malaria eradication: vaccines. PLoS Med. 2011;8(1):e1000398.
4. Amino R, Thiberge S, Martin B, Celli S, Shorte S, Frischknecht F, Ménard R. Quantitative imaging of *Plasmodium* transmission from mosquito to mammal. Nat Med. 2006;12(2):220–4.
5. Sturm A, Graewe S, Franke-Fayard B, Retzlaff S, Bolte S, Roppenser B, Aepfelbacher M, Janse C, Heussler V. Alteration of the parasite plasma

membrane and the parasitophorous vacuole membrane during exo-erythrocytic development of malaria parasites. Protist. 2009;160(1):51–63.

6. Frischknecht F, Baldacci P, Martin B, Zimmer C, Thiberge S, Olivo-Marin JC, Shorte SL, Ménard R. Imaging movement of malaria parasites during transmission by *Anopheles* mosquitoes. Cell Microbiol. 2004;6(7):687–94.

7. Charoenvit Y, Sedegah M, Yuan L, Gross M, Cole C, Bechara R, Leef M, Robey F, Lowell G, Beaudoin R. Active and passive immunization against *Plasmodium yoelii* sporozoites. Bull World Health Organ. 1990;68(Suppl):26.

8. Sack BK, Miller JL, Vaughan AM, Douglass A, Kaushansky A, Mikolajczak S, Coppi A, Gonzalez-Aseguinolaza G, Tsuji M, Zavala F. Model for *in vivo* assessment of humoral protection against malaria sporozoite challenge by passive transfer of monoclonal antibodies and immune serum. Infect Immun. 2014;82(2):808–17.

9. White MT, Verity R, Griffin JT, Asante KP, Owusu-Agyei S, Greenwood B, Drakeley C, Gesase S, Lusingu J, Ansong D. Immunogenicity of the RTS, S/AS01 malaria vaccine and implications for duration of vaccine efficacy: secondary analysis of data from a phase 3 randomised controlled trial. Lancet Infect Dis. 2015;15(12):1450–8.

10. Chelimo K, Ofulla AV, Narum DL, Kazura JW, Lanar DE, John CC. Antibodies to *Plasmodium falciparum* antigens vary by age and antigen in children in a malaria-holoendemic area of Kenya. Pediatr Infect Dis J. 2005;24(8):680–4.

11. John CC, Zickafoose JS, Sumba PO, King CL, Kazura JW. Antibodies to the *Plasmodium falciparum* antigens circumsporozoite protein, thrombospondin-related adhesive protein, and liver-stage antigen 1 vary by ages of subjects and by season in a highland area of Kenya. Infect Immun. 2003;71(8):4320–5.

12. Casares S, Brumeanu T-D, Richie TL. The RTS, S malaria vaccine. Vaccine. 2010;28(31):4880–94.

13. Olotu A, Moris P, Mwacharo J, Vekemans J, Kimani D, Janssens M, Kai O, Jongert E, Lievens M, Leach A. Circumsporozoite-specific T cell responses in children vaccinated with RTS, S/AS01 E and protection against *P falciparum* clinical malaria. PLoS One. 2011;6(10):e25786.

14. Clinical Trial Partnerships RTSS. Efficacy and safety of RTS, S/AS01 malaria vaccine with or without a booster dose in infants and children in Africa: final results of a phase 3, individually randomised, controlled trial. Lancet. 2015;386(9988):31–45.

15. Hopp CS, Chiou K, Ragheb DR, Salman A, Khan SM, Liu AJ, Sinnis P. Longitudinal analysis of *Plasmodium* sporozoite motility in the dermis reveals component of blood vessel recognition. elife. 2015;4:e07789.

16. Ishino T, Yano K, Chinzei Y, Yuda M. Cell-passage activity is required for the malarial parasite to cross the liver sinusoidal cell layer. PLoS Biol. 2004;2(1):e4.

17. Vanderberg JP, Frevert U. Intravital microscopy demonstrating antibody-mediated immobilisation of *Plasmodium berghei* sporozoites injected into skin by mosquitoes. Int J Parasitol. 2004;34(9):991–6.

18. Okitsu SL, Silvie O, Westerfeld N, Curcic M, Kammer AR, Mueller MS, Sauerwein RW, Robinson JA, Genton B, Mazier D. A virosomal malaria peptide vaccine elicits a long-lasting sporozoite-inhibitory antibody response in a phase 1a clinical trial. PLoS One. 2007;2(12):e1278.

19. Hollingdale MR, Nardin EH, Tharavanij S, Schwartz A, Nussenzweig R. Inhibition of entry of *Plasmodium falciparum* and *P. vivax* sporozoites into cultured cells; an in vitro assay of protective antibodies. J Immunol. 1984;132(2):909–13.

20. Behet MC, Foquet L, van Gemert G-J, Bijker EM, Meuleman P, Leroux-Roels G, Hermsen CC, Scholzen A, Sauerwein RW. Sporozoite immunization of human volunteers under chemoprophylaxis induces functional antibodies against pre-erythrocytic stages of *Plasmodium falciparum*. Malar J. 2014;13(1):1.

21. Merle NS, Church SE, Fremeaux-Bacchi V, Roumenina LT. Complement system part I - molecular mechanisms of activation and regulation. Front Immunol. 2015;6:262.

22. Hommel M, Elliott SR, Soma V, Kelly G, Fowkes FJ, Chesson JM, Duffy MF, Bockhorst J, Avril M, Mueller I. Evaluation of the antigenic diversity of placenta-binding *Plasmodium falciparum* variants and the antibody repertoire among pregnant women. Infect Immun. 2010;78(5):1963–78.

23. Dent AE, Chelimo K, Sumba PO, Spring MD, Crabb BS, Moormann AM, Tisch DJ, Kazura JW. Temporal stability of naturally acquired immunity to Merozoite Surface Protein-1 in Kenyan adults. Malar J. 2009;8(1):162.

24. Chelimo K, Embury PB, Sumba PO, Vulule J, Ofulla AV, Long C, Kazura JW, Moormann AM. Age-related differences in naturally acquired T cell memory to *Plasmodium falciparum* merozoite surface protein 1. PLoS One. 2011;6(9):e24852.

25. Michon P, Cole-Tobian JL, Dabod E, Schoepflin S, Igu J, Susapu M, Tarongka N, Zimmerman PA, Reeder JC, Beeson JG. The risk of malarial

infections and disease in Papua New Guinean children. Am J Trop Med Hyg. 2007;76(6):997–1008.

26. McCallum FJ, Persson KE, Mugyenyi CK, Fowkes FJ, Simpson JA, Richards JS, Williams TN, Marsh K, Beeson JG. Acquisition of growth-inhibitory antibodies against blood-stage *Plasmodium falciparum*. PLoS One. 2008;3(10):e3571.

27. McCall MB, Wammes LJ, Langenberg MC, van Gemert G-J, Walk J, Hermsen CC, Graumans W, Koelewijn R, Franetich J-F, Chishimba S. Infectivity of *Plasmodium falciparum* sporozoites determines emerging parasitemia in infected volunteers. Sci Transl Med. 2017;9(395):eaag2490.

28. Ishizuka AS, Lyke KE, DeZure A, Berry AA, Richie TL, Mendoza FH, Enama ME, Gordon IJ, Chang L-J, Sarwar UN. Protection against malaria at 1 year and immune correlates following PfSPZ vaccination. Nat Med. 2016;22(6):614–23.

29. Stanisic DI, Richards JS, McCallum FJ, Michon P, King CL, Schoepflin S, Gilson PR, Murphy VJ, Anders RF, Mueller I. Immunoglobulin G subclass-specific responses against *Plasmodium falciparum* merozoite antigens are associated with control of parasitemia and protection from symptomatic illness. Infect Immun. 2009;77(3):1165–74.

30. Zang M, Mandraju R, Rai U, Shiratsuchi T, Tsuji M. Monoclonal Antibodies against *Plasmodium falciparum* Circumsporozoite Protein. Antibodies. 2017;6(3):30.

31. Mershon KL, Morrison SL. Antibody–complement interaction. Ther Monoclonal Antibodies. 2009;16:371–83.

32. Diebolder CA, Beurskens FJ, de Jong RN, Koning RI, Strumane K, Lindorfer MA, Voorhorst M, Ugurlar D, Rosati S, Heck AJ. Complement is activated by IgG hexamers assembled at the cell surface. Science. 2014;343(6176):1260–3.

33. Ishizaka K, Ishizaka T, Sugahara T. Biological activity of soluble antigen-antibody complexes VII. Role of an antibody fragment in the induction of biological activities. J Immunol. 1962;88(6):690–701.

34. Fujita T. The activation mechanism of human complement system by immune precipitate formed with rabbit IgG antibody. Microbiol Immunol. 1979;23(10):1023–31.

35. Cleary KL, Chan HC, James S, Glennie MJ, Cragg MS. Antibody distance from the cell membrane regulates antibody effector mechanisms. J Immunol. 2017;198(10):3999–4011.

36. Radin K, Clement F, Jongert E, Sterckx YG, Ockenhouse C, Regules J, Lemiale F, Leroux-Roels G. A monoclonal antibody-based immunoassay to measure the antibody response against the repeat region of the circumsporozoite protein of *Plasmodium falciparum*. Malar J. 2016;15(1):543.

37. Boyle MJ, Reiling L, Feng G, Langer C, Osier FH, Aspeling-Jones H, Cheng YS, Stubbs J, Tetteh KK, Conway DJ, et al. Human antibodies fix complement to inhibit *Plasmodium falciparum* invasion of erythrocytes and are associated with protection against Malaria. Immunity. 2015;42(3):580–90.

38. Ishino T, Chinzei Y, Yuda M. A *Plasmodium* sporozoite protein with a membrane attack complex domain is required for breaching the liver sinusoidal cell layer prior to hepatocyte infection†. Cell Microbiol. 2005; 7(2):199–208.

39. Yilmaz B, Portugal S, Tran TM, Gozzelino R, Ramos S, Gomes J, Regalado A, Cowan PJ, d'Apice AJ, Chong AS. Gut microbiota elicits a protective immune response against malaria transmission. Cell. 2014;159(6):1277–89.

40. Ong GL, Mattes MJ. Mouse strains with typical mammalian levels of complement activity. J Immunol Methods. 1989;125(1–2):147–58.

41. McCoy ME, Golden HE, Doll TA, Yang Y, Kaba SA, Burkhard P, Lanar DE. Mechanisms of protective immune responses induced by the *Plasmodium falciparum* circumsporozoite protein-based, self-assembling protein nanoparticle vaccine. Malaria J. 2013;12(1):136.

42. Foquet L, Hermsen CC, van Gemert G-J, Van Braeckel E, Weening KE, Sauerwein R, Meuleman P, Leroux-Roels G. Vaccine-induced monoclonal antibodies targeting circumsporozoite protein prevent *Plasmodium falciparum* infection. J Clin Invest. 2014;124(1):140.

43. Deal C, Balazs AB, Espinosa DA, Zavala F, Baltimore D, Ketner G. Vectored antibody gene delivery protects against *Plasmodium falciparum* sporozoite challenge in mice. Proc Natl Acad Sci U S A. 2014;111(34):12528–32.

44. Hoffman SL, Oster CN, Plowe CV, Woollett GR, Beier JC, Chulay JD, Wirtz RA, Hollingdale MR, Mugambi M. Naturally acquired antibodies to sporozoites do not prevent malaria: vaccine development implications. Science. 1987; 237(4815):639–42.

45. Webster H, Brown A, Chuenchitra C, Permpanich B, Pipithkul J. Characterization of antibodies to sporozoites in Plasmodium falciparum malaria and correlation with protection. J Clin Microbiol. 1988;26(5):923–7.

46. John CC, Moormann AM, Pregibon DC, Sumba PO, McHugh MM, Narum DL, Lanar DE, Schluchter MD, Kazura JW. Correlation of high levels of antibodies to multiple pre-erythrocytic *Plasmodium falciparum* antigens and protection from infection. Am J Trop Med Hyg. 2005;73(1):222–8.

47. John CC, Tande AJ, Moormann AM, Sumba PO, Lanar DE, Min XM, Kazura JW. Antibodies to pre-erythrocytic *Plasmodium falciparum* antigens and risk of clinical malaria in Kenyan children. J Infect Dis. 2008;197(4):519–26.

12

Methods used in the spatial analysis of tuberculosis epidemiology

Debebe Shaweno[1,2][*] (iD), Malancha Karmakar[2,3], Kefyalew Addis Alene[4,5], Romain Ragonnet[1,6], Archie CA Clements[7], James M. Trauer[2,8], Justin T. Denholm[2,3] and Emma S. McBryde[1,9]

Abstract

Background: Tuberculosis (TB) transmission often occurs within a household or community, leading to heterogeneous spatial patterns. However, apparent spatial clustering of TB could reflect ongoing transmission or co-location of risk factors and can vary considerably depending on the type of data available, the analysis methods employed and the dynamics of the underlying population. Thus, we aimed to review methodological approaches used in the spatial analysis of TB burden.

Methods: We conducted a systematic literature search of spatial studies of TB published in English using Medline, Embase, PsycInfo, Scopus and Web of Science databases with no date restriction from inception to 15 February 2017. The protocol for this systematic review was prospectively registered with PROSPERO (CRD42016036655).

Results: We identified 168 eligible studies with spatial methods used to describe the spatial distribution ($n = 154$), spatial clusters ($n = 73$), predictors of spatial patterns ($n = 64$), the role of congregate settings ($n = 3$) and the household ($n = 2$) on TB transmission. Molecular techniques combined with geospatial methods were used by 25 studies to compare the role of transmission to reactivation as a driver of TB spatial distribution, finding that geospatial hotspots are not necessarily areas of recent transmission. Almost all studies used notification data for spatial analysis (161 of 168), although none accounted for undetected cases. The most common data visualisation technique was notification rate mapping, and the use of smoothing techniques was uncommon. Spatial clusters were identified using a range of methods, with the most commonly employed being Kulldorff's spatial scan statistic followed by local Moran's I and Getis and Ord's local Gi(d) tests. In the 11 papers that compared two such methods using a single dataset, the clustering patterns identified were often inconsistent. Classical regression models that did not account for spatial dependence were commonly used to predict spatial TB risk. In all included studies, TB showed a heterogeneous spatial pattern at each geographic resolution level examined.

Conclusions: A range of spatial analysis methodologies has been employed in divergent contexts, with all studies demonstrating significant heterogeneity in spatial TB distribution. Future studies are needed to define the optimal method for each context and should account for unreported cases when using notification data where possible. Future studies combining genotypic and geospatial techniques with epidemiologically linked cases have the potential to provide further insights and improve TB control.

Keywords: Spatial analysis, Tuberculosis, Genotypic cluster

* Correspondence: debebesh@gmail.com
[1]Department of Medicine, University of Melbourne, Melbourne, Victoria, Australia
[2]Victorian Tuberculosis Program at the Peter Doherty Institute for Infection and Immunity, Melbourne, Victoria, Australia
Full list of author information is available at the end of the article

Background

Mycobacterium tuberculosis (*Mtb*) transmission often occurs within a household or small community because prolonged duration of contact is typically required for infection to occur, creating the potential for localised clusters to develop [1]. However, geospatial TB clusters are not always due to ongoing person-to-person transmission but may also result from reactivation of latent infection in a group of people with shared risk factors [1, 2]. Spatial analysis and identification of areas with high TB rates (clusters), followed by characterisation of the drivers of the dynamics in these clusters, have been promoted for targeted TB control and intensified use of existing TB control tools [3, 4].

TB differs from other infectious diseases in several ways that are likely to influence apparent spatial clustering. For example, its long latency and prolonged infectious period allow for significant population mobility between serial cases [5]. Thus, *Mtb* infection acquired in a given location may progress to TB disease in an entirely different region, such that clustering of cases may not necessarily indicate intense transmission but could rather reflect aggregation of population groups at higher risk of disease, such as migrants [6]. Similarly, *Mtb* infection acquired from workplaces and other congregate settings can be wrongly attributed to residential exposure, as only an individual's residence information is typically recorded on TB surveillance documents in many settings [7, 8].

Identifying heterogeneity in the spatial distribution of TB cases and characterising its drivers can help to inform targeted public health responses, making it an attractive approach [9]. However, there are practical challenges in appropriate interpretation of spatial clusters of TB. Of particular importance is that the observed spatial pattern of TB may be affected by factors other than genuine TB transmission or reactivation, including the type and resolution of data and the spatial analysis methods used [10]. For instance, use of incidence data versus notification data could give considerably different spatial pattern [11], as the latter misses a large number of TB cases and could be skewed towards areas with better access to health care in high-burden settings [12, 13]. Thus, spatial analysis using notification data alone in such settings could result in misleading conclusions.

Similarly, the type of model used and the spatial unit of data analysis are important determinants of the patterns identified and their associations [14–16]. That is, different spatial resolutions could lead to markedly different results for the same dataset regardless of the true extent of spatial correlation [15, 17, 18] and the effect observed at a regional level may not hold at the individual level (an effect known as the ecological fallacy) [19]. Therefore, we aimed to review methodological approaches used in the spatial analysis of TB burden. We also considered how common issues in data interpretation were managed, including sparse data, false-positive identification of clustering and undetected cases.

Methods

Data source and search strategy

Our search strategy aimed to identify peer-reviewed studies of the distribution and determinants of TB that employed spatial analysis methods. In this review, studies were considered spatial if they incorporated any spatial approaches (e.g. geocoding, spatial analysis units, cluster detection methods, spatial risk modelling) into the design and analysis of the distribution, determinants and outcomes of TB [20]. We searched Medline, Embase, Web of Science, Scopus and PsycInfo databases from their inception to 15 February 2017 using a combination of keywords and medical subject headings (MeSH) pertaining to our two central concepts: tuberculosis and space. We refined search terms related to the latter concept after reviewing key studies, including a previous systematic review not limited to TB [21]. The full search strategy was adapted to the syntax of the individual database from the following conceptual structure: (tuberculosis OR multidrug-resistant tuberculosis) AND (spatial analysis OR geographic mapping OR spatial regression OR spatiotemporal analysis OR spatial autocorrelation analysis OR geography OR geographic distribution OR geographic information system OR geographically weighted regression OR space-time clustering OR 'spati*' OR 'hotspots' OR cluster analysis) and is provided in the Appendix. Studies targeted to special populations (e.g. homeless, migrants, HIV-infected persons) and that considered the entire population of a region were permitted. Additional papers were also identified through hand searching the bibliographies of retrieved articles and from suggestions from experts in the field.

Eligibility, and inclusion and exclusion criteria

We included peer-reviewed papers that incorporated the spatial analysis approaches described above in the study of TB. After exclusion of duplicates, titles and abstracts were screened by two researchers (DS and MK) to identify potentially eligible studies. Of these papers, articles were excluded hierarchically on the basis of article type, whether the method used could be considered spatial or not and the outcomes assessed. No exclusions were made on the basis of the outcome reported, with studies that considered incidence, prevalence or any TB-related health outcome included. Studies were excluded if the language of the publication was not English, the report was a letter, conference abstract or a review or only reported the temporal (trend) of TB. Spatial studies of non-tuberculous mycobacteria, non-human diseases and population immunological profiles were also excluded. Full-text articles were excluded if they did not provide sufficient information on the spatial analysis techniques employed. There were no exclusions based on study setting or anatomical site of disease.

Data extraction and synthesis

Three independent reviewers (DS, MK, KAA) performed data extraction using pretested data extraction forms and stored these in a Microsoft Excel 2016 spreadsheet (Microsoft Corporation, Redmond, Washington, USA). Disagreements were resolved by consensus. The following information was extracted from each paper: country, publication year, study aim, data type (notifications or survey), type of TB disease (smear-positive pulmonary, smear-negative pulmonary and extrapulmonary), geographic level, spatial methods (map types, cluster detection methods, statistical regression methods, spatial lag, spatial error, spatial smoothing techniques), time scale and outcomes reported (whether quantification of TB cases or TB-related health outcomes, such as mortality, default from care, disability-adjusted life years (DALYs) and key conclusions). In studies which combined geospatial methods with genotypic clustering methods, we also extracted the genotypic cluster identification methods. Spatial analysis techniques were categorised as either visualisation (mapping), exploration (using statistical tests to identify spatial clusters) or statistical modelling [19, 22]. Counts and proportions were primarily used to summarise study findings. The protocol for this systematic review was prospectively registered with PROSPERO (CRD42016036655). Although we adhered to our original published protocol, here we additionally describe the importance of genotypic methods and the application of spatial methods in informing public health interventions in response to requests during peer review.

Results

Study characteristics

A total of 2350 records were identified from the electronic searches, of which 252 full-text articles were assessed. Of these, 168 articles met all inclusion criteria and were included in the final narrative synthesis (Fig. 1). Using a cutoff of 100 TB cases per 100,000 population in reported incidence in 2016, 111 (66%) of the studies were from low-incidence settings.

All references returned by the search strategy were from the period 1982 to 2017, with 71% published from 2010 onwards (Additional file 1: Figure S1). Earlier studies (predominantly in the 1980s and 1990s) tended to be descriptive visualisations, while studies in the last two decades frequently incorporated cluster detection and risk prediction. More recently, a range of statistical techniques including Bayesian statistical approaches and geographically weighted regression have become increasingly popular.

Key objectives of included studies

Spatial analysis was applied to address a range of objectives (Table 1), with the commonest ones including description of the distribution ($n = 135$), statistical analysis of spatial clustering ($n = 73$) and analysis of risk factors and risk prediction ($n = 64$). Spatial methods were also used to determine the relative importance of transmission by comparison to reactivation as a driver of TB incidence ($n = 25$), the effect of TB interventions ($n = 2$), barriers to TB service uptake ($n = 2$), spatial distribution of TB-related health outcomes (mortality, default, hospitalisation) ($n = 5$), spatial pattern of TB incidence among people living with HIV (PLHIV) ($n = 4$), HIV-related TB mortality ($n = 4$), multidrug-resistant TB (MDR-TB) drivers ($n = 1$), TB outbreak detection ($n = 3$) and drivers of spatial clustering (including the role of congregate settings, such as social drinking venues and schools) ($n = 30$).

Types of TB disease analysed

Spatial analysis was most commonly conducted on data for all types of TB (i.e. without distinction between pulmonary or extrapulmonary; $n = 121$), followed by pulmonary TB only ($n = 28$) and smear-positive pulmonary TB only ($n = 13$). Spatial analysis of multidrug-resistant TB (MDR-TB) and extensively drug-resistant TB (XDR-TB) was reported in 15 studies and one study respectively.

Data used and scale of analysis

Nearly all studies used retrospective TB program data (notifications), with the exception of five studies that used prevalence surveys and two prospectively collected data. None of the studies using notification data accounted for undetected/unreported cases. In all included studies, spatial analysis of TB was based on the individual's residence, except for three studies that explored the effect of exposure from social gathering sites.

Spatial analysis was generally done using data aggregated over administrative spatial units ($n = 131$), but the scale of aggregation differed markedly. Common spatial scales included census tract ($n = 20$), district ($n = 15$), postal code ($n = 15$), county ($n = 15$), neighbourhood ($n = 10$), health area ($n = 7$), municipality ($n = 11$), state ($n = 7$), province ($n = 6$), local government area (LGA) ($n = 4$) and ward ($n = 4$). Data were analysed at the individual level in 37 studies, while three studies were reported at a continent and country scale.

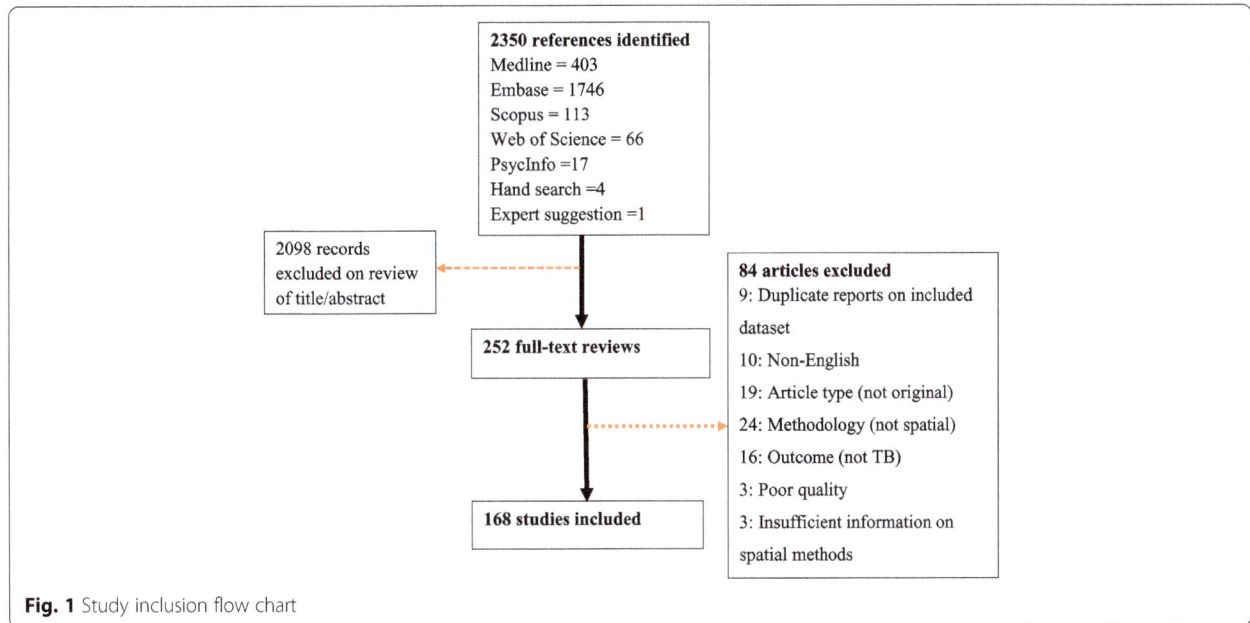

Fig. 1 Study inclusion flow chart

Table 1 Application areas of spatial methods in TB studies

Spatial method application areas	Methods used	References
Spatial TB distribution or spatial clustering	Dot maps, rate maps, thematic maps, Moran's *I*, GetisOrd statistic, NNI Besag and Newel statistic, *k*-functions, spatial scan statistic	[1, 2, 7, 8, 12, 16, 23–41, 44–49, 51–54, 57–72, 75, 93–95, 99, 100, 102–176]
Risk factors	Bayesian CAR models, regression models (with or without including spatial terms), GWR, PCA, mixture models, spatial lag models	[8, 12, 33, 36, 38, 40, 42–44, 46–52, 58, 59, 62, 70, 71, 93, 94, 99–102, 104, 111, 112, 116, 117, 120, 123, 125, 127–129, 131, 136, 137, 141–143, 145, 148, 149, 156, 161, 164, 176–189]
Monitoring spatiotemporal TB trends	Temporal trend maps	[27, 36–39]
Intervention evaluation	Distance map, kernel density map	[73, 74]
Barriers to TB care	Rate map, dot map, travel time map, distance map	[12, 187]
TB program performance	Map (time to detection)	[184]
HIV-related TB incidence	Rate map, dot map, spatial scan statistic	[40, 166, 186, 190]
TB treatment outcomes	Spatial empirical Bayes smoothing, kernel density maps, spatial scan statistic, spatial regression	[152, 155, 179, 183, 191]
Mortality related to TB/HIV coinfection	Rate map, thematic maps, Moran's *I* and spatial regression	[42, 43, 174, 192]
Transmission	Dot maps (congregate settings)	[54, 55, 193]
	Dot maps (cases)	[7, 8]
	Geospatial and genotypic clustering methods	[1, 2, 25, 28, 47, 57, 59–72, 93–95, 169, 194]
Methodological	Spatial scan statistic	[25]
TB outbreak detection	Spatial scan statistic	[1, 25, 28]
Prevalence estimation	Model-based geostatistics	[80]
Drivers of MDR-TB	*k*-function	[35]

NNI nearest neighbourhood index, *CAR models* conditional autoregressive models, *GWR* geographically weighted regression, *PCA* principal component analysis, *HIV* human immunodeficiency virus, *MDR-TB* multidrug-resistant TB

Methods in the spatial analysis of TB

Table 2 shows the range of spatial methods used. Spatial analysis was used to visualise patterns ($n = 154$), explore spatial clusters ($n = 73$) and identify risk factors for clustering ($n = 64$), with risk prediction undertaken by 11 studies. Of the included studies, six did not explicitly report any of these methods but reported statistical results that implied the use of these methods.

Data visualisation

Data visualisation was the most consistently applied technique, with 154 of the studies using at least one data visualisation method to present TB distribution and/or risk factor patterns across space (Table 1). The TB incidence rate was the commonest indicator mapped ($n = 63$), followed by event maps ($n = 37$), which were smoothed using kernel density in seven studies. Data visualisation was based on standardised morbidity ratios

(SMR) in 12 studies. Five studies reported maps of trends in TB incidence over time, and thematic maps were used in nine to consider the impact of risk factors on TB incidence by displaying the spatial distribution of other variables. Variables plotted included climate ($n = 1$), socioeconomic factors ($n = 5$), diabetes ($n = 1$) and obesity ($n = 1$).

Approaches used to account for data sparseness

TB is a relatively rare disease at the population level, and burden is typically expressed in terms of cases per 100,000 population. Various approaches were used to account for this sparseness in the number of cases, such as aggregating cases over administrative geographic levels and over time periods (ranging from 1 to 25 years).

An alternative approach was rate smoothing, although this practice was rare, despite the fact that TB rates were the commonest indicators mapped. In the included

Table 2 Spatial methods used in spatial analysis of tuberculosis ($n = 168$)

Method category	Method	Number	References
Visualisation	Rate map	63	[12, 16, 23, 26, 27, 29–34, 37, 41, 44–46, 48, 51, 52, 57, 58, 60, 61, 70, 100, 102, 103, 105, 106, 120, 123–146, 164, 165, 170, 173–176, 195, 196]
	Dot map	37	[2, 7, 8, 35, 40, 47, 53, 54, 59, 66, 67, 72, 73, 75, 95, 107–122, 158, 166, 169, 178, 191, 197]
	SMR map	12	[38, 49, 99, 100, 124, 126, 127, 129, 138, 142, 148, 149]
	Kernel density map	7	[35, 37, 62, 93, 120, 147, 171]
	Case counts maps	3	[108, 167, 172]
	Others*	17	[16, 24, 50, 60, 62, 63, 68, 71, 99, 100, 103, 104, 116, 148, 166, 168, 185, 198]
Spatial cluster analysis	Global Moran's I	28	[16, 26, 34, 37, 39, 44, 48, 49, 51, 58, 65, 93, 100, 102, 123, 126, 128, 131, 133, 135, 138, 139, 145, 150, 161, 180, 188, 199]
	Local Moran's I	14	[16, 41, 44, 49, 51, 93, 100, 123, 126, 131, 135, 138, 145, 192]
	Kulldorff's spatial scan statistic	43	[1, 2, 23–32, 40, 57, 63, 64, 70, 71, 94, 109–111, 119, 120, 130, 135, 138, 139, 141, 151–160, 163, 164, 166, 191]
	GetisOrd statistic	12	[2, 16, 26, 39, 49, 54, 65, 93, 104, 131, 139, 161]
	k-NN	8	[35, 53, 69, 72, 93, 114, 122, 163]
	k-function	6	[35, 62, 93, 116, 117, 147]
	Besag and Newell statistic	2	[125, 145]
Statistical modelling	Bayesian CAR models	7	[38, 44, 49, 99, 101, 127, 148]
	Geographically weighted regression	6	[16, 50, 93, 102–104]
	Mixture modelling	2	[142, 149]
	Conventional logistic	15	[8, 40, 70, 71, 94, 95, 111, 112, 120, 141, 161, 177, 178, 187, 189]
	Conventional Poisson	5	[46, 125, 136, 145, 156]
	Conventional linear	5	[12, 47, 129, 137, 176]
	Negative binomial	1	[164]
	Factor analysis	6	[50, 103, 117, 143, 146, 170]
	Regression models with spatial terms	9	[42, 48, 51, 58, 100, 116, 128, 131, 188]
	Spatial prediction	11	[38, 42, 43, 62, 80, 99, 101, 127, 131, 148, 181]

SMR standardised morbidity ratio, *k-NN* k-nearest neighbourhood test, *CAR* conditional autoregressive
*Includes maps of disability-adjusted life years (DALYs), survival time, factor scores, probability maps, proportion of cases and regression coefficients

studies, smoothed rates were used in six (4%) studies. Similarly, of 12 studies that analysed SMRs, smoothed SMRs were presented in seven. In the included studies, several different data smoothing techniques were used, including fully Bayesian ($n = 8$), empirical Bayes ($n = 4$) and spatial empirical Bayes ($n = 5$). A significant number of visualisation reports ($n = 30$) were not complemented by hypothesis testing, either by exploration methods or modelling approaches. In 12 studies (7%), maps were not presented, but a narrative description of TB burden or a tabular presentation of TB distribution by administrative unit was described.

Spatial cluster (hotspot) identification

Use of at least one spatial cluster identification method was reported in 73 (43%) studies, with Kulldorff's spatial scan statistic used most frequently ($n = 43$), followed by Local Moran test ($n = 14$) and Getis and Ord's local Gi(d) statistic ($n = 12$). Nearest neighbour index (NNI), k-function and Besag and Newell methods were reported in eight, six and two studies respectively (Table 1). The presence of overall area-wide heterogeneity was assessed most often using global Moran I ($n = 28$). In three studies, no globally significant spatial autocorrelation was seen, although there was spatial clustering locally. Although studies used data aggregated over various spatial scales, only one evaluated the impact of spatial scale on the hotspot detection performance of the spatial scan statistic. Use of individual address-level data improved

the sensitivity of the spatial scan statistic compared to data aggregated at the administrative level.

Simultaneous use of two spatial cluster detection methods was reported in 11 studies and showed differences in hotspot identification that ranged from complete disagreement to some degree of similarity (Table 3).

False-positive clustering

Not all spatial clusters are true clusters. False-positive clusters can arise from various sources, including data and methods used, and unmeasured confounding. Given that notification data were by far the most commonly used data source in the spatial analyses reviewed here, it could not be determined if these clusters represented true clusters of tuberculosis incidence or if they were caused by factors such as pockets of improved case detection. The role of differential TB detection has been documented in some studies from low-income settings, where increased spatial TB burden was linked to improved health care access [12].

In addition, rate was the commonest disease indicator used for disease mapping, as well as cluster detection in this study. As described earlier, rates are liable to stochasticity and can lead to false-positive clustering. However, rate smoothing and stability (sensitivity) analysis of clusters identified using rates was done in only a few studies [23, 24]. This remains an important area of consideration in the future spatial analysis of TB.

Table 3 Comparisons of spatial clusters from multiple cluster identification methods

Author, year	Methods	Outcome	Conclusion
Alene, K, 2017 [49]	Local Moran's I Getis and Ord	Clustered Clustered	50% similarity (two non-significant clusters identified by LISA)
Álvarez-Hernández, G., et al. 2010 [145]	Local Moran's I Besag and Newell	No significant Clustered	Widely conflicting
Dangisso M, et al. 2015 [26]	Getis and Ord Spatial scan statistic	Clustered Clustered	Similar overall pattern, but marked differences by years
Feske, M., et al. 2011 [93, 178]	Getis and Ord GWR residuals	Clustered Heterogeneous	Similar overall pattern, but some local differences
Ge E, et al. 2016 [139]	Getis and Ord Spatial scan statistic	Clustered Clustered	Similar overall pattern, but differences in some locations and across time
Haase I, et al. 2007 [2]	Hotspot analysis SaTScan	Clustered Clustered	Similar overall pattern, but some local differences
Hassarangsee S, et al. 2015 [138]	LISA Spatial scan statistic	Clustered Clustered	Very similar, but not identical
Li L, et al. 2016 [135]	LISA Spatial scan statistic	No significant cluster, Clustered	Widely conflicting
Maceiel ELN, et al. 2010 [131]	LISA, Getis and Ord Model prediction	Clustered Heterogeneous	Widely conflicting
Wubuli A, et al. 2015 [16]	LISA Getis and Ord	Clustered Clustered	Similar overall pattern, but some local differences
Wang T, et al 2016 [102]	Spatial scan statistic Getis and Ord	Clustered Clustered	Similar overall pattern, but some local differences

GWR geographically weighted regression; *LISA* local indicators of spatial association

Spatiotemporal analysis
Temporal scale
In the spatial analysis of TB, the time window is an important dimension that influences the spatial pattern of TB [25]. As TB is relatively a rare disease at the population level and has a long incubation period, detection of apparent spatial clusters requires a longer time scale than for acute infectious diseases that may form spatial clusters within days of the start of outbreak. Because of this, the included studies were based on cases that accumulated over considerable time periods, ranging from 1 to 25 years, with use of data aggregated over 5 years being the most frequent practice (20%).

Approaches
Generally, two approaches were used in the space-time cluster analysis of TB. The first uses classical space-time clustering using algorithms which scan space over a changing time window, such as Kulldorff's spatial scan statistic [23, 25–29]. The second approach is to account for the temporal dimension by repeating the spatial analysis for each time unit [26, 30–35]. In some studies, spatial patterns in temporal trends of TB incidence were determined as increasing or decreasing [27, 36–39].

Spatial statistical modelling
Different statistical modelling approaches were used to describe the relationship between TB and ecological factors in 65 (39%) studies, including nine spatially explicit models using Bayesian approaches. Conditional autoregressive (CAR) models were used in nine models to account for spatial correlation. Classical regression models were used in 33, while non-Bayesian spatial regression models were reported in 12.

Of the regression models that evaluated the effect on model fit of including spatial structure (spatial error or spatial lag), the inclusion of spatial structure improved the performance of the model in seven studies and failed to do so in two (based on deviance information criteria). Spatial lag was explicitly modelled in seven studies and highlighted the significant influence of neighbouring locations on TB distribution.

Traditional models including a Bayesian approach assumed a stationary relationship between TB and its spatial covariates and hence imposed a single (global) regression model on the entire study area. Only six studies used a geographically weighted regression (a local regression model) to accommodate variation in the association between TB and its risk factors from place to place and showed spatially varying (non-stationary) effects (n = 6). Other models used included mixture modelling (n = 2) and factor analysis using principal component analysis (PCA) (n = 4).

Results from spatial analysis
Geographic distribution of TB
The geographic distribution of TB was heterogeneous in all included studies both from low- and high-incidence settings, although no formal hypothesis testing was presented in 55 (33%). An exception was one study from South Africa that reported no significant clustering of cases among HIV patients on ART [40]. Spatial analysis was also used to describe the drivers of drug-resistant tuberculosis, with tighter spatial aggregation of MDR-TB cases compared with non-MDR cases taken as evidence of transmission of MDR-TB [41].

Spatial analyses into both HIV and TB investigated outcomes including HIV-associated TB incidence (n = 4) and spatial patterns of TB/HIV-related mortality (n = 4). All such studies revealed significant spatial heterogeneity. TB/HIV-related mortality in children was linked to areas with low socio-economic status and maternal deaths [42, 43].

Spatial methods used to study the impact of community-based TB treatment showed marked improvement in access compared to health facility-based treatment approaches (n = 1), and similar studies demonstrated travel time and distance to be important barriers to TB control (n = 2).

Correlations with social and environmental factors
The observed spatial patterns of TB were consistently linked to areas with poverty (n = 14), overcrowding and non-standard housing (n = 9), ethnic minority populations (n = 3), population density (n = 2), low education status (n = 2), health care access (n = 3) and immigrant populations (n = 5). However, a minority of studies have also found conflicting or non-significant associations between TB and poverty [44–46], population density [47–49] and unemployment [45, 47].

Four studies (including three from China) examined the correlation of climatic factors with TB incidence, with conflicting results. Two province-level studies in China using data from different time periods found TB burden to be associated with increasing annual average temperature [33, 50], although correlation with humidity was conflicting. Positive associations were observed with average precipitation [33, 50] and with air pressure [33] in these studies, while inverse associations were observed with sun exposure [50] and with wind speed [33]. In contrast, a county-level study which used average monthly climate data within a single province of China found the reverse, with temperature, precipitation, wind speed and sunshine exposure showing associations in the opposite direction [51]. A study that compared TB incidence between regions with different climatic conditions showed higher incidence at dry regions and low incidence in humid regions [52].

Space-time analysis to detect TB outbreaks

Studies reporting the application of the spatial methods in the early identification of TB outbreak were uncommon. Space-time TB studies using retrospective surveillance data in the USA found that the spatial scan statistic and other methods could effectively detect outbreaks months before local public authorities became aware of the problem [25, 28]. However, as space-time clusters of TB can be due to either ongoing transmission or reactivation, characterising the drivers that resulted in the spatial clustering is essential. Findings from studies which compared the timeliness and accuracy of space-time clusters in identifying TB outbreaks varied with spatial resolution and the background population, with two studies from the USA detecting ongoing outbreaks [25, 28], in contrast to false alarms due to reactivation TB among immigrants in a study from Canada [1].

Spatial analysis of the source of TB infection

Spatial methods were also used to determine the role of households and congregate settings (e.g. social gathering venues, schools) on TB transmission risk (Table 1). The role of the household was determined by cross-referencing child and adolescent TB infection or disease with adult TB in two studies [7, 8]. In these studies, the importance of household exposure declined with the age of the child, such that TB disease or infection was related to residential exposure to adult TB in younger children but not adolescents.

Congregate settings, which pose increased transmission risk, were identified using multiple techniques that included linking TB cases to social gathering places [53] and mapping the distribution of rebreathed air volume (RAV) [54] (including grading these settings based on TB transmission principles [55]). These approaches identified schools and social gathering sites as high-risk areas.

Identifying local drivers

Recent transmission is a critical mechanism driving local TB epidemiology in high-burden settings, while reactivation of remotely acquired infection is thought to predominate in most low-endemic settings [4, 56]. Geospatial clusters may reflect increased disease risk due to geographic proximity, which may correspond to recent transmission, or reactivation of latent TB infection in an aggregate of individuals infected elsewhere or both [57]. In the reviewed studies, spatial methods coupled with other methods were used to identify which of these two mechanisms drives local TB epidemiology in the following three ways.

Combining spatial clusters with cohort clustering: TB clustering can occur from ongoing transmission or from reactivation of latent infection among high-risk subgroups due to shared characteristics such as similar country of birth rather than a shared transmission network, a phenomenon known as cohort clustering. Cohort cluster analysis is used to identify selected high-risk population subgroups for targeted interventions based on the relative TB incidence they bear. The Lorenz curve is a simple visualisation tool that compares the clustering (inequality) in the subgroup of interest across regions and over time. One study, which combined such cohort (birth country) cluster analysis using the Lorenz curve of inequality with spatial cluster analysis [31] revealed colocation of these cluster types, suggesting the presence of both transmission and reactivation. Spatial clusters among foreign-born persons covered too large an area compared to clusters among the locally born to be consistent with direct person-to-person transmission. In addition, spatial modelling was also applied to differentiate the role of transmission from reactivation by assessing spatial dependence. The presence of spatial dependence (autocorrelation) was taken to indicate transmission, while its absence was considered to indicate reactivation [58].

Combining spatial and genotype clustering: Genotypic clustering of TB may be used as a proxy for recent transmission, such that geospatial clusters in which cases are genotypically clustered may be taken as stronger evidence for locations where recent transmission has occurred. These approaches were combined to quantify the role of recent transmission and determine geographical locations of such transmission in 25 studies. This was done either by determining the spatial distribution of genotypic clusters [25, 28, 59–69] or by assessing the genotypic similarity of cases contained within geospatial clusters [2, 57, 65, 70, 71].

The findings from these studies varied considerably by the country and sub-population studied (locally born versus immigrants) (Table 4). Genotypic clusters were spatially clustered in many studies, providing evidence of recent local transmission. In some studies, cases in geospatial clusters were less likely to be dominated by genotypically similar cases (i.e. were dominated by unique strains) than cases outside the geospatial clusters, implying spatial aggregation of reactivation TB [57]. This finding highlights that geospatial hotspots in low TB incidence settings are not necessarily areas of recent transmission and spatial clustering may be primarily mediated by social determinants, such as migration, HIV and drug abuse [57].

Table 4 Overlap between spatial and molecular clustering

Authors	Country	Genotyping methods	Findings
Bishai WR, et al. 1998 [95]	USA	IS6110-RFLP and PGRS	Genotypic clusters with epidemiologic links were spatially clustered but 76% of DNA clustered cases lack epidemiologic links.
Mathema B, et al. 2002 [169]	USA	IS6110-RFLP and spoligotyping	Genotypic clusters showed spatial aggregation
Richardson M, et al. 2002 [72]	South Africa	IS6110-RFLP and spoligotyping	Spatial aggregation of genotypic clusters was limited
Nguyen D, et al. 2003 [69]	Canada	IS6110-RFLP and spoligotyping	Genotypically similar cases were not more spatially clustered than genotypically unique cases
Moonan P, et al. 2004 [61]	USA	IS6110-RFLP and spoligotyping	Genotypic clusters were spatially heterogeneous
Jacobson L, et al. 2005 [59]	Mexico	IS6110-RFLP and spoligotyping	Spatial patterns were similar for both cases categorised as reactivation or recent transmission
Haase I, et al. 2007 [2]	Canada	IS6110-RFLP and spoligotyping	In spatial TB clusters of immigrants, there was significant genotype similarity
Higgs B, et al. 2007 [25]	USA	IS6110-RFLP and PGRS	Space-time clusters contained genotypic clusters
Feske ML, et al. 2011 [93, 178]	USA	IS6110-RFLP and spoligotyping	Genotypically clustered cases were randomly distributed across space
Evans JT, et al. 2011 [66]	UK	Spoligotyping and MIRU-VNTR	Genotypic clusters showed spatial aggregation
Nava-Aguilera E, et al. 2011 [67]	Mexico	Spoligotyping	Genotypic clusters were not spatially aggregated
Prussing C, et al. 2013 [57]	USA	Spoligotyping and 12- MIRU-VNTR	Cases in geospatial clusters were equally or less likely to share similar genotypes than cases outside geospatial clusters
Tuite AR, et al. 2013 [94]	Canada	Spoligotyping and 24-MIRU-VNTR	The proportion of cases in genotypic clusters was five times that seen in spatial clusters (23% vs 5%)
Kammerer JS, et al. 2013 [28]	USA	Spoligotyping and 12-MIRU-VNTR	Genotypically similar cases were spatially clustered
Verma A, et al. 2014 [1]	Canada	IS6110-RFLP and Spoligotyping	Space-time clusters contained few or no genotypically similar cases
Izumi K, et al. 2015 [65]	Japan	IS6110-RFLP	Both genotypically similar and unique strains formed spatial hotspots
Chamie G, et al. 2015 [194]	Uganda	Spoligotyping	Genotypic clusters shared social gathering sites (clinic, place of worship, market or bar)
Chan-Yeung M, et al. 2005 [47]	Hong Kong	IS6110-RFLP	Spatial locations of genotypic clusters and unique cases did not differ by their sociodemographic characteristics
Gurjav U, et al. 2016 [70]	Australia	24-MIRU-VNTR	Spatial hotspots were characterised by a high proportion of unique strains; less than 4% of cases in spatial clusters were genotypically similar
Ribeiro FK, et al. 2016 [62]	Brazil	IS6110-RFLP and Spoligotyping	Genotypic clusters were spatially clustered
Saavedra-Campos M, et al. 2016 [71]	England	24-MIRU-VNTR	10% of cases clustered spatially and genotypically
Seraphin MN, et al. 2016 [64]	USA	Spoligotyping and 24-MIRU-VNTR	22% of cases among USA-born and 5% among foreign-born clustered spatially and genotypically
Yuen CM, et al. 2016 [68]	USA	Spoligotyping and 24-MIRU-VNTR	Genotype clustered cases were spatially heterogeneous
Yeboah-Manu D, et al. 2016 [63]	Ghana	IS6110 and rpoB PCR	Genotypic clusters showed spatial aggregation
Zelner J, et al. 2016 [60]	Peru	24-MIRU-VNTR	Genotypic clusters showed spatial aggregation

PGRS polymorphic GC-rich repetitive sequence

Combinations of multiple methods were typically used for genotyping, with the commonest being IS6110 restriction fragment length polymorphism (IS6110-RFLP) and spoligotyping ($n = 9$), followed by mycobacterial interspersed repetitive unit variable number tandem repeat (MIRU-VNTR) and spoligotyping ($n = 5$), although use of a single method was reported in six studies (Table 4). No identified studies reported use of whole genome sequencing.

Temporal distribution of genotypically clustered cases

The temporal pattern of genotypic clustering could provide insights to distinguish between transmission and reactivation. In some studies, the temporal distribution of genotypically clustered cases indicated periods of 1 to more than 8 years between the genotypically clustered cases [1, 72], implying reactivation TB could also show genotypic similarity.

Use of spatial methods to inform public health interventions

In addition to their use in characterising the spatial distribution and determinants of TB, spatial methods have been used to inform TB-related public health interventions. In these studies, spatial analysis methods have proved to be attractive in guiding public health interventions, although their application to TB care beyond research is not well documented. For instance, spatial analysis techniques have been used to identify locations with a high density of TB cases (termed hotspots, although this definition was not based on spatial statistical tests). Community screening was then conducted in these areas, and its yield was compared to that from routine service provision. This GIS-guided screening was found to considerably improve the detection of individuals with latent TB infection and other infectious diseases [73]. Similarly, a study from South Africa highlighted the potential for using GIS to promote community-based DOTS by locating and geographically linking TB patients to their nearest supervision sites, although programmatic implementation of this approach was not reported [74].

The potential for spatial methods to be used for the early detection of TB outbreaks has also been described, although the findings widely varied based on the background population [1, 28]. Spatial cluster analysis using data at higher geographic resolutions improves the method's performance in cluster detection [25].

Discussion

While a range of methodologies has been employed in divergent contexts, we found that essentially all geospatial studies of TB have demonstrated significant heterogeneity in spatial distribution. Spatial analysis was applied to improve understanding of a range of TB-related issues, including the distribution and determinants of TB, the mechanisms driving the local TB epidemiology, the effect of interventions and the barriers to TB service uptake. Recently, geospatial methods have been combined with genotypic clustering techniques to understand the drivers of local TB epidemiology, although most such studies remain limited to low-endemic settings.

In almost all reviewed studies, retrospective program data (notifications) were used. Notification data, especially from resource-scarce settings, suffer from the often large proportion of undetected cases and are heavily dependent on the availability of diagnostic facilities [12]. None of the spatial studies of TB that used notification data accounted for undetected cases, such that patterns in the spatial distribution and clustering could be heavily influenced by case detection performance [11]. Hence, distinguishing the true incidence pattern

from the detection pattern has rarely been undertaken, despite its importance in interpretation.

The problems of undetected cases could be compounded in the spatial analysis of drug-resistant forms of TB, especially in resource-scarce settings where testing for drug-resistant TB is often additionally conditional on the individual's risk factors for drug resistance [75]. However, recently, there have been some attempts to account for under-detection in the spatial analysis of TB. A Bayesian geospatial modelling approach presented a framework to estimate TB incidence and case detection rate for any spatial unit and identified previously unreported spatial areas of high burden [11]. Another approach is to estimate incidence using methods such as capture-recapture [76, 77] and mathematical modelling [78]. If case detection rate is truly known for a defined region, incidence can be calculated as notifications divided by case detection rate, although this is rarely if ever the case. Spatial analysis using prevalence data could also be considered in areas where such data are available.

In relation to the data problems outlined above, spatial analysis of TB could benefit from the use of model-based geostatistics, which is commonly used in other infectious diseases [79], although there are few studies that consider *Mtb* [80]. In particular, measurement of TB prevalence is impractical to perform at multiple locations due to logistic reasons. Therefore, model-based geostatistics can be used to predict disease prevalence in areas that have not been sampled from prevalence values at nearby locations at low or no cost, producing smooth continuous surface estimates.

Mapping of notification rates was the most commonly used data visualisation technique, in which TB cases were categorised at a particular administrative spatial level. This approach has the advantage of easy interpretability, although it can introduce bias because the size of the regions and the locations of their boundaries typically reflect administrative requirements, which may not reflect the spatial distribution of epidemiological factors [19, 22]. In addition, patterns observed across regions may depend on the spatial scale chosen, an effect known as the modifiable areal unit problem (MAUP) [17]. Because the choice of spatial scale mainly depends on the limitations of available data [81], only one study was able to provide a systematic evaluation of the effect of scale on spatial patterns, demonstrating improved performance of Kulldorff's spatial scan statistic method at a high geographic resolution [25]. Different spatial resolutions could lead to markedly different results for the same dataset regardless of the true extent of correlation, due to averaging (aggregation effect) or other spatial processes operating at different scales

[15, 17, 18]. Assessing the presence of this effect should be a priority for future studies using aggregated data in spatial TB studies.

Bayesian smoothing techniques can mitigate the problems of stochastically unstable rates from areas with small population [81], although such techniques were not widely used in the included studies and so false spatial clustering remains an important consideration. The less frequent use of rate smoothing techniques in the spatial analysis of TB could have various explanations, including lack of software packages that are easily accessible to the wider user (although GeoDa spatial software currently provides an accessible platform to people with limited statistical or mathematical backgrounds [82]). It may also be that most spatial analyses of TB are based on data aggregated over larger geographic areas from several years, such that the problem of statistical stochasticity may not be a major problem, although this was not explicitly discussed in the included studies.

In all studies that applied spatial cluster identification tools, TB cases were clustered irrespective of whether the setting was low or high endemic. However, in studies that incorporated more than one cluster identification method, areas identified as hotspots were not identical, with the extent of agreement between the alternative methods highly variable. This could be partly attributable to different methods testing separate hypotheses, such that these results may correctly support one hypothesis while refuting another. However, there is no consensus on how to interpret these findings appropriately and consistently [82, 83], and method selection did not typically appear to be based on such considerations [84, 85]. Thus, caution is required when considering interventions assessing clusters with one method only, as is frequently undertaken in TB spatial analysis [22].

Use of multiple cluster detection methods and requiring their overlap to represent a truly high-risk area is increasingly recommended [82, 84, 86]. However, this approach could also increase the risk of false-positive spatial clustering when different methods are used serially until significant clusters are observed [85]. Sensitivity analysis of spatial clustering [87, 88] and cluster validation using geostatistical simulations [23, 89, 90] can help identify robust clusters. While methods that adjust for confounding are generally preferred [91], further investigative strategies including data collection and cluster surveillance are required to validate an observed spatial cluster before introducing interventions [84, 85]. Although the focus of this study is TB, several methodological considerations outlined here would remain true for many infectious diseases.

In several studies, presence of spatial clustering or spatial autocorrelation in TB distribution was considered to reflect ongoing TB transmission, while its absence was taken to indicate reactivation [58]. Recently, molecular techniques have been combined with geospatial methods to understand the drivers of local TB epidemiology, although findings from these studies vary by country and the subset of the population studied. While spatial clustering of genotypically related cases was reported in several studies and likely reflected intense local TB transmission [61, 65], spatial clusters were dominated by genotypically unique strains in some studies, implying that reactivation was the dominant process [47, 72]. Hence, the combination of genotypic and geospatial techniques can improve understanding of the relative contribution of reactivation and transmission and other local contributors to burden.

Notwithstanding the general principles outlined above, not all spatial clusters of genotypically related cases will necessarily result from recent transmission, as simultaneous reactivation of remotely acquired infection and limited genetic variation in the pathogen population can also lead to genotypic similarity of spatially clustered cases [2, 92]. In some studies, the time between the first and last diagnosis of the cases in the genetic cluster ranged from 1 to more than 8 years [1, 72], suggesting that genotypic clustering could occur from spatially clustered reactivation. Similarly, limited spatial aggregation of genotypically clustered cases [72, 93, 94] and lack of epidemiological links between genotypically clustered cases in some studies may reflect migration of the human population over the extended time scale over which TB clusters occur [95], although casual transmission creating spatially diffuse clusters is an alternative explanation.

The extent of genotypic similarity between cases also depends on the discriminatory power of the genotyping method and the diversity of the pathogen population. Compared to whole genome sequencing, standard molecular genotyping (spoligotyping, MIRU-VNTR and IS6110) methods generally overestimate TB transmission with a false-positive clustering rate of 25 to 75% based on strain prevalence in the background population [92, 96]. The accuracy of these tests in distinguishing ongoing transmission from genetically closely related strains is very low among immigrants from high TB incidence settings with limited pathogen diversity [92, 97]. Thus, care should be taken when interpreting the genotypic similarity of cases among immigrant groups, as independent importation of closely related strains is possible. The frequent finding of more extensive genotypic than spatial clusters [71, 94] may reflect overestimation by the genotypic methods [98]. On the other hand, TB transmission might not result in apparent spatial clustering due to reasons that include population movement, poor surveillance and unmeasured confounding.

Regression models used for spatial analysis of TB were either conventional regression models or models that incorporated spatial effects. Although the former was more commonly employed, the majority of models incorporating spatial effects confirmed that accounting for spatial correlation improved model fit [11, 33, 44, 58, 99–101]. Conventional regression models assume spatial independence of model residuals and so ignore the potential presence of spatial autocorrelation, such that non-spatial models may lead to false conclusions regarding covariate effects.

The use of the conventional regression models described above may be appropriate for spatial analysis and spatial prediction, in the case that spatial dependence in residuals has been ruled out. Under this approach, the standard procedure is to start with classical ordinary least squares (OLS) regression models and then look for spatial dependence in the residuals, which implies the need for a spatially explicit regression model [82]. Several of the models reviewed here did not appear to adopt this approach, and so, caution is required when interpreting the findings from such analyses.

Most regression models treat the association between TB rates and ecological factors as global and are unable to capture local variation in the estimates of the association. However, geographically weighted regression (GWR) estimates coefficients for all spatial units included [22] and has often found the effect of risk factors on TB incidence to be spatially variable [16, 102–104], implying that global models may be inadequate to consider locally appropriate interventions. Few studies were able to perform explicit Bayesian spatial modelling incorporating information from nearby locations, thereby producing stable and robust estimates for areas with small populations and robust estimates of the effects of covariates [91].

While our review focused on methodological issues, several consistent observations were noted. Most importantly, all studies included in this review demonstrated that TB displayed a heterogeneous spatial pattern across various geographic resolutions. This reflects the underlying tendency for spatial dependence that can be caused by person-to-person transmission, socio-economic aggregation [49] and environmental effects [58, 93]. However, in nearly all included studies, spatial analyses of TB were based on the individual's residence, although considerable TB infection is acquired from workplaces and other social gathering sites [8, 54]. Such studies could wrongly attribute TB acquired from such sites to residential exposure, leading to resource misallocation.

Several models have shown significant associations between TB rates and demographic, socioeconomic and risk-factor variables, although it is difficult to rule out publication bias favouring studies with positive findings. However, associations observed between TB rates and different factors such as population density, unemployment and poverty at the population level varied across studies. These were recognised as important individual-level risk factors, highlighting the potential for ecological fallacy.

We did not perform individual study level analysis of bias in this review. Analyses in the reviewed studies involved counts and proportions across different spatial distributions, rather than comparisons across different treatment/exposure groups. Standard tools of bias analysis predominantly focus on different treatment groups within cohorts (absent from our included studies) and hence are not applicable to this review. We have however discussed many potential sources of bias in the studies included in our review.

Most of the reviewed studies were from high-income settings, which may either reflect publication bias or a focus of research efforts on such settings. In high-incidence settings, the more limited use of spatial analysis methods could reflect a lack of access to resources (e.g. georeferenced data and spatial software packages) or insufficient expertise in these settings. However, it is these high-transmission settings which stand to gain the most from an improved understanding of TB spatial patterns and also these settings in which geospatial clustering may be most important epidemiologically.

Conclusions

A range of spatial analysis methodologies have been employed in divergent contexts, with virtually all studies demonstrating significant heterogeneity in spatial TB distribution regardless of geographic resolution. Various spatial cluster detection methods are available, although there is no consensus on how to interpret the considerable inconsistencies in the outputs of these methods applied to the same dataset. Further studies are needed to determine the optimal method for each context and research question and should also account for unreported cases when using notifications as input data where possible. Combining genotypic and geospatial techniques with epidemiologically linkage of cases has the potential to improve understanding of TB transmission.

Appendix
Search strings
Search terms used in Embase, Medline, PsycInfo, Scopus and Web of Science
The exp refers to explode which means include all subheadings underneath spatial analysis. When exploded, it contains geographic mapping, spatial regression and spatiotemporal analysis.

Brackets () denote subject headings (MeSH in Medline and Emtree in Embase) terms highlighted by the database.

Medline and PsycInfo

1. (exp spatial analysis) OR (Geographic information systems) OR (Space-time clustering) OR geographic* analys*.mp OR spati*regres*.mp OR spat*temp*.mp OR spat* analys*.mp OR spat* temp* analys*.mp OR spat* temp* pattern*.mp OR geography* distribut*.mp OR spat* temp* distribut*.mp OR heterogen* distribut.mp OR spacetime cluster*mp OR space-time cluster*mp OR hotspot.mp Or hot spots. mp OR GIS OR spati*
2. (tuberculosis) OR (tuberculosis, multidrug resistant) OR TB.mp
3. 1 AND 2

Embase

1. (spatial analysis) OR (geographic mapping) OR (spatial regression) OR (Spatiotemporal analysis OR (spatial autocorrelation analysis) OR (geography) OR (geographic distribution) OR (geographically weighted regression) OR (geographic information systems) OR (cluster analysis) OR geographic* analys*.mp OR spati*regres*.mp OR spat*temp*.mp OR spat* analys*.mp OR spat* temp* analys*.mp OR spat* temp* pattern*.mp OR geography* distribut*.mp OR spat* temp* distribut*.mp OR heterogen* distribut.mp OR spacetime cluster*mp OR space-time cluster*mp OR hotspot.mp Or hot spots. mp OR GIS OR spati*
2. (tuberculosis) OR (multidrug resistant tuberculosis) OR TB.mp
3. 1 AND 2

Scopus
("Spatial analysis" OR
  "Spatio-temporal analysis" OR
  "Geographic Information System" OR
  "Geographic Mapping" OR
  "geographic distribution" OR
  "spatial regression" OR
  "spatial autocorrelation analysis" OR
  "Spatiotemporal analysis" OR
  hotspot OR
  "hot spot" AND tuberculosis/TB

Web of science
[(Spatial analysis) OR
  (Spatio-temporal analysis) OR
  (Geographic Information System) OR
  (Geographic Mapping) OR
  (geographic distribution) OR
  (spatial regression) OR

(spatial autocorrelation analysis) OR
(Spatiotemporal analysis) OR
(hotspot) OR
(hot spot)] AND (Tuberculosis)

Abbreviations
CAR models: Conditional autoregressive models; GIS: Geographic information system; GWR: Geographically weighted regression; HIV: Human immunodeficiency virus; LISA: Local indicators of spatial association; NNI: Nearest neighbourhood index; PCA: Principal component analysis; TB: Tuberculosis

Acknowledgements
The authors are grateful to the University of Melbourne librarians for their extensive assistance in sourcing articles.

Funding
We did not receive funding for this study. Debebe Shaweno is the recipient of the Melbourne International Research Scholarship and Melbourne International Fee Remission Scholarship. James Trauer is a recipient of an Early Career Fellowship from the NHMRC (APP1142638).

Authors' contributions
DS and EM conceived the study, which was refined by JD and JT. DS developed data extraction checklist, and DS, MK and KA extracted the data. DS drafted the manuscript, and all authors provided input into revisions and approved the final draft for submission.

Competing interests
The authors declare that they have no competing interests.

Author details
[1]Department of Medicine, University of Melbourne, Melbourne, Victoria, Australia. [2]Victorian Tuberculosis Program at the Peter Doherty Institute for Infection and Immunity, Melbourne, Victoria, Australia. [3]Department of Microbiology and Immunology, University of Melbourne, Melbourne, Victoria, Australia. [4]Research School of Population Health, College of Health and Medicine, The Australian National University, Canberra, Australia. [5]Institute of Public Health, College of Medicine and Health Sciences, University of Gondar, Gondar, Ethiopia. [6]Burnet Institute, Melbourne, Australia. [7]Curtin University, Bentley, Western Australia, Australia. [8]School of Public Health and Preventive Medicine, Monash University, Melbourne, Australia. [9]Australian Institute of Tropical Health and Medicine, James Cook University, Townsville, Queensland, Australia.

References

1. Verma A, Schwartzman K, Behr MA, Zwerling A, Allard R, Rochefort CM, Buckeridge DL. Accuracy of prospective space-time surveillance in detecting tuberculosis transmission. Spatial Spatio-Temp Epidemiol. 2014;8:47–54.
2. Haase I, Olson S, Behr MA, Wanyeki I, Thibert L, Scott A, Zwerling A, Ross N, Brassard P, Menzies D, et al. Use of geographic and genotyping tools to characterise tuberculosis transmission in Montreal. Int J Tuber Lung Dis. 2007;11(6):632–8.
3. Theron G, Jenkins HE, Cobelens F, Abubakar I, Khan AJ, Cohen T, Dowdy DW. Data for action: collection and use of local data to end tuberculosis. Lancet. 2015;386(10010):2324–33.
4. Yates TA, Khan PY, Knight GM, Taylor JG, McHugh TD, Lipman M, White RG, Cohen T, Cobelens FG, Wood R, et al. The transmission of Mycobacterium tuberculosis in high burden settings. Lancet Infect Dis. 2016;16(2):227–38.
5. Dye C, Loyd K. Tuberculosis. In: Jamison DTBJ, Measham AR, editors. Disease control priorities in developing countries. 2nd ed. Washington DC: WorldBank; 2006.
6. McBryde ES, Denholm JT. Risk of active tuberculosis in immigrants: effects of age, region of origin and time since arrival in a low-exposure setting. Med J Aust. 2012;197(8):458–61.
7. Middelkoop K, Bekker LG, Morrow C, Zwane E, Wood R. Childhood tuberculosis infection and disease: a spatial and temporal transmission analysis in a South African township. Samj South Afr Med J. 2009;99(10): 738–43.
8. Middelkoop K, Bekker LG, Morrow C, Lee N, Wood R. Decreasing household contribution to TB transmission with age: a retrospective geographic analysis of young people in a South African township. BMC Infect Dis. 2014; 14:221.
9. Keshavjee S, Dowdy D, Swaminathan S. Stopping the body count: a comprehensive approach to move towards zero tuberculosis deaths. Lancet. 2015;386(10010):e46–7.
10. Sasson C, Cudnik MT, Nassel A, Semple H, Magid DJ, Sayre M, Keseg D, Haukoos JS, Warden CR. Identifying high-risk geographic areas for cardiac arrest using three methods for cluster analysis. Acad Emerg Med. 2012;19(2): 139–46.
11. Shaweno D, Trauer JM, Denholm JT, McBryde ES. A novel Bayesian geospatial method for estimating tuberculosis incidence reveals many missed TB cases in Ethiopia. BMC Infect Dis. 2017;17(1):662.
12. Dangisso MH, Datiko DG, Lindtjorn B. Accessibility to tuberculosis control services and tuberculosis programme performance in southern Ethiopia. Glob Health Action. 2015;8:29443.
13. World Health Organization. Global tuberculosis report 2016: World Health Organization; 2016.
14. Clements ACA, Lwambo NJS, Blair L, Nyandindi U, Kaatano G, Kinung'hi S, Webster JP, Fenwick A, Brooker S. Bayesian spatial analysis and disease mapping: tools to enhance planning and implementation of a schistosomiasis control programme in Tanzania. Tropical Med Int Health. 2006;11(4):490–503.
15. Lai P-C, So F-M, Chan K-W. Spatial epidemiological approaches in disease mapping and analysis: CRC Press; 2008.
16. Wubuli A, Xue F, Jiang D, Yao X, Upur H, Wushouer Q. Socio-demographic predictors and distribution of pulmonary tuberculosis (TB) in Xinjiang, China: a spatial analysis. PLoS One. 2015;10(12).
17. Manley D, Flowerdew R, Steel D. Scales, levels and processes: studying spatial patterns of British census variables. Comput Environ Urban Syst. 2006;30(2):143–60.
18. Cressie N. Statistics for spatial data. Terra Nova. 1992;4(5):613–7.
19. Pfeiffer D. Spatial analysis in epidemiology. Oxford ; New York: Oxford University Press; 2008.
20. Kirby RS, Delmelle E, Eberth JM. Advances in spatial epidemiology and geographic information systems. Ann Epidemiol. 2017;27(1):1–9.
21. Smith CM, Le Comber SC, Fry H, Bull M, Leach S, Hayward AC. Spatial methods for infectious disease outbreak investigations: systematic literature review. Eurosurveillance. 2015;20(39):1–21.
22. Durr PA, Gatrell AC. GIS and spatial analysis in veterinary science: Cabi; 2004.
23. Nunes C. Tuberculosis incidence in Portugal: spatiotemporal clustering. Int J Health Geogr [Electronic Resource]. 2007;6:30.
24. Bhatt V, Tiwari N. A spatial scan statistic for survival data based on Weibull distribution. Stat Med. 2014;33(11):1867–76.
25. Higgs BW, Mohtashemi M, Grinsdale J, Kawamura LM. Early detection of tuberculosis outbreaks among the San Francisco homeless: trade-offs between spatial resolution and temporal scale. PLoS One [Electronic Resource]. 2007;2(12):e1284.
26. Dangisso MH, Datiko DG, Lindtjorn B. Spatio-temporal analysis of smear-positive tuberculosis in the Sidama Zone, Southern Ethiopia. PLoS One. 2015;10(6).
27. Areias C, Briz T, Nunes C. Pulmonary tuberculosis space-time clustering and spatial variation in temporal trends in Portugal, 2000-2010: an updated analysis. Epidemiol Infect. 2015;143(15):3211–9.
28. Kammerer JS, Shang N, Althomsons SP, Haddad MB, Grant J, Navin TR. Using statistical methods and genotyping to detect tuberculosis outbreaks. Int J Health Geogr. 2013;12:15.
29. Wang T, Xue F, Chen Y, Ma Y, Liu Y. The spatial epidemiology of tuberculosis in Linyi City, China, 2005-2010. BMC Public Health. 2012;12(1).
30. Silva AP, Souza WV, Albuquerque Mde F. Two decades of tuberculosis in a city in Northeastern Brazil: advances and challenges in time and space. Rev Soc Bras Med Trop. 2016;49(2):211–21.
31. Roth D, Otterstatter M, Wong J, Cook V, Johnston J, Mak S. Identification of spatial and cohort clustering of tuberculosis using surveillance data from British Columbia, Canada, 1990–2013. Soc Sci Med. 2016;168:214–22.
32. Gurjav U, Burneebaatar B, Narmandakh E, Tumenbayar O, Ochirbat B, Hill-Cawthorne GA, Marais BJ, Sintchenko V. Spatiotemporal evidence for cross-border spread of MDR-TB along the Trans-Siberian Railway line. Int J Tuber Lung Dis. 2015;19(11):1376–82.
33. Cao K, Yang K, Wang C, Guo J, Tao LX, Liu QR, Gehendra M, Zhang YJ, Guo XH. Spatial-temporal epidemiology of tuberculosis in Mainland China: an analysis based on Bayesian theory. Int J Environ Res Public Health. 2016;13(5).
34. de Queiroga RP, de Sa LD, Nogueira Jde A, de Lima ER, Silva AC, Pinheiro PG, Braga JU. Spatial distribution of tuberculosis and relationship with living conditions in an urban area of Campina Grande--2004 to 2007. Rev Bras Epidemiol. 2012;15(1):222–32.
35. Lin H, Shin S, Blaya JA, Zhang Z, Cegielski P, Contreras C, Asencios L, Bonilla C, Bayona J, Paciorek CJ, et al. Assessing spatiotemporal patterns of multidrug-resistant and drug-sensitive tuberculosis in a South American setting. Epidemiol Infect. 2011;139(11):1784–93.
36. Davidow AL, Marmor M, Alcabes P. Geographic diversity in tuberculosis trends and directly observed therapy, New York City, 1991 to 1994. Am J Respir Crit Care Med. 1997;156(5):1495–500.
37. Venâncio TS, Tuan TS, Nascimento LFC. Incidence of tuberculosis in children in the state of São Paulo, Brazil, under spatial approach. Cien Saude Colet. 2015;20(5):1541–7.
38. Jafari-Koshki T, Arsang-Jang S, Raei M. Applying spatiotemporal models to study risk of smear-positive tuberculosis in Iran, 2001-2012. Int J Tuber Lung Dis. 2015;19(4):469–74.
39. Jia ZW, Jia XW, Liu YX, Dye C, Chen F, Chen CS, Zhang WY, Li XW, Cao WC, Liu HL, et al. Spatial analysis of tuberculosis cases in migrants and permanent residents, Beijing, 2000-2006. Emerg Infect Dis. 2008;14(9):1413–20.
40. Houlihan CF, Mutevedzi PC, Lessells RJ, Cooke GS, Tanser FC, Newell ML. The tuberculosis challenge in a rural South African HIV programme. BMC Infect Dis. 2009;10 (no pagination)(23).
41. Jenkins HE, Plesca V, Ciobanu A, Crudu V, Galusca I, Soltan V, Serbulenco A, Zignol M, Dadu A, Dara M, et al. Assessing spatial heterogeneity of multidrug-resistant tuberculosis in a high-burden country. Eur Respir J. 2013; 42(5):1291–301.
42. Musenge E, Vounatsou P, Collinson M, Tollman S, Kahn K. The contribution of spatial analysis to understanding HIV/TB mortality in children: a structural equation modelling approach. Glob Health Action. 2013;6:19266.
43. Musenge E, Vounatsou P, Kahn K. Space-time confounding adjusted determinants of child HIV/TB mortality for large zero-inflated data in rural South Africa. Spatial Spatio-Temporal Epidemiol. 2011;2(4):205–17.
44. Harling G, Castro MC. A spatial analysis of social and economic determinants of tuberculosis in Brazil. Health Place. 2014;25:56–67.
45. De Castro DB, Pinto RC, De Albuquerque BC, Sadahiro M, Braga JU. The socioeconomic factors and the indigenous component of tuberculosis in amazonas. PLoS One. 2016;11(6) (no pagination)(e0158574).
46. Wong MK, Yadav R-P, Nishikiori N, Eang MT. The association between household poverty rates and tuberculosis case notification rates in Cambodia, 2010. Western Pacific Surveill Response J. 2013;4(1):25–33.

47. Chan-Yeung M, Yeh AGO, Tam CM, Kam KM, Leung CC, Yew WW, Lam CW. Socio-demographic and geographic indicators and distribution of tuberculosis in Hong Kong: a spatial analysis. Int J Tuber Lung Dis. 2005; 9(12):1320–6.

48. Shaweno D, Shaweno T, Trauer JM, Denholm JT, McBryde ES. Heterogeneity of distribution of tuberculosis in Sheka Zone, Ethiopia: drivers and temporal trends. Int J Tuber Lung Dis. 2017;21(1):79–85 and i.

49. Alene KA, Viney K, McBryde ES, Clements ACA. Spatial patterns of multidrug resistant tuberculosis and relationships to socioeconomic, demographic and household factors in northwest Ethiopia. PLoS One. 2017;12(2) (no pagination)(e0171800).

50. Li XX, Wang LX, Zhang J, Liu YX, Zhang H, Jiang SW, Chen JX, Zhou XN. Exploration of ecological factors related to the spatial heterogeneity of tuberculosis prevalence in P. China. Glob Health Action. 2014;7:23620.

51. Rao HX, Zhang X, Zhao L, Yu J, Ren W, Zhang XL, Ma YC, Shi Y, Ma BZ, Wang X, et al. Spatial transmission and meteorological determinants of tuberculosis incidence in Qinghai Province, China: a spatial clustering panel analysis. Infect Dis Pov. 2016;5(1) (no pagination)(45).

52. Beiranvand R, Karimi A, Delpisheh A, Sayehmiri K, Soleimani S, Ghalavandi S. Correlation assessment of climate and geographic distribution of tuberculosis using geographical information system (GIS). Iran J Public Health. 2016;45(1):86–93.

53. Munch Z, Van Lill S, Booysen C, Zietsman H, Enarson D, Beyers N. Tuberculosis transmission patterns in a high-incidence area: a spatial analysis. Int J Tuber Lung Dis. 2003;7(3):271–7.

54. Patterson B, Morrow CD, Kohls D, Deignan C, Ginsburg S, Wood R. Mapping sites of high TB transmission risk: integrating the shared air and social behaviour of TB cases and adolescents in a South African township. Sci Total Environ. 2017;05.

55. Murray EJ, Marais BJ, Mans G, Beyers N, Ayles H, Godfrey-Faussett P, Wallman S, Bond V. A multidisciplinary method to map potential tuberculosis transmission 'hot spots' in high-burden communities. Int J Tuber Lung Dis. 2009;13(6):767–74.

56. Ricks PM, Cain KP, Oeltmann JE, Kammerer JS, Moonan PK. Estimating the burden of tuberculosis among foreign-born persons acquired prior to entering the U.S., 2005–2009. PLOS One. 2011;6(11):e27405.

57. Prussing C, Castillo-Salgado C, Baruch N, Cronin WA. Geo-epidemiologic and molecular characterization to identify social, cultural, and economic factors where targeted tuberculosis control activities can reduce incidence in Maryland, 2004-2010. Public Health Rep. 2013;128(Suppl 3):104–14.

58. Ng IC, Wen TH, Wang JY, Fang CT. Spatial dependency of tuberculosis incidence in Taiwan. PLoS One. 2012;7(11).

59. Jacobson LM, Garcia-Garcia Ma DL, Hernandez-Avila JE, Cano-Arellano B, Small PM, Sifuentes-Osornio J, Ponce-De-Leon A. Changes in the geographical distribution of tuberculosis patients in Veracruz, Mexico, after reinforcement of a tuberculosis control programme. Trop Med Int Health. 2005;10(4):305–11.

60. Zelner JL, Murray MB, Becerra MC, Galea J, Lecca L, Calderon R, Yataco R, Contreras C, Zhang ZB, Manjourides J, et al. Identifying hotspots of multidrug-resistant tuberculosis transmission using spatial and molecular genetic data. J Infect Dis. 2016;213(2):287–94.

61. Moonan PK, Bayona M, Quitugua TN, Oppong J, Dunbar D, Jost KC, Burgess G, Singh KP, Weis SE. Using GIS technology to identify areas of tuberculosis transmission and incidence. Int J Health Geogr. 2004;3(1):23.

62. Ribeiro FK, Pan W, Bertolde A, Vinhas SA, Peres RL, Riley L, Palaci M, Maciel EL. Genotypic and spatial analysis of Mycobacterium tuberculosis transmission in a high-incidence urban setting. Clin Infect Dis. 2015;61(5):758–66.

63. Yeboah-Manu D, Asare P, Asante-Poku A, Otchere ID, Osei-Wusu S, Danso E, Forson A, Koram KA, Gagneux S. Spatio-temporal distribution of Mycobacterium tuberculosis complex strains in Ghana. PLoS One. 2016;11(8) (no pagination)(e0161892).

64. Seraphin MN, Lauzardo M, Doggett RT, Zabala J, Morris JG Jr, Blackburn JK. Spatiotemporal clustering of Mycobacterium tuberculosis complex genotypes in Florida: genetic diversity segregated by country of birth. PLoS One [Electronic Resource]. 2016;11(4):e0153575.

65. Izumi K, Ohkado A, Uchimura K, Murase Y, Tatsumi Y, Kayebeta A, Watanabe Y, Ishikawa N. Detection of tuberculosis infection hotspots using activity spaces based spatial approach in an urban Tokyo, from 2003 to 2011. PLoS One. 2015;10(9).

66. Evans JT, Wani RL, Anderson L, Gibson AL, Smith EG, Wood A, Olowokure B, Abubakar I, Mann JS, Gardiner S, et al. A geographically-restricted but prevalent Mycobacterium tuberculosis strain identified in the West Midlands region of the UK between 1995 and 2008. PLoS One. 2011;6(3) (no pagination)(e17930).

67. Nava-Aguilera E, Lopez-Vidal Y, Harris E, Morales-Perez A, Mitchell S, Flores-Moreno M, Villegas-Arrizon A, Legorreta-Soberanis J, Ledogar R, Andersson N. Clustering of Mycobacterium tuberculosis cases in Acapulco: spoligotyping and risk factors. Clin Dev Immunol. 2011;2011:408375.

68. Yuen CM, Kammerer JS, Marks K, Navin TR, France AM. Recent transmission of tuberculosis—United States, 2011–2014. PLoS One. 2016;11(4):e0153728.

69. Nguyen D, Brassard P, Westley J, Thibert L, Proulx M, Henry K, Schwartzman K, Menzies D, Behr MA. Widespread pyrazinamide-resistant Mycobacterium tuberculosis family in a low-incidence setting. J Clin Microbiol. 2003;41(7):2878–83.

70. Gurjav U, Jelfs P, Hill-Cawthorne GA, Marais BJ, Sintchenko V. Genotype heterogeneity of Mycobacterium tuberculosis within geospatial hotspots suggests foci of imported infection in Sydney, Australia. Infect Genet Evol. 2016;40:346–51.

71. Saavedra-Campos M, Welfare W, Cleary P, Sails A, Burkitt A, Hungerford D, Okereke E, Acheson P, Petrovic M. Identifying areas and risk groups with localised Mycobacterium tuberculosis transmission in northern England from 2010 to 2012: spatiotemporal analysis incorporating highly discriminatory genotyping data. Thorax. 2016;71(8):742–8.

72. Richardson M, van Lill SW, van der Spuy GD, Munch Z, Booysen CN, Beyers N, van Helden PD, Warren RM. Historic and recent events contribute to the disease dynamics of Beijing-like Mycobacterium tuberculosis isolates in a high incidence region. Int J Tuber Lung Dis. 2002;6(11):1001–11.

73. Goswami ND, Hecker EJ, Vickery C, Ahearn MA, Cox GM, Holland DP, Naggie S, Piedrahita C, Mosher A, Torres Y, et al. Geographic information system-based screening for TB, HIV, and syphilis (GIS-THIS): a cross-sectional study. PLoS One. 2012;7 (10) (no pagination)(e46029).

74. Tanser F, Wilkinson D. Spatial implications of the tuberculosis DOTS strategy in rural South Africa: a novel application of geographical information system and global positioning system technologies. Trop Med Int Health. 1999;4(10):634–8.

75. Manjourides J, Lin HH, Shin S, Jeffery C, Contreras C, Cruz JS, Jave O, Yagui M, Asencios L, Pagano M, et al. Identifying multidrug resistant tuberculosis transmission hotspots using routinely collected data. Tuberculosis. 2012; 92(3):273–9.

76. Stephen C. Capture-recapture methods in epidemiological studies. Infect Control Hospital Epidemiol. 1996;17(4):262–6.

77. Guernier V, Guégan J-F, Deparis X. An evaluation of the actual incidence of tuberculosis in French Guiana using a capture-recapture model. Microbes Infect. 2006;8(3):721–7.

78. WHO. Technical appendix - methods used to estimate the global burden of disease caused by TB, vol. 2015; 2014.

79. Clements AC, Firth S, Dembelé R, Garba A, Touré S, Sacko M, Landouré A, Bosqué-Oliva E, Barnett AG, Brooker S. Use of Bayesian geostatistical prediction to estimate local variations in Schistosoma haematobium infection in western Africa. Bull World Health Organ. 2009;87(12):921–9.

80. Li XX, Wang LX, Zhang H, Jiang SW, Fang Q, Chen JX, Zhou XN. Spatial variations of pulmonary tuberculosis prevalence co-impacted by socio-economic and geographic factors in People's Republic of China, 2010. BMC Public Health. 2014;14:257.

81. Rytkönen MJ. Not all maps are equal: GIS and spatial analysis in epidemiology. Int J Circumpolar Health. 2004;63(1):9–24.

82. Nassel AF, Root ED, Haukoos JS, McVaney K, Colwell C, Robinson J, Eigel B, Magid DJ, Sasson C. Multiple cluster analysis for the identification of high-risk census tracts for out-of-hospital cardiac arrest (OHCA) in Denver, Colorado. Resuscitation. 2014;85(12):1667–73.

83. Wheeler DC. A comparison of spatial clustering and cluster detection techniques for childhood leukemia incidence in Ohio, 1996–2003. Int J Health Geogr. 2007;6(1):13.

84. Wartenberg D, Greenberg M. Solving the cluster puzzle: clues to follow and pitfalls to avoid. Stat Med. 1993;12(19–20):1763–70.

85. Wartenberg D. Investigating disease clusters: why, when and how? J Royal Stat Soc. 2001;164(1):13–22.

86. Burra T, Jerrett M, Burnett RT, Anderson M. Conceptual and practical issues in the detection of local disease clusters: a study of mortality in Hamilton, Ontario. Can Geographer/Le Géographe Canadien. 2002;46(2):160–71.

87. Anselin L. Exploring spatial data with GeoDaTM: a workbook. Urbana. 2004; 51:61801.

88. Anselin L, Syabri I, Kho Y. GeoDa: an introduction to spatial data analysis. In: Handbook of applied spatial analysis; 2010. p. 73–89.

89. Goovaerts P, Jacquez GM. Accounting for regional background and population size in the detection of spatial clusters and outliers using geostatistical filtering and spatial neutral models: the case of lung cancer in Long Island, New York. Int J Health Geogr. 2004;3(1):14.

90. Goovaerts P, Jacquez GM. Detection of temporal changes in the spatial distribution of cancer rates using local Moran's I and geostatistically simulated spatial neutral models. J Geogr Syst. 2005;7(1):137–59.

91. Aamodt G, Samuelsen SO, Skrondal A. A simulation study of three methods for detecting disease clusters. Int J Health Geogr. 2006;5(1):15.

92. Stucki D, Ballif M, Egger M, Furrer H, Altpeter E, Battegay M, Droz S, Bruderer T, Coscolla M, Borrell S. Standard genotyping overestimates transmission of Mycobacterium tuberculosis among immigrants in a low-incidence country. J Clin Microbiol. 2016;54(7):1862–70.

93. Feske ML, Teeter LD, Musser JM, Graviss EA. Including the third dimension: a spatial analysis of TB cases in Houston Harris County. Tuberculosis. 2011; 91(SUPPL. 1):S24–33.

94. Tuite AR, Guthrie JL, Alexander DC, Whelan MS, Lee B, Lam K, Ma J, Fisman DN, Jamieson FB. Epidemiological evaluation of spatiotemporal and genotypic clustering of Mycobacterium tuberculosis in Ontario, Canada. Int J Tuber Lung Dis. 2013;17(10):1322–7.

95. Bishai WR, Graham NM, Harrington S, Pope DS, Hooper N, Astemborski J, Sheely L, Vlahov D, Glass GE, Chaisson RE. Molecular and geographic patterns of tuberculosis transmission after 15 years of directly observed therapy. JAMA. 1998;280(19):1679–84.

96. Roetzer A, Diel R, Kohl TA, Rückert C, Nübel U, Blom J, Wirth T, Jaenicke S, Schuback S, Rüsch-Gerdes S, et al. Whole genome sequencing versus traditional genotyping for investigation of a Mycobacterium tuberculosis outbreak: a longitudinal molecular epidemiological study. PLoS Med. 2013; 10(2):e1001387.

97. Wampande EM, Mupere E, Debanne SM, Asiimwe BB, Nsereko M, Mayanja H, Eisenach K, Kaplan G, Boom HW, Gagneux S, et al. Long-term dominance of Mycobacterium tuberculosis Uganda family in peri-urban Kampala-Uganda is not associated with cavitary disease. BMC Infect Dis. 2013;13:484.

98. Streicher EM, Warren RM, Kewley C, Simpson J, Rastogi N, Sola C, van der Spuy GD, van Helden PD, Victor TC. Genotypic and phenotypic characterization of drug-resistant Mycobacterium tuberculosis isolates from rural districts of the Western Cape Province of South Africa. J Clin Microbiol. 2004;42(2):891–4.

99. Souza WV, Carvalho MS, Albuquerque MDFPM, Barcellos CC, Ximenes RAA. Tuberculosis in intra-urban settings: a Bayesian approach. Trop Med Int Health. 2007;12(3):323–30.

100. Erazo C, Pereira SM, Da Conceição N. Costa M, Evangelista-Filho D, Braga JU, Barreto ML. Tuberculosis and living conditions in Salvador, Brazil: a spatial analysis. Rev Panamericana de Salud Publica/Pan American Journal of Public Health. 2014;36(1):24–30.

101. da Roza DL, Caccia-Bava Mdo C, Martinez EZ. Spatio-temporal patterns of tuberculosis incidence in Ribeirao Preto, state of Sao Paulo, southeast Brazil, and their relationship with social vulnerability: a Bayesian analysis. Rev Soc Bras Med Trop. 2012;45(5):607–15.

102. Wang W, Jin YY, Yan C, Ahan A, Cao MQ: Local spatial variations analysis of smear-positive tuberculosis in Xinjiang using geographically weighted regression model. BMC Public Health 2016, 16.

103. Sun W, Gong J, Zhou J, Zhao Y, Tan J, Ibrahim AN, Zhou Y. A spatial, social and environmental study of tuberculosis in China using statistical and GIS technology. Int J Environ Res Public Health [Electronic Resource]. 2015;12(2):1425–48.

104. Liu Y, Jiang S, Liu Y, Wang R, Li X, Yuan Z, Wang L, Xue F. Spatial epidemiology and spatial ecology study of worldwide drug-resistant tuberculosis. Int J Health Geogr. 2011;10.

105. Jenkins HE, Gegia M, Furin J, Kalandadze I, Nanava U, Chakhaia T, Cohen T. Geographical heterogeneity of multidrug-resistant tuberculosis in Georgia, January 2009 to June 2011. Eurosurveillance. 2014;19(11).

106. Gaudette LA, Ellis E. Tuberculosis in Canada: a focal disease requiring distinct control strategies for different risk groups. Tubercle Lung Dis. 1993; 74(4):244–53.

107. Froggatt K. Tuberculosis: spatial and demographic incidence in Bradford, 1980-2. J Epidemiol Community Health. 1985;39(1):20–6.

108. Zorzenon dos Santos RM, Amador A, de Souza WV, de Albuquerque MF, Ponce Dawson S, Ruffino-Netto A, Zarate-Blades CR, Silva CL. A dynamic analysis of tuberculosis dissemination to improve control and surveillance. PLoS One [Electronic Resource]. 2010;5(11):e14140.

109. Touray K, Adetifa IM, Jallow A, Rigby J, Jeffries D, Cheung YB, Donkor S, Adegbola RA, Hill PC. Spatial analysis of tuberculosis in an urban west

African setting: is there evidence of clustering? Tropical Med Int Health. 2010;15(6):664–72.

110. Tadesse T, Demissie M, Berhane Y, Kebede Y, Abebe M. The clustering of smear-positive tuberculosis in Dabat, Ethiopia: a population based cross sectional study. PLoS One [Electronic Resource]. 2013;8(5):e65022.

111. Shah L, Choi HW, Berrang-Ford L, Henostroza G, Krapp F, Zamudio C, Heymann SJ, Kaufman JS, Ciampi A, Seas C, et al. Geographic predictors of primary multidrug-resistant tuberculosis cases in an endemic area of Lima, Peru. Int J Tuber Lung Dis. 2014;18(11):1307–14.

112. Lin HH, Shin SS, Contreras C, Asencios L, Paciorek CJ, Cohen T. Use of spatial information to predict multidrug resistance in tuberculosis patients, Peru. Emerg Infect Dis. 2012;18(5):811–3.

113. Lai PC, Low CT, Tse WS, Tsui CK, Lee H, Hui PK. Risk of tuberculosis in high-rise and high density dwellings: an exploratory spatial analysis. Environ Pollution (Barking, Essex : 1987). 2013;183:40–5.

114. Kolifarhood G, Khorasani-Zavareh D, Salarilak S, Shoghli A, Khosravi N. Spatial and non-spatial determinants of successful tuberculosis treatment outcomes: an implication of geographical information systems in health policy-making in a developing country. J Epidemiol Glob Health. 2015;5(3):221–30.

115. Hino P, Villa TC, Sassaki CM, Nogueira Jde A, dos Santos CB. Geoprocessing in health area. Rev Latino-Am Enfermagem. 2006;14(6):939–43.

116. Ge E, Lai PC, Zhang X, Yang X, Li X, Wang H, Wei X. Regional transport and its association with tuberculosis in the Shandong province of China, 2009-2011. J Transp Geogr. 2015;46:232–43.

117. Dragioevio S, Schuurman N, Fitzgerald J. The utility of exploratory spatial data analysis in the study of tuberculosis incidences in an urban Canadian population. Cartographica. 2004;39(2):29–39.

118. Dominkovics P, Granell C, Pérez-Navarro A, Casals M, Orcau À, Caylà JA. Development of spatial density maps based on geoprocessing web services: application to tuberculosis incidence in Barcelona, Spain. Int J Health Geogr. 2011;10.

119. Dogba JB, Cadmus SI, Olugasa BO. Mapping of Mycobacterium tuberculosis cases in post-conflict Liberia, 2008-2012: a descriptive and categorical analysis of age, gender and seasonal pattern. Afr J Med Med Sci. 2014;(43 Suppl):117–24.

120. De Abreu E Silva M, Di Lorenzo Oliveira C, Teixeira Neto RG, Camargos PA. Spatial distribution of tuberculosis from 2002 to 2012 in a midsize city in Brazil. BMC Public Health. 2016;16(1).

121. Cegielski JP, Griffith DE, McGaha PK, Wolfgang M, Robinson CB, Clark PA, Hassell WL, Robison VA, Walker KP Jr, Wallace C. Eliminating tuberculosis one neighborhood at a time.[Reprint in Rev Panam Salud Publica. 2013 Oct; 34(4):284-94 Note: Original is in English and republished one is in Spanish.; PMID: 24301742], [Reprint in Am J Public Health. 2014 Apr;104 Suppl 2:S214-33; PMID: 24899457]. Am J Public Health. 2013;103(7):1292–300.

122. Cadmus SI, Akingbogun AA, Adesokan HK. Using geographical information system to model the spread of tuberculosis in the University of Ibadan, Nigeria. Afr J Med Med Sci. 2010;39(Suppl):193–9.

123. Zhou H, Yang X, Zhao S, Pan X, Xu J. Spatial epidemiology and risk factors of pulmonary tuberculosis morbidity in Wenchuan earthquake-stricken area. J Evid-Based Med. 2016;9(2):69–76.

124. Yeh YP, Chang HJ, Yang J, Chang SH, Suo D, Chen THH. Incidence of tuberculosis in mountain areas and surrounding townships: dose-response relationship by geographic analysis. Ann Epidemiol. 2005;15(7):526–32.

125. Yang X, Liu Q, Zhang R. Epidemiology of pulmonary tuberculosis in Wenchuan earthquake stricken area: population-based study. J Evid-Based Med. 2013;6(3):149–56.

126. Uthman OA. Spatial and temporal variations in incidence of tuberculosis in Africa, 1991 to 2005. World Health Popul. 2008;10(2):5–15.

127. Randremanana RV, Richard V, Rakotomanana F, Sabatier P, Bicout DJ. Bayesian mapping of pulmonary tuberculosis in Antananarivo, Madagascar. BMC Infect Dis. 2010;10 (no pagination)(21).

128. Pereira AG, Medronho Rde A, Escosteguy CC, Valencia LI, Magalhaes Mde A. Spatial distribution and socioeconomic context of tuberculosis in Rio de Janeiro, Brazil. Rev Saude Publica. 2015;49:48.

129. Pang PTT, Leung CC, Lee SS. Neighbourhood risk factors for tuberculosis in Hong Kong. Int J Tuber Lung Dis. 2010;14(5):585–92.

130. Nana Yakam A, Noeske J, Dambach P, Bowong S, Fono LA, Ngatchou-Wandji J. Spatial analysis of tuberculosis in Douala, Cameroon: clustering and links with socio-economic status. Int J Tuber Lung Dis. 2014;18(3):292–7.

131. Maciel ELN, Pan W, Dietze R, Peres RL, Vinhas SA, Ribeiro FK, Palaci M, Rodrigues RR, Zandonade E, Golub JE. Spatial patterns of pulmonary

tuberculosis incidence and their relationship to socio-economic status in Vitoria, Brazil. Int J Tuber Lung Dis. 2010;14(11):1395–402.

132. Lopez De Fede A, Stewart JE, Harris MJ, Mayfield-Smith K. Tuberculosis in socio-economically deprived neighborhoods: missed opportunities for prevention. Int J Tuber Lung Dis. 2008;12(12):1425–30.

133. Liu Y, Li X, Wang W, Li Z, Hou M, He Y, Wu W, Wang H, Liang H, Guo X. Investigation of space-time clusters and geospatial hot spots for the occurrence of tuberculosis in Beijing. Int J Tuber Lung Dis. 2012;16(4): 486–91.

134. Lim JR, Gandhi NR, Mthiyane T, Mlisana K, Moodley J, Jaglal P, Ramdin N, Brust JCM, Ismail N, Rustomjee R, et al. Incidence and geographic distribution of extensively drug-resistant tuberculosis in KwaZulu-Natal Province, South Africa. PLoS One. 2015;10(7).

135. Li L, Xi YL, Ren F. Spatio-temporal distribution characteristics and trajectory similarity analysis of tuberculosis in Beijing, China. Int J Environ Res Public Health. 2016;13(3).

136. Kistemann T, Munzinger A, Dangendorf F. Spatial patterns of tuberculosis incidence in Cologne (Germany). Soc Sci Med. 2002;55(1):7–19.

137. Kakchapati S, Choonpradub C, Lim A. Spatial and temporal variations in tuberculosis incidence, Nepal. Southeast Asian J Trop Med Public Health. 2014;45(1):95.

138. Hassarangsee S, Tripathi NK, Souris M. Spatial pattern detection of tuberculosis: a case study of Si Sa Ket province, Thailand. Int J Environ Res Public Health. 2015;12(12):16005–18.

139. Ge E, Zhang X, Wang X, Wei X. Spatial and temporal analysis of tuberculosis in Zhejiang Province, China, 2009–2012. Infect Dis Poverty. 2016;5(1) (no pagination)(11).

140. Fluegge KR. Using spatial disease patterns and patient-level characteristics to describe prevalence elastic behavior in treatment for latent tuberculosis infection (LTBI). Public Health Nurs. 2015;32(5):517–31.

141. Couceiro L, Santana P, Nunes C. Pulmonary tuberculosis and risk factors in Portugal: a spatial analysis. Int J Tuber Lung Dis. 2011;15(11):1445–54.

142. Chandrasekaran SK, Arivarignan G. Disease mapping using mixture distribution. Indian J Med Res. 2006;123(6):788–98.

143. Burgess L. Tuberculosis and urban ecological structure: the Derby case, 1979–83. East Midland Geogr. 1986;9(1–2):9–20.

144. Beyers N, Gie RP, Zietsman HL, Kunneke M, Hauman J, Tatley M, Donald PR. The use of a geographical information system (GIS) to evaluate the distribution of tuberculosis in a high-incidence community. South Afr Med J Suid-Afrikaanse Tydskrif Vir Geneeskunde. 1996;86(1):40–1 44.

145. Alvarez-Hernandez G, Lara-Valencia F, Reyes-Castro PA, Rascon-Pacheco RA. An analysis of spatial and socio-economic determinants of tuberculosis in Hermosillo, Mexico, 2000-2006. Int J Tuber Lung Dis. 2010;14(6):708–13.

146. Acevedo-Garcia D. Zip code-level risk factors for tuberculosis: neighborhood environment and residential segregation in New Jersey, 1985-1992. Am J Public Health. 2001;91(5):734–41.

147. Pinto ML, da Silva TC, Gomes LCF, Bertolozzi MR, Villavicencio LMM, Azevedo KMFA, de Figueiredo TMRM. Occurrence of tuberculosis cases in Crato, Ceará, from 2002 to 2011: a spatial analisys of specific standards. Rev Brasil Epidemiol. 2015;18(2):313–25.

148. Srinivasan R, Venkatesan P. Bayesian spatio-temporal model for tuberculosis in India. Indian J Med Res. 2015;142(April):478–80.

149. Schlattmann P, Dietz E, Bohning D. Covariate adjusted mixture models and disease mapping with the program DismapWin. Stat Med. 1996;15(7–9): 919–29.

150. Zhao F, Cheng S, He G, Huang F, Zhang H, Xu B, Murimwa TC, Cheng J, Hu D, Wang L. Space-time clustering characteristics of tuberculosis in China, 2005-2011. PLoS One. 2013, 8(12).

151. Zaragoza Bastida A, Hernandez Tellez M, Bustamante Montes LP, Medina Torres I, Jaramillo Paniagua JN, Mendoza Martinez GD, Ramirez Duran N. Spatial and temporal distribution of tuberculosis in the State of Mexico, Mexico. Thescientificworldjournal. 2012;2012:570278.

152. Yamamura M, de Freitas IM, Santo Neto M, Chiaravalloti Neto F, Popolin MA, Arroyo LH, Rodrigues LB, Crispim JA, Arcencio RA. Spatial analysis of avoidable hospitalizations due to tuberculosis in Ribeirao Preto, SP, Brazil (2006-2012). Rev Saude Publica. 2016(50):20.

153. Tiwari N, Kandpal V, Tewari A, Rao KRM, Tolia VS. Investigation of tuberculosis clusters in Dehradun city of India. Asian Pac J Trop Med. 2010; 3(6):486–90.

154. Tiwari N, Adhikari CM, Tewari A, Kandpal V. Investigation of geo-spatial hotspots for the occurrence of tuberculosis in Almora district, India,

155. Santos Neto M, Yamamura M, Garcia MC, Popolin MP, Rodrigues LB, Chiaravalloti Neto F, Fronteira I, Arcencio RA. Pulmonary tuberculosis in Sao Luis, State of Maranhao, Brazil: space and space-time risk clusters for death (2008-2012). Rev Soc Bras Med Trop. 2015;48(1):69–76.

156. Randremanana RV, Sabatier P, Rakotomanana F, Randriamanantena A, Richard V. Spatial clustering of pulmonary tuberculosis and impact of the care factors in Antananarivo City. Tropical Med Int Health. 2009;14(4):429–37.

157. Rakotosamimanana S, Mandrosovololona V, Rakotonirina J, Ramamonjisoa J, Ranjalahy JR, Randremanana RV, Rakotomanana F. Spatial analysis of pulmonary tuberculosis in Antananarivo Madagascar: tuberculosis-related knowledge, attitude and practice. PLoS One. 2014;9(11).

158. Onozuka D, Hagihara A. Geographic prediction of tuberculosis clusters in Fukuoka, Japan, using the space-time scan statistic. BMC Infect Dis. 2007;7.

159. Olfatifar M, Karami M, Hosseini SM, Parvin M. Clustering of pulmonary tuberculosis in Hamadan province, west of Iran: a population based cross sectional study (2005-2013). J Res Health Sci. 2016;16(3):166–9.

160. Gomez-Barroso D, Rodriguez-Valin E, Ramis R, Cano R. Spatio-temporal analysis of tuberculosis in Spain, 2008-2010. Int J Tuber Lung Dis. 2013;17(6): 745–51.

161. Tsai PJ, Lin ML, Chu CM, Perng CH. Spatial autocorrelation analysis of health care hotspots in Taiwan in 2006. BMC Public Health. 2009;9.

162. Mokrousov I. Genetic geography of Mycobacterium tuberculosis Beijing genotype: a multifacet mirror of human history? Infect Genet Evol. 2008;8(6): 777–85.

163. Brassard P, Henry KA, Schwartzman K, Jomphe M, Olson SH. Geography and genealogy of the human host harbouring a distinctive drug-resistant strain of tuberculosis. Infect Genet Evol. 2008;8(3):247–57.

164. Li T, He XX, Chang ZR, Ren YH, Zhou JY, Ju LR, Jia ZW. Impact of new migrant populations on the spatial distribution of tuberculosis in Beijing. Int J Tuber Lung Dis. 2011;15(2):163–8.

165. Wallace D. The resurgence of tuberculosis in New York City: a mixed hierarchically and spatially diffused epidemic. Am J Public Health. 1994; 84(6):1000–2.

166. Wei W, Wei-Sheng Z, Ahan A, Ci Y, Wei-Wen Z, Ming-Qin C. The characteristics of TB epidemic and TB/HIV co-infection epidemic: a 2007– 2013 retrospective study in Urumqi, Xinjiang Province, China. PloS One. 2016;11(10):e0164947.

167. Egunjobi L. Spatial distribution of mortality from leading notifiable diseases in Nigeria. Soc Sci Med. 1993;36(10):1267–72.

168. Marlow MA, Maciel EL, Sales CM, Gomes T, Snyder RE, Daumas RP, Riley LW. Tuberculosis DALY-gap: spatial and quantitative comparison of disease burden across urban slum and non-slum census tracts. J Urban Health. 2015;92(4):622–34.

169. Mathema B, Bifani PJ, Driscoll J, Steinlein L, Kurepina N, Moghazeh SL, Shashkina E, Marras SA, Campbell S, Mangura B, et al. Identification and evolution of an IS6110 low-copy-number Mycobacterium tuberculosis cluster. J Infect Dis. 2002;185(5):641–9.

170. Souza WV, Ximenes R, Albuquerque MFM, Lapa TM, Portugal JL, Lima MLC, Martelli CMT. The use of socioeconomic factors in mapping tuberculosis risk areas in a city of northeastern Brazil. Rev Panamericana de Salud Publica/ Pan American Journal of Public Health. 2000;8(6):403–10.

171. Yamamura M, Santos-Neto M, dos Santos RA, Garcia MC, Nogueira JA, Arcencio RA. Epidemiological characteristics of cases of death from tuberculosis and vulnerable territories. Rev Latino-Am Enfermagem. 2015; 23(5):910–8.

172. Perri BR, Proops D, Moonan PK, Munsiff SS, Kreiswirth BN, Kurepina N, Goranson C, Ahuja SD. Mycobacterium tuberculosis cluster with developing drug resistance, New York, New York, USA, 2003-2009. Emerg Infect Dis. 2011;17(3):372–8.

173. Terlikbayeva A, Hermosilla S, Galea S, Schluger N, Yegeubayeva S, Abildayev T, Muminov T, Akiyanova F, Bartkowiak L, Zhumadilov Z, et al. Tuberculosis in Kazakhstan: analysis of risk determinants in national surveillance data. BMC Infect Dis. 2012;12 (no pagination)(262).

174. Lima MD, Martins-Melo FR, Heukelbach J, Alencar CH, Boigny RN, Ramos AN. Mortality related to tuberculosis-HIV/AIDS co-infection in Brazil, 2000-2011: epidemiological patterns and time trends. Cadernos Saude Publica. 2016;32(10):e00026715.

175. Santos Neto M, Yamamura M, Garcia MCC, Popolin MP, Rodrigues LBB, Chiaravalloti Neto F, Fronteira I, Arcêncio RA. Pulmonary tuberculosis in São

Luis, State of Maranhão, Brazil: space and space-time risk clusters for death (2008-2012). Rev Soc Bras Med Trop. 2015;48(1):69–76.

176. Sousa P, Oliveira A, Gomes M, Gaio AR, Duarte R. Longitudinal clustering of tuberculosis incidence and predictors for the time profiles: the impact of HIV. Int J Tuber Lung Dis. 2016;20(8):1027–32.

177. Crisan A, Wong HY, Johnston JC, Tang P, Colijn C, Otterstatter M, Hiscoe L, Parker R, Pollock SL, Gardy JL. Spatio-temporal analysis of tuberculous infection risk among clients of a homeless shelter during an outbreak. Int J Tuber Lung Dis. 2015;19(9):1033–8.

178. Feske ML, Teeter LD, Musser JM, Graviss EA. Giving TB wheels: public transportation as a risk factor for tuberculosis transmission. Tuberculosis. 2011;91(Suppl 1):S16–23.

179. Herrero MB, Arrossi S, Ramos S, Braga JU. Spatial analysis of the tuberculosis treatment dropout, Buenos Aires, Argentina. Rev Saude Publica. 2015;49.

180. Jacob BJ, Krapp F, Ponce M, Gottuzzo E, Griffith DA, Novak RJ. Accounting for autocorrelation in multi-drug resistant tuberculosis predictors using a set of parsimonious orthogonal eigenvectors aggregated in geographic space. Geospat Health. 2010;4(2):201–17.

181. Kang J, Zhang N, Shi R. A Bayesian nonparametric model for spatially distributed multivariate binary data with application to a multidrug-resistant tuberculosis (MDR-TB) study. Biometrics. 2014;70(4):981–92.

182. Leung CC, Yew WW, Tam CM, Chan CK, Chang KC, Law WS, Wong MY, Au KF. Socio-economic factors and tuberculosis: a district-based ecological analysis in Hong Kong. Int J Tuber Lung Dis. 2004;8(8):958–64.

183. Nunes C, Duarte R, Veiga AM, Taylor B. Who are the patients that default tuberculosis treatment? - space matters! Epidemiol Infect. 2017:1–5.

184. Nunes C, Taylor BM. Modelling the time to detection of urban tuberculosis in two big cities in Portugal: a spatial survival analysis. Int J Tuber Lung Dis. 2016;20(9):1219–25.

185. Obasanya J, Abdurrahman ST, Oladimeji O, Lawson L, Dacombe R, Chukwueme N, Abiola T, Mustapha G, Sola C, Dominguez J, et al. Tuberculosis case detection in Nigeria, the unfinished agenda. Tropical Med Int Health. 2015;20(10):1396–402.

186. Rodrigues AL Jr, Ruffino-Netto A, de Castilho EA. Spatial distribution of M. tuberculosis-HIV coinfection in Sao Paulo State, Brazil, 1991-2001. [Portuguese, English]. Rev Saude Publica. 2006;40(2):265–70.

187. Ross JM, Cattamanchi A, Miller CR, Tatem AJ, Katamba A, Haguma P, Handley MA, Davis JL. Investigating barriers to tuberculosis evaluation in Uganda using geographic information systems. Am J Trop Med Hyg. 2015;93(4):733–8.

188. Tipayamongkholgul M, Podang J, Siri S. Spatial analysis of social determinants for tuberculosis in Thailand. J Med Assoc Thailand = Chotmaihet Thangphaet. 2013;96(Suppl 5):S116–21.

189. Wanyeki I, Olson S, Brassard P, Menzies D, Ross N, Behr M, Schwartzman K. Dwellings, crowding, and tuberculosis in Montreal. Soc Sci Med. 2006;63(2):501–11.

190. Rodrigues-Junior AL, Ruffino-Netto A, de Castilho EA. Spatial distribution of the human development index, HIV infection and AIDS-tuberculosis comorbidity: Brazil, 1982-2007. Rev Brasil Epidemiol. 2014;17(Suppl 2):204–15.

191. Santos-Neto M, Yamamura M, Garcia MC, Popolin MP, Silveira TR, Arcencio RA. Spatial analysis of deaths from pulmonary tuberculosis in the city of Sao Luis, Brazil. J Bras Pneumol. 2014;40(5):543–51.

192. Uthman OA, Yahaya I, Ashfaq K, Uthman MB. A trend analysis and sub-regional distribution in number of people living with HIV and dying with TB in Africa, 1991 to 2006. Int J Health Geogr [Electronic Resource]. 2009;8:65.

193. Carter A, Zwerling A, Olson S, Tannenbaum T-N, Schwartzman K. Tuberculosis and the city. Health Place. 2009;15(3):807–13.

194. Chamie G, Wandera B, Marquez C, Kato-Maeda M, Kamya MR, Havlir DV, Charlebois ED. Identifying locations of recent TB transmission in rural Uganda: a multidisciplinary approach. Trop Med Int Health. 2015;20(4):537–45.

195. McGuigan MA, Yamada J. The geographic distribution of tuberculosis and pyridoxine supply in Ontario. Can J Hospital Pharm. 1995;48(6):348–51.

196. Strauss R, Fulop G, Pfeifer C. Tuberculosis in Austria 1995-99: geographical distribution and trends. Euro surveillance. 2003;8(1):19–26.

197. Smith CM, Hayward AC. DotMapper: an open source tool for creating interactive disease point maps. BMC Infect Dis. 2016;16:145.

198. MRC Tuberculosis and chest Diseases Unit. The geographical distribution of tuberculosis notifications in a national survey of England and Wales (1978–79). Report from the Medical Research Council Tuberculosis and Chest Diseases Unit. Tubercle. 1982;63(2):75–88.

199. Bai J, Zou G, Mu S, Ma Y. Using spatial analysis to identify tuberculosis transmission and surveillance. In: Lecture Notes in Electrical Engineering, vol. 277: LNEE; 2014. p. 337–44.

13

Association of longitudinal alcohol consumption trajectories with coronary heart disease

Dara O'Neill[1]* iD, Annie Britton[2], Mary K. Hannah[3], Marcel Goldberg[4], Diana Kuh[2,5], Kay Tee Khaw[6] and Steven Bell[7]

Abstract

Background: Studies have shown that alcohol intake trajectories differ in their associations with biomarkers of cardiovascular functioning, but it remains unclear if they also differ in their relationship to actual coronary heart disease (CHD) incidence. Using multiple longitudinal cohort studies, we evaluated the association between long-term alcohol consumption trajectories and CHD.

Methods: Data were drawn from six cohorts (five British and one French). The combined analytic sample comprised 35,132 individuals (62.1% male; individual cohorts ranging from 869 to 14,247 participants) of whom 4.9% experienced an incident (fatal or non-fatal) CHD event. Alcohol intake across three assessment periods of each cohort was used to determine participants' intake trajectories over approximately 10 years. Time to onset for (i) incident CHD and (ii) fatal CHD was established using surveys and linked medical record data. A meta-analysis of individual participant data was employed to estimate the intake trajectories' association with CHD onset, adjusting for demographic and clinical characteristics.

Results: Compared to consistently moderate drinkers (males: 1–168 g ethanol/week; females: 1–112 g ethanol/week), inconsistently moderate drinkers had a significantly greater risk of incident CHD [hazard ratio (HR) = 1.18, 95% confidence interval (CI) = 1.02–1.37]. An elevated risk of incident CHD was also found for former drinkers (HR = 1.31, 95% CI = 1.13–1.52) and consistent non-drinkers (HR = 1.47, 95% CI = 1.21–1.78), although, after sex stratification, the latter effect was only evident for females. When examining fatal CHD outcomes alone, only former drinkers had a significantly elevated risk, though hazard ratios for consistent non-drinkers were near identical. No evidence of elevated CHD risk was found for consistently heavy drinkers, and a weak association with fatal CHD for inconsistently heavy drinkers was attenuated following adjustment for confounding factors.

Conclusions: Using prospectively recorded alcohol data, this study has shown how instability in drinking behaviours over time is associated with risk of CHD. As well as individuals who abstain from drinking (long term or more recently), those who are inconsistently moderate in their alcohol intake have a higher risk of experiencing CHD. This finding suggests that policies and interventions specifically encouraging consistency in adherence to lower-risk drinking guidelines could have public health benefits in reducing the population burden of CHD. The absence of an effect amongst heavy drinkers should be interpreted with caution given the known wider health risks associated with such intake.

Trial registration: ClinicalTrials.gov, NCT03133689.

Keywords: Alcohol, Coronary heart disease, IPD meta-analysis, Longitudinal design

* Correspondence: d.oneill@ucl.ac.uk
[1]CLOSER, Department of Social Science, Institute of Education, University College London, London, UK
Full list of author information is available at the end of the article

Background

The relationship between alcohol consumption and coronary heart disease (CHD) is of scientific and public health interest, yet it remains a subject of debate. Studies have found evidence both for and against the possibility of an association [1, 2]. The concept of a potentially cardio-protective effect of moderate drinking compared to non-drinking or heavier consumption, termed the U/J-shaped curve, has been particularly controversial [3–5]. Some clinical evidence suggests that alcohol may affect different pathways thought to influence CHD risk, including hypertension [6, 7], body mass index (BMI) [8] and lipid levels [9, 10]. However, this purported effect continues to be disputed [11], which poses challenges in the formation of health-care policy and can hinder wider public understanding of the health impact of lifestyle choices.

Much of the discussion around the evidence base for the alcohol–CHD association has focussed on design limitations in observational studies, such as the failure to distinguish between non-drinkers and former drinkers [12, 13]. The decision to stop drinking could be influenced by the onset of ill health, and such sick quitters could potentially bias estimates of disease risk in lifelong abstainers if not analysed independently [14]. Studies have most commonly used single baseline measures of alcohol intake and that drinking behaviours can change over time has, therefore, not typically been reflected in the alcohol epidemiology literature [15, 16].

Recent efforts have been made to establish long-term trajectories of alcohol intake, enabling differentiation between patterns of drinking that fluctuate over time. Different trajectories have been found to have distinct patterns of association with intermediate markers of cardiovascular health, including carotid intima media thickness [17], pulse wave velocity [18] and inflammatory markers [19], but this work has yet to link these drinking typologies to CHD events directly. More commonly, studies with longitudinal assessments of drinking have used average intake, typically between only two measurement occasions, in evaluations of CHD risk [20], but such aggregation can mask consumption variation over time. The importance of capturing variability is evident from previous work that has shown how isolated episodes of heavy drinking can offset the potentially protective effects of moderate drinking [2]. Failure to account for stability in alcohol intake levels may bias risk estimates [21]. In the current study, we have used an alcohol intake trajectory approach, previously employed in the study of intermediate CHD markers [17–19], to address this research gap. We have drawn data from multiple cohort studies to investigate whether longitudinal trajectories of alcohol consumption differ in their association with total CHD incidence (fatal or non-fatal). Furthermore, since research has suggested that the cardio-protective effect of moderate drinking may be less evident with fatal CHD outcomes [22], particularly in comparison to heavier intake [23], a secondary aim of this work was to examine how the longitudinal trajectories are specifically associated with mortality due to CHD.

Methods

Sample, design and cohort selection

Data were obtained from five British cohort studies: the European Prospective Investigation of Cancer, Norfolk Cohort (EPIC-N) [24]; the Medical Research Council's National Survey of Health and Development 1946 (NSHD) [25]; West of Scotland Twenty-07: 1930s (T07-1930s) [26]; West of Scotland Twenty-07: 1950s (T07-1950s) [26] and Whitehall II (WII) [27]. Further data were obtained from an additional French cohort: Gaz et Electricité (GAZEL) [28]. Descriptions of each cohort are provided in Fig. 1 and complete cohort profiles are available via the above citations. The cohorts were chosen for their coverage of relevant variables and design similarity. They each included prospective alcohol intake data across three assessments covering an approximate 10-year interval, as well as pertinent covariate and verified CHD outcome data. Prior to commencement of the analysis, additional harmonisation was performed for all cohort datasets to maximise consistency in variable names and definitions. The study design was pre-registered on ClinicalTrials.gov (identifier NCT03133689), and a STROBE statement is provided in Additional file 1 (Section S1).

The combined dataset initially comprised 62,799 participant records in total (cohort-specific counts are provided in Fig. 1). The exposure variable was measured across three assessment points covering a decade on average, with the last assessment point treated as the study baseline from which time-to-event outcomes were measured. Of the initial sample, 19,277 participants were excluded due to attrition or having experienced a CHD event prior to the study baseline. A further 8390 participants were not included due to incomplete data linkage. Following these exclusion criteria (further details of which are provided in Fig. 1), a sample of 35,132 (62.1% male) participants remained and these comprised the analytic sample.

Measures

Outcomes

The primary endpoint was CHD incidence, as ascertained from linked health records and survey data. Non-fatal CHD data were available for NSHD, but the time to event from the end of the exposure period was not ascertainable, so this study was omitted from the analysis of the incident CHD end point. Mortality due to CHD was examined as a secondary outcome in supplementary analyses, and all cohorts contributed data to this analysis. CHD events were previously coded using the codebook of the International Statistical Classification of Diseases and Related Health

	EPIC-N	GAZEL	NSHD	T07-1930s	T07-1950s	WII
Cohort Description						
Recruitment date	1993-1997	1989	1946	1987-1988	1987-1988	1985-1988
Cohort type	Regional cohort	Occupational cohort (utility workers)	National birth cohort	Regional cohort	Regional cohort	Occupational cohort (civil servants)
Sampling location	Norfolk, UK	France-wide	UK-wide	Western Scotland, UK	Western Scotland, UK	London, UK
Sex	42.5% Male	74.1% Male	49.2% Male	42.6% Male	44.3% Male	67.8% Male
Exposure assessment period	1993-1997 to 2006-2011	1992 to 2002	1982 to 1999	1987-1988 to 1995-1997	1987-1988 to 1995-1997	1985-1988 to 1997-1999
Participant Selection						
Cohort samples at initial exposure assessment	25,639	20,535	3,322	1,551	1,444	10,308
Sample excluded due to attrition or CHD event before end of exposure assessment period	16,347	281	331	602	258	1,458
Sample excluded due to unavailability of outcome follow-up data	1,830	6,007	12	80	184	277
Analysis sample	7,462	14,247	2,979	869	1,002	8,573

Fig. 1 Cohort description and participant selection flowchart. CHD coronary heart disease, EPIC-N European Prospective Investigation of Cancer, Norfolk, GAZEL Gaz et Electricité, T07-1930s West of Scotland Twenty-07 Study 1930s, T07-1950s West of Scotland Twenty-07 Study 1950s, WII Whitehall II

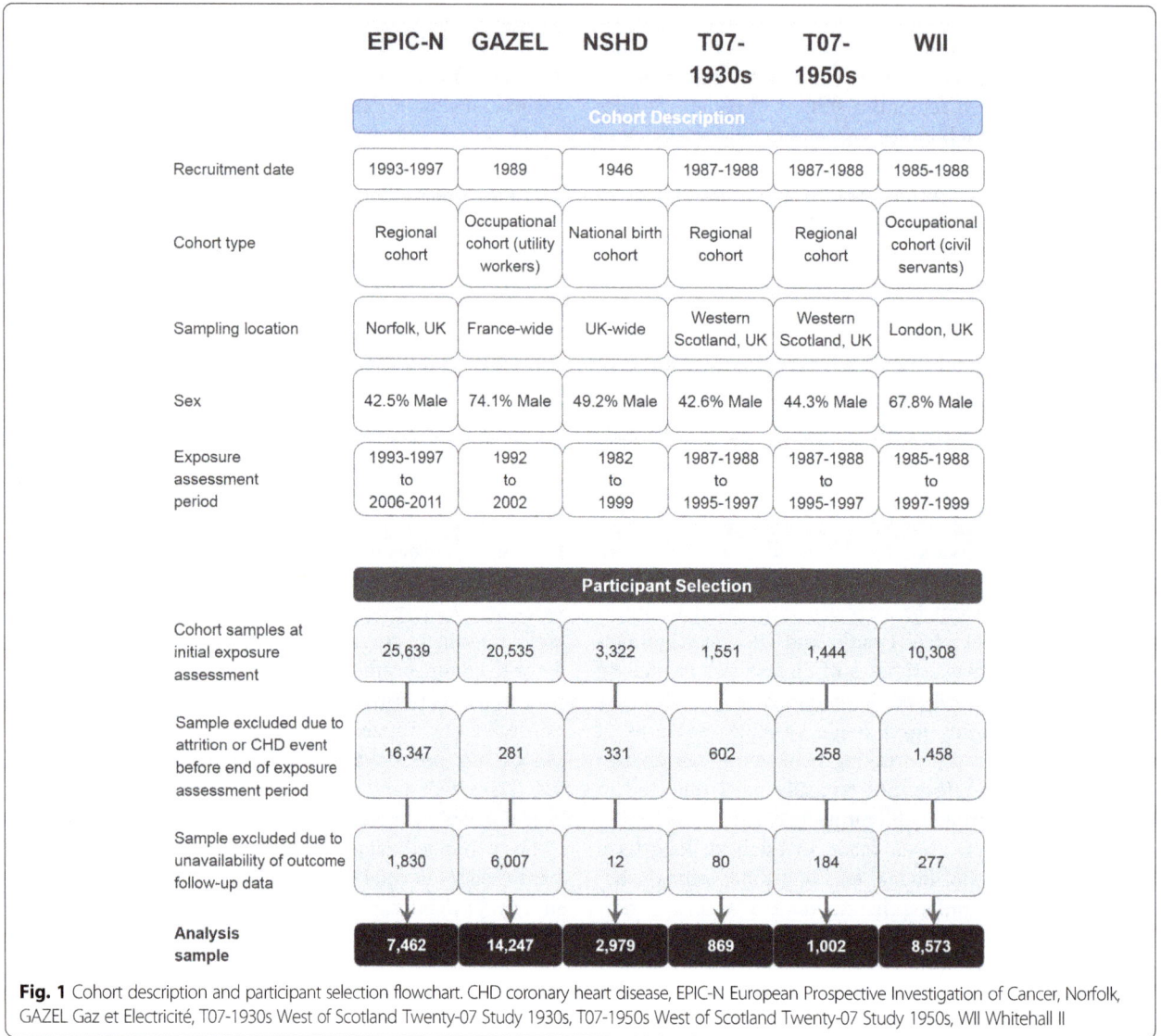

Problems (ICD) [29]: ICD-9: 410–414 Ischaemic heart disease and ICD-10: I20-I25 Ischaemic heart diseases. For the Twenty-07 cohorts, non-fatal CHD events were identified using the Royal College of General Practitioners' codebook [30] (codes 1940, 1945 and 1950). Survival time was calculated for all participants as time (in years) between the end of the alcohol assessment period and date of CHD event, death from non-CHD causes, study dropout or last date of data linkage (study specific), whichever occurred first. Additional details of study enrolment and follow-up procedures are available in Additional file 1 (Section S10).

Exposure

Trajectories of self-reported alcohol intake were derived using weekly alcohol intake measurements collected across three consecutive waves of each cohort study. The resultant trajectories comprised a decade of follow-up on average. Standard drink definitions were used to define alcohol

(ethanol) content in reported drinks (half-pints of beer or cider, small glasses of wine, and single servings of spirits): 8 g ethanol in the British cohort data and 10 g in the French GAZEL data [31, 32]. Reported consumption at each measurement occasion was categorised according to UK drinking guidelines at the time of data collection, which recommended a maximum intake level for lower-risk drinking of 168 g of ethanol a week for males and 112 g of ethanol a week for females [33]. Although recently published UK guidelines have proposed identical thresholds for males and females [34], the analytic report upon which they are based identified risk functions for both CHD morbidity and mortality that notably differed between males and females [35], particularly at higher levels of consumption [23]. The focus in the present study was on stability of adherence to lower-risk drinking guidelines over time, and we consequently categorised participants according to longitudinal profiles as defined in Table 1. Consistently moderate

Table 1 Drinker type definitions with observed counts and percentages (within sex and overall)

Drinker type	Weekly alcohol intake	N (%)		
		Male	Female	Total
Consistent non-drinker	0 g at each wave of data collection	807 (4.6)	1335 (12.4)	2142 (7.5)
Former drinker	0 g at last wave but intake >0 g at any earlier wave	1831 (10.4)	2249 (21.0)	4080 (14.4)
Consistently moderate	Male: 1–168 g at each wave	7249 (41.0)	4161 (38.8)	11,410 (40.2)
	Female: 1–112 g at each wave			
Inconsistently moderate	Male: 1–168 g for most but not all waves	3599 (20.4)	2037 (19.0)	5636 (19.8)
	Female: 1–112 g for most but not all waves			
Consistently heavy	Male: >168 g at each wave	2216 (12.5)	349 (3.3)	2565 (9.0)
	Female: >112 g at each wave			
Inconsistently heavy	Male: >168 g for most but not all waves	1979 (11.2)	598 (5.6)	2577 (9.1)
	Female: >112 g for most but not all waves			

drinkers were used as the reference category [14]. Drinkers with inconsistent levels of alcohol intake were defined according to their modal intake, i.e. their most frequent level of intake. For example, where a participant had an equal number of heavy and moderate drinking periods, they were categorised as inconsistently heavy drinkers. This ensured that participants who occasionally drank heavily were not grouped with participants who consistently adhered to lower-risk drinking guidelines.

Covariates

Known demographic and lifestyle risk factors for CHD were selected for inclusion in the modelling, including sex and age. Socioeconomic position was defined using the participant's occupational status, categorised as low (non-skilled or semi-skilled), intermediate (mid-level) or high (professional or executive) [36]. Smoking status was assessed, with participants categorised as current, ex- or non-smokers. To account for variability in the alcohol intake assessment interval, the time difference between initial and final assessments was calculated for each participant. Additional clinical data were obtained on BMI (measured as kg/m^2) and self-reported high blood pressure or use of antihypertensive medication (yes/no). All of the covariates were assessed at the commencement of the follow-up period for CHD (the occasion of the third and final alcohol assessment), which we have defined as the current study's baseline.

Statistical analysis

Prior to undertaking inferential analyses, multiple imputation by chained equations was completed using the R 'mice' package (v2.30) to address missing covariate and exposure data. Altogether, 100 imputations were performed for both the incident and fatal CHD analyses, ensuring congruence between the imputation and substantive models. Outcome data with the Nelson–Aalen hazard [37] were used but not imputed.

The modelling was performed as individual participant data (IPD) meta-analyses, accounting for the clustering of participants within each cohort. Both one- and two-step approaches are available and can give comparable results under particular conditions [38]. However, the one-step approach, in which all data are analysed simultaneously with clustering incorporated as a random effect term, is thought to be less prone to bias in pooled effect estimates and standard errors [39] and to be the preferred approach where covariate adjustments are required or where inter-study heterogeneity may be present [40, 41]. Consequently, one-step IPD meta-analysis was performed using hierarchical (mixed effects) Cox regression modelling incorporating a random effect term for cohort membership with maximum likelihood estimations. Models were developed iteratively: an initial model accounting for age, sex and intake assessment interval (partially adjusted for confounding), followed by an extended model that additionally included smoking status and socioeconomic status covariates (maximally adjusted for confounding). Supplementary modelling extended the adjustment further, including potential mediators, to examine clinical pathways (maximally adjusted for confounding and mediation). Schoenfeld residuals were plotted to ascertain that the proportional hazards assumption had not been violated (available in Additional file 1: Section S2).

Given most existing work in this area has employed single one-off measures of alcohol intake, for comparative purposes, an initial IPD meta-analysis was undertaken in this study using participants' final intake measurement prior to the outcome follow-up period (i.e. at this study's baseline). This single measure categorisation allowed a distinction to be made between different intake levels (none, moderate or heavy), but not stability of intake over time or discontinuation of drinking. This analysis was followed by the modelling of the primary exposure, the longitudinal drinking trajectory categorisation. Additional stratified analyses were also completed to explore specific characteristics of the alcohol–CHD relationship. Research has suggested that the association of alcohol with cardiovascular risk may differ between older and younger populations [42], so age-stratified modelling of the longitudinal drinker typology was also performed (aged ≤55 vs >55 years at this study's baseline). Further stratified analyses were undertaken to explore sex-specific effects. Finally, sensitivity analyses were conducted to determine the impact of modelling assumptions on this study's main results.

The statistical analyses were performed in R (v3.4.1; R Foundation for Statistical Computing, Vienna, Austria). All statistical significance testing was two-tailed, using an inference threshold of $p < 0.05$.

Results

Sample characteristics

Descriptive statistics, for the overall sample and stratified by drinker type, are presented in Table 2. Additional descriptive statistics, stratified by cohort, are provided in Additional file 1 (Section S3). Statistics on data missingness are also reported in Table 2, and further detail is provided in Additional file 1 (Section S4).

Across the drinker types, mean age ranged from 57.1 years (standard deviation, SD = 6.4) for the inconsistently moderate drinkers to 61.9 (SD = 9.1) for the former drinkers. Heavy drinkers were most likely to be male (consistently heavy 86.4%; inconsistently heavy 76.8%), whereas abstainers were more likely to be female (consistent non-drinker 62.3%; former drinker 55.1%). Heavy drinkers had the highest proportion reporting past or current smoking (consistently heavy 50.7%; inconsistently heavy 50.4%). Consistently moderate drinkers were most likely to be of high socioeconomic position (47.8%), followed by both consistently and inconsistently heavy drinkers (45.9% and 46.5%). Conversely, consistent non-drinkers had the highest proportion in a low socioeconomic position (23.9%). BMI showed little variation between drinker types (all had means of 26 kg/m^2). Known hypertension was least common amongst consistently moderate drinkers (26.2%) and most common amongst inconsistently heavy drinkers (31.6%) and former drinkers (31.7%). The mean assessment interval covered by the drinking trajectories was similar across all drinker types (range 10.7–11.8 years).

Crude outcome statistics are also provided in Table 2. In the pooled sample, 4.9% of participants experienced an incident CHD (fatal or non-fatal) event during the follow-up. This was lowest for consistently heavy drinkers (3.8%) and highest for former-drinkers (6.1%). The mean follow-up time was 12.6 years (SD = 4.3). In total, 397,264.4 person-years at risk were captured, with mean person-years varying from 11.0 years (former drinkers) to 13.9 years (consistently heavy drinkers). The

overall CHD incidence rate was 4.3 CHD cases per 1000 person-years.

The proportion of individuals dying due to CHD during the follow-up was 0.9%. This varied between drinker types, from 0.6% for the consistently heavy group to 1.3% amongst consistent non-drinkers. The mean follow-up time was 13.7 years (SD = 4.1). In combination, 480,124.7 person-years were captured for this outcome, with the mean person-years again lowest for former drinkers (11.9 years) but highest for inconsistently moderate drinkers (14.8 years). The overall rate of fatal CHD was 0.7 cases per 1000 person-years.

Single intake measure categorisation

In a series of hierarchical Cox regression models with alcohol intake defined according to a single intake measurement just prior to the outcome follow-up period, no discernible difference in incident CHD risk was observed between heavy and moderate drinkers. However, those who reported no intake at this most recent measurement point had an increased risk of CHD compared to those who drank but did so within the recommended limits [model maximally adjusted for confounding: hazard ratio (HR) = 1.26, 95% confidence interval (CI) = 1.11–1.43]. The estimates are illustrated in Fig. 2 and reported in full in Additional file 1 (Section S5a).

Longitudinal intake trajectories

When modelling overall CHD risk using the longitudinal intake typology with adjustment for age, sex and intake assessment interval, both consistent non-drinkers (HR = 1.51, 95% CI = 1.25–1.82) and former drinkers (HR = 1.35, 95% CI = 1.16–1.57) showed greater risk of incident CHD compared to participants who reported persistently moderate intake. A smaller but still significant effect was also found for inconsistently moderate drinkers (HR = 1.21, 95% CI = 1.04–1.40). The effects remained statistically significant after additional adjustment for smoking status and socioeconomic position (detailed in Fig. 3). No differences in risk for heavy drinking, consistent or otherwise, were found.

When potential mediators, BMI and hypertension, were included in the modelling, the drinker type effects were attenuated, with the effect for inconsistently moderate drinkers becoming non-significant (HR = 1.16, 95% CI = 1.00–1.34). Full details of the modelling steps are provided in Additional file 1 (Section S5a), including the associations of each covariate with CHD onset risk. Older age, male sex, history (current or past) of smoking, higher BMI and

Table 2 Descriptive results: overall sample

Variable	Level	Drinker type							Overall
		Consistent non-drinker	Former drinker	Consistently moderate drinker	Inconsistently moderate drinker	Consistently heavy drinker	Inconsistently heavy drinker	Unknown	
Record count, N		2142	4080	11,410	5636	2565	2577	6722	35,132
Age, Mean (SD)		58.9 (8.1)	61.9 (9.1)	59.7 (8.1)	57.1 (6.4)	58.0 (5.7)	57.9 (6.6)	58.6 (7.3)	59.1 (7.7)
Sex, N (%)	Male	807 (37.7)	1831 (44.9)	7249 (63.5)	3599 (63.9)	2216 (86.4)	1979 (76.8)	4140 (61.6)	21,821 (62.1)
	Female	1335 (62.3)	2249 (55.1)	4161 (36.5)	2037 (36.1)	349 (13.6)	598 (23.2)	2582 (38.4)	13,311 (37.9)
Smoker, N (%)	No	1351 (63.1)	2383 (58.4)	6933 (60.8)	3124 (55.4)	1218 (47.5)	1234 (47.9)	2280 (33.9)	18,523 (52.7)
	Current smoker	321 (15.0)	494 (12.1)	1008 (8.8)	764 (13.6)	540 (21.1)	473 (18.4)	1022 (15.2)	4622 (13.2)
	Ex-smoker	407 (19.0)	1129 (27.7)	3322 (29.1)	1630 (28.9)	759 (29.6)	825 (32.0)	1335 (19.9)	9407 (26.8)
	Unknown	63 (2.9)	74 (1.8)	147 (1.3)	118 (2.1)	48 (1.9)	45 (1.7)	2085 (31.0)	2580 (7.3)
Socioeconomic position, N (%)	High	510 (23.8)	1353 (33.2)	5454 (47.8)	2279 (40.4)	1178 (45.9)	1198 (46.5)	2400 (35.7)	14,372 (40.9)
	Intermediate	1104 (51.5)	1953 (47.9)	4924 (43.2)	2708 (48.0)	1184 (46.2)	1158 (44.9)	3005 (44.7)	16,036 (45.6)
	Low	512 (23.9)	733 (18.0)	980 (8.6)	612 (10.9)	190 (7.4)	207 (8.0)	1263 (18.8)	4497 (12.8)
	Unknown	16 (0.7)	41 (1.0)	52 (0.5)	37 (0.7)	13 (0.5)	14 (0.5)	54 (0.8)	227 (0.6)
BMI, mean (SD)		26.2 (4.9)	26.3 (4.4)	25.6 (3.5)	26.0 (3.9)	26.1 (3.3)	26.2 (3.7)	26.5 (4.1)	26 (3.9)
High blood pressure, N (%)	No	1498 (69.9)	2784 (68.2)	8409 (73.7)	4010 (71.1)	1790 (69.8)	1759 (68.3)	3376 (50.2)	23,626 (67.2)
	Yes	641 (29.9)	1292 (31.7)	2990 (26.2)	1620 (28.7)	774 (30.2)	815 (31.6)	1551 (23.1)	9683 (27.6)
	Unknown	3 (0.1)	4 (0.1)	11 (0.1)	6 (0.1)	1 (~0.0)	3 (0.1)	1795 (26.7)	1823 (5.2)
Intake interval, mean (SD)		11.4 (2.6)	11.8 (2.4)	11.4 (2.2)	11.2 (2.4)	10.7 (1.7)	11.1 (2.3)	12.6 (2.8)	11.5 (2.4)
CHD (all) during follow-up, N (%)	No	1803 (84.2)	3549 (87.0)	10,260 (89.9)	4775 (84.7)	2375 (92.6)	2229 (86.5)	4748 (70.6)	29,739 (84.6)
	Yes	129 (6.0)	250 (6.1)	560 (4.9)	264 (4.7)	98 (3.8)	107 (4.2)	310 (4.6)	1718 (4.9)
	Unknown	210 (9.8)	281 (6.9)	590 (5.2)	597 (10.6)	92 (3.6)	241 (9.4)	1664 (24.8)	3675 (10.5)
CHD (all) person years, mean (SD)		12.7 (4.5)	11.0 (4.7)	12.4 (4.4)	13.8 (3.7)	13.9 (3.4)	13.5 (3.8)	12.1 (4.5)	12.6 (4.3)
CHD (fatal) during follow-up, N (%)	No	2113 (98.6)	4031 (98.8)	11,328 (99.3)	5593 (99.2)	2549 (99.4)	2550 (99.0)	6630 (98.6)	34,794 (99.0)
	Yes	27 (1.3)	49 (1.2)	78 (0.7)	40 (0.7)	15 (0.6)	25 (1.0)	91 (1.4)	325 (0.9)
	Unknown	2 (0.1)	0 (0.0)	4 (~0.0)	3 (0.1)	1 (~0.0)	2 (0.1)	1 (~0.0)	13 (~0.0)
CHD (fatal) person years, mean (SD)		13.9 (4.2)	11.9 (4.6)	13.2 (4.3)	14.8 (3.2)	14.6 (3.1)	14.3 (3.5)	13.9 (4.0)	13.7 (4.1)

BMI body mass index, kg/m2 kilogram per metre squared, CHD coronary heart disease, SD standard deviation, N count

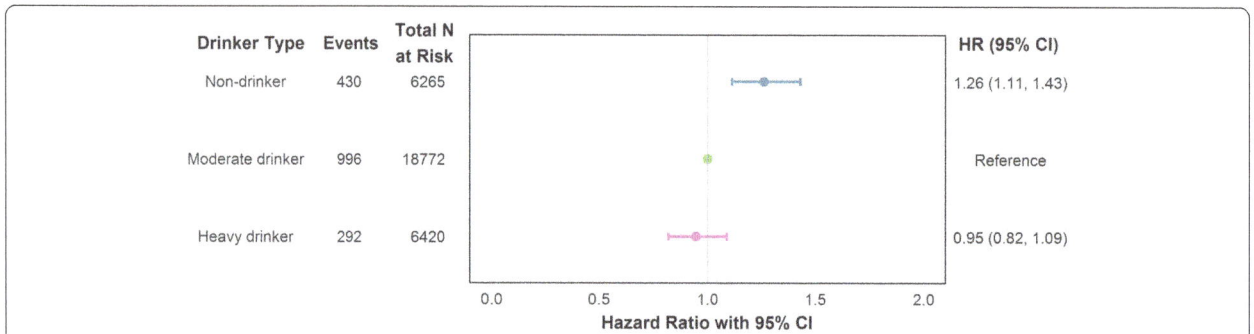

Fig. 2 Association of drinker type (single intake measurement) with incident (fatal or non-fatal) CHD using maximal adjustment for confounding. Adjustment variables comprised age, sex (reference category: male), socioeconomic position (reference category: intermediate), smoker status (reference category: non-smoker) and intake assessment interval. CHD coronary heart disease, CI confidence interval, HR hazard ratio

high blood pressure were all significantly associated with increased risk of CHD.

Stratified analyses

In age-stratified analyses of the longitudinal trajectory exposure, participants aged up to 55 years and those aged above showed comparable associations with the incident CHD outcome (visualised in Fig. 4). Consistent non-drinkers (aged ≤55: HR = 1.97, 95% CI = 1.29–3.02; aged > 55: HR = 1.38, 95% CI = 1.11–1.71) and former drinkers (aged ≤55: HR = 1.60, 95% CI = 1.09–2.37; aged > 55: HR = 1.27, 95% CI = 1.08–1.51) both demonstrated significantly greater CHD risk compared to consistently moderate drinkers. However, inconsistently moderate drinkers in the older age group also had an increased risk of incident CHD (HR = 1.25, 95% CI = 1.06–1.48), a

finding not replicated in the younger subsample. Further details are provided in Additional file 1 (Section S6a).

Further stratified analyses were performed to assess if the alcohol–CHD association differed by sex, again using the longitudinal intake categories (illustrated in Fig. 5). Amongst male participants, former drinkers were at significantly greater risk of incident CHD compared to consistently moderate drinkers after maximal adjustment for confounding factors (HR = 1.29, 95% CI = 1.06–1.56). After equivalent adjustment in the female stratum, both former drinkers (HR = 1.38, 95% CI = 1.07–1.78) and consistent non-drinkers (HR = 1.91, 95% CI = 1.43–2.55) showed increased risk compared to their consistently moderate counterparts. A full table of results is provided in Additional file 1 (Section S7a).

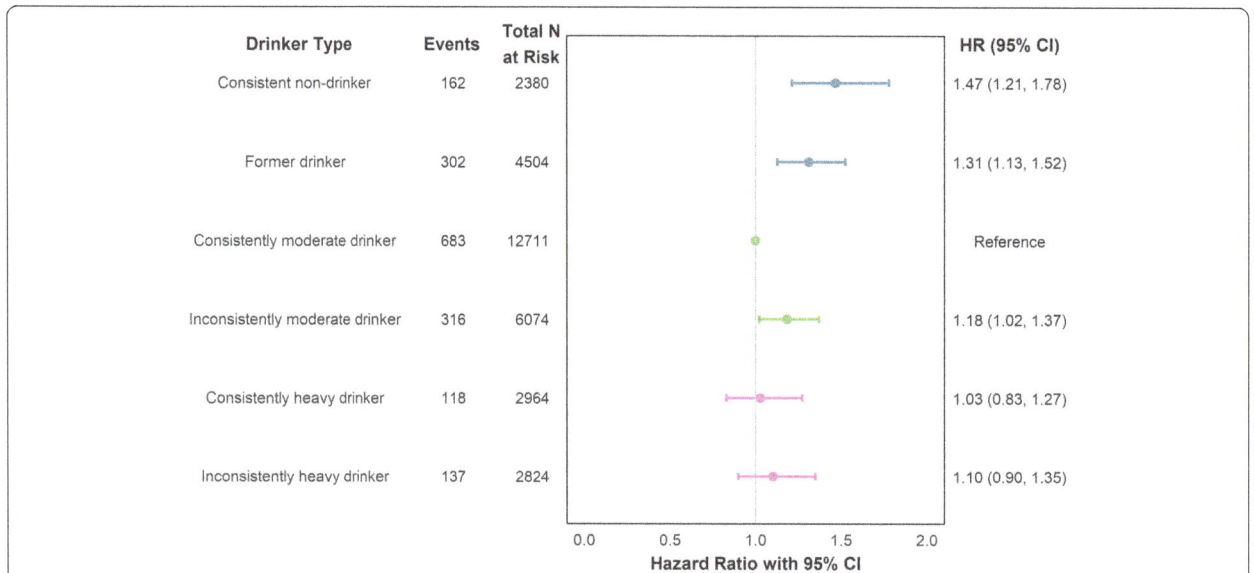

Fig. 3 Association of drinker type (longitudinal intake measurement) with incident (fatal or non-fatal) CHD using maximal adjustment for confounding. Adjustment variables comprised age, sex (reference category: male), socioeconomic position (reference category: intermediate), smoker status (reference category: non-smoker) and intake assessment interval. CHD coronary heart disease, CI confidence interval, HR hazard ratio

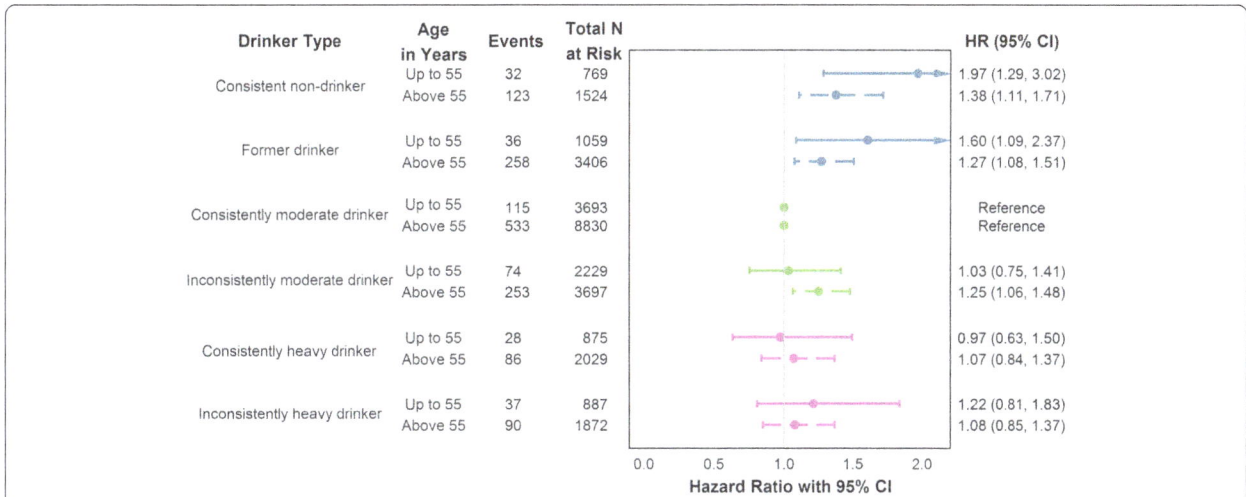

Drinker Type	Age in Years	Events	Total N at Risk		HR (95% CI)
Consistent non-drinker	Up to 55	32	769		1.97 (1.29, 3.02)
	Above 55	123	1524		1.38 (1.11, 1.71)
Former drinker	Up to 55	36	1059		1.60 (1.09, 2.37)
	Above 55	258	3406		1.27 (1.08, 1.51)
Consistently moderate drinker	Up to 55	115	3693		Reference
	Above 55	533	8830		Reference
Inconsistently moderate drinker	Up to 55	74	2229		1.03 (0.75, 1.41)
	Above 55	253	3697		1.25 (1.06, 1.48)
Consistently heavy drinker	Up to 55	28	875		0.97 (0.63, 1.50)
	Above 55	86	2029		1.07 (0.84, 1.37)
Inconsistently heavy drinker	Up to 55	37	887		1.22 (0.81, 1.83)
	Above 55	90	1872		1.08 (0.85, 1.37)

Fig. 4 Age-stratified association of drinker type (longitudinal intake measurement) with incident (fatal or non-fatal) CHD using maximal adjustment for confounding. Adjustment variables comprised age, sex (reference category: male), socioeconomic position (reference category: intermediate), smoker status (reference category: non-smoker) and intake assessment interval. CHD coronary heart disease, CI confidence interval, HR hazard ratio

CHD mortality

When analyses were replicated using fatal CHD as the outcome, most results were comparable to those obtained when using all incident CHD events. For the longitudinal intake trajectories, and in contrast to the incident CHD analysis, inconsistently moderate drinkers did not have a greater CHD mortality risk compared to the consistently moderate reference group (HR = 1.04, 95% CI = 0.72–1.52). Only former drinkers had a significantly elevated risk of fatal CHD (HR = 1.54, 95% CI = 1.07–2.22) after maximal adjustment for confounding factors, but the HR for consistent non-drinkers was near identical (HR = 1.52, 95% CI = 0.97–2.38), implying that again both drinker types were at

elevated risk of fatal CHD. Inconsistently heavy drinkers did show some evidence of having an increased risk of experiencing a fatal CHD event in the lesser-adjusted model (HR = 1.53, 95% CI = 0.99–2.37), but it did not achieve statistical significance and was attenuated after additional adjustment for smoking status and socioeconomic status (HR = 1.36, 95% CI = 0.87–2.11). Full model details are provided in Additional file 1 (Section S5b).

Age-stratified analyses revealed similar patterns of association as with the pooled (non-stratified) analysis. In sex-stratified analyses, however, some differences were observed, with only female consistent non-drinkers having an elevated risk of fatal CHD after adjustment for covariates

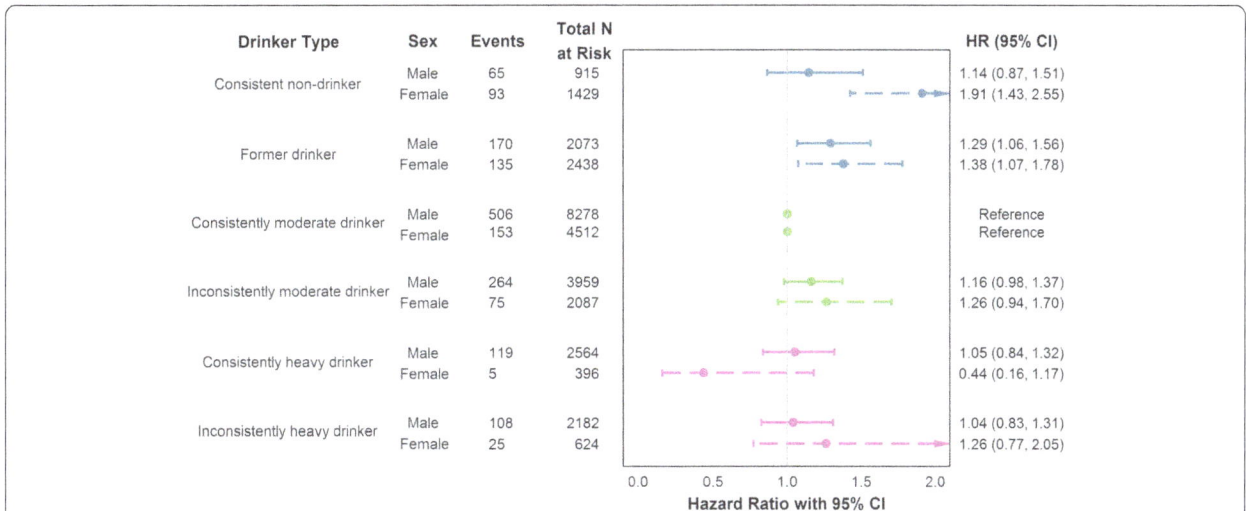

Drinker Type	Sex	Events	Total N at Risk		HR (95% CI)
Consistent non-drinker	Male	65	915		1.14 (0.87, 1.51)
	Female	93	1429		1.91 (1.43, 2.55)
Former drinker	Male	170	2073		1.29 (1.06, 1.56)
	Female	135	2438		1.38 (1.07, 1.78)
Consistently moderate drinker	Male	506	8278		Reference
	Female	153	4512		Reference
Inconsistently moderate drinker	Male	264	3959		1.16 (0.98, 1.37)
	Female	75	2087		1.26 (0.94, 1.70)
Consistently heavy drinker	Male	119	2564		1.05 (0.84, 1.32)
	Female	5	396		0.44 (0.16, 1.17)
Inconsistently heavy drinker	Male	108	2182		1.04 (0.83, 1.31)
	Female	25	624		1.26 (0.77, 2.05)

Fig. 5 Sex-stratified association of drinker type (longitudinal intake measurement) with incident (fatal or non-fatal) CHD using maximal adjustment for confounding. Adjustment variables comprised age, socioeconomic position (reference category: intermediate), smoker status (reference category: non-smoker) and intake assessment interval. CHD coronary heart disease, CI confidence interval, HR hazard ratio

(HR = 2.62, 95% CI = 1.25–5.49). Additional detail on age-stratified and sex-stratified analyses are included in Additional file 1 (Sections S6b and S7b, respectively).

Sensitivity analyses

As the GAZEL cohort was the only non-UK data source included in this study, the longitudinal modelling was replicated with this cohort's data omitted to verify that its inclusion did not introduce bias. Results obtained using only UK data sources were essentially unchanged from the findings attained when all cohorts were included (details are provided in Additional file 1: Section S8). To identify the impact of the imputation model implemented in the primary analyses, the modelling was also performed using complete case data only. The point estimates and significance of effects were essentially unchanged from the imputed data modelling (see Additional file 1: Section S9).

Discussion

In this study, we utilised prospectively collected longitudinal data on alcohol consumption from six cohorts to examine the association of 10-year drinking trajectories and risk of developing and/or dying from CHD. Through iterative modelling that accounted for heterogeneity across the datasets and potential confounders of the alcohol–CHD association, our work has shown that incident CHD risk is significantly higher amongst both non-drinkers and former drinkers compared to drinkers who always adhered to lower-risk intake guidelines. We have also demonstrated that the stability of such adherence is pertinent. Participants who mostly drank moderately, but not persistently so, had greater risk of incident CHD compared to their consistently moderate drinking counterparts. In terms of CHD mortality, former drinkers and consistent non-drinkers were again found to be at higher risk, although the effect for the persistent abstainers was somewhat attenuated after adjustment for smoking status and socioeconomic status. We found no evidence that heavy drinking was associated with risk of CHD, and reasons for this are discussed below. Overall, the findings from this study support the notion of a cardioprotective effect of moderate alcohol intake relative to non-drinking. However, crucially, stability in the level of alcohol consumption over time appears to be an important modifier of this association.

The use of repeat measurements of alcohol consumption in lieu of a one-time assessment has enabled us to measure the stability of consumption over time and to address the call for research on the role of intake trajectories in CHD onset [43]. Through this approach, we have demonstrated how intermittent adherence to lower-risk drinking guidelines, i.e. an inconsistently moderate intake, is associated with an increased risk of incident CHD. This provides some support for the proposal that variability in alcohol intake levels can offset the potential protective effects of moderate drinking [2, 20]. An association was found between inconsistently heavy drinkers and fatal CHD, although the wide confidence bounds and weakening of the association following maximal adjustment for confounding factors limits interpretation of this effect. It may be that unstable drinking patterns reflect wider lifestyle changes across the life course, and possibly even the impact of periods of ill health or life stress. The effects were further attenuated when adjustment was made for clinical characteristics, namely BMI and hypertension, suggesting that these may both act as potential pathways through which unstable drinking trajectories are associated with CHD. The impact of BMI could also reflect the role of other lifestyle choices, such as diet and exercise.

Access to prospectively recorded alcohol intake data across multiple assessment times has also allowed the current study to distinguish recent abstainers from longer-term non-drinkers in a manner that helps reduce the potential for recall bias. Such bias can occur where drinking behaviour is retrospectively measured at a single time point [44], a technique commonly used in alcohol epidemiology research. In line with the sick-quitter hypothesis [14], former drinkers were found in the present study to have an elevated risk of both incident and fatal CHD. These effects were attenuated following adjustment for the clinical covariates, suggesting that poor health may explain former drinkers' increased likelihood of developing CHD and perhaps may even have motivated the decision to abstain itself. Consistent non-drinkers, however, did also have a significant risk of incident CHD after adjustment for potential confounders, and although the error bounds were wider, their CHD mortality estimate was equivalent to that of former drinkers, implying that short- and long-term abstinence are both associated with an increased risk of CHD.

Despite our finding of parity in CHD risk amongst non-drinkers and former drinkers in the pooled sample analyses, previous research has suggested that there may be age-dependent differences in this association. However, this observation was based on studies in which abstinence was determined retrospectively from a single baseline assessment [42], in contrast to the repeated measures design used in the current study. When we stratified our sample by age, the associations between both abstainer groups and incident CHD risk was comparable for younger (≤55 years) and older (>55 years) participants. As similar results were also observed for risk of fatal CHD, our findings challenge the argument that there are age-dependent differences between long-term and more recent abstainers, yet the wide confidence bounds around the fatal CHD risk estimates for those aged 55 or below arguably restricts such inferences. A divergence between the age groups was found for inconsistently moderate drinkers. Such drinkers in the older subsample had a significantly elevated risk of incident CHD, an effect that was not evident in the younger group. Older participants may have been more likely to experience lifestyle changes that influenced their drinking habits. Retirement, for example, is known to co-occur with increases in alcohol intake [45, 46], particularly amongst existing drinkers [47].

It has also been suggested that the J-shaped association between alcohol consumption and CHD may be more pronounced in women than men [23], a theory that our study supports in part. Whilst both male and female former drinkers had significantly increased risk of incident CHD, only female consistent non-drinkers showed such an elevated risk. Female non-drinkers (both long term and more recent abstainers) were similarly at risk of fatal CHD, even after maximal adjustment for confounding factors. Research has also suggested that alcohol intake may increase oestrogen levels in women, which in turn act as a protective factor against CHD [48]. Male former drinkers also showed significantly greater risk of CHD mortality than consistently moderate drinkers after accounting for age and other characteristics, but this difference was attenuated once the estimates were adjusted for lifestyle behaviours such as smoking. This suggests that these additional covariates may play a greater role than drinking in the occurrence of fatal CHD events for males. Previous literature has proposed that smoking can offset any alcohol-related differences in CHD mortality risk amongst men [49].

In the present study, no association with CHD risk was found for consistently heavy drinkers. Stable patterns of heavy drinking may reflect continued good health across the assessment interval [50], the converse of the sick quitter type. Statistically significant associations between high levels of alcohol intake and CHD onset risk have been observed in some previous research [21, 51], but not persistently so [52–54]. Although our study identified heavy drinkers across all cohorts, only a limited number were in the female sample, potentially limiting statistical power in their analysis, and by extension, in the non-stratified analysis. This issue of small counts for female heavy drinkers has similarly constrained earlier work in this area [1]. Particularly heavy drinkers may be under-represented in the datasets utilised in this study, which could have biased downwards the estimate of association between heavy intake and cardiovascular risk. If further data are available, it may be possible to explore alternative intake thresholds and validate the present study's findings. Similarly, additional data may enable the disaggregation of CHD phenotypes, which could provide more nuanced insights into how heavy drinking is associated with different variants of the disease [55]. Consequently, the interpretation of the absence of an effect amongst heavy drinkers in the current study should be done cautiously, particularly in light of the known wider health impact of heavy alcohol intake levels [56].

There are additional limitations to our study that warrant consideration. For example, selection bias may have occurred [57], in which participants dropped out of the cohort studies before the outcome assessment period. It is possible that some heavy drinkers could have experienced adverse health outcomes at a younger age and discontinued their research participation. Particularly heavy drinkers are already known to be under-sampled in population-level surveys [32, 58], so caution is required in drawing inferences about such elevated intake levels. Similarly, information on alcohol intake prior to the exposure assessment period was not consistently available, so the long-term abstainers modelled in this current study may include some participants who ceased drinking prior to recruitment. Given that the current work included only cohort studies for which we had access to individual-level data, the concept of availability bias [59] is also pertinent. Access to additional datasets may help further validate our findings. Such increased sample sizes would also permit more detailed examination than was possible in the current study into the intake variance that occurs amongst drinkers who are inconsistent in their adherence to lower-risk drinking guidelines. Relatedly, the identification of drinking trajectories in the present study was based on drinking volume only and so we were not equipped to look at the role of episodic heavy drinking [60]. Further clarification of the alcohol–CHD association may be achieved where sufficient data are available on other characteristics of consumption, such as drinking frequency. All cohorts included in the current study used self-report for determining alcohol intake; although this is vulnerable to estimation errors, research has shown that drinking data collected through this method remains valid and reliable [44, 61]. A further design consideration in interpreting the current study's results is the harmonisation of data across the different cohort datasets. Establishing equivalent variable definitions in the harmonisation of data constrains the level of detail and raises the possibility of residual confounding. For example, it was not possible to establish a more nuanced smoking variable due to data availability and so there is a possibility of residual confounding by smoking intensity. Relatedly, although an equal number of intake measurements was used across cohorts to establish intake trajectories, the observed time intervals varied (see Section S2 of Additional file 1). While adjustment was made through inclusion of assessment interval length in the regression modelling, it remains possible that limitations in the cohort data harmonisation may have introduced bias. Although country-specific drink conversions were used to calculate alcohol intake [31], there remains potential differences between GAZEL and the other cohorts, such as the possible influence of dietary differences for which residual confounding could also have occurred [62]. The French paradox, for example, implies that that there is an inverse relationship between saturated fat intake and CHD onset risk that is specific to France [63], a relationship in which alcohol debatably plays a role [64]. However, sensitivity analyses showed that the exclusion of GAZEL data did not modify the current study findings. Moreover, the use throughout this study of mixed-effects modelling has helped account for data clustering and thereby helped improve the validity of the results obtained.

Conclusions

In summary, the present study has utilised longitudinal alcohol intake data pooled from multiple cohort sources to establish trajectories of drinking behaviour and assess their association with risk of incident and fatal CHD. The study has demonstrated that recent and more long-term abstainers are at elevated risk of developing CHD, although the effect for persistent abstainers may be confined to females only. The trajectory approach used in this work has also enabled us to show that stability of alcohol intake levels amongst those who do not abstain is pertinent to risk of CHD onset. Drinkers who mostly, but inconsistently, adhered to moderate drinking levels, particularly if aged over 55 years, were found to have elevated risk of incident CHD. There was also some indication that variability in drinking levels amongst heavier drinkers were associated with increased likelihood of CHD mortality, although that effect was attenuated by adjustment for other demographic and lifestyle characteristics. No evidence of elevated risk amongst consistently heavy drinkers was found but this was potentially attributable to under-representation of such drinkers in the sampled data. These findings, nonetheless, illustrate that longitudinal alcohol trajectories have added utility in identifying at-risk drinker types beyond what is possible with single assessments of alcohol consumption. Our findings provide additional insight into the potential cardioprotective effect of moderate alcohol intake, and indicate that consistency of intake levels is a relevant consideration in cardiovascular risk assessments, and in related health education efforts.

Abbreviations

BMI: Body mass index; CHD: Coronary heart disease; CI: Confidence interval; EPIC-N: European Prospective Investigation of Cancer, Norfolk; GAZEL: Gaz et Electricité; HR: Hazard ratio; ICD: International Statistical Classification of Diseases and Related Health Problems; IPD: Individual participant data; NSHD: Medical Research Council's National Survey of Health and Development 1946; SD: Standard deviation; T07-1930s: West of Scotland Twenty-07 Study 1930s; T07-1950s: West of Scotland Twenty-07 Study 1950s; WII: Whitehall II

Acknowledgments

We thank all participants, researchers and support staff involved in the EPIC-N, NSHD, West of Scotland Twenty-07, WII and GAZEL studies.

Funding

This work has been undertaken as part of the Alcohol Life-course Project (http://www.ucl.ac.uk/alcohol-lifecourse), which is funded by the UK Medical Research Council/Alcohol Research UK (MR/M006638/1) and the European Research Council (ERC-StG-2012-309337_AlcoholLifecourse).
EPIC-N is supported by programme grants from the UK Medical Research Council (G0401527 and G1000143) and Cancer Research United Kingdom (C864/A8257) with additional support from the Stroke Association, British Heart Foundation, Research Into Ageing and the Academy of Medical Science.
GAZEL was partly supported by Agence Nationale De La Recherché (ANR-08-BLAN-0028-01), Agence Française de Sécurité Sanitaire de l'Environnement et du Travail (AFSSET-EST08–35), Electricité de France-Gaz de France and the TGIR Cohortes Santé 2008 Program.
NSHD is supported by the UK Medical Research Council (MR_UC_12019/01). Twenty-07 is funded by the UK Medical Research Council (MC_A540_53462 and MC_UU_12017/13). WII is supported by the UK Medical Research Council (MR/K013351/1 and G0902037), the British Heart Foundation (RG/13/2/30098) and the US National Institutes of Health (R01HL36310 and R01AG013196). The funding bodies had no role in the design of this study, the collection, analysis, and interpretation of the data, or in writing the manuscript.

Authors' contributions

DON, AB and SB devised the study, designed the study protocol, analysed the data, interpreted the output and wrote the manuscript. MKH, MG, DK and KTK provided data access and critical revisions of the manuscript. All authors read and approved the final version.

Competing interests

The authors declare that they have no competing interests.

Author details

[1]CLOSER, Department of Social Science, Institute of Education, University College London, London, UK. [2]Research Department of Epidemiology and Public Health, University College London, London, UK. [3]MRC/CSO Social and Public Health Sciences Unit, Institute of Health and Wellbeing, University of Glasgow, Glasgow, UK. [4]Inserm UMS 011, Villejuif, France and Paris Descartes University, Villejuif, France. [5]UK MRC Unit for Lifelong Health & Ageing at UCL, London, UK. [6]Cambridge Institute of Public Health, University of Cambridge, Cambridge, UK. [7]Department of Public Health and Primary Care, University of Cambridge, Cambridge, UK.

References

1. Roerecke M, Rehm J. Chronic heavy drinking and ischaemic heart disease: a systematic review and meta-analysis. Open Heart. 2014;1:e000135.
2. Ruidavets J-B, Ducimetière P, Evans A, Montaye M, Haas B, Bingham A, et al. Patterns of alcohol consumption and ischaemic heart disease in culturally divergent countries: the prospective epidemiological study of myocardial infarction (PRIME). BMJ. 2010;341:c6077.
3. Stockwell T, Chikritzhs T. Commentary: another serious challenge to the hypothesis that moderate drinking is good for health? Int J Epidemiol. 2013; 42:1792–4.
4. Thompson PL. J-curve revisited: cardiovascular benefits of moderate alcohol use cannot be dismissed. Med J Aust. 2013;198:419–22.
5. de Gaetano G, Costanzo S. Alcohol and health: Praise of the J curves. J Am Coll Cardiol. 2017;70:923 LP–925.
6. Roerecke M, Kaczorowski J, Tobe SW, Gmel G, Hasan OSM, Rehm J. The effect of a reduction in alcohol consumption on blood pressure: a systematic review and meta-analysis. Lancet Public Health. 2017;2:e108–20.
7. Chen L, Davey Smith G, Harbord RM, Lewis SJ, Smith GD, Harbord RM, et al. Alcohol intake and blood pressure: a systematic review implementing a Mendelian randomization approach. PLoS Med. 2008;5:0461–71.
8. Cho Y, Shin S-Y, Won S, Relton CL, Davey Smith G, Shin M-J. Alcohol intake and cardiovascular risk factors: a Mendelian randomisation study. Sci Rep. 2015;5:18422.
9. Holmes MV, Asselbergs FW, Palmer TM, Drenos F, Lanktree MB, Nelson CP, et al. Mendelian randomization of blood lipids for coronary heart disease. Eur Heart J. 2015;36:539–50.
10. Tabara Y, Ueshima H, Takashima N, Hisamatsu T, Fujiyoshi A, Zaid M, et al. Mendelian randomization analysis in three Japanese populations supports a causal role of alcohol consumption in lowering low-density lipid cholesterol levels and particle numbers. Atherosclerosis. 2016;254:242–8.
11. Caetano R. Does a little drinking make your heart grow stronger? J Stud Alcohol Drugs. 2017;78:341–3.
12. Fillmore KM, Kerr WC, Stockwell T, Chikritzhs T, Bostrom A. Moderate alcohol use and reduced mortality risk: systematic error in prospective studies. Addict Res Theory. 2006;14:101–32.
13. Rimm EB, Moats C. Alcohol and coronary heart disease: drinking patterns and mediators of effect. Ann Epidemiol. 2007;17:S3–7.
14. Rehm J, Irving H, Ye Y, Kerr WC, Bond J, Greenfield TK. Are lifetime abstainers the best control group in alcohol epidemiology? On the stability and validity of reported lifetime abstention. Am J Epidemiol. 2008;168:866–71.
15. Roerecke M. On bias in alcohol epidemiology and the search for the perfect study. Addiction. 2017;112:217–8.
16. Knott CS, Bell S, Britton A. The stability of baseline-defined categories of alcohol consumption over the adult life course: a 28-year prospective cohort study. Addiction. 2018;113:34–43.
17. Britton A, Hardy R, Kuh D, Deanfield J, Charakida M, Bell S. Twenty-year trajectories of alcohol consumption during midlife and atherosclerotic thickening in early old age: findings from two British population cohort studies. BMC Med. 2016;14:111.
18. O'Neill D, Britton A, Brunner EJ, Bell S. Twenty-five-year alcohol consumption trajectories and their association with arterial aging: a prospective cohort study. J Am Heart Assoc. 2017;6:e005288.
19. Bell S, Mehta G, Moore K, Britton A. Ten-year alcohol consumption typologies and trajectories of C-reactive protein, interleukin-6 and interleukin-1 receptor antagonist over the following 12 years: a prospective cohort study. J Intern Med. 2017;281:75–85.
20. Emberson JR, Shaper AG, Wannamethee SG, Morris RW, Whincup PH. Alcohol intake in middle age and risk of cardiovascular disease and mortality: accounting for intake variation over time. Am J Epidemiol. 2005;161:856–63.
21. Britton A, Marmot MG, Shipley MJ. How does variability in alcohol consumption over time affect the relationship with mortality and coronary heart disease? Addiction. 2010;105:639–45.
22. Rehm J, Sempos CT, Trevisan M. Average volume of alcohol consumption, patterns of drinking and risk of coronary heart disease - a review. J Cardiovasc Risk. 2003;10:15–20.
23. Roerecke M, Rehm J. The cardioprotective association of average alcohol consumption and ischaemic heart disease: a systematic review and meta-analysis. Addiction. 2012;107:1246–60.
24. Day N, Oakes S, Luben R, Khaw K-T, Bingham S, Welch A, et al. EPIC-Norfolk: study design and characteristics of the cohort. Br J Cancer. 1999;80(Suppl 1):95–103.
25. Kuh D, Pierce M, Adams J, Deanfield J, Ekelund U, Friberg P, et al. Cohort profile: updating the cohort profile for the MRC National Survey of health and development: a new clinic-based data collection for ageing research. Int J Epidemiol. 2011;40:e1–9.
26. Benzeval M, Der G, Ellaway A, Hunt K, Sweeting H, West P, et al. Cohort profile: west of Scotland Twenty-07 study: health in the community. Int J Epidemiol. 2009;38:1215–23.
27. Marmot M, Brunner E. Cohort profile: the Whitehall II study. Int J Epidemiol. 2005;34:251–6.
28. Goldberg M, Leclerc A, Zins M. Cohort profile update: The GAZEL cohort study. Int J Epidemiol. 2015;44:77g.
29. World Health Organization. The ICD-10 classification of mental and behavioural disorders: clinical descriptions and diagnostic guidelines. Geneva: World Health Organization; 1992.
30. The Royal College of General Practitioners. The classification and analysis of general practice data. Occasional paper no. 26. 2nd ed. London: The Royal College of General Practitioners; 1986.
31. Kalinowski A, Humphreys K. Governmental standard drink definitions and low-risk alcohol consumption guidelines in 37 countries. Addiction. 2016; 111:1293–8.
32. Britton A, O'Neill D, Bell S. Underestimating the alcohol content of a glass of wine: the implications for estimates of mortality risk. Alcohol Alcohol. 2016; 51:609–14.
33. Royal Colleges of Physicians Psychiatrists and General Practitioners. Alcohol and the heart in perspective: Sensible limits reaffirmed. J R Coll Physicians Lond. 1995;29:266–71.
34. Department of Health. UK chief medical officers' low risk drinking guidelines. London: Department of Health; 2016.
35. Holmes J, Angus C, Buykx P, Ally AK, Stone T, Meier P, et al. Mortality and morbidity risks from alcohol consumption in the UK: analyses using the Sheffield alcohol policy model (v.2.7) to inform the UK chief medical officers' review of the UK lower risk drinking guidelines. Sheffield: ScHARR, University of Sheffield; 2016.
36. Office for National Statistics. Standard occupational classification 2010. Basingstoke: Palgrave Macmillan; 2010.
37. White IR, Royston P. Imputing missing covariate values for the cox model. Stat Med. 2009;28:1982–98.
38. Thompson S, Kaptoge S, White I, Wood A, Perry P, Danesh J, et al. Statistical methods for the time-to-event analysis of individual participant data from multiple epidemiological studies. Int J Epidemiol. 2010;39:1345–59.
39. Debray TPA, Moons KGM, van Valkenhoef G, Efthimiou O, Hummel N, Groenwold RHH, et al. Get real in individual participant data (IPD) meta-analysis: a review of the methodology. Res Synth Methods. 2015;6:293–309.
40. Thomas D, Radji S, Benedetti A. Systematic review of methods for individual patient data meta-analysis with binary outcomes. BMC Med Res Methodol. 2014;14:79.
41. Tierney JF, Vale C, Riley R, Smith CT, Stewart L, Clarke M, et al. Individual participant data (IPD) meta-analyses of randomised controlled trials: guidance on their use. PLoS Med. 2015;12:e1001855.
42. Zhao J, Stockwell T, Roemer A, Naimi T, Chikritzhs T. Alcohol consumption and mortality from coronary heart disease: an updated meta-analysis of cohort studies. J Stud Alcohol Drugs. 2017;78:375–86.
43. Maggs JL, Staff J. No benefit of light to moderate drinking for mortality from coronary heart disease when better comparison groups and controls included: a commentary on Zhao et al. (2017). J Stud Alcohol Drugs. 2017; 78:387–8.
44. Bell S, Britton A. Reliability of a retrospective decade-based life-course alcohol consumption questionnaire administered in later life. Addiction. 2015;110:1563–73.
45. Zins M, Guéguen A, Kivimaki M, Singh-Manoux A, Leclerc A, Vahtera J, et al. Effect of retirement on alcohol consumption: longitudinal evidence from the French GAZEL cohort study. PLoS One. 2011;6:e26531.
46. Halonen JI, Stenholm S, Pulakka A, Kawachi I, Aalto V, Pentti J, et al. Trajectories of risky drinking around the time of statutory retirement: a longitudinal latent class analysis. Addiction. 2017;112:1163–70.
47. Wang X, Steier JB, Gallo WT. The effect of retirement on alcohol consumption: results from the US health and retirement study. Eur J Pub Health. 2014;24:485–9.

48. Grønbæk M. The positive and negative health effects of alcohol- and the public health implications. J Intern Med. 2009;265:407–20.

49. Xu W-H, Zhang X-L, Gao Y-T, Xiang Y-B, Gao L-F, Zheng W, et al. Joint effect of cigarette smoking and alcohol consumption on mortality. Prev Med. 2007;45:313–9.

50. Ng Fat L, Cable N, Shelton N. Worsening of health and a cessation or reduction in alcohol consumption to special occasion drinking across three decades of the life course. Alcohol Clin Exp Res. 2015;39:166–74.

51. Bobak M, Malyutina S, Horvat P, Pajak A, Tamosiunas A, Kubinova R, et al. Alcohol, drinking pattern and all-cause, cardiovascular and alcohol-related mortality in Eastern Europe. Eur J Epidemiol. 2016;31:21–30.

52. Dai J, Mukamal KJ, Krasnow RE, Swan GE, Reed T. Higher usual alcohol consumption was associated with a lower 41-y mortality risk from coronary artery disease in men independent of genetic and common environmental factors: the prospective NHLBI twin study. Am J Clin Nutr. 2015;102:31–9.

53. Huang C, Zhan J, Liu Y-J, Li D-J, Wang S-Q, He Q-Q. Association between alcohol consumption and risk of cardiovascular disease and all-cause mortality in patients with hypertension: a meta-analysis of prospective cohort studies. Mayo Clin Proc. 2014;89:1201–10.

54. Bell S, Daskalopoulou M, Rapsomaniki E, George J, Britton A, Bobak M, et al. Association between clinically recorded alcohol consumption and initial presentation of 12 cardiovascular diseases: population based cohort study using linked health records. BMJ. 2017;356:j909.

55. Bell S, Hemingway H. Alcohol and cardiovascular disease: Author's response. BMJ. 2017;356:j1340.

56. Molina PE, Gardner JD, Souza-smith FM, Annie M, Molina PE, Gardner JD, et al. Alcohol abuse: critical pathophysiological processes and contribution to disease burden. Physiology. 2014;29:203–15.

57. Naimi TS, Stockwell T, Zhao J, Xuan Z, Dangardt F, Saitz R, et al. Selection biases in observational studies affect associations between 'moderate' alcohol consumption and mortality. Addiction. 2017;112:207–14.

58. Britton A, Ben-Shlomo Y, Benzeval M, Kuh D, Bell S. Life course trajectories of alcohol consumption in the United Kingdom using longitudinal data from nine cohort studies. BMC Med. 2015;13:47.

59. Riley RD. Commentary: like it and lump it? Meta-analysis using individual participant data. Int J Epidemiol. 2010;39:1359–61.

60. Roerecke M, Greenfield TK, Kerr WC, Bondy S, Cohen J, Rehm J. Heavy drinking occasions in relation to ischaemic heart disease mortality - an 11–22 year follow-up of the 1984 and 1995 US national alcohol surveys. Int J Epidemiol. 2011;40:1401–10.

61. Batty GD, Shipley M, Tabák A, Singh-Manoux A, Brunner E, Britton A, et al. Generalizability of occupational cohort study findings. Epidemiology. 2014; 25:932–3.

62. Zhang X-Y, Shu L, Si C-J, Yu X-L, Liao D, Gao W, et al. Dietary patterns, alcohol consumption and risk of coronary heart disease in adults: a meta-analysis. Nutrients. 2015;7:6582–605.

63. Chiva-Blanch G, Arranz S, Lamuela-Raventos RM, Estruch R. Effects of wine, alcohol and polyphenols on cardiovascular disease risk factors: evidences from human studies. Alcohol Alcohol. 2013;48:270–7.

64. Biagi M, Bertelli AAE. Wine, alcohol and pills: what future for the French paradox? Life Sci. 2015;131:19–22.

14

Clinical utility of the S3-score for molecular prediction of outcome in non-metastatic and metastatic clear cell renal cell carcinoma

Florian Büttner[1,2], Stefan Winter[1,2], Steffen Rausch[3], Jörg Hennenlotter[3], Stephan Kruck[3], Arnulf Stenzl[3], Marcus Scharpf[4], Falko Fend[4], Abbas Agaimy[5], Arndt Hartmann[5], Jens Bedke[3,6], Matthias Schwab[1,2,6,7,8*†] and Elke Schaeffeler[1,2*†]

Abstract

Background: Stratification of cancer patients to identify those with worse prognosis is increasingly important. Through in silico analyses, we recently developed a gene expression-based prognostic score (S3-score) for clear cell renal cell carcinoma (ccRCC), using the cell type-specific expression of 97 genes within the human nephron. Herein, we verified the score using whole-transcriptome data of independent cohorts and extend its application for patients with metastatic disease receiving tyrosine kinase inhibitor treatment. Finally, we sought to improve the signature for clinical application using qRT-PCR.

Methods: A 97 gene-based S3-score ($S3_{97}$) was evaluated in a set of 52 primary non-metastatic and metastatic ccRCC patients as well as in 53 primary metastatic tumors of sunitinib-treated patients. Gene expression data of The Cancer Genome Atlas ($n = 463$) was used for platform transfer and development of a simplified qRT-PCR-based 15-gene S3-score ($S3_{15}$). This $S3_{15}$-score was validated in 108 metastatic and non-metastatic ccRCC patients and ccRCC-derived metastases including in part several regions from one metastasis. Univariate and multivariate Cox regression stratified by T, N, M, and G were performed with cancer-specific and progression-free survival as primary endpoints.

Results: The $S3_{97}$-score was significantly associated with cancer-specific survival (CSS) in 52 ccRCC patients (HR 2.9, 95% CI 1.0–8.0, $P_{\text{Log-rank}} = 3.3 \times 10^{-2}$) as well as progression-free survival in sunitinib-treated patients (2.1, 1.1–4.2, $P_{\text{Log-rank}} = 2.2 \times 10^{-2}$). The qRT-PCR based $S3_{15}$-score performed similarly to the $S3_{97}$-score, and was significantly associated with CSS in our extended cohort of 108 patients (5.0, 2.1–11.7, $P_{\text{Log-rank}} = 5.1 \times 10^{-5}$) including metastatic (9.3, 1.8–50.0, $P_{\text{Log-rank}} = 2.3 \times 10^{-3}$) and non-metastatic patients (4.4, 1.2–16.3, $P_{\text{Log-rank}} = 1.6 \times 10^{-2}$), even in multivariate Cox regression, including clinicopathological parameters (7.3, 2.5–21.5, $P_{\text{Wald}} = 3.3 \times 10^{-4}$). Matched primary tumors and metastases revealed similar $S3_{15}$-scores, thus allowing prediction of outcome from metastatic tissue. The molecular-based qRT-PCR $S3_{15}$-score significantly improved prediction of CSS by the established clinicopathological-based SSIGN score ($P = 1.6 \times 10^{-3}$).

Conclusion: The S3-score offers a new clinical avenue for ccRCC risk stratification in the non-metastatic, metastatic, and sunitinib-treated setting.

Keywords: Renal cell carcinoma, Prognostic marker, Survival, ccRCC, Metastases, Sunitinib

* Correspondence:
matthias.schwab@ikp-stuttgart.de; elke.schaeffeler@ikp-stuttgart.de
†Matthias Schwab and Elke Schaeffeler contributed equally to this work.
[1]Dr. Margarete Fischer-Bosch Institute of Clinical Pharmacology, Auerbachstrasse 112, 70376 Stuttgart, Germany
Full list of author information is available at the end of the article

Background

Clear cell renal cell carcinoma (ccRCC) is the most common subtype of renal cell carcinoma, with a currently increasing incidence [1–3]. Approximately 30% of patients develop metastases and, despite the implementation of targeted therapies, the 5 year survival rate of patients with metastatic disease remains below 20%. Thus, stratification of patients with ccRCC into different molecularly defined groups to identify patients at risk of worse outcome is increasingly important in the perspective of personalized medicine. With this in mind, several prognostic scores have been developed based on, for example, pathological features, gene expression, or DNA methylation status [4–6]. One of the most widely applied score established on clinicopathological data is the SSIGN (stage, size, grade, and necrosis) score [7, 8], whereas the ClearCode34 score, which predicts two ccRCC subtypes (ccA/ccB), has been suggested for prediction of survival using gene expression data [9, 10]. Moreover, Rini et al. [11] proposed a 16-gene score to predict recurrence in ccRCC patients. In general, prognostic signatures using RNA-seq data hold great promise for precision oncology, as previously demonstrated for lung adenocarcinoma [12]. We recently developed an in silico prediction score (named S3-score) for ccRCC, based on the gene expression of 97 signature genes and the similarity of gene expression between tumor cells and their proposed normal cell of origin in the nephron [13]. The S3-score outperforms several other scores [13], including the ClearCode34 model, and significantly improves the predictive value of the SSIGN score and the original ccA/ccB assignment based on clustering [14]. Moreover, compared with the ccA/ccB signature, the S3-score is slightly less dependent on the tumor section investigated [13] and, in consequence displays little intra-tumor heterogeneity. This is of importance because, in a recent study investigating the ccA/ccB signature [10], approximately one-quarter of metastatic tumors (two of nine patients) displayed intra-tumor heterogeneity and, in 43% of the cases, patient-matched primary and metastatic tumors displayed different molecular ccA/ccB subtypes. In this context, a recent multiregion sampling process using a protein-based prognostic model was described, enabling the study of the impact of intra-tumor heterogeneity on risk stratification of sunitinib-treated metastatic patients [15].

As our S3-score was evaluated only in silico using data from The Cancer Genome Atlas (TCGA), we now intended to verify the performance of the score using newly generated whole transcriptome data of an independent cohort of ccRCC patients, including metastases derived from ccRCC, to determine the concordance of the score prediction in primary tumors and ccRCC-derived metastases. Moreover, we evaluated whether the score predicts outcome in sunitinib-treated ccRCC patients. Finally, our objective was to improve the clinical applicability of the S3-score by reducing the number of genes necessary for calculation of the score and by using the more cost-effective real-time PCR technology.

Methods

Study cohorts

The study investigated different ccRCC cohorts listed in Table 1 and Additional file 1: Figure S1.

First, our 97 gene-based S3-score ($S3_{97}$), which was developed using publically available gene expression data of a ccRCC cohort from TCGA (n = 463) (Table 1) [16] was evaluated in a set of 52 primary ccRCC patients (ccRCC cohort 1). These 52 primary tumor samples were collected from non-metastatic and metastatic patients with ccRCC histology, treated at the Department of Urology, University Hospital Tuebingen, Germany. Patient characteristics are provided in Table 1. The use of the tissue was approved by the ethics committee of the University of Tuebingen and informed written consent was provided by each subject prior to surgical resection. Cancer-specific survival (CSS) was used as the endpoint in the survival analysis of these ccRCC patients.

In addition, publicly available gene expression data from an independent cohort of primary tumors obtained from sunitinib-treated ccRCC patients (n = 53, sunitinib-treated cohort) (Table 1) [17] were used in the analysis. This cohort consisted of ccRCC patients with synchronous or metachronous metastases, who received first-line sunitinib treatment (dosing schedule: 50 mg/day, 4 weeks on/2 weeks off; at least one 28-day cycle of sunitinib treatment completed; prior cytokine therapy allowed) [17]. Primary ccRCC tissue samples were collected from patients undergoing nephrectomy prior to sunitinib treatment [17]. Further details of these study patients are outlined in Beuselinck et al. [17]. Progression-free survival was used as the endpoint in the survival analysis of sunitinib-treated ccRCC patients.

Next, publicly available gene expression data of TCGA [16] from the cohort of ccRCC patients (n = 463) (Table 1) were used as a development cohort to define a modified S3-score, which requires a reduced number of genes for clinical application. This $S3_{15}$-score was validated in an extended cohort of 108 metastatic and non-metastatic ccRCC patients treated at the Department of Urology, University Hospital Tuebingen, Germany (extended ccRCC cohort 2, n = 108) (Table 1). CSS was used as endpoint in the survival analysis. Kaplan–Meier curves of CSS for ccRCC cohorts 1 and 2, as well as for the TCGA cohort are shown in Additional file 1: Figure S2.

Table 1 Patient demographics and clinical characteristics of The Cancer Genome Atlas (TCGA) clear cell renal cell carcinoma (ccRCC) cohort (*n* = 463 with available RNA-Seq data), as well as our cohorts (*n* = 52 with available microarray data; *n* = 108 with available RT-PCR data) and a sunitinib-treated cohort published by Beuselinck et al. [17][a] (*n* = 53)

		ccRCC TCGA (*n* = 463)		ccRCC cohort 1 (*n* = 52)		Sunitinib treated cohort[a] (*n* = 53)		Extended ccRCC cohort 2[b] (*n* = 108)	
		n, value	%	*n*, value	%	*n*, value	%	*n*, value	%
Sex	Male	297	64.15%	35	67.3%	37	69.81%	63	58.33%
	Female	166	35.85%	17	32.69%	16	30.19%	45	41.67%
Age (year)	Median (range)	61 (26–90)		64 (37–90)		58 (44–80)		65 (34–90)	
T	T1	226	48.81%	17	32.69%	NA	NA	51	47.22%
	T2	59	12.74%	4	7.69%	NA	NA	10	9.26%
	T3	168	36.29%	31	59.62%	NA	NA	47	43.52%
	T4	10	2.16%	0	0.00%	NA	NA	0	0.00%
N	N0	215	46.44%	46	88.46%	NA	NA	97	89.81%
	N1	15	3.24%	4	7.69%	NA	NA	8	7.41%
	N2	0	0.00%	2	3.85%	NA	NA	3	2.78%
	NX	233	50.32%	0	0.00%	NA	NA	0	0.00%
M	M0	374	80.78%	41	78.85%	NA	NA	92	85.19%
	M1	76	16.41%	10	19.23%	NA	NA	15	13.89%
	MX	13	2.81%	1	1.92%	NA	NA	1	0.93%
G	G1	7	1.51%	9	17.31%	NA	NA	24	22.22%
	G2	200	43.20%	30	57.69%	NA	NA	60	55.56%
	G2–G3	0	0.00%	1	1.92%	NA	NA	2	1.85%
	G3	183	39.52%	11	21.15%	NA	NA	20	18.52%
	G4	72	15.55%	1	1.92%	NA	NA	1	0.93%
	GX	1	0.22%	0	0.00%	NA	NA	0	0.00%
	NA	0	0.00%	0	0.00%	NA	NA	1	0.93%
Necrosis	Present	218	47.08%	10	19.23%	NA	NA	17	15.74%
	Absent	245	52.92%	42	80.77%	NA	NA	91	84.26%
Follow-up time (years)	Median (range)	3.1 (0.0–10.0)		3.0 (0.0–10.0)		1.0 (0.1–4.9)		3.4 (0.0–11.1)	
Overall survival	Deceased	152	32.83%	17	32.69%	NA	NA	29	26.85%
	Alive	311	67.17%	35	67.31%	NA	NA	79	73.15%
Cancer-specific survival	Cancer-related death	104	22.46%	15	28.85%	NA	NA	21	19.44%
	Alive/non-cancer-related death	359	77.54%	37	71.15%	NA	NA	87	80.56%
Progression free survival under sunitinib therapy	Yes	–	–	–	–	14	26.4%	–	–
	No	–	–	–	–	39	73.6%	–	–

T primary tumor, *N* regional lymph node, *M* distant metastasis present at diagnosis, *G* grading, *NA* not available

[a]ccRCC cohort published by Beuselinck et al. [17]; descriptive data were not available

[b]This extended ccRCC cohort 2 includes the 52 patients from ccRCC cohort 1

In addition, metastases samples (*n* = 22) derived from 15 patients treated at the Department of Urology, University Hospital Tuebingen, Germany, were collected, including matched primary tumor and metastases samples from five patients of our ccRCC cohorts 1 and 2 (Additional file 1: Table S1 and S5). In part, several regions from one metastasis were collected. Further details about metastases are given in Additional file 1: Table S1 and S5. Use of the tissue was approved by the ethics committee of the University of Tuebingen and informed written consent was provided by each subject prior to surgical resection.

Additional file 1: Figure S1 shows an overview about the workflow of data analyses including the different cohorts and technologies used in the present study.

Gene expression analyses and S3-score calculation

Total RNA was isolated from fresh-frozen ccRCC and metastasis tissue using the mirVana™ miRNA Isolation

Kit (Life Technologies) as previously described [18, 19]. Genome-wide transcriptome analyses were performed using Human Transcriptome Array HTA 2.0 (Affymetrix) according to the manufacturer's protocol. Further processing of microarray data were performed as previously described [18] (Additional file 1: Supplementary methods). Gene expression data (generated using HuGene 1.0ST Affymetrix array) from 53 sunitinib-treated ccRCC patients were downloaded from ArrayExpress (E-MTAB-3267).

Quantitative real-time PCR (qRT-PCR) was performed using TaqMan technology on a BioMARK System (Fluidigm) as described previously [18, 19]. TaqMan gene expression assays for 97 genes of the S3-score, as well as five genes used for normalization were purchased from Life Technologies. Further details about calculation of the S3-score based on interprofile correlations and development of a S3-score calculation model for use of qRT-PCR data are provided in the Additional file 1: Supplementary methods.

ClearCode34 and SSIGN calculation

The SSIGN score was calculated as denoted in Zigeuner et al. [8]. The ClearCode34 classifier, as introduced by Brooks et al. [9], was applied on the set of matched primary tumors and metastases of our present cohort for which genome-wide expression data measured by HTA 2.0 microarrays were available (Additional file 1: Supplementary methods).

Statistical analyses

All statistical analyses were performed with R-3.3.3, including additional packages (Additional file 1: Supplementary methods) [20]. Survival analyses for endpoints CSS or progression-free survival were conducted by Kaplan–Meier curves and corresponding log-rank tests as well as uni- and multivariate Cox models. Comparisons of Cox models were performed by analysis of deviance. All statistical tests were two sided. Statistical significance was defined as $P < 0.05$ (Additional file 1: Supplementary methods).

Results

Evaluation of the S3-score in ccRCC primary tumors and primary tumors of patients treated with sunitinib

We previously developed the S3-score in silico using RNA-seq data from the TCGA (Table 1) [13]. The S3-score was calculated based on 97 genes by correlating tumor expression to the expression in the eight nephron regions. In the present work, we first evaluated this 97 gene-based S3-score ($S3_{97}$) in our own cohort, consisting of 52 ccRCC samples (ccRCC cohort1) (Table 1) for which genome-wide expression data using transcriptome arrays were generated. Partitioning of the ccRCC samples by means of the cut-off value that was established in our previous work [13] resulted in two groups with significantly varying CSS (Fig. 1a);

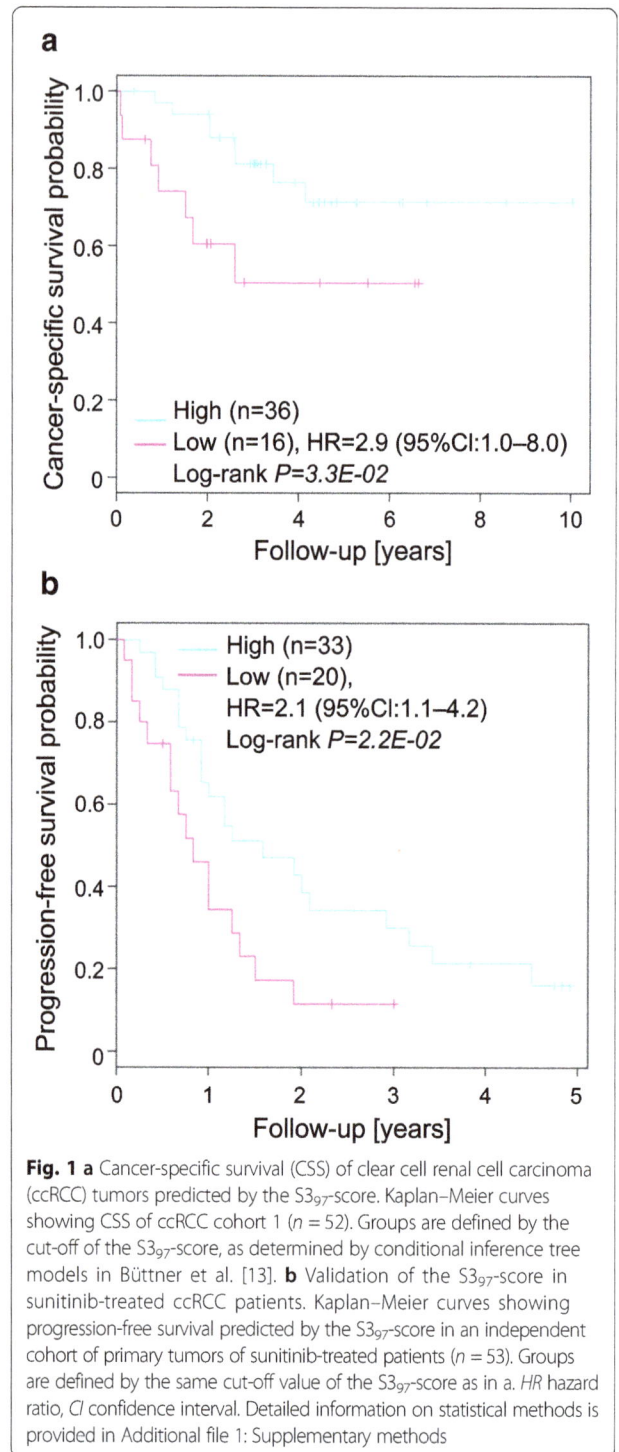

Fig. 1 a Cancer-specific survival (CSS) of clear cell renal cell carcinoma (ccRCC) tumors predicted by the $S3_{97}$-score. Kaplan–Meier curves showing CSS of ccRCC cohort 1 ($n = 52$). Groups are defined by the cut-off of the $S3_{97}$-score, as determined by conditional inference tree models in Büttner et al. [13]. **b** Validation of the $S3_{97}$-score in sunitinib-treated ccRCC patients. Kaplan–Meier curves showing progression-free survival predicted by the $S3_{97}$-score in an independent cohort of primary tumors of sunitinib-treated patients ($n = 53$). Groups are defined by the same cut-off value of the $S3_{97}$-score as in a. *HR* hazard ratio, *CI* confidence interval. Detailed information on statistical methods is provided in Additional file 1: Supplementary methods

i.e. patients with a high $S3_{97}$-score had an decreased risk for cancer-related death compared to patients with low $S3_{97}$-scores. Furthermore, univariate Cox regression including evaluation of the predictive ability according to Harrell's c-index indicated a significant association of the $S3_{97}$-score with patient survival (HR 2.9, 95% CI 1.0–8.0, $P_{\text{Log-rank}} = 3.3 \times 10^{-2}$) (Additional file 1: Table S2).

Since survival prediction might be majorly influenced by treatment with, for example, sunitinib, we next investigated whether prediction of survival is possible in sunitinib-treated patients. Using a cohort of 53 sunitinib-treated metastatic ccRCC patients with publically available microarray data [17], we calculated the S3-score based on the 97 signature genes. Partitioning of the sunitinib-treated patients by means of our established cut-off value resulted in two groups with significantly varying progression-free survival (Fig. 1b); i.e., patients with a high $S3_{97}$-score had increased progression-free survival probability after sunitinib treatment compared with patients with a low $S3_{97}$-score. Furthermore, univariate Cox regression including evaluation of the predictive ability according to Harrell's c-index, indicated a significant association of the $S3_{97}$-score with patient survival after treatment with sunitinib (HR 2.1, 95% CI 1.1–4.2, $P_{\text{Log-rank}} = 2.2 \times 10^{-2}$) (Additional file 1: Table S2).

Refinement of the 97 gene-based $S3_{97}$-score for clinical application

Based on our results, the $S3_{97}$-score has the ability to significantly predict not only CSS in ccRCC patients, but also the progression-free survival in sunitinib-treated individuals. However, calculation of the score was currently based on gene expression data of 97 marker genes, generated through genome-wide transcriptome analyses (RNA-seq or microarray). Thus, for clinical application and utility of the S3-score, expression analyses using quantitative real-time PCR (qRT-PCR), as well as a reduced number of genes, would be more appropriate. Therefore, we aimed to develop a new calculation model of the S3-score. First, the expression of the 97 signature genes, which constituted the basis for the development of the new prediction approach, and the expression of five normalization genes, was quantified by qRT-PCR in our extended ccRCC cohort of 108 non-metastatic and metastatic samples (ccRCC cohort 2) (Table 1). In order to ensure minimum failure rates in future applications, all assays that failed at least once were excluded. Moreover, we considered only genes that were (after normalization) comparable with respect to mean expression and variation of expression between the RNA-seq data from the TCGA cohort and the RT-PCR values (Additional file 1: Supplementary methods and Additional file 1: Figure S3). In total, the resulting set of variables used for model selection included 41 genes. Subsequently, a linear model using RNA-seq data from the TCGA cohort was created that reconstructs the correlation-based S3-scores.

The resulting model identified by model selection included 15 genes (Additional file 1: Table S3) and showed good correlation with microarray-based values in our

cohort (Spearman's rank correlation coefficient = 0.91) (Additional file 1: Figure S4). Thus, including the five normalization genes, $S3_{15}$-score determination based on qRT-PCR requires only 20 genes to be measured. Univariate Cox regression indicated that the $S3_{15}$-score was significantly associated with CSS in our extended ccRCC cohort 2 ($n = 108$) (Table 2). CSS was significantly different between patients with a high and low $S3_{15}$-score in the cohort ($n = 108$, HR 5.0, 95% CI 2.1–11.7, $P_{\text{Log-rank}} = 5.15 \times 10^{-5}$) (Fig. 2a). Moreover, similarly to the 97 gene-based $S3_{97}$-score we could confirm the ability of the $S3_{15}$-score to predict CSS in non-metastatic (HR 4.4, 95% CI 1.2–16.3, $P_{\text{Log-Rank}} = 1.6 \times 10^{-2}$) as well as metastatic patients (HR 9.3, 95% CI 1.8–50.0, $P_{\text{Log-rank}} = 2.3 \times 10^{-3}$) (Fig. 2b).

As expected, a higher incidence of advanced stage tumors as well as metastatic tumors occurred in the $S3_{15}$-low group with poor survival (Additional file 1: Figure S5 and Table S4). Next, we compared the $S3_{15}$-score with clinicopathological prediction factors (T, N, M, G). Multivariate Cox regression indicated that the $S3_{15}$-score is able to significantly improve the predictive ability of the clinicopathological parameters (Table 3). Additionally, the multivariate Cox model outperformed the univariate model (TNMG vs. TNMG+S3: $P_{\chi2} = 3.98 \times 10^{-4}$). Moreover, the $S3_{15}$-score significantly improved CSS prediction when added to the Cox model initially including only the clinicopathologic-based SSIGN score ($P_{\chi2} = 1.6 \times 10^{-3}$) (Fig. 2c).

Evaluation of the $S3_{97}$-score and $S3_{15}$-score in metastases derived from ccRCC patients

Tumor heterogeneity of the original S3-score has been previously evaluated to assess whether a single tumor sample is sufficient for prediction of survival [13]. We now aimed to investigate the $S3_{97}$-score and $S3_{15}$-score in metastases in order to evaluate the concordance between primary tumors and metastases. First, we analyzed the $S3_{97}$-score in metastases using microarray data. For a total of 15 ccRCC patients, genome-wide expression data were generated from metastases samples, including five metastatic patients from our ccRCC cohorts with matched primary tumor and metastases samples, as well as three patients for whom several metastases were available. Calculation of the $S3_{97}$-score individually for tumor and metastases resulted in similar risk prediction (Fig. 3a). One patient (P4) was assigned to the high risk group (low $S3_{97}$-score) with worse prognosis using either metastases or tumor tissue (Additional file 1: Table S5). Three patients (P1, P3, P5) showed a high $S3_{97}$-score in tumor as well as metastasis tissue (Additional file 1: Table S5). S3-score was discordant between the primary tumor and its metastasis in only one sample (P2). For different metastases derived from the same patient (P7,

Table 2 Univariate Cox regression for cancer-specific survival in the extended clear cell renal cell carcinoma cohort 2 ($n = 108$)

Univariate analyses	Variable	Level	No. of cases	HR (95% CI)	P value (Log-rank test)	c-index
All patients	$S3_{15}$-score	high	87	1 (Ref.)	5.15×10^{-5}	0.69
		low	21	4.96 (2.10–11.72)		
M0	$S3_{15}$-score	high	77	1 (Ref.)	1.62×10^{-2}	0.68
		low	15	4.37 (1.17–16.29)		
M1	$S3_{15}$-score	high	9	1 (Ref.)	2.31×10^{-3}	0.71
		low	6	9.32 (1.75–49.58)		

CI confidence interval, HR hazard ratio, Ref. reference level

$S3_{15}$-scores were determined based on gene expression data measured by RT-PCR; tumors with metastasis status MX were disregarded

P8), as well as for four regions of one metastasis (P6), the $S3_{97}$-score values were also comparable (Fig. 3a). Using the ClearCode34 signature, recently used also for metastatic tissue [10], revealed similar results and classification of tumor/metastases pairs into different molecular subtypes as the $S3_{97}$-score (Additional file 1: Table S5). We additionally performed qRT-PCR quantification and calculation of the $S3_{15}$-score in a subset of metastases samples. Regarding the five metastatic patients from our ccRCC cohorts for whom primary tumors as well as metastases were available, we found that, except for one case, the $S3_{97}$-score tendency was preserved using the improved $S3_{15}$-score (Fig. 3b).

Discussion

Several risk scores based on gene expression data have been developed for prediction of patient survival in ccRCC [4]. We recently developed a novel prediction score, named the S3-score, based on the similarity of gene expression in the tumor to its cell of origin in the nephron region [13, 21]. Thus, in contrast to other scores, risk prediction using the S3-score is related to biologic alterations of the cell of origin of ccRCC. The S3-score outperformed other scores or signatures based on gene expression data or clinicopathological variables [13, 21] and was even able to improve the predictive value of the clinically validated SSIGN score [7, 8]. Moreover, evaluation of tumor heterogeneity of our S3-score showed that only a few samples displayed heterogeneity [13], which indicates that risk prediction with our score is largely independent from the tumor region investigated.

Generally, most of the scores developed using gene expression data are thus far not introduced into clinical practice because they have not been generated to evaluate individual patients. Thus, for clinical application, the prediction scores need to be validated in several studies defining optimal cut-off values for classification of individual patients into subtypes. Moreover, prediction scores, typically developed using genome-wide gene expression data, need to be evaluated using different technologies and gene expression platforms. Since our S3-score, which is based on the expression of 97 signature genes, was originally developed using RNA-seq data from the TCGA, we first evaluated its predictive ability in the present work using gene expression data generated through microarray technology in our own ccRCC cohort. Here, we showed not only that a platform transfer to microarray data is possible, but also that the $S3_{97}$-score significantly predicts CSS in our cohort.

In contrast to other prediction scores such as the 16-gene signatures [11], the 97 marker genes were not selected based on pathway analyses (e.g., including genes related to inflammation or immune response) and subsequent optimization for prediction of prognosis, but were originally selected to show that tumor aggressiveness in RCC correlates with the level of divergence from its cell of origin within the nephron region. Noticeably, we observe an overlap of one vascular pathway gene (PPAP2B) in the 97 marker genes and those genes from the 16-gene signature described by Rini et al. [11]. Further studies are warranted to compare the predictive ability of both scores.

Because metastases might represent the most aggressive phenotypes of a heterogeneous tumor, herein, we were interested in inter-tumor or metastases heterogeneity, using gene expression data generated by microarray technology once again. Interestingly, the predictive $S3_{97}$-score was comparable between matched tumor and metastases, or matched metastases pairs. In only one case (Additional file 1: Table S5) classification differed between metastases and tumors.

Since data on treatment outcome are limited in the TCGA cohort originally used to develop the S3-score, we were not previously able to evaluate the effect of tyrosine kinase inhibitor (TKI) treatment on outcome prediction. Therefore, herein, we investigated the $S3_{97}$-score using microarray data from a cohort of sunitinib-treated ccRCC patients. In this cohort, the $S3_{97}$-score was significantly associated with progression-free survival of patients, indicating that our score enables even prediction of sunitinib outcome. Whether the same holds true for immunotherapy

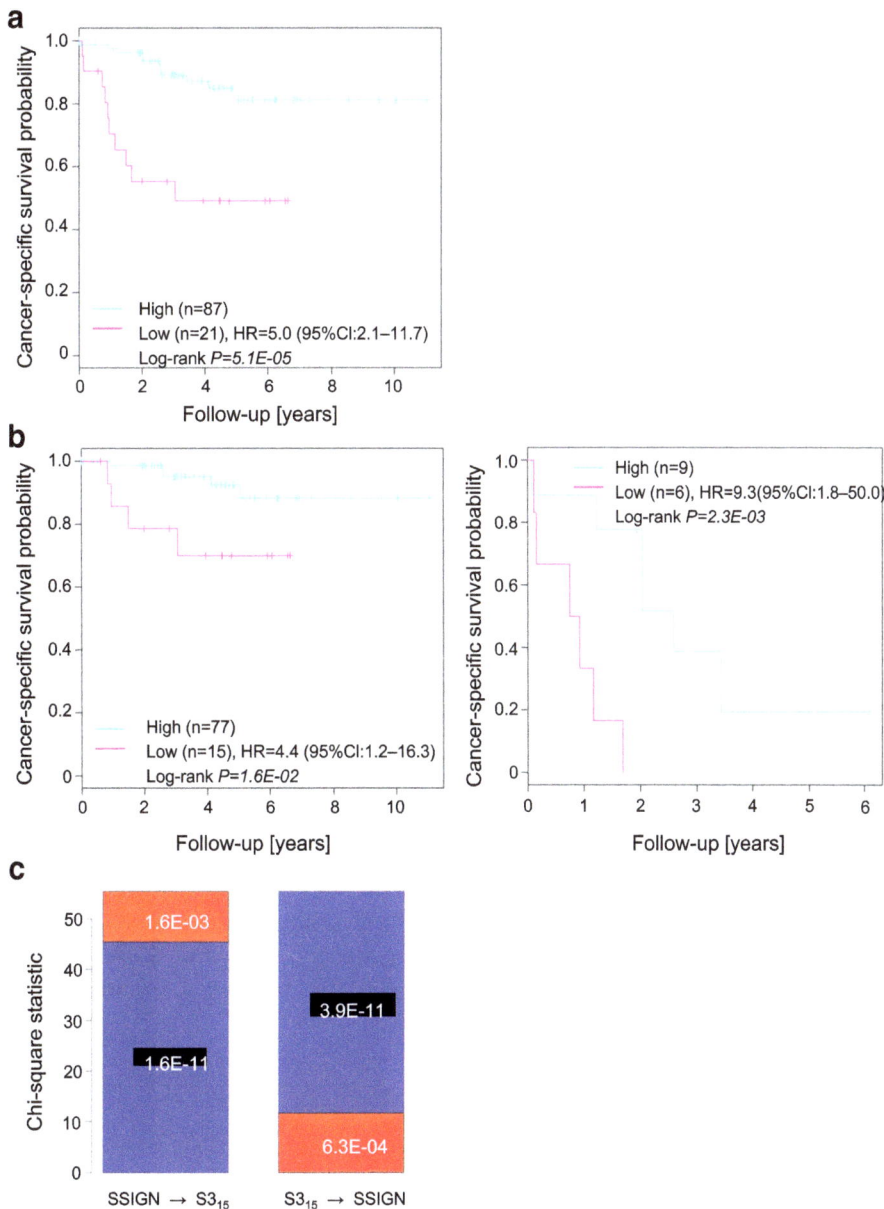

Fig. 2 Cancer-specific survival (CSS) of clear cell renal cell carcinoma (ccRCC) tumors of our validation cohort predicted by the simplified RT-PCR-based $S3_{15}$-score. Kaplan–Meier curves showing CSS of (**a**) the extended ccRCC cohort 2 ($n = 108$) and (**b**) the non-metastatic ($n = 92$) and metastatic subsets ($n = 15$) of this cohort. Groups are defined by the cut-off of the $S3_{15}$-score, as determined by conditional inference tree models. **c** $S3_{15}$-score significantly improves the established SSIGN prediction score. χ^2 statistic values depict the improvement of the model likelihood when risk classification based on the $S3_{15}$-score (red) was added to the Cox model initially including only the SSIGN score (blue; left) or vice versa (right). χ^2 test P values are shown in the bars. *HR* hazard ratio, *CI* confidence interval. Detailed information on statistical methods is provided in Additional file 1: Supplementary methods

in the form of T cell immune checkpoint inhibitors like nivolumab needs to be investigated in future studies. Preliminary investigation of the $S3_{97}$-score in metastatic RCC patients treated with nivolumab [22] shows that the $S3_{97}$-score did not differ significantly in pre- and post-treatment biopsies (Additional file 1: Figure S6), indicating that there was no influence of treatment with nivolumab on the S3-score.

Taken together, we provide evidence that the $S3_{97}$-score is more widely applicable than originally intended. To provide a more cost-effective approach for clinical application of the S3-score in individual patient samples, such as even formalin-fixed paraffin-embedded samples, we improved the $S3_{97}$-score by reducing the number of signature genes from 97 to 15 especially for expression analyses through RT-PCR. Our improved

Table 3 Multivariate Cox regression for cancer-specific survival in the extended ccRCC cohort 2 ($n = 108$)

Multivariate analyses	variable	level	P-value (Wald test)	HR (95%CI)
Including T,N,M,G and S3$_{15}$-score	S3$_{15}$-score	high		1 (Ref.)
		low	0.00033	7.3 (2.5–21.5)
	Primary tumor	T1		1 (Ref.)
		T2	0.37	3.0 (0.3–35.0)
		T3	0.01	6.0 (1.5–24.3)
	Lymph Nodes	N0		1 (Ref.)
		N1	0.25	0.5 (0.1–1.7)
		N2	0.45	0.4 (0.0–3.9)
	Distant metastasis	M0		1 (Ref.)
		M1	0.00001	23.5 (6.0–92.2)
	Fuhrman grade	G1		1 (Ref.)
		G2	0.73	1.5 (0.2–14.1)
		G3	0.93	0.9 (0.1–10.3)

Abbreviations: *CI* confidence interval, *HR* hazard ratio, *Ref.* reference level. S3$_{15}$-scores were determined based on gene expression data measured by RT-PCR; T, primary tumor; N, regional lymph node; M, distant metastasis present at diagnosis; G, grading; tumors with grade "G2–3" and "G4" were added to "G3". Tumors with no grading information or metastasis status "MX" were disregarded

S3$_{15}$-score was validated using RT-PCR technology in a cohort of 108 ccRCC cases, clearly indicating that the S3$_{15}$-score was associated with CSS in the complete cohort, as well as non-metastatic and metastatic subsets. Moreover, the S3$_{15}$-score improves prediction of CSS by the currently clinically applied SSIGN score, which is based on clinical parameters and pathologic features. Finally, the S3$_{15}$-score allows risk prediction in tumor and metastases tissue.

In summary, we found that our score enables valid prediction of patient outcome even if applied to different sample types (e.g., primary and metastatic tissue) and independent cohorts (e.g., patients treated with TKIs). Moreover, different platforms (RNA-seq, microarray) and technologies more appropriate for clinical utility (qRT-PCR) can be used for prediction of patient risk by the S3-score. Further prospective studies are warranted to assess the implementation

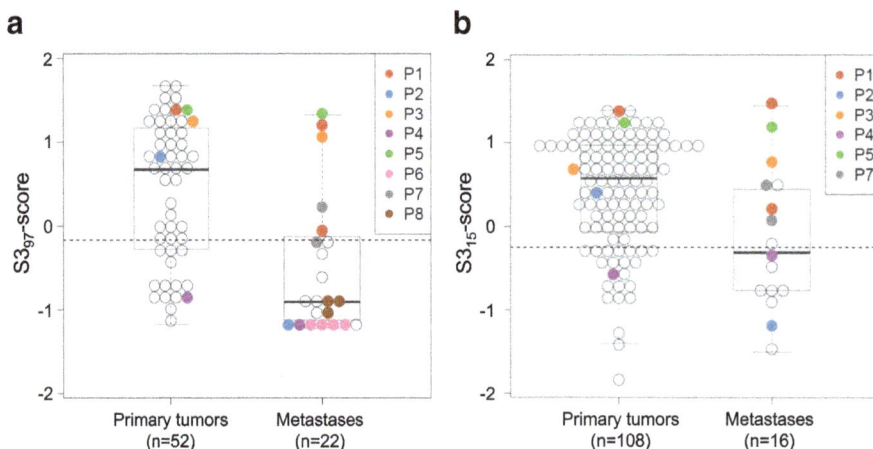

Fig. 3 a S3$_{97}$-score prediction in primary tumors and metastases samples derived from clear cell renal cell carcinoma (ccRCC) patients. Identical colors indicate primary and metastatic tissues derived from the same patient; for one patient (P6), four regions of one metastasis were analyzed. The dashed horizontal line indicates the S3$_{97}$-score cut-off. **b** S3$_{15}$-score in primary tumors and metastases, indicating similar scores in matched primary tumors and metastases except for one case. The dashed horizontal line indicates the S3$_{15}$-score cut-off. Detailed information on statistical methods is provided in Additional file 1: Supplementary methods

of the score into clinical practice with consequences on personalized patient care.

Conclusions

Since the stratification of patients to identify those with worse prognosis is increasingly important, especially for treatment selection, the molecular subtyping through gene expression signatures may be promising for ccRCC patients. In the present work, the clinical utility of the gene expression-based S3-score, which reflects the similarity of the tumor to its cell of origin in the nephron, was assessed in independent cohorts. The 97 gene-based $S3_{97}$-score and a simplified 15-gene RT-PCR-based $S3_{15}$-score are significantly associated with CSS or progression-free survival in non-metastatic and metastatic ccRCC patients, as well as in TKI-treated patients. As a result, this score, as a promising, cost-effective, and robust diagnostic tool, enables the risk stratification of patients with ccRCC in clinical practice in the non-metastatic, metastatic, and sunitinib-treated setting.

Acknowledgements
We gratefully acknowledge Andrea Jarmuth and Ursula Waldherr for their excellent technical assistance, as well as Heidi Köhler for figure preparation. The results shown here are in part based upon data generated by the TCGA Research Network. We would like to thank The Cancer Genome Atlas (TCGA) initiative, all tissue donors, and the investigators who contributed to the acquisition and analyses of the samples used in this study. Information about TCGA and the investigators and institutions who constitute the TCGA research network can be found at http://cancergenome.nih.gov/.

Funding
This work was supported by the Robert Bosch Foundation (Stuttgart, Germany), the DFG SFB grant [DFG SFB685 C05], Ferdinand-Eisenberger-grant of the German Society of Urology [RaS1/FE-14], and the ICEPHA Graduate School Tuebingen-Stuttgart. None of the mentioned funding organizations were involved in experimental/clinical work, data analyses, nor preparation of the manuscript.

Authors' contributions
Conception and design: FB, MSchwab, ES. Development of methodology: FB, SW. Acquisition of data: FB, SW, SR, JH, AA, AH, MSchwab, FF. Statistical analyses: FB, SW. Analysis and interpretation of data: FB, SW, AA, AH, MSchwab, FF, SR, SK, AS, JB, ES, MSchwab. Writing, review, and/or revision of the manuscript: FB, SW, AA, AH, MSchwab, FF, SR, SK, JB, JH, AS, ES, MSchwab. Study supervision: JB, MSchwab. All authors read and approved the final manuscript.

Competing interests
JB: consultancies, honoraria or study participation from Bayer, BMS, GSK, Immatics, Novartis, Pfizer, and Roche. AS: consultancies, honoraria or study participation from Bayer, BMS, Immatics, Novartis, Pfizer, and Roche. All other authors declare that they have no competing interests.

Author details
[1]Dr. Margarete Fischer-Bosch Institute of Clinical Pharmacology, Auerbachstrasse 112, 70376 Stuttgart, Germany. [2]University of Tuebingen, Tuebingen, Germany. [3]Department of Urology, University Hospital Tuebingen, Tuebingen, Germany. [4]Institute of Pathology and Neuropathology, University Hospital Tuebingen, Tuebingen, Germany. [5]Institute of Pathology, Friedrich-Alexander University Erlangen-Nuernberg, University Hospital Erlangen-Nuernberg, Erlangen, Germany. [6]German Cancer Consortium (DKTK) and German Cancer Research Center (DKFZ), Heidelberg, Germany. [7]Department of Clinical Pharmacology, University Hospital Tuebingen, Tuebingen, Germany. [8]Department of Pharmacy and Biochemistry, University of Tuebingen, Tuebingen, Germany.

References
1. Hsieh JJ, Purdue MP, Signoretti S, Swanton C, Albiges L, Schmidinger M, et al. Renal cell carcinoma. Nat Rev Dis Primers. 2017;3:17009. https://doi.org/10.1038/nrdp.2017.9.
2. Moch H, Cubilla AL, Humphrey PA, Reuter VE, Ulbright TM. The 2016 WHO classification of tumours of the urinary system and male genital organs-part a: renal, penile, and Testicular Tumours. Eur Urol. 2016;70:93–105. https://doi.org/10.1016/j.eururo.2016.02.029.
3. Shuch B, Amin A, Armstrong AJ, Eble JN, Ficarra V, Lopez-Beltran A, et al. Understanding pathologic variants of renal cell carcinoma: distilling therapeutic opportunities from biologic complexity. Eur Urol. 2015;67:85–97. https://doi.org/10.1016/j.eururo.2014.04.029.
4. Gulati S, Martinez P, Joshi T, Birkbak NJ, Santos CR, Rowan AJ, et al. Systematic evaluation of the prognostic impact and intratumour heterogeneity of clear cell renal cell carcinoma biomarkers. Eur Urol. 2014; 66:936–48. https://doi.org/10.1016/j.eururo.2014.06.053.
5. Malouf GG, Su X, Zhang J, Creighton CJ, Ho TH, Lu Y, et al. DNA methylation signature reveals cell ontogeny of renal cell carcinomas. Clin Cancer Res. 2016; 22:6236–46. https://doi.org/10.1158/1078-0432.CCR-15-1217.
6. van Vlodrop IJH, Joosten SC, de MT, Smits KM, Van Neste L, Melotte V, et al. A four-gene promoter methylation marker panel consisting of GREM1, NEURL, LAD1, and NEFH predicts survival of clear cell renal cell Cancer patients. Clin Cancer Res. 2017;23:2006–18. https://doi.org/10.1158/1078-0432.CCR-16-1236.
7. Parker WP, Cheville JC, Frank I, Zaid HB, Lohse CM, Boorjian SA, et al. Application of the stage, size, grade, and necrosis (SSIGN) score for clear cell renal cell carcinoma in contemporary patients. Eur Urol. 2017;71:665–73. https://doi.org/10.1016/j.eururo.2016.05.034.
8. Zigeuner R, Hutterer G, Chromecki T, Imamovic A, Kampel-Kettner K, Rehak P, et al. External validation of the Mayo Clinic stage, size, grade, and necrosis (SSIGN) score for clear-cell renal cell carcinoma in a single European Centre applying routine pathology. Eur Urol. 2010;57:102–9. https://doi.org/10.1016/j.eururo.2008.11.033.
9. Brooks SA, Brannon AR, Parker JS, Fisher JC, Sen O, Kattan MW, et al. ClearCode34: a prognostic risk predictor for localized clear cell renal cell carcinoma. Eur Urol. 2014;66:77–84. https://doi.org/10.1016/j.eururo.2014.02.035.
10. Serie DJ, Joseph RW, Cheville JC, Ho TH, Parasramka M, Hilton T, et al. Clear cell type a and B molecular subtypes in metastatic clear cell renal cell

carcinoma: tumor heterogeneity and aggressiveness. Eur Urol. 2016;67:979–85. https://doi.org/10.1016/j.eururo.2016.11.018.

11. Rini B, Goddard A, Knezevic D, Maddala T, Zhou M, Aydin H, et al. A 16-gene assay to predict recurrence after surgery in localised renal cell carcinoma: development and validation studies. Lancet Oncol. 2015;16:676–85. https://doi.org/10.1016/S1470-2045(15)70167-1.

12. Shukla S, Evans JR, Malik R, Feng FY, Dhanasekaran SM, Cao X, et al. Development of a RNA-Seq based prognostic signature in lung adenocarcinoma. J Natl Cancer Inst. 2017;109(1):djw200. https://doi.org/10.1093/jnci/djw200.

13. Büttner F, Winter S, Rausch S, Reustle A, Kruck S, Junker K, et al. Survival prediction of clear cell renal cell carcinoma based on gene expression similarity to the proximal tubule of the nephron. Eur Urol. 2015;68:1016–20. https://doi.org/10.1016/j.eururo.2015.05.045.

14. Brannon AR, Reddy A, Seiler M, Arreola A, Moore DT, Pruthi RS, et al. Molecular stratification of clear cell renal cell carcinoma by consensus clustering reveals distinct subtypes and survival patterns. Genes Cancer. 2010;1:152–63. https://doi.org/10.1177/1947601909359929.

15. Lubbock ALR, Stewart GD, O'Mahony FC, Laird A, Mullen P, O'Donnell M, et al. Overcoming intratumoural heterogeneity for reproducible molecular risk stratification: a case study in advanced kidney cancer. BMC Med. 2017;15:118. https://doi.org/10.1186/s12916-017-0874-9.

16. Cancer Genome Atlas Research Network. Comprehensive molecular characterization of clear cell renal cell carcinoma. Nature. 2013;499:43–9. https://doi.org/10.1038/nature12222.

17. Beuselinck B, Job S, Becht E, Karadimou A, Verkarre V, Couchy G, et al. Molecular subtypes of clear cell renal cell carcinoma are associated with sunitinib response in the metastatic setting. Clin Cancer Res. 2015;21:1329–39. https://doi.org/10.1158/1078-0432.CCR-14-1128.

18. Winter S, Fisel P, Büttner F, Rausch S, D'Amico D, Hennenlotter J, et al. Methylomes of renal cell lines and tumors or metastases differ significantly with impact on pharmacogenes. Sci Rep. 2016;6:29930. https://doi.org/10.1038/srep29930.

19. Fisel P, Kruck S, Winter S, Bedke J, Hennenlotter J, Nies AT, et al. DNA methylation of the SLC16A3 promoter regulates expression of the human lactate transporter MCT4 in renal cancer with consequences for clinical outcome. Clin Cancer Res. 2013;19:5170–81. https://doi.org/10.1158/1078-0432.CCR-13-1180.

20. R Core Team. R: a language and environment for statistical computing. Vienna: R Foundation for Statistical Computing; 2014.

21. Fenner A. Kidney cancer: Tumour versus nephron gene expression yields survival score. Nat Rev Urol 2015;12:415. doi:https://doi.org/10.1038/nrurol.2015.155.

22. Choueiri TK, Fishman MN, Escudier B, McDermott DF, Drake CG, Kluger H, et al. Immunomodulatory activity of Nivolumab in metastatic renal cell carcinoma. Clin Cancer Res. 2016;22:5461–71. https://doi.org/10.1158/1078-0432.CCR-15-2839.

15

Dementia subtype and living well: results from the Improving the experience of Dementia and Enhancing Active Life (IDEAL) study

Yu-Tzu Wu[1,3*], Linda Clare[1], John V. Hindle[1], Sharon M. Nelis[1], Anthony Martyr[1], Fiona E. Matthews[2] and on behalf of the Improving the experience of Dementia and Enhancing Active Life study

Abstract

Background: The heterogeneity of symptoms across dementia subtypes has important implications for clinical practice and dementia research. Variation in subtypes and associated symptoms may influence the capability to live well for people with dementia and carers. The aim of this study is to investigate the potential impact of dementia subtypes on the capability to live well for both people with dementia and their carers.

Methods: The analysis was based on the 1283 dyads of community-dwelling people with dementia and carers in the Improving the experience of Dementia and Enhancing Active Life (IDEAL) project, a large cohort study in Great Britain. Capability to live well was defined using three measures: quality of life, life satisfaction and wellbeing. Structural equation modelling was used to investigate capability to live well in seven dementia subtypes: Alzheimer's disease (AD), Vascular dementia (VaD), mixed AD/VaD, frontotemporal dementia (FTD), Parkinson's disease dementia (PDD), Lewy body dementia (LBD) and unspecified/other, accounting for dyadic data structure and adjusting for age and sex, type of relationship between person with dementia and their carer and the number of chronic conditions.

Results: The major subtypes in this study population were AD (56%), VaD (11%) and mixed AD/VaD (21%). Compared to participants with AD, people with non-AD subtypes generally reported a lower capability to live well. Carers for people with PDD (− 1.71; 95% confidence interval (CI) − 3.24, − 0.18) and LBD (− 2.29; 95% CI − 3.84, − 0.75) also reported a lower capability to live well than carers for people with AD. After adjusting for demographic factors and comorbidity, PDD (− 4.28; 95% CI − 5.65, − 2.91) and LBD (− 3.76; 95% CI − 5.14, − 2.39) continued to have the strongest impact on both people with dementia and their carers.

Conclusions: This study suggests a variation in capability to live well across dementia subtypes. It is important for care providers to consider different needs across subtypes. Health professionals who provide post-diagnostic support may need to pay more attention to the complex needs of people living with PDD and LBD and their carers.

Keywords: Dementia, Subtype, Quality of life, Wellbeing, Life satisfaction, Caregiving

* Correspondence: yu-tzu.wu@kcl.ac.uk
[1]REACH: The Centre for Research in Ageing and Cognitive Health, St Luke's Campus, University of Exeter Medical School, Exeter EX1 2LU, UK
[3]Present address: Health Service and Population Research Department, Institute of Psychiatry, Psychology and Neuroscience, King's College London, David Goldberg Centre, De Crespigny Park, Denmark Hill, London SE5 8AF, UK
Full list of author information is available at the end of the article

Background

Dementia is a key priority area in health and social care planning across the world, with an increasing emphasis on timely diagnosis and appropriate support throughout the trajectory of the condition [1, 2]. To support the large number of people living with dementia and their carers to live well and manage the condition, provision of effective post-diagnostic care has become an important issue for health services and clinical practice [3]. For example, in the UK the current National Health Service (NHS) strategy to improve dementia care includes encouraging general practitioners to play a leading role in the coordination and continuity of care for people with dementia [4]. Yet there is a lack of evidence-based guidance to enable health professionals to identify high-risk groups who might experience poor quality of life due to dementia-related symptoms and need additional support to live well with their condition.

Living well with chronic illness has been defined as the best achievable state of physical, mental and social health and wellbeing, indexed by a self-perceived level of comfort, function and contentment with life [5]. The concept of 'living well' with dementia has been largely equated to a good quality of life. However, living well can mean more than a score on quality of life measured at a specific time point. The concept should encompass other inter-related constructs such as the experience of satisfaction with life and a sense of subjective wellbeing [6].

The heterogeneity of symptoms across dementia subtypes has been a key topic in clinical practice and relevant research [7, 8]. Variation in the symptoms associated with different subtypes may influence quality of life and wellbeing in people with dementia and their carers. Needs for post-diagnostic support and care may also vary across different subtypes. Indeed, previous studies have highlighted the potential impact of dementia subtypes on quality of life in people with dementia and on the burden of caregiving. Compared to Alzheimer's disease (AD), people with Lewy body dementia (LBD) tend to report a worse quality of life [9–11]. Family carers for people with frontotemporal dementia (FTD) and LBD have been found to experience a greater caregiving burden than carers for people with AD [11–13]. However, most existing studies were based on a relatively small number of participants recruited from clinical or residential settings and focused on specific subtypes and variation in people with dementia or carers separately. To address limitations in the existing studies, the aim of this study is to investigate the potential impact of dementia subtypes on the capability to live well using 1283 dyads of community-dwelling people with dementia and their carers in Great Britain.

Methods

Study population

The Improving the experience of Dementia and Enhancing Active Life (IDEAL) project is a longitudinal cohort study of community-dwelling people with dementia and their carers across England, Scotland and Wales. The study was set up to investigate social, psychological and economic factors that support people living well with dementia. The participants were recruited through a network of 29 NHS sites between July 2014 and August 2016. Eligible participants needed to have a clinical diagnosis of dementia and a Mini-Mental State Examination (MMSE) score of 15 or above on entry into the study. Primary carers, who provided practical or emotional unpaid support for people with dementia, were also invited to take part where possible. For those who agreed to take part, researchers visited participants and completed structured interviews to collect data. The study protocol has been published elsewhere [14]. The IDEAL study was approved by the Wales Research Ethics Committee 5 (reference 13/WA/0405) and the Ethics Committee of the School of Psychology, Bangor University (reference 2014-11684). IDEAL is registered with the UK Clinical Research Network, number 16593.

The IDEAL cohort at baseline included 1547 people with dementia and 1283 carers. This analysis focused on the 1283 dyads of person with dementia and their carer.

Measurements

Capability to live well was defined using three individual measures for quality of life, life satisfaction and wellbeing for the person with dementia and the carer. For people with dementia, self-rated life satisfaction was measured by the Satisfaction with Life Scale (SwLS; score range 5–35), which is designed to measure global judgements of satisfaction with life [15]; wellbeing was measured by the World Health Organization Five Well-being Index (WHO-5; score range 0–100), which includes items on positive mood, vitality and general interests [16]; and quality of life was measured by the Quality of Life in Alzheimer's Disease (QOL-AD; score range 13–52), which is a dementia-specific measure of quality of life, incorporating multiple aspects of mood, health status, interpersonal relationships and financial situation [17]. The same measures for life satisfaction and wellbeing were used in the carer interview, but quality of life was measured using the World Health Organization Quality of Life-Brief (WHOQOL-BREF), which includes two single indicators (overall quality of life and general health) and four domains (physical health, psychological health, social relationships and environment) [18]. WHOQOL-BREF is designed to measure multiple components related to quality of life and does not have a total score. To provide an overall score for quality of life in carers, a factor analysis was conducted to estimate factor scores for those with complete data. The mean and standard deviation (SD) of the WHOQOL-BREF factor score was 0.0 (SD = 2.1) with a range between − 7.9 and 4.7. More detailed information is provided in Additional file 1.

The interviews collected information on age, sex, dementia subtypes and the type of relationship between the person with dementia and the carer. Age was divided into five groups: < 65, 65–69, 70–74, 75–79 and ≥ 80 for both people with dementia and carers. Dementia diagnoses were obtained from medical records of the participants and classified in seven groups: Alzheimer's disease (AD), vascular dementia (VaD), mixed AD and VaD, frontotemporal dementia (FTD), Parkinson's disease dementia (PDD), Lewy body dementia (LBD) and other/unspecified. For those who selected other or an unspecified diagnosis in the interviews, open-ended text descriptions provided by the interviewer were reviewed by two clinicians and re-categorised into the six empirical groups where possible. The type of relationship between the person with dementia and carer was categorised into two groups: spouse/partner and family/friend such as daughters, sons and grandchildren. Due to the small numbers of friends serving as carers ($N = 12$), this group was combined with family carers. As poor health status has been related to poor quality of life and wellbeing, the number of chronic conditions was used to indicate the general physical health of people with dementia and was measured using the Charlson Comorbidity Index [19].

Analytical strategy

Before conducting the dyadic analysis, the associations between subtypes and the three living well measures in people with dementia and carers were investigated using multivariate modelling. Structural equation modelling (SEM) was used to build two latent factors including three living well measures in people with dementia (SwLS, WHO-5 and QOL-AD) and carers (SwLS, WHO-5 and WHOQOL-BREF factor score), and SwLS was fixed at 1 in the latent factors. Covariance of their error terms was estimated to account for the dyadic structure (Fig. 1). The dyadic relationships between subtypes and living well latent factors (P and C in Fig. 1) were also examined in SEM adjusting for the age and sex of people with dementia and carers as well as the type of relationship between persons with dementia and their carers. Further adjustment for number of chronic conditions was conducted to account for physical health conditions in people with dementia. The estimation method of maximum likelihood with missing values was used in the modelling in order to account for missing data [20]. To investigate whether the associations between dementia subtypes and capability to live well were different in those without carers, a sensitivity analysis was conducted to test the model in all IDEAL participants ($N = 1547$). This study was based on the IDEAL baseline data version 2.0. All analyses were conducted using Stata 14.2.

Results

Descriptive information on the 1283 dyads is reported in Table 1. The median age was 77 (interquartile range (IQR) = 12.0) for people with dementia and 71 (IQR = 14.0) for carers. More than half of people with dementia were men, while nearly 70% of the carers were women. Most carers were spouses or partners (81%) of the person with dementia. Nearly 56% of the participants had AD, 11% had VaD and 21% had a diagnosis of mixed AD and VaD. A relatively small percentage of participants

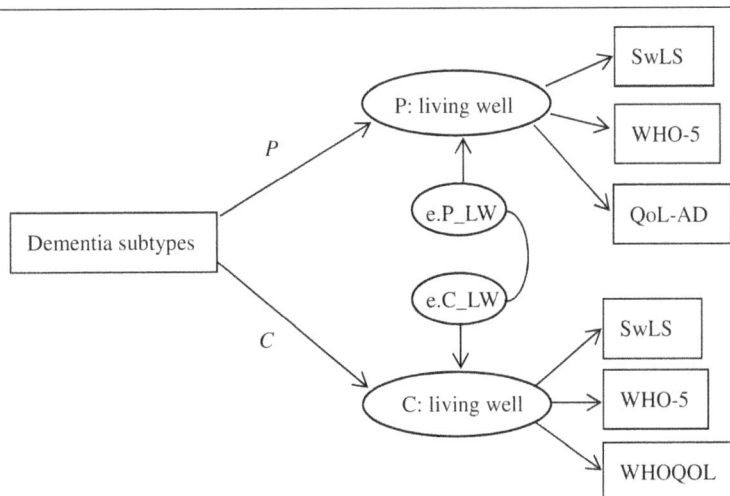

Fig. 1 Dyadic relationship between subtypes and capability to live well in people with dementia (*P*) and carers (*C*)

Table 1 Descriptive information on the study population (*N* = 1283)

	People with dementia: *N*(%)	Carers: *N*(%)
Age		
80+	482 (37.6)	216 (16.8)
75–79	306 (23.9)	223 (17.4)
70–74	232 (18.1)	267 (20.8)
65–69	160 (12.5)	208 (16.2)
< 65	103 (8.0)	369 (28.8)
Sex		
Men	755 (58.9)	402 (31.3)
Women	528 (41.1)	881 (68.7)
Dementia subtype		
Alzheimer's disease (AD)	715 (55.7)	
Vascular dementia (VaD)	142 (11.1)	
Mixed AD and VaD	263 (20.5)	
Frontotemporal dementia (FTD)	45 (3.5)	
Parkinson's disease dementia (PDD)	43 (3.4)	
Lewy body dementia (LBD)	43 (3.4)	
Other/unspecified	32 (2.5)	
Type of relationship		
Spouse/partner	1039 (81.0)	
Family/friend	244 (19.0)	
Chronic conditions (missing = 89)		
1–2	611 (51.2)	
3–4	426 (35.7)	
5+	157 (13.1)	

had FTD (3.5%), PDD (3.4%) and LBD (3.4%); the other/unspecified category accounted for 2.5%. The median MMSE score of people with dementia was 23 (IQR = 6.0), and 27% of people with dementia and 22% of the carers had no educational qualification. Approximately one-third of people with dementia (35%) and carers (30%) reported fair or poor self-rated health.

Table 2 reports the means and standard deviations of the three living well measures in people with dementia and carers across subtypes. People with dementia generally reported higher scores for life satisfaction and well-being than their carers, but the patterns across subtypes were similar in people with dementia and carers. The mean scores were generally higher in AD and lower in PDD and LBD.

Table 2 Mean scores and standard deviation of living well measures in people with dementia and carers across subtypes

	People with dementia			Carers		
	SwLS	WHO-5	QOL-AD	SwLS	WHO-5	WHOQOL-BREF[a]
AD	27.3 (5.5)	64.2 (19.5)	37.7 (5.5)	24.1 (6.4)	56.6 (19.6)	0.1 (2.0)
VaD	25.6 (6.3)	58.6 (21.2)	35.9 (6.5)	23.4 (6.3)	53.0 (19.3)	−0.1 (2.1)
Mixed AD/VaD	26.3 (5.9)	59.8 (21.0)	36.3 (5.8)	24.4 (6.5)	55.2 (19.9)	0.0 (2.1)
FTD	25.7 (5.9)	61.0 (20.5)	38.7 (5.4)	21.9 (7.2)	53.2 (21.8)	−0.2 (2.2)
PDD	22.0 (6.8)	47.9 (20.4)	33.1 (5.7)	21.5 (5.6)	50.1 (19.0)	−0.4 (1.8)
LBD	23.7 (5.2)	50.7 (17.8)	33.0 (6.3)	20.4 (7.9)	47.7 (20.9)	−0.7 (2.1)
Other	26.2 (7.6)	58.5 (24.8)	34.7 (8.1)	23.2 (6.4)	56.9 (18.3)	−0.4 (2.2)

AD Alzheimer's disease, *VaD* vascular dementia, *FTD* frontotemporal dementia, *PDD* Parkinson's disease dementia, *LBD* Lewy body dementia, *SwLS* Satisfaction with Life Scale, *WHO-5* World Health Organization Five Well-being Index, *QOL-AD* Quality of Life in Alzheimer's Disease,
[a]WHOQOL-BREF factor score estimated from six domains

In people with dementia, loadings of the living well latent factors (SwLS fixed at 1) were estimated to be 3.82 (95% confidence interval (CI) 3.52, 4.13) for WHO-5 and 1.21 (95% CI 1.12, 1.31) for QOL-AD. In carers, loading estimates were 3.37 (95% CI 3.11, 3.62) for WHO-5 and 0.41 (95% CI 0.38, 0.44) for the WHOQOL-BREF factor score. The two living well latent factors were correlated, and the estimated covariance was 5.62 (95% CI 4.22, 7.03).

Table 3 reports dyadic associations between subtypes and capability to live well in people with dementia and carers (P and C in Fig. 1). Participants with non-AD subtypes reported a lower capability to live well than those with AD. Significant differences were found for VaD (− 1.69; 95% CI − 2.52, − 0.87), mixed AD/VaD (− 1.34; 95% CI − 1.99, − 0.70), PDD (− 4.39; 95% CI − 5.80, − 2.97), LBD (− 3.81; 95% CI − 5.23, − 2.40) and other (− 1.98; 95% CI − 3.59, − 0.38) after adjusting for age, sex and type of relationship. For carers, the variations across subtypes were relatively small, but lower capability to live well was also found for carers of people with PDD (− 1.55; 95% CI − 3.06, − 0.03) and LBD (− 1.77; 95% CI − 3.29, − 0.25) compared to carers of people with AD. Further adjustment for the number of chronic conditions in people with dementia attenuated the difference in VaD (− 0.96; 95% CI − 1.77, − 0.15) and mixed AD/VaD (− 0.87; 95% CI − 1.50, − 0.24) for people with dementia, but the effect sizes for PDD and LBD remained similar in both. The association between subtypes and capability to live well was similar for all people with dementia, including those without carers. More detailed information on the sensitivity analysis is provided in Additional file 1.

Based on the adjusted results, Fig. 2a–c shows estimated scores for the three living well measures across subtypes in people with dementia and their carers. Carers had systematically lower scores than people with dementia, but estimates for SwLS and WHO-5 were similar in those with PDD and LBD.

Discussion
Main findings
Using dyadic analysis methods, this study suggest a potential impact of subtype diagnosis on capability to live well in both people with dementia and carers. People with non-AD subtypes, including VaD, mixed VaD/AD, PDD and LBD, had a lower capability to live well than those with AD. For carers, those caring for people with PDD and LBD reported lower scores on living well measures than carers of people with AD. Further adjustment for comorbidity attenuated differences between AD, VaD and mixed AD/VaD, but PDD and LBD continued to have a particularly strong impact on capability to live well in both people with dementia and carers.

Strengths and limitations
The IDEAL study included a large number of community-dwelling people with dementia and their carers across Great Britain. In addition to major subtypes (AD and VaD), people with rare subtypes were also recruited and were represented by at least 40 dyads in this study population. The interviews included multiple measures of living well, including aspects of quality of life, life satisfaction and wellbeing for both people with dementia and their carers. The method of dyadic analysis was used to investigate the association between subtypes and capability to live well in both people with dementia and carers and to take into account correlations within dyads.

To be eligible to take part, participants needed to have a clinical diagnosis of dementia and a MMSE score of 15 or above. People with severe dementia were not included in the study, and the dyadic association between subtypes and capability to live well might be different in this group compared to the current study population focusing on mild to moderate dementia. Given our interest in the dyadic relationship, this analysis mainly focused on

Table 3 Results of structural equation model: dyadic associations between subtypes and capability to live well in people with dementia and carers (N = 1283)

	Unadjusted		Adjusted 1		Adjusted 2	
	Person with dementia (P)	Carer (C)	Person with dementia (P)	Carer (C)	Person with dementia (P)	Carer (C)
AD	(Reference)	(Reference)	(Reference)	(Reference)	(Reference)	(Reference)
VaD	−1.64 (−2.47, −0.82)	−0.72 (−1.62, 0.17)	− 1.69 (− 2.52, − 0.87)	−0.58 (− 1.47, 0.31)	−0.96 (− 1.77, − 0.15)	−0.22 (− 1.12, 0.68)
Mixed AD/VaD	− 1.14 (− 1.78, − 0.50)	−0.17 (− 0.87, 0.54)	−1.34 (− 1.99, − 0.70)	−0.19 (− 0.89, 0.50)	−0.87 (− 1.50, − 0.24)	0.05 (− 0.66, 0.75)
FTD	−0.13 (− 1.49, 1.23)	−0.83 (− 2.34, 0.68)	0.39 (− 0.99, 1.78)	−0.30 (− 1.80, 1.20)	0.17 (−1.16, 1.50)	−0.42 (− 1.92, 1.07)
PDD	−4.26 (−5.68, −2.85)	−1.71 (− 3.24, − 0.18)	−4.39 (− 5.80, − 2.97)	− 1.55 (− 3.06, − 0.03)	− 4.28 (− 5.65, − 2.91)	− 1.51 (− 3.02, − 0.01)
LBD	−3.72 (− 5.14, −2.31)	−2.29 (− 3.84, − 0.75)	−3.81 (− 5.23, − 2.40)	− 1.77 (− 3.29, − 0.25)	−3.76 (− 5.14, − 2.39)	−1.77 (− 3.28, − 0.26)
Other	− 1.88 (− 3.48, − 0.27)	− 0.84 (− 2.61, 0.93)	−1.98 (− 3.59, − 0.38)	− 0.97 (− 2.72, 0.78)	−1.98 (− 3.54, − 0.43)	−0.99 (− 2.72, 0.75)

AD Alzheimer's disease, *VaD* vascular dementia, *FTD* frontotemporal dementia, *PDD* Parkinson's disease dementia, *LBD* Lewy body dementia, *Adjusted 1* age and sex in people with dementia and carers, type of relationship between the person with dementia and carer, *Adjusted 2* all factors in Adjusted 1 and number of chronic conditions in people with dementia

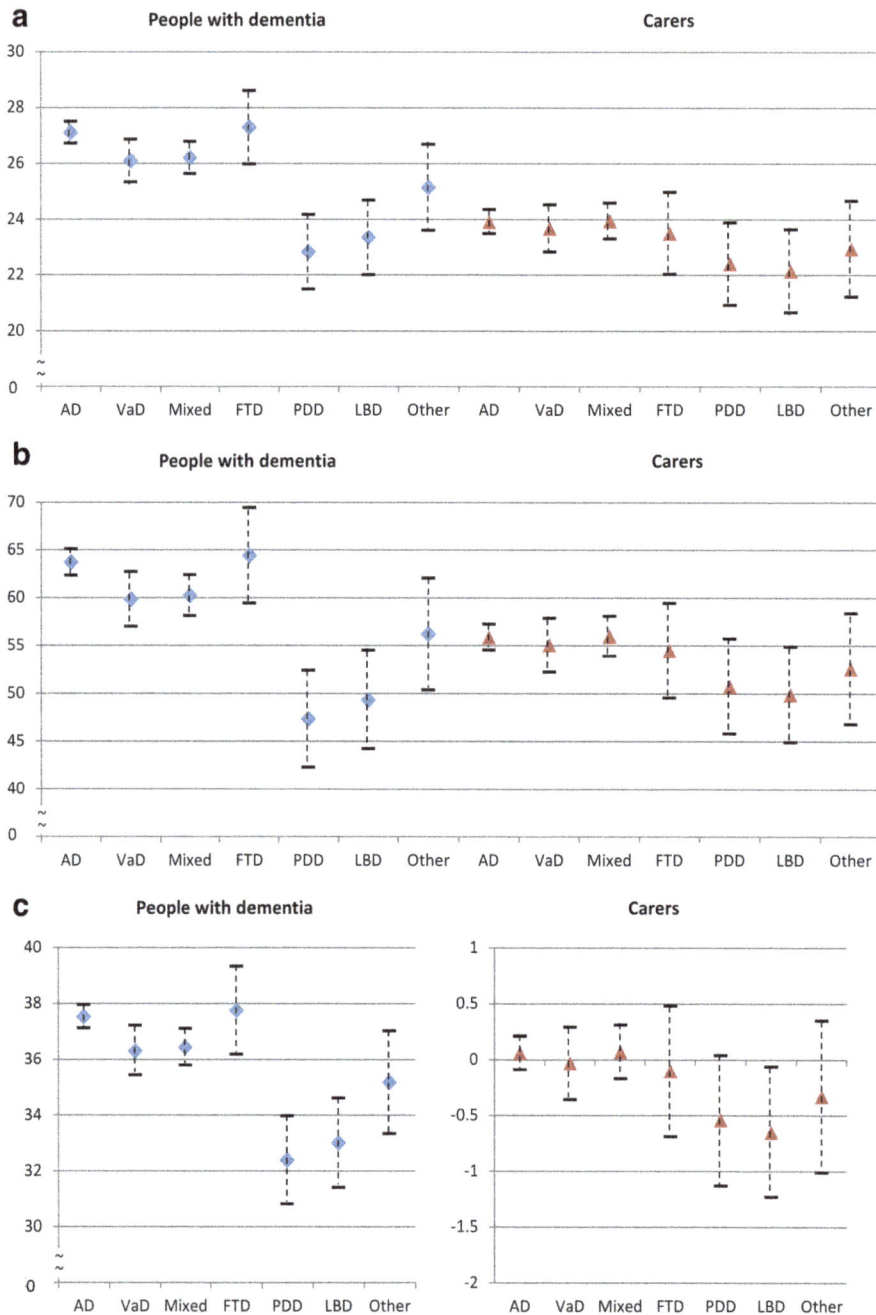

Fig. 2 Estimated scores of living well measures across subtypes (adjusted for age, sex, type of relationship and number of chronic conditions in people with dementia) (**a**) Life satisfaction (SwLS) (**b**) Well-being (WHO-5) (**c**) Quality of life (QOL-AD) for people with dementia, WHOQOL-BREF factor score for carers

participants with carers. Since those without carers might have better health status and functional ability and in some cases might not need a carer, the association between subtypes and capability to live well might be different in this group. Nevertheless, similar results were found in sensitivity analyses including all participants irrespective of carer involvement ($N = 1547$); therefore, this should have a minimal impact on the main findings.

The diagnoses of dementia subtypes were made by different clinicians across the country. Variation in clinical practice and potential diagnostic misclassification could not be addressed in this analysis. However, a clinical diagnosis reflects the experience of people with dementia and their carers attending health services and leads to selection of particular treatments and disease management plans. Different measures for quality of life were used in people with dementia and the carers, and therefore changes in quality of life scores were not directly comparable. To generate an overall score for quality of life in carers, six independent domains in WHOQOL-BREF were combined using factor analysis. Although measures for quality of life were different for people with dementia and carers, this study mainly focused on relative differences, and similar patterns were found in these two quality of life measures.

Interpretation of results

People with non-AD subtypes had a lower capability to live well than those with AD. When further adjusting for comorbidity, the difference between AD, VaD and mixed AD/VaD reduced considerably. This suggests that the burden of chronic conditions might explain much of the observed differences across these subtypes. Although the diagnosis of VaD is based on cerebrovascular pathology and small vessel disease, people with VaD might also experience physical disabilities as well as language and visuospatial deficits due to stroke and heart attack and thus may have poor quality of life and wellbeing [8].

People with PDD and LBD continued to show a particularly poor capability to live well, even when we further adjusted for the number of chronic conditions. This corresponds to findings from previous studies [9–11]. These two subtypes are closely related, and the differential diagnosis is largely based on when symptoms first appear. The core symptoms of LBD, including fluctuating cognition, visual hallucinations and spontaneous features of Parkinsonism [8], may have a relatively large impact on daily life compared to the major symptoms of memory loss in AD. A higher number of autonomic symptoms such as fatigue, postural dizziness and mucosal dryness have also been reported in PDD and LBD than in AD [21]. PDD is also associated with high comorbidity [22, 23], and the mix of physical, emotional and cognitive changes might have a negative impact on quality of life for the person with dementia as well as their carer. Carers of people with PDD and LBD have been reported to experience a higher level of stress than carers of those with AD and VaD [24]. This might be due to the challenges of responding to symptoms such as hallucinations, motor disability and functional impairment in PDD and LBD [11].

The literature has suggested a greater burden of care in FTD [12, 13]. FTD generally occurs in younger age groups (< 65) and includes symptoms related to changes in personality, behaviour and function [7]. Although these symptoms may plausibly increase the burden of caregiving and cause poor quality of life and wellbeing, this study did not find a difference in the capability to live well between carers of people with FTD and AD. A previous study from Australia has reported variation in caregiving burden across different FTD variants [12].

Although carers of persons with behavioural variant FTD (bvFTD) did report a particularly high burden, carers for people with other FTD variants, including semantic dementia and progressive non-fluent aphasia, had similar levels of burden to carers of people with AD. Indeed, the mean scores for living well measures were found to be lower for the 10 IDEAL carers of people with bvFTD than for carers of people with other FTD variants. However, it is not possible to test differences within this subtype based on such a small sample size and limited statistical power. In addition, this study population only included those with mild to moderate dementia and did not include those with advanced FTD.

Dyadic modelling was used to consider the capability to live well in both people with dementia and carers and to account for correlations within dyads. In addition to relative differences across subtype, this study also reveals baseline differences between people with dementia and carers through this dyadic analysis approach. Capability to live well was clearly not independent in these dyads, but relative difference across subtype, a dyad-level measure, was not considerably affected by this correlation. However, absolute scores on living well measures were lower for carers than for people with dementia. Despite variation across subtypes, baseline scores for life satisfaction and wellbeing in carers were close to those for participants with PDD and LBD, who had the worst capability to live well. This indicates that carers generally reported a poorer capability to live well than people with dementia, regardless of subtype.

Clinical implications and future research directions

Variation in capability to live well was found across dementia subtypes, particularly PDD and LBD. Guidelines for dementia care may need to be tailored for different subtypes and provide additional support for these high-risk groups. Since the impact of living with VaD and mixed AD/VaD may be related to comorbidity, treatment of hypertension and vascular diseases is important for those with these subtypes. Health professionals who provide post-diagnostic support and care may need to pay more attention to the PDD and LBD subtypes and consider potential approaches to improve quality of life and wellbeing for both people with dementia and their carers [25]. In addition to medical treatments, some non-pharmacological interventions might support those living with PDD and LBD to maintain daily function. For example, a recent pilot randomised controlled trial focusing on 29 people with PDD and LBD has suggested that cognitive rehabilitation, an individualised approach addressing personally relevant goals, can be effective in managing the impact of the cognitive difficulties on daily life and in improving quality of life [26]. Future intervention studies may extend this approach to include the physical symptoms seen in PDD and LBD and reduce the combined impact of cognitive and physical symptoms on the capability to live well with these conditions. Carers reported relatively low scores on living well measures across all dementia subtypes. Burden of caregiving appears to be an important issue, and appropriate support for family carers is vital [1].

To reduce the impact of subtype diagnosis, future research may focus on identifying specific factors related to the quality of life and wellbeing in PDD and LBD and developing potential interventions to improve disease management in people with dementia and carers. In addition to medications, psychosocial and rehabilitative interventions may play an important role in addressing neuropsychiatric and behavioural symptoms and general physical, psychological and social health [27].

Conclusions

The findings of this study suggest important differences in the capability to live well across dementia subtypes. Dementia care and health professionals who provide post-diagnostic support should consider different needs across subtypes, in particular the complex needs of people living with PDD and LBD and their carers.

Abbreviations

AD: Alzheimer's disease; bvFTD: Behavioural variant frontotemporal dementia; CI: Confidence interval; FTD: Frontotemporal dementia; IDEAL: Improving the experience of Dementia and Enhancing Active Life; IQR: Interquartile range; LBD: Lewy body dementia; MMSE: Mini-Mental State Examination; PDD: Parkinson's disease dementia; QOL-AD: Quality of Life in Alzheimer's Disease; SD: Standard deviation; SEM: Structural equation modelling; SwLS: Satisfaction with Life Scale; VaD: Vascular dementia; WHO-5: World Health Organization Five Well-being Index; WHOQOL-BREF: World Health Organization Quality of Life-Brief

Acknowledgements

We are grateful to the three UK research networks, the National Institute for Health Research (NIHR) Clinical Research Network in England, the Scottish Dementia Network (SDN) and Health and Care Research Wales, for supporting the study. We thank the local principal investigators and staff at our NHS sites, the IDEAL study participants and their families, the members of the ALWAYs group and the Project Advisory Group.

Funding

This work was supported by the Economic and Social Research Council (UK) and the National Institute for Health Research (UK) through grant ES/L001853/2 'Improving the experience of dementia and enhancing active life: living well with dementia' (investigators: L. Clare, I.R. Jones, C. Victor, J.V. Hindle, R.W. Jones, M. Knapp, M. Kopelman, R. Litherland, A. Martyr, F.E. Matthews, R.G. Morris, S.M. Nelis, J. Pickett, C. Quinn, J. Rusted, J.

Thom). The funders had no role in study design, data collection and analysis, decision to publish or preparation of the manuscript.

Authors' contributions

YTW and FEM developed the original idea and designed the approach. YTW conducted the data analysis, and FEM supervised the analysis. YTW, LC, JVH, SMN, AM and FEM contributed to manuscript writing. All authors read and approved the final manuscript.

Competing interests

The authors declare that they have no competing interests.

Author details

[1]REACH: The Centre for Research in Ageing and Cognitive Health, St Luke's Campus, University of Exeter Medical School, Exeter EX1 2LU, UK. [2]Institute of Health and Society, Newcastle University, The Baddiley-Clark Building, Richardson Road, Newcastle Upon Tyne NE4 5PL, UK. [3]Present address: Health Service and Population Research Department, Institute of Psychiatry, Psychology and Neuroscience, King's College London, David Goldberg Centre, De Crespigny Park, Denmark Hill, London SE5 8AF, UK.

References

1. World Health Organization. Dementia: a public health priority. Geneva: World Health Organization; 2012.
2. Alzheimer's Society. Dementia UK. 2014. https://www.alzheimers.org.uk/info/20025/policy_and_influencing/251/dementia_uk. Accessed 01 Aug 2018.
3. UK government, Department of Health. Prime Minister's challenge on dementia. 2020:2015. www.gov.uk/government/publications/prime-ministers-challenge-on-dementia-2020. Accessed 01 Aug 2018
4. National Health Services England. The well pathway for dementia. 2016. www.england.nhs.uk/mentalhealth/wp-content/uploads/sites/29/2016/03/dementia-well-pathway.pdf. Accessed 01 Aug 2018.
5. Institute of Medicine. Living well with chronic illness: a call for public health action. Washington: National Academies Press; 2012.
6. Martyr A, Nelis SM, Quinn C, Wu Y-T, Lamont RA, Henderson C, et al. Living well with dementia: a systematic review and correlational meta-analysis of factors associated with quality of life, well-being and life satisfaction in people with dementia. Psychol Med. 2018; https://doi.org/10.1017/S0033291718000405.
7. Hughes JC. Alzheimer's and other dementias. Oxford: Oxford Press; 2011.
8. Robinson L. Dementia: timely diagnosis and early intervention. BMJ 2015; 350:h3029. doi:https://doi.org/10.1136/bmj.h3029.
9. Bostrom F, Jonsson L, Minthon L, Londos E. Patients with dementia with Lewy bodies have more impaired quality of life than patients with Alzheimer disease. Alzheimer Dis Assoc Disord. 2007;21:150–4.
10. Thomas P, Lalloue F, Preux P-M, Hazif-Thomas C, Pariel S, Inscale R, Belmin J, Clement J-P. Dementia patients caregivers quality of life: the PIXEL study. Int J Geriatr Psychiatry. 2006;21:50–6.
11. Zweig YR, Galvin JE. Lewy body dementia: the impact on patients and caregivers. Alzheimers Res Ther. 2014;6:21.
12. Mioshi E, Foxe D, Leslie F, Savage S, Hsieh S, Miller L, Hodges JR, Piguet O. The impact of dementia severity on caregiver burden in frontotemporal dementia and Alzheimer disease. Alzheimer Dis Assoc Disord. 2013;27:68–73.

13. Riedijk SR, De Vugt ME, Duivenvoorden HJ, Niermeijer MF, Van Swieten JC, Verhey FR, Tibben A. Caregiver burden, health-related quality of life and coping in dementia caregivers: a comparison of frontotemporal dementia and Alzheimer's disease. Dement Geriatr Cogn Disord. 2006;22:405–12.

14. Clare L, Nelis SM, Quinn C, Martyr A, Henderson C, Hindle JV, et al. Improving the experience of dementia and enhancing active life—living well with dementia: study protocol for the IDEAL study. Health Qual Life Outcomes. 2014;12:164.

15. Diener E, Emmons RA, Larsen RJ, Griffin S. The satisfaction with life scale. J Pers Assess. 1985;49:71–5.

16. Bech P. Measuring the dimension of psychological general well-being by the WHO-5. Qual Life Newslett. 2004;32:15–6.

17. Logsdon RG, Gibbons LE, McCurry SM, Teri L. Quality of life in Alzheimer's disease: patient and caregiver reports. New York: Springer; 2000. p. 17–30.

18. Skevington SM, Lotfy M, O'Connell KA. The World Health Organization's WHOQOL-BREF quality of life assessment: psychometric properties and results of the international field trial. A report from the WHOQOL group. Qual Life Res. 2004;13:299–310.

19. Charlson ME, Charlson RE, Peterson JC, Marinopoulos SS, Briggs WM, Hollenberg JP. The Charlson comorbidity index is adapted to predict costs of chronic disease in primary care patients. J Clin Epidemiol. 2008;61:1234–40.

20. Stata structural equation modeling reference manual, Release 13. StataCorp LP. 2013. https://www.stata.com/manuals13/sem.pdf. Accessed 01 Aug 2018.

21. Allan L, McKeith I, Ballard C, Kenny RA. The prevalence of autonomic symptoms in dementia and their association with physical activity, activities of daily living and quality of life. Dement Geriatr Cogn Disord. 2006;22:230–7.

22. Clague F, Mercer SW, Mclean G, Reynish E, Guthrie B. Comorbidity and polypharmacy in people with dementia: insights from a large, population-based cross-sectional analysis of primary care data. Age Ageing. 2017;46:33–9.

23. McLean G, Hindle JV, Guthrie B, Mercer SW. Co-morbidity and polypharmacy in Parkinson's disease: insights from a large Scottish primary care database. BMC Neurol. 2017;17:126.

24. Lee DR, McKeith I, Mosimann U, Ghosh-Nodyal A, Thomas AJ. Examining carer stress in dementia: the role of subtype diagnosis and neuropsychiatric symptoms. Int J Geriatr Psychiatry. 2013;28:135–41.

25. National Health Services England. Dementia diagnosis and management. A brief pragmatic resource for general practitioners. https://www.england.nhs.uk/wp-content/uploads/2015/01/dementia-diag-mng-ab-pt.pdf. Accessed 01 Aug 2018.

26. Hindle JV, Watermeyer TJ, Roberts J, Brand A, Hoare Z, Martyr A, Clare L. Goal-orientated cognitive rehabilitation for dementias associated with Parkinson's disease-A pilot randomised controlled trial. Int J Geriatr Psychiatry. 2018;33(5):718–28.

27. Morhardt D, Weintraub S, Khayum B, Robinson J, Medina J, O'Hara M, Mesulam M, Rogalski EJ. The CARE pathway model for dementia: psychosocial and rehabilitative strategies for care in young-onset dementias. Psychiatr Clin North Am. 2015;38:333–52.

16

Genotype-guided versus traditional clinical dosing of warfarin in patients of Asian ancestry

Nicholas L. Syn[1,2†], Andrea Li-Ann Wong[1,2†], Soo-Chin Lee[1,2], Hock-Luen Teoh[3], James Wei Luen Yip[4], Raymond CS Seet[3,13], Wee Tiong Yeo[4], William Kristanto[4], Ping-Chong Bee[5], LM Poon[1], Patrick Marban[1], Tuck Seng Wu[6], Michael D. Winther[7], Liam R. Brunham[8,9], Richie Soong[2,10], Bee-Choo Tai[11] and Boon-Cher Goh[1,2,12*]

Abstract

Background: Genotype-guided warfarin dosing has been shown in some randomized trials to improve anticoagulation outcomes in individuals of European ancestry, yet its utility in Asian patients remains unresolved.

Methods: An open-label, non-inferiority, 1:1 randomized trial was conducted at three academic hospitals in South East Asia, involving 322 ethnically diverse patients newly indicated for warfarin (NCT00700895). Clinical follow-up was 90 days. The primary efficacy measure was the number of dose titrations within the first 2 weeks of therapy, with a mean non-inferiority margin of 0.5 over the first 14 days of therapy.

Results: Among 322 randomized patients, 269 were evaluable for the primary endpoint. Compared with traditional dosing, the genotype-guided group required fewer dose titrations during the first 2 weeks (1.77 vs. 2. 93, difference −1.16, 90% CI −1.48 to −0.84, $P < 0.001$ for both non-inferiority and superiority). The percentage of time within the therapeutic range over 3 months and median time to stable international normalized ratio (INR) did not differ between the genotype-guided and traditional dosing groups. The frequency of dose titrations (incidence rate ratio 0.76, 95% CI 0.67 to 0.86, $P = 0.001$), but not frequency of INR measurements, was lower at 1, 2, and 3 months in the genotype-guided group. The proportions of patients who experienced minor or major bleeding, recurrent venous thromboembolism, or out-of-range INR did not differ between both arms. For predicting maintenance doses, the pharmacogenetic algorithm achieved an $R^2 = 42.4\%$ ($P < 0.001$) and mean percentage error of −7.4%.

Conclusions: Among Asian adults commencing warfarin therapy, a pharmacogenetic algorithm meets criteria for both non-inferiority and superiority in reducing dose titrations compared with a traditional dosing approach, and performs well in prediction of actual maintenance doses. These findings imply that clinicians may consider applying a pharmacogenetic algorithm to personalize initial warfarin dosages in Asian patients.

Trial registration: ClinicalTrials.gov NCT00700895. Registered on June 19, 2008.

Keywords: Pharmacogenetics, Pharmacogenomics, Precision medicine, CYP2C9, Cytochrome P450, VKORC1, Warfarin, Anticoagulants, Anticoagulation, Polymorphism

* Correspondence: phcgbc@nus.edu.sg
†Nicholas L. Syn and Andrea Li-Ann Wong contributed equally to this work.
[1]Department of Haematology-Oncology, National University Cancer Institute, Singapore, Singapore
[2]Cancer Science Institute of Singapore, National University of Singapore, Singapore, Singapore
Full list of author information is available at the end of the article

Background

While effective in preventing thromboembolic events, clinical application of warfarin is characterized by a narrow therapeutic index and often requires multiple dose titrations especially during the first few weeks of therapy. Well-managed warfarin therapy is associated with a reduction in the risk of complications [1], yet the majority of patients do not achieve long-term stable international normalized ratio (INR) within the therapeutic range [2], indicating the difficulty in identifying an optimal maintenance dose for individual patients. A growing body of evidence has emerged indicating that the cytochrome P450 2C9 (*CYP2C9*) and Vitamin K epoxide reductase complex subunit 1 (*VKORC1*) genotypes are associated with maintenance dose requirements, accounting for up to 40–45% of the inter-individual variability, depending on the populations and specific polymorphisms studied [3–5]. Accordingly, since 2007, the United States Food and Drug Administration product label for warfarin has been updated to reflect the potential value of incorporating genetic information into dose selection. Most major contemporary clinical trials and meta-analyses comparing genotype-guided dosing to routine clinical practice or clinically guided algorithms have employed surrogate outcomes and were not powered to demonstrate a difference in clinical endpoints [6–13].

To date, the utility of genotype-guided dosing remains unresolved, particularly in Asian populations, since most randomized studies have thus far been performed in predominantly Caucasian cohorts. Variation in the epidemiology of *VKORC1* and *CYP2C9* genetic polymorphisms across different ancestral populations could impact the performance of pharmacogenetically tailored dosing strategies [6, 7, 14]. The *VKORC1* H1/H1 haplotype, which confers high sensitivity to warfarin, is present in 74%, 42%, and 7% of self-identified Chinese, Malay, and Indian patients, respectively, while the *CYP2C9**3 allele, which is associated with the poor metabolizer phenotype, is present in 7%, 9%, and 18% of patients, respectively [15]. On average, Asian patients homozygous for less-sensitive *VKORC1* haplotypes (H7, H8, or H9) and wild-type for *CYP2C9* will require more than 3.5 times the maintenance dosage needed by patients with the *VKORC1* H1/H1 haplotype and a copy of the *CYP2C9**3 allele [15], highlighting a potential pitfall of empirical dose initiation and titration. Consequently, the application of pharmacogenetics to provide tailored doses to patients of Asian ancestry is particularly compelling. Accordingly, this randomized trial was conducted to test whether a pharmacogenetically based dosing algorithm, which was developed from a racially diverse Asian cohort [16], is non-inferior to traditional clinical dosing.

Methods

The ethics review committees at participating centers approved the study protocol (Additional file 1). The study was conducted in accordance with Good Clinical Practice guidelines, and patients provided written informed consent prior to enrollment. All serious adverse events were reported to the Domain Specific Review Board and the Medical Clinical Research Committee, Ministry of Health, in accordance with published guidelines. The study is registered at ClinicalTrials.gov (Identifier: NCT00700895).

Study design

This open-label, non-inferiority, randomized trial was conducted in three large tertiary hospitals in South East Asia. Randomization was computer generated with a 1:1 allocation ratio, and patients were allocated to the treatment arms by means of sequentially numbered, opaque, and sealed envelopes.

Eligibility criteria were age 18 years or older, a new indication for long-term anticoagulation with warfarin, and transaminases less than three times the upper limit of normal and bilirubin within normal range. Exclusion criteria were uncontrolled hypertension, peptic ulcer disease, previous history of liver disease, malabsorption syndrome or chronic diarrheal conditions, or any other medical conditions deemed unfit for warfarin administration based on the clinical judgment of primary treating physicians. Patients were not allowed to start warfarin before enrolment in the study. Demographic, clinical, and laboratory measurements were collected at baseline. Patient genotypes were determined through pyrosequencing as previously described [15, 16], and data on race or ethnicity was self-reported.

Intervention

The study intervention period comprised of a dose initiation period (first 3 days) and a dose adjustment period (remainder of study). All patients were initiated on low-molecular weight heparins at the point of randomization. The expected turnaround time for genotyping was 2 days and warfarin was initiated on the third day in both groups. Patients randomized to the genotype-guided dosing strategy received their tailored dose for 3 consecutive days. This was calculated using an algorithm which takes into account the presence of the *CYP2C9**3 allele, *VKORC1* 381 genotype, age, and weight [16]. The *VKORC1* 381 T > C single nucleotide polymorphism is in complete linkage disequilibrium with −1639G > A, and has been shown to discriminate the H1 and H7 haplotypes in Asian individuals [15, 16]. If genotype results were unavailable by the first scheduled dose of warfarin (day 1), the patient would be treated with the traditional dosing approach. Patients randomized to the traditional dosing approach were initiated using a standardized loading dose regimen used by the National University Hospital Anticoagulation Clinic consisting of per os warfarin 5 mg on days 1 and 2, followed by 3 mg on day 3. If the patient was more than 75 years of age, the dose on day 2 was lowered to 4 mg (Additional file 1). To account for instances when a different dose than that pre-specified was administered during the warfarin initiation period, deviations from the protocol-specified dose were considered as dose adjustments. During the first 14 days, there were three mandatory INR checks on day 6, between days 7 and 9, and between days 12 and 14. Based on these INR measurements, warfarin dose titrations in both groups as well as decisions to stop low-molecular weight heparin treatment were made according to usual clinical practice and centralized at the anticoagulation clinics (Additional file 1: Appendices 1 and 2). Included patients were followed up until day 90 after warfarin initiation. The number and frequency of follow-up visits were according to dosing tables that simulate real-world clinical practice (Additional file 1). If urgent anticoagulation was needed, patients on both study arms received low molecular weight heparin till INR reached the therapeutic range of 1.9 to 3.1 to avoid warfarin-induced thrombosis due to inhibition of Protein S and C. To avoid variability from different warfarin sources, Marevan° tablets supplied by GlaxoSmithKline (Douglas Manufacturing Ltd., AK, NZ) were used throughout this study.

Outcomes

The primary outcome was the number of dose titrations performed up to end of week 2 (day 14). Patients censored prior to day 14 were excluded from the modified intention-to-treat set due to insufficient data on dose titrations, INR, and other anticoagulation parameters for the evaluation of primary and secondary endpoints.

Secondary outcomes were time to stable INR, defined as the number of days from warfarin initiation to attaining therapeutic INR (≥ 1.9 and ≤ 3.1) for the latter of two consecutive measurements that are at least 7 days apart; percentage of time spent within the therapeutic range (PTTR), which was estimated using the linear interpolation method of Rosendaal et al. [17]; incidence of dose adjustments and INR monitoring during follow-up; and the proportions of patients who had a bleeding episode (classified as minor or major [18]), recurrent venous thromboembolism, and any measured INR value < 1.9 or > 3.1. The PTTR was included in June 2016 as a secondary outcome by way of protocol amendment following a meeting with the Scientific Review Committee for the Surveillance and Pharmacogenomics Initiative for Adverse Drug Reactions (SAPhIRE) program, who recommended that reporting of this endpoint would facilitate between-trial comparisons and enable meta-analyses of similar trials.

Statistical analysis

The trial was powered to establish whether genotype-guided warfarin dose administration was non-inferior to traditional clinical dosing for the primary endpoint of number of dose titrations within the first 2 weeks of therapy. Based on previous data [19], the sample size was estimated assuming a conservative between-group mean difference of 1.0 and a common standard deviation of 1.4 dose titrations. Therefore, with 80% power and a one-sided type I error of 5%, a sample size of 270 would be able to demonstrate non-inferiority of the genotype-guided group for a predefined non-inferiority margin of 0.5 dose titrations. Assuming up to 15% loss to follow-up before day 14, a minimum of 320 patients was deemed necessary. If the upper bound of the 90% confidence interval (CI) of the difference in treatment (genotype-guided vs. traditional dosing) was lesser than 0.5, the null hypothesis would be rejected, which would signify that the genotype-guided strategy was non-inferior to the traditional dosing approach. When non-inferiority was proven, a two-tailed t test with an alpha value of 0.05 was used for superiority testing.

All other secondary endpoints were tests of superiority of genotype-guided dosing versus traditional dosing, and significance was defined as a two-tailed nominal $P < 0.05$. Time to stable INR was evaluated using the Kaplan–Meier method, and the log-rank test was used to compare differences. Percentage of time within the therapeutic range was compared using two-sample t tests. Mixed effects Poisson regression models were used to estimate incidence rate ratios (IRRs) for comparing the number of dose adjustments and INR measurements between interventions, while accounting for possible intra-subject correlation of count data which were measured at 1, 2, and 3 months. To account for the reduced follow-up time among patients who withdrew or discontinued the trial before day 90, we used an exposure variable in the Poisson regression for the number of days on trial. Predicted incidences of dose adjustments and INR measurements were estimated via Stata's post-estimation command, immediately after fitting Poisson regression models. Differences in the proportions of patients who experienced minor or major bleeding, recurrent venous thromboembolism, and INR < 1.9 or > 3.1 were quantified using relative risks, with P values provided by Fisher's exact test, and 95% CIs obtained from exact binomial distributions. Finally, the performance of the genotype-guided warfarin dosing model was evaluated using the Pearson's product-moment correlation, with 95% CIs computed based on Fisher's transformation, mean percentage error, root mean squared error, and Bland–Altman analysis.

All analyses were performed on a modified intention-to-treat basis and without imputation. Statistical analyses were performed in Stata version 13.0 (STATA Corp., College Station, TX, USA).

Results

From May 11, 2007, through July 14, 2016, a total of 334 patients were screened, of whom 322 were randomized (159 to the genotype-guided group and 163 to the traditional dosing group) (Fig. 1). Baseline characteristics and genotypic distributions were well-balanced between both groups. Patients had a median age of 60 years (range, 19–89), and the majority of patients were male (58.4%) and of Chinese race (61.2%) (Table 1). Genotype results were available within the first 4 days for 147 of 159 (92.5%) patients randomized to the pharmacogenetics arm, and therefore these patients successfully received the first genotype-tailored dose on days 3 or 4 as scheduled in the protocol. Specifically, 88 (55.3%), 34 (21.4%), 14 (8.8%), and 11 (6.9%) patients had genotype results returned on days 1 through 4, respectively. The remaining 12 patients (7.5%) randomized to the pharmacogenetics arm were switched to traditional dosing as genotype results were not available by day 5.

In the primary analysis only patients who received warfarin treatment for at least 14 days were included. Thus, 133 (83.6%) and 136 (83.4%) patients from the genotype-guided and traditional dosing groups, respectively, were included in the modified intention-to-treat set (reasons for censoring are shown in Fig. 1). Clinical demographics and genotypic frequencies among patients who discontinued warfarin before 14 days of therapy are detailed in Additional file 2: Table S1, and baseline characteristics were relatively similar as compared to the overall population. The causes of death of four patients in the traditional dosing group were cardiac arrest, retroperitoneal bleed, hospital-associated pneumonia, and advanced cancer. Median duration of warfarin therapy was comparable between the two groups, and was 90.0 days (interquartile range (IQR) 83.8–90.0 days) in the traditional dosing group and 90.0 days (IQR 77.0–90.0 days) in the genotype-guided group.

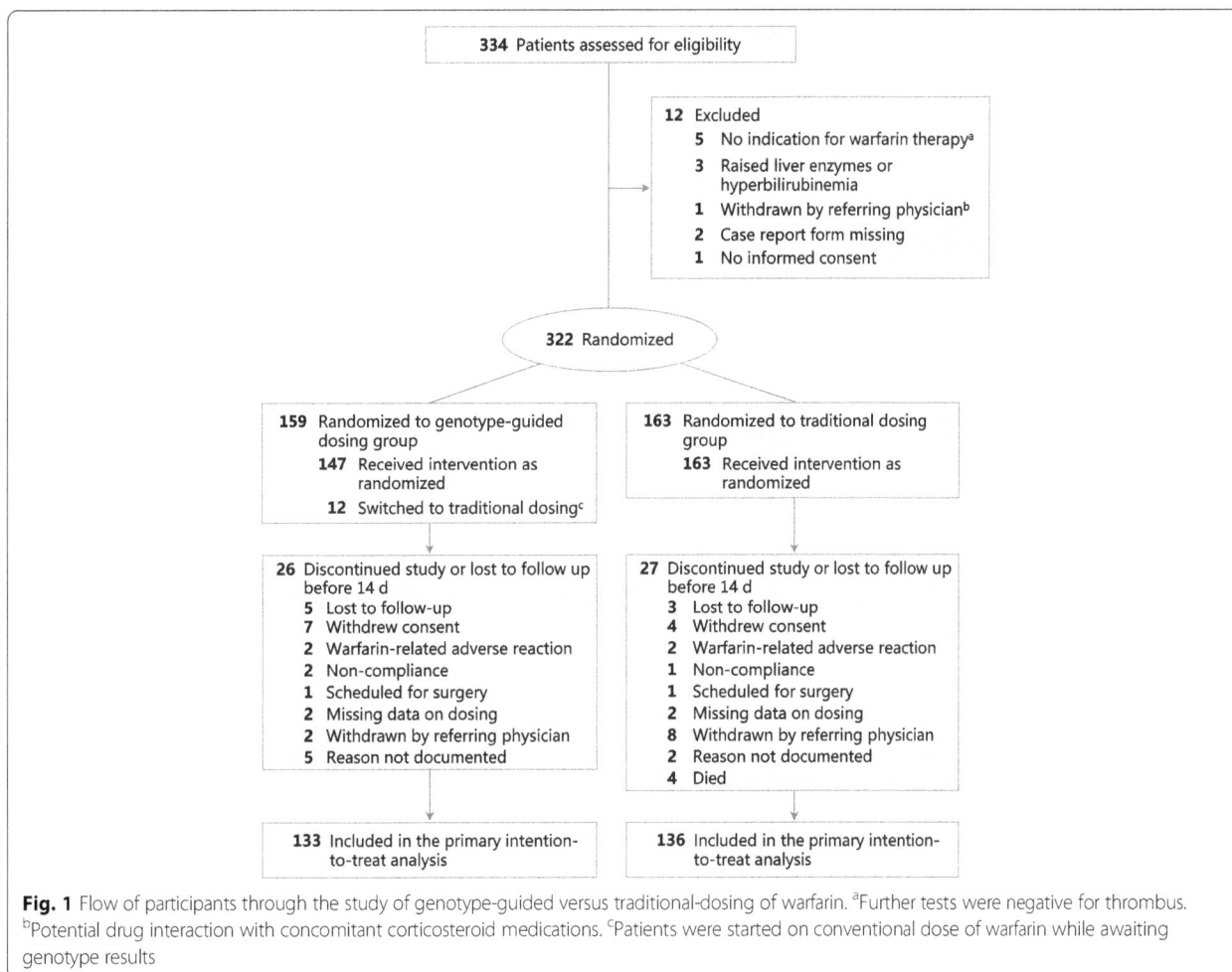

Fig. 1 Flow of participants through the study of genotype-guided versus traditional-dosing of warfarin. [a]Further tests were negative for thrombus. [b]Potential drug interaction with concomitant corticosteroid medications. [c]Patients were started on conventional dose of warfarin while awaiting genotype results

Table 1 Baseline clinical characteristics and demographics

	Traditional dosing ($n = 163$)	Genotype-guided dosing ($n = 159$)
Age, mean (SD), years	59.4 (14.5)	58.4 (14.3)
Male, No. (%)	88 (54.0)	100 (62.9)
Weight, mean (SD), kg	66.9 (16.8)	67.3 (14.1)
Race, No. (%)		
Chinese	98 (60.1)	99 (62.3)
Malay	39 (23.9)	32 (20.1)
Indian	17 (10.4)	14 (8.8)
Others	9 (5.5)	14 (8.8)
CYP2C9 genotype, No./total (%)		
Presence of *3 allele	11/160 (6.9)	7/158 (4.4)
VKORC1–381 genotype, No./total (%)		
C/C	91/162 (56.2)	97/159 (61.0)
C/T	47/162 (29.0)	43/159 (27.0)
T/T	24/162 (14.8)	19/159 (12.0)
Indication, No./total (%)		
Atrial fibrillation	55/160 (34.4)	61/156 (39.1)
Stroke	11/160 (6.9)	11/156 (7.1)
Deep vein thrombosis	44/160 (27.5)	42/156 (26.9)
Pulmonary embolism	19/160 (11.9)	17/156 (10.9)
Left ventricular thrombus	17/160 (10.6)	18/156 (11.5)
Others	26/160 (16.3)	14/156 (9.0)
Amiodarone, No./total (%)	3/159 (1.9)	7/156 (4.5)
Low-molecular weight heparins, No./total (%)	78/159 (49.1)	88/157 (56.1)
Medical history, No./total (%)		
Stroke	16/160 (10.0)	10/157 (6.4)
Deep vein thrombosis	7/160 (4.4)	4/157 (2.6)
Pulmonary embolism	2/160 (1.3)	3/157 (1.9)
Myocardial infarction	8/160 (5.0)	17/157 (10.8)
Congestive heart failure	21/160 (13.1)	18/157 (11.5)
Hypertension	86/160 (53.8)	92/157 (58.6)
Type 2 diabetes mellitus	58/160 (36.3)	56/157 (35.7)
Centre, No. (%)		
National University Hospital, Singapore	144 (88.3)	144 (90.6)
University of Malaya Medical Centre, Malaysia	15 (9.2)	15 (9.4)
Tan Tock Seng Hospital, Singapore	4 (2.5)	0 (0.0)

Primary outcome

The average number of dose titrations performed up to the 14th day was 1.77 (95% CI 1.55 to 2.00) in the genotype-guided group versus 2.93 (95% CI 2.63 to 3.24) in the traditional dosing group (mean difference –1.16, 90% CI –1.48 to –0.84). Thus, both non-inferiority ($P < 0.001$), according to the pre-specified definition, and superiority ($P < 0.001$) of the genotype-guided dosing algorithm over the traditional dosing algorithm was established (Fig. 2). This difference in mean number of

dose titrations corresponds to an IRR of 0.60 (95% CI 0.51 to 0.70, two-sided $P < 0.001$) in favor of the genotype-guided dosing algorithm.

Secondary outcomes

The effect of warfarin therapy on INR trajectories is depicted in Fig. 3a. The median time to stable INR, defined as the number of days from randomization to the latter of two consecutive measurements that are at least 7 days apart, was 36 days (IQR 20–74 days) in the

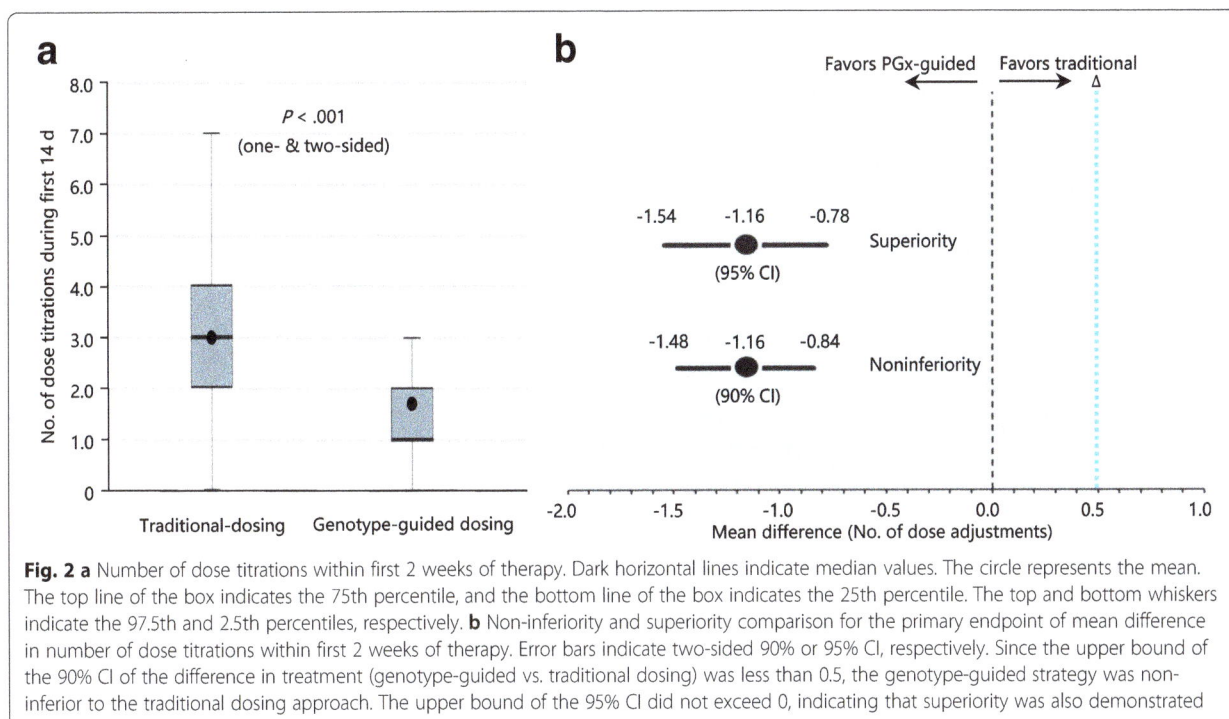

Fig. 2 a Number of dose titrations within first 2 weeks of therapy. Dark horizontal lines indicate median values. The circle represents the mean. The top line of the box indicates the 75th percentile, and the bottom line of the box indicates the 25th percentile. The top and bottom whiskers indicate the 97.5th and 2.5th percentiles, respectively. **b** Non-inferiority and superiority comparison for the primary endpoint of mean difference in number of dose titrations within first 2 weeks of therapy. Error bars indicate two-sided 90% or 95% CI, respectively. Since the upper bound of the 90% CI of the difference in treatment (genotype-guided vs. traditional dosing) was less than 0.5, the genotype-guided strategy was non-inferior to the traditional dosing approach. The upper bound of the 95% CI did not exceed 0, indicating that superiority was also demonstrated

genotype-guided group versus 37 days (IQR 22–76 days) in the traditional dosing group. A total of 103 (77.4%) patients in the genotype-guided group achieved stable INR as compared with 108 (79.4%) in the traditional dosing groups, and the rate of attaining stable INR was not statistically different between groups (genotype-guided vs. traditional dosing HR 1.00, 95% CI 0.76 to 1.31, $P = 0.99$) (Fig. 3b). There was no evidence of difference in the percentage of time in the therapeutic range (based on the pre-specified INR target of 1.9–3.1) over the follow-up period (Fig. 3a). The percentage of time in the pre-specified therapeutic range were 60.0% (95% CI 56.1% to 64.0%) in the genotype-guided group compared with 57.1% (95% CI 53.2% to 61.0%) in the traditional dosing group (mean difference 2.9%, 95% CI −2.6% to 8.4%, $P = 0.29$). Based on a post-hoc target INR range of 2.0–3.0, the percentage of time in the therapeutic range was 52.5% (95% CI 48.5% to 56.5%) in the genotype-guided group compared with 47.1% (95% CI 43.0% to 51.1%) in the traditional dosing group (mean difference 5.4%, 95% CI −0.2% to 11.1%, $P = 0.059$).

The number of dose adjustments and INR measurements generally decreased over the first through third months of treatment (Fig. 3c, d). The frequency of dose adjustments was significantly lower in the genotype-guided group over the entire duration of treatment (4.51 ± 2.20 vs. 6.06 ± 2.93, IRR 0.76, 95% CI 0.67 to 0.86, $P = 0.001$) compared to the traditional dosing group, after accounting for variation in between-individual exposure time and within-individual correlations in repeated measurements using a log-linear mixed effects Poisson model. The frequency of INR

measurements did not differ significantly between the genotype-guided group versus the traditional dosing group over the follow-up period (8.63 ± 4.26 vs. 9.48 ± 4.05, IRR 0.91, 95% CI 0.82 to 1.01, $P = 0.076$).

Minor bleeding complications occurred in 8/132 (6.1%, 95% CI 2.7% to 11.6%) patients in the genotype-guided group versus 8/135 (5.9%, 95% CI 2.6% to 11.3%) patients in the traditional dosing group (RR 1.02, 95% CI 0.40 to 2.64, $P = 0.96$); major bleeding complications occurred in 5/133 (3.8%, 95% CI 1.2% to 8.6%) and 5/136 (3.7%, 95% CI 1.2% to 8.4%) patients, respectively (RR 1.02, 95% CI 0.30 to 3.45; $P = 0.97$); and recurrent venous thromboembolism was documented in 2/132 (1.5%, 95% CI 0.2% to 5.4%) and 1/135 (0.7%, 95% CI 0.02% to 4.1%) patients, respectively (RR 2.05, 95% CI 0.19 to 22.3, $P = 0.55$). Furthermore, an INR value of less than 1.9 was recorded at least once in 129/132 (97.7%, 95% CI 93.5% to 99.5%) in the genotype-guided group versus 128/135 (94.8%, 95% CI 89.6% to 97.9%) in the traditional dosing group (RR 1.03, 95% CI 0.98 to 1.08, $P = 0.21$), whereas a measured INR of greater than 3.1 occurred in 59/132 (44.7%, 95% CI 36.0% to 53.6%) and 60/135 (44.4%, 95% CI 35.9% to 53.2%), respectively (RR 1.01, 95% CI 0.77 to 1.31, $P = 0.97$). Thus, no significant differences in these safety outcomes were detected between the genotype-guided and traditional dosing regimens.

The predictive performance of the pharmacogenetic maintenance dose model was also evaluated (Fig. 4a). Based on available data, the predicted daily maintenance dosages correlated positively with actual documented

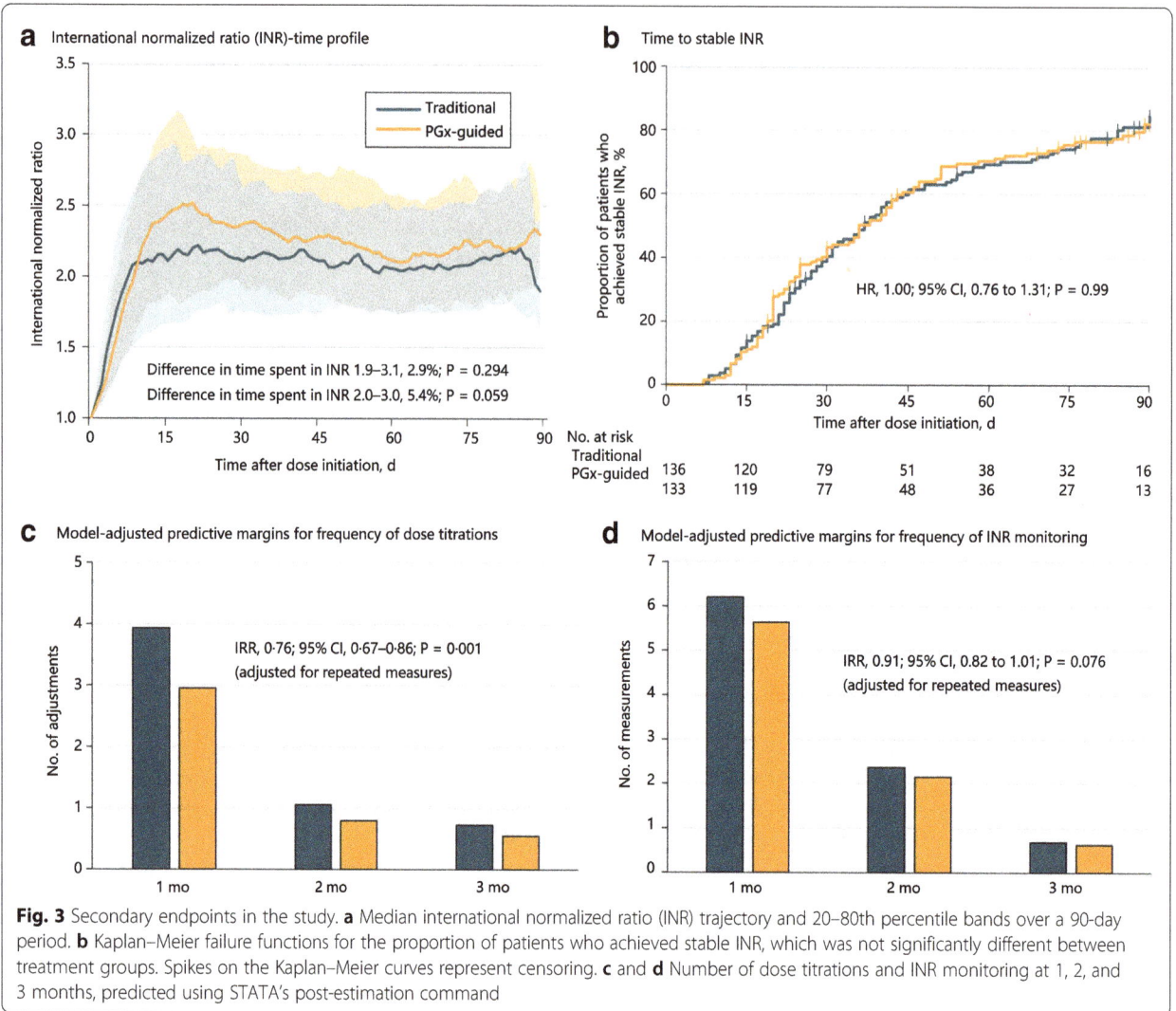

Fig. 3 Secondary endpoints in the study. **a** Median international normalized ratio (INR) trajectory and 20–80th percentile bands over a 90-day period. **b** Kaplan–Meier failure functions for the proportion of patients who achieved stable INR, which was not significantly different between treatment groups. Spikes on the Kaplan–Meier curves represent censoring. **c** and **d** Number of dose titrations and INR monitoring at 1, 2, and 3 months, predicted using STATA's post-estimation command

stable dosages ($R^2 = 42.4\%$, 95% CI 31.9% to 52.4%, $P <$ 0.001) with a root mean-squared error of 1.10 mg and a mean percentage error of −7.4% (Fig. 4b), indicating a low level of positive forecast bias and a respectable level of predictive accuracy.

Discussion

Warfarin and its analogues have been used as oral anticoagulants for more than 60 years, and many institutions worldwide still employ an empirical dose initiation protocol despite the known inter-individual variability in dose requirements and anticoagulation outcomes. In this study involving patients with a new indication for warfarin therapy, the number of dose titrations in the first 2 weeks, and also throughout the follow-up period, was lower in the genotype-guided group than in the traditional dosing group. Furthermore, the genotype dosing algorithm accurately predicted the maintenance dose requirements in patients who achieved stable INR. Our findings are

consistent with results from the COUMAGEN-I trial [10], which showed a similar advantage for accurate prediction of stable doses and frequency of dosing adjustments in the pharmacogenetically guided arm, but similar outcomes in terms of anticoagulation control parameters such as the fraction of out-of-range INRs.

The finding that percentage of time spent within the therapeutic range (PTTR) was not statistically different between the two groups was similar to that observed in the recent COAG trial [6], but different from that in the EU-PACT [7], COUMAGEN-II [8], and GIFT trials [13]. Although widely interpreted as failure of genotype-guided dosing, a major confounder when interpreting these endpoints are the incidence of dose adjustments and INR monitoring performed in the genotype-guided group and in the control group. Given that dosing titrations were performed more frequently in our control arm than in the genotype-guided arm, this could have inflated the PTTR in the traditional dosing group and diminished any

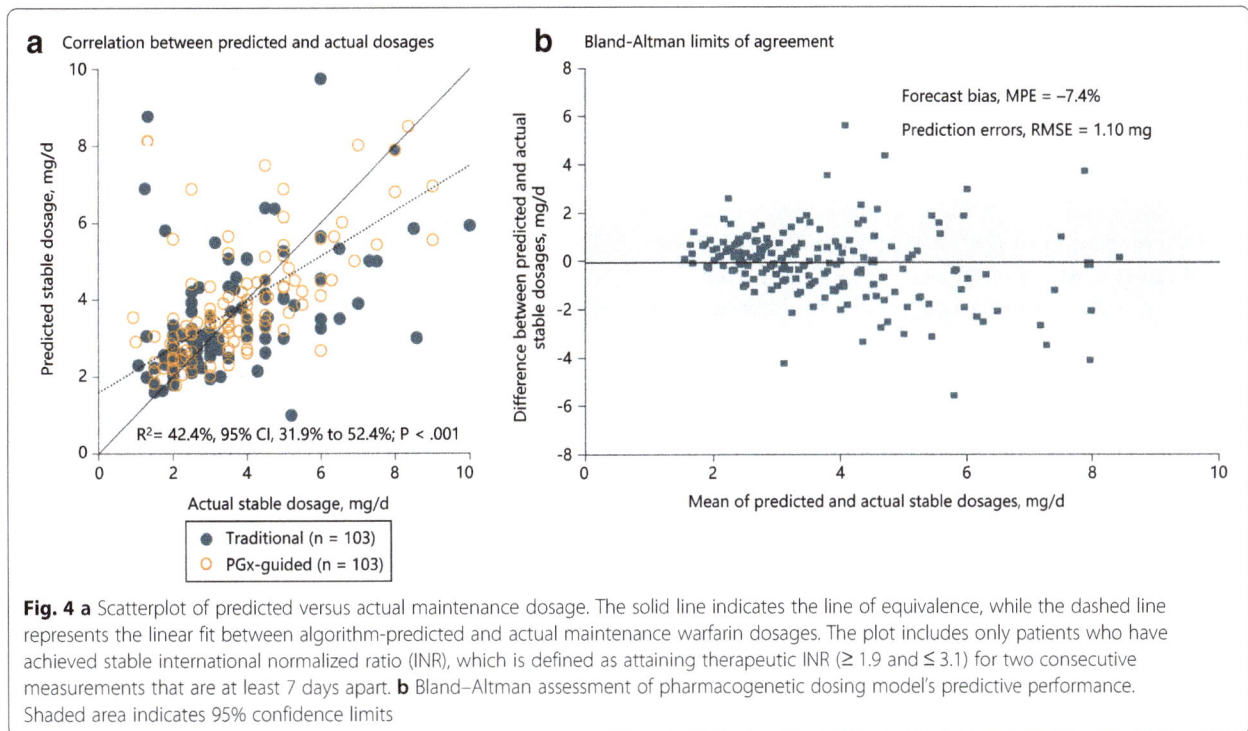

Fig. 4 a Scatterplot of predicted versus actual maintenance dosage. The solid line indicates the line of equivalence, while the dashed line represents the linear fit between algorithm-predicted and actual maintenance warfarin dosages. The plot includes only patients who have achieved stable international normalized ratio (INR), which is defined as attaining therapeutic INR (≥ 1.9 and ≤ 3.1) for two consecutive measurements that are at least 7 days apart. **b** Bland–Altman assessment of pharmacogenetic dosing model's predictive performance. Shaded area indicates 95% confidence limits

apparent benefit of genotype-guided dosing. Notwithstanding, our trial was not designed to answer whether genotype-guided dosing improves anticoagulation control when controlled for the number of dose adjustments. Future trials may therefore consider incorporating this potential confounder as an adjustment or stratification variable into their statistical analysis plans.

Some investigators have advocated that warfarin dosing algorithms should be population specific and evaluated in populations similar to those from which they were developed [14, 20]. Therefore, although several genotype-based dosing algorithms have been proposed [21–25], a strength of this study is the selection of an algorithm [16] developed and validated in a cohort that is racially comparable to the current study population.

The use of clinical algorithms for dose initiation and dose adjustment were applied in the EU-PACT and COAG studies, which enrolled predominantly Caucasian and Black populations. These dosing algorithms have not been validated in Asian populations, and therefore were not used in this study. Moreover, the fact that PTTR of the control group was comparable between our study and the clinical algorithm dosing groups in the Western studies would suggest no difference in outcomes with application of clinical algorithm-based dosing in this study.

From the viewpoint of clinical applicability, the findings of this study are representative of and generalizable to an ethnogeographically diverse Asian population; the Chinese and Indian patients in these studies are mostly migrants from China and South India, and the Malay patients are

indigenous to the islands of the Indonesian archipelago, including Malaya, Sumatra, and Java [15, 16]. Reduction of frequency of dose titrations (the primary endpoint) using genotype-based algorithms is highly desirable in the context of Asia, where long distances from rural or suburban areas to healthcare facilities poses a barrier to optimal anticoagulation therapy.

The use of a non-inferiority design in this study deserves mention. Firstly, no comparative data about the capability of a genotype-guided dosing strategy in reducing the number of dose titrations was available at the time of conceptualization, although early observational and retrospective studies suggested that genotyping may have value in informing dose selection [26]. Considering that, at the time this trial was conceived, there was no prospective data comparing pharmacogenetically guided dosing versus traditional dosing, it was arguably a reasonable concern that pharmacogenetically guided dosing could be worse than traditional dosing in terms of the number of dose adjustments required in the first 2 weeks. As such, a non-inferiority null hypothesis that genotype-guided dosing could be worse than traditional dosing was arguably justifiable and valid at that time. Therefore, the trial was designed to demonstrate that pharmacogenetically guided dosing was not less efficacious than conventional dosing, and as secondary endpoints, to test whether a genotype-guided algorithm accurately predicts maintenance dose requirements and improves other markers of anticoagulation control.

There are several limitations of this study. Firstly, we did not evaluate a combination of a loading-dose algorithm and dose-revision algorithm in the genotype-guided arm, which may be responsible for the PTTR advantage observed in the EU-PACT study [7]. Simulations integrating a pharmacokinetic-pharmacodynamic model [27, 28] and genotype frequencies present in a Han-Chinese cohort in fact suggests that the deployment of genetically informed loading doses and dose revisions is superior to a clinically guided dosing regimen [29]. Nevertheless, this study was not designed to test a difference in the PTTR, which as mentioned earlier, may be confounded by imbalance in the number of dose titrations performed in the two groups, nor was it powered to detect differences in the outcome of bleeding and re-thrombosis. Other limitations include the lack of adjustment for multiplicity among the secondary endpoints; its open-label design, which potentially introduces ascertainment bias; and a lack of pre-specified adjusted or subgroup analyses, for example, assessment of endpoints according to ethnic grouping, which may have afforded further information on the utility of genotype-guided warfarin dosing. Furthermore, approximately 16% of patients were excluded because they did not continue warfarin for 14 days, although it should be noted that this attrition rate is in line with the expected dropout rate of approximately 15% that was accounted for in our sample size calculations. Moreover, the study was designed as a multicenter clinical trial yet the majority (86.7%) of patients were enrolled at a single tertiary care center due to slow accrual in the other centers. This therefore limits the generalizability of our results.

Conclusions

In this randomized, non-inferiority clinical trial that included 322 adults of South East Asian ancestry, genotype-guided dosing reduced the number of dose titrations during the first 2 weeks compared to traditional dosing (1.77 vs. 2.93) while maintaining similar INR time within therapeutic ranges. The reduction in frequency of dose revisions persisted over the 90-day follow-up period (incidence rate ratio 0.76). The genotype-guided algorithm also accurately predicted maintenance dose requirements. These findings imply that clinicians treating Asian patients may consider applying a pharmacogenetic algorithm to personalize initial warfarin dosages.

Abbreviations

CYP2C9: cytochrome P450 2C9; INR: International normalized ratio; PTTR: percentage of time spent in therapeutic range; VKORC1: Vitamin K epoxide reductase complex 1

Acknowledgements

We are grateful to Hiarul Fariz Hairol, Jesinda Pauline, Swee Siang Ng, King Xin Koh, Mohamed Hafiz Ridhwan Bin Yahy, Zuan Yu Mok, Michelle Rozario, Sili Tan, and Fei Fei Gan for technical and administrative support.

Funding

This investigator-initiated trial was funded by the Singapore Ministry of Health's National Medical Research Council (NMRC/CSA/021/2010 and NMRC/CSA/0048/2013). The Surveillance and Pharmacogenomics Initiative for Adverse Drug Reactions (SAPhIRE) program is supported by a Strategic Position Funds Grant (SPF2014/001) from the Biomedical Research Council of the Agency for Science, Technology and Research (A*STAR). This research is also supported by the National Research Foundation Singapore and the Singapore Ministry of Education under their Research Centres of Excellence Initiative.

Authors' contributions

Concept and design: BCG, BCT, NLS, SCL. Acquisition, analysis, or interpretation of data: NLS, ALW, BCG, BCT, SCL, PM, HLT, GY, WTY, MLP, TSW, LB, MW, PCB, RS, RCSS, WK. Drafting of the manuscript: NLS, BCG, SCL, BCT, LB, ALW. Critical revision of the manuscript for important intellectual content: BCG, SCL, BCT, NLS, LB, ALW. Statistical analysis: NLS, BCT. Administrative, technical, or material support: PM, TSW, MW. Study supervision: BCG, SCL. All authors read and approved the final manuscript.

Competing interests

The authors declare that they have no competing interests.

Author details

[1]Department of Haematology-Oncology, National University Cancer Institute, Singapore, Singapore. [2]Cancer Science Institute of Singapore, National University of Singapore, Singapore, Singapore. [3]Division of Neurology, Department of Medicine, National University Health System, Singapore, Singapore. [4]Department of Cardiology, National University Heart Centre, Singapore, Singapore. [5]Department of Medicine, University of Malaya Medical Centre, Kuala Lumpur, Malaysia. [6]Department of Pharmacy, National University Hospital, Singapore, Singapore. [7]Genome Institute of Singapore, Agency for Science, Technology and Research, Singapore, Singapore. [8]Translational Laboratory in Genetic Medicine, Agency for Science, Technology and Research, Singapore, Singapore. [9]Department of Medicine, Centre for Heart Lung Innovation, University of British Columbia, Vancouver, Canada. [10]Department of Pathology, Yong Loo Lin School of Medicine, National University Health System, Singapore, Singapore. [11]Saw Swee Hock School of Public Health, National University of Singapore, Singapore, Singapore. [12]Department of Pharmacology, Yong Loo Lin School of Medicine, National University Health System, Singapore 119228, Singapore. [13]Department of Medicine, Yong Loo Lin School of Medicine, National University of Singapore, Singapore, Singapore.

References

1. Passman R. Time in therapeutic range in warfarin-treated patients: is very good good enough? JAMA. 2016;316:872.
2. Pokorney SD, Simon DN, Thomas L, Gersh BJ, Hylek EM, Piccini JP, et al. Stability of international normalized ratios in patients taking long-term warfarin therapy. JAMA. 2016;316:661.
3. Jonas DE, McLeod HL. Genetic and clinical factors relating to warfarin dosing. Trends Pharmacol Sci. 2009;30:375–86.
4. Johnson JA, Cavallari LH. Warfarin pharmacogenetics. Trends Cardiovasc Med. 2015;25:33–41.
5. Syn NL-X, Yong W-P, Lee S-C, Goh B-C. Genetic factors affecting drug disposition in Asian cancer patients. Expert Opin Drug Metab Toxicol. 2015;11:1879–92.
6. Kimmel SE, French B, Kasner SE, Johnson JA, Anderson JL, Gage BF, et al. A pharmacogenetic versus a clinical algorithm for warfarin dosing. N Engl J Med. 2013;369:2283–93.
7. Pirmohamed M, Burnside G, Eriksson N, Jorgensen AL, Toh CH, Nicholson T, et al. A randomized trial of genotype-guided dosing of warfarin. N Engl J Med. 2013;369:2294–303.
8. Anderson JL, Horne BD, Stevens SM, Woller SC, Samuelson KM, Mansfield JW, et al. A randomized and clinical effectiveness trial comparing two pharmacogenetic algorithms and standard care for individualizing warfarin dosing (CoumaGen-II). Circulation. 2012;125:1997–2005.
9. Brensinger CM, Kimmel SE. Genetic warfarin dosing tables versus algorithms. JACC. 2011;57:612–8. http://dx.doi.org/10.1016/j.jacc.2010.08.643
10. Anderson JL, Horne BD, Stevens SM, Grove AS, Barton S, Nicholas ZP, et al. Randomized trial of genotype-guided versus standard warfarin dosing in patients initiating oral anticoagulation. Circulation. 2007;116:2563–70.
11. Stergiopoulos K, Brown DL. Genotype-guided vs clinical dosing of warfarin and its analogues. JAMA Intern Med. 2014;174:1330.
12. Dahal K, Sharma SP, Fung E, Lee J, Moore JH, Unterborn JN, et al. Meta-analysis of randomized controlled trials of genotype-guided vs standard dosing of warfarin. Chest. 2015;148:701–10.
13. Gage BF, Bass AR, Lin H, Woller SC, Stevens SM, Al-Hammadi N, et al. Effect of genotype-guided warfarin dosing on clinical events and anticoagulation control among patients undergoing hip or knee arthroplasty. JAMA. 2017;318:1115.
14. Limdi NA, Brown TM, Yan Q, Thigpen JL, Shendre A, Liu N, et al. Race influences warfarin dose changes associated with genetic factors. Blood. 2015;126:539–45.
15. Lee S-C, Ng S-S, Oldenburg J, Chong P-Y, Rost S, Guo J-Y, et al. Interethnic variability of warfarin maintenance requirement is explained by VKORC1 genotype in an Asian population. Clin Pharmacol Ther. 2006;79:197–205.
16. Tham L-S, Goh B-C, Nafziger A, Guo J-Y, Wang L-Z, Soong R, et al. A warfarin-dosing model in Asians that uses single-nucleotide polymorphisms in vitamin K epoxide reductase complex and cytochrome P450 2C9. Clin Pharmacol Ther. 2006;80:346–55.
17. Rosendaal FR, Cannegieter SC, Van Der Meer FJM, Briet E. A method to determine the optimal intensity of oral anticoagulant therapy. Thromb Haemost. 1993;69:236–9.
18. Levine M, Gent M, Hirsh J, Leclerc J, Anderson D, Weitz J, et al. A comparison of low-molecular-weight heparin administered primarily at home with unfractionated heparin administered in the hospital for proximal deep-vein thrombosis. N Engl J Med. 1996;334:677–81.
19. Kovacs MJ, Rodger M, Anderson DR, Morrow B, Kells G, Kovacs J, et al. Comparison of 10-mg and 5-mg warfarin initiation nomograms together with low-molecular-weight heparin for outpatient treatment of acute venous thromboembolism. A randomized, double-blind, controlled trial. Ann Intern Med. 2003;138:714–9.
20. Kubo K, Ohara M, Tachikawa M, Cavallari LH, Lee MTM, Wen MS, et al. Population differences in S-warfarin pharmacokinetics among African Americans, Asians and whites: their influence on pharmacogenetic dosing algorithms. Pharmacogenomics J. 2017;17(6):494–500.
21. Gage BF, Eby C, Milligan PE, Banet GA, Duncan JR, McLeod HL. Use of pharmacogenetics and clinical factors to predict the maintenance dose of warfarin. Thromb Haemost. 2003;91:87–94.
22. Sconce EA, Khan TI, Wynne HA, Avery P, Monkhouse L, King BP, et al. The impact of CYP2C9 and VKORC1 genetic polymorphism and patient characteristics upon warfarin dose requirements: proposal for a new dosing regimen. Blood. 2005;106:2329–33.
23. International Warfarin Pharmacogenetics Consortium, Klein TE, Altman RB, Eriksson N, Gage BF, Kimmel SE, Lee MT, Limdi NA, Page D, Roden DM, Wagner MJ, JJ CMD. Estimation of the warfarin dose with clinical and pharmacogenetic data. N Engl J Med. 2009;360:753–64.
24. Lenzini P, Wadelius M, Kimmel SE, Anderson JL. Integration of genetic, clinical, and INR data to refine warfarin dosing. Clin Pharmacol Ther. 2010;87:572–8.
25. Avery PJ, Jorgensen A, Hamberg AK, Wadelius M, Pirmohamed M, Kamali F. A proposal for an individualized pharmacogenetics-based warfarin initiation dose regimen for patients commencing anticoagulation therapy. Clin Pharmacol Ther. 2011;90:701–6.
26. Voora D, Eby C, Linder MW, Milligan PE, Bukaveckas BL, McLeod HL, et al. Prospective dosing of warfarin based on cytochrome P-450 2C9 genotype. Thromb Haemost. 2005;93:700–5.
27. Hamberg a-K, Dahl M-L, Barban M, Scordo MG, Wadelius M, Pengo V, et al. A PK-PD model for predicting the impact of age, CYP2C9, and VKORC1 genotype on individualization of warfarin therapy. Clin Pharmacol Ther. 2007;81:529–38.
28. Hamberg a-K, Wadelius M, Lindh JD, Dahl ML, Padrini R, Deloukas P, et al. A pharmacometric model describing the relationship between warfarin dose and INR response with respect to variations in CYP2C9, VKORC1, and age. Clin Pharmacol Ther. 2010;87:727–34.
29. Syn NL-X, Lee S-C, Brunham LR, Goh B-C. Pharmacogenetic versus clinical dosing of warfarin in individuals of Chinese and African-American ancestry: assessment using data simulation. Pharmacogenet Genomics. 2015;25:491–500.

17

Modulation of innate immune responses at birth by prenatal malaria exposure and association with malaria risk during the first year of life

Hamtandi Magloire Natama[1,2,3], Gemma Moncunill[4†], Eduard Rovira-Vallbona[1†], Héctor Sanz[4], Hermann Sorgho[2], Ruth Aguilar[4], Maminata Coulibaly-Traoré[2], M. Athanase Somé[2], Susana Scott[5], Innocent Valéa[2], Petra F. Mens[6], Henk D. F. H. Schallig[6], Luc Kestens[1,3], Halidou Tinto[2,7], Carlota Dobaño[4†] and Anna Rosanas-Urgell[1*†] (iD)

Abstract

Background: Factors driving inter-individual differences in immune responses upon different types of prenatal malaria exposure (PME) and subsequent risk of malaria in infancy remain poorly understood. In this study, we examined the impact of four types of PME (i.e., maternal peripheral infection and placental acute, chronic, and past infections) on both spontaneous and toll-like receptors (TLRs)-mediated cytokine production in cord blood and how these innate immune responses modulate the risk of malaria during the first year of life.

Methods: We conducted a birth cohort study of 313 mother-child pairs nested within the COSMIC clinical trial (NCT01941264), which was assessing malaria preventive interventions during pregnancy in Burkina Faso. Malaria infections during pregnancy and infants' clinical malaria episodes detected during the first year of life were recorded. Supernatant concentrations of 30 cytokines, chemokines, and growth factors induced by stimulation of cord blood with agonists of TLRs 3, 7/8, and 9 were measured by quantitative suspension array technology. Crude concentrations and ratios of TLR-mediated cytokine responses relative to background control were analyzed.

Results: Spontaneous production of innate immune biomarkers was significantly reduced in cord blood of infants exposed to malaria, with variation among PME groups, as compared to those from the non-exposed control group. However, following TLR7/8 stimulation, which showed higher induction of cytokines/chemokines/growth factors than TLRs 3 and 9, cord blood cells of infants with evidence of past placental malaria were hyper-responsive in comparison to those of infants not-exposed. In addition, certain biomarkers, which levels were significantly modified depending on the PME category, were independent predictors of either malaria risk (GM-CSF TLR7/8 crude) or protection (IL-12 TLR7/8 ratio and IP-10 TLR3 crude, IL-1RA TLR7/8 ratio) during the first year of life.

Conclusions: These findings indicate that past placental malaria has a profound effect on fetal immune system and that the differential alterations of innate immune responses by PME categories might drive heterogeneity between individuals to clinical malaria susceptibility during the first year of life.

Keywords: Malaria in pregnancy, Prenatal malaria exposure, Innate immunity, Cytokines, Toll-like receptor, Malaria in infancy

---

* Correspondence: arosanas@itg.be
†Gemma Moncunill, Eduard Rovira-Vallbona, Carlota Dobaño and Anna Rosanas-Urgell contributed equally to this work.
[1]Department of Biomedical Sciences, Institute of Tropical Medicine, B 2000 Antwerp, Belgium
Full list of author information is available at the end of the article

Background

Despite the widespread implementation of Intermittent Preventive Treatment with sulfadoxine-pyrimethamine (IPTp-SP) to prevent malaria during pregnancy, infants in endemic countries are often born to mothers with placental malaria (PM). This is likely to increase their risk of a malaria infection in early childhood [1–7]. Factors explaining the association between PM and risk of malaria infection during infancy are still not well understood, but this association has been correlated with changes in malaria-specific fetal immunity [8]. Cord blood mononuclear cells of neonates born to mothers with PM can specifically respond to plasmodial asexual blood stage antigens, impacting on immune response to *Plasmodium falciparum* infection during infancy [9–15]. This prenatal exposure to malaria-infected erythrocytes or their soluble products can lead to fetal immune priming to malaria blood stage antigens or to fetal immune tolerance in some infants [11, 16–20]. Nonetheless, factors that lead to this inter-individual difference in immune responses to malaria antigens upon prenatal exposure are unknown.

In early infancy, innate immunity is the main defense barrier of the host, as newborns have a naïve adaptive immune system [21, 22]. The immune cellular response starts with the recognition of pathogen molecules known as pathogen-associated-molecular patterns (PAMPs) by cells of the innate immune system through pattern recognition receptors (PRRs). Among these receptors, it has been shown that toll-like receptors (TLRs) are key initiators of innate immunity and promoters of adaptive immunity via direct and indirect mechanisms [23–25]. Ligands binding to TLRs generate intracellular signals, activate gene expression, and enhance the release of cytokines and chemokines [26, 27], which are important players in the pathogenesis of and protection against malaria [28]. Therefore, in early life, protection from infections relies extensively on innate immunity, and hence, factors that modulate the development of fetal innate immunity may drive variation in susceptibility to malaria between individuals in early infancy.

A few studies have reported that history of *P. falciparum* infections during pregnancy may have an effect on neonatal innate immune responses upon TLRs stimulation with implications for the outcome of newly encountered infections in early life [11, 29, 30]. Cytokine responses upon TLRs stimulation of cord blood cells have been found to be profoundly affected by either maternal peripheral infections occurring late in pregnancy [29, 30] or past PM [11]. In addition, it has been shown that exposure to malarial antigens in utero has different effects on the immune environment at birth, such as the number and/or activation status of immune cell populations, including antigen-presenting cells, regulatory, and effector CD4+ T cells, depending on the type of exposure [10–15]. Overall, these data indicate that maternal peripheral and placental infections during pregnancy have an impact on cord blood cytokine responses to TLR agonists and that time and type of malaria exposure can skew cytokine responses towards a regulatory/tolerogenic or to a proinflammatory profile. In this regard, a tolerogenic profile would render infants more susceptible to malaria infections during the first year of life, whereas a proinflammatory profile can lead to more severe malaria episodes, whereas a Th1/Th17 profile could be protective.

Human TLRs that are known to be stimulated by malaria parasite-derived molecules include TLR2 (by glycosylphosphatidylinositol), TLR4 (by hemozoin), and TLR9 (by hemozoin and parasite DNA) [31–34]. However, the clinical relevance of TLR-mediated immune responses in the susceptibility to malaria has been mainly reported for endosomal PRRs such as TLR3, TLR7/8, and TLR9 in African children. Indeed, higher TLR3- and TLR7/8-mediated interleukin (IL)-10 responses at birth were found to be associated with a significant increased risk of *P. falciparum* infection in infants in Benin [30], whereas polymorphisms in TLR9 gene were associated with difference in susceptibility to malaria in Burundian and Ghanaian children [35, 36].

In this study, we assessed the effect of different types of prenatal malaria exposure (PME) on endosomal TLR-mediated cytokine responses in cord blood samples collected at birth, and we investigated the subsequent risk of malaria during the first year of life in a highly seasonal malaria endemic area of Burkina Faso.

Methods

Study design and participants

A prospective birth cohort study was nested within the COSMIC trial (NCT01941264). In brief, COSMIC was a cluster randomized controlled trial investigating the protective efficacy of adding community-scheduled screening and treatment of malaria during pregnancy (CSST) to the standard IPTp-SP (CSST/IPTp-SP; intervention arm) compared to IPTp-SP alone (control arm) in Burkina Faso, Benin, and The Gambia [37]. The CSST extension strategy was implemented through monthly screening using rapid diagnostic tests (RDTs) and treatment of malaria infections with artemether-lumefantrine (AL). Pregnant women in both arms who experienced clinical malaria during pregnancy were also treated with AL. In addition, all pregnant women in the two arms were further screened for malaria during antenatal care (ANC) booking using light microscopy (LM). Furthermore, additional blood spots on filter papers during community screening (CSST/IPTp-SP arm) and at each ANC visit (both CSST/IPTp-SP and IPTp-SP arms) were collected for posterior malaria diagnostic by quantitative real-time polymerase chain reaction (qPCR). At the time of delivery, placenta biopsies and cord blood samples in heparin containing tubes were collected from mother-child pairs. Placenta histology was performed later on within the parent COSMIC trial, while cord blood samples were immediately processed. Of the 734 mother-child pairs enrolled in the birth cohort in Burkina Faso, a subgroup of 313 mothers and their offspring were included for the present study. Those mother-child pairs were selected based on the history of malaria infection during pregnancy (using LM and RDT results) and the availability of cord blood samples for immunological assays at delivery (Fig. 1). The study was conducted in the rural health district of Nanoro, a high and seasonal malaria transmission area in Centre-West of Burkina Faso [38].

Recruitment and follow-up

The recruitment procedure of the mother-child pairs and details of the 1-year follow-up of infants included in the birth cohort study have been previously described [39, 40]. Shortly, pregnant women from Nanoro participating in the COSMIC trial were asked at antenatal care visits to participate in the birth cohort study prior to delivery. At delivery, healthy newborns with their mothers were enrolled after informed consent was obtained. Exclusion criteria were presence of major congenital malformation, chronic disease, or signs of cerebral asphyxia. Clinical malaria episodes in infants were monitored by passive case detection, for which mothers were encouraged to seek care in peripheral health centers at any time their child felt sick. At each attendance to health facilities, a clinical examination was performed and mothers were asked for previous health events. In the case of fever (axillary temperature ≥ 37.5 °C) or history of fever in the previous 24 h, a malaria RDT was

performed and positive infants were treated according to national guidelines.

Sample collection

Sample collection procedures have been described elsewhere [41]. In brief, at time of delivery, approximately 200 μL of maternal peripheral blood was obtained by finger-prick for blood smear preparation and blood spot on filter paper. A placental tissue section was collected from the maternal side and preserved in 10% neutral buffer formalin at 4 °C for histology examination. In addition, cord blood (approximately 10 mL) was collected in heparin-containing tubes by venipuncture of the umbilical vein for TLRs stimulation assays. The remaining cord blood in the heparinized tube was transferred from the peripheral health centers to the laboratory at the Clinical Research Unit of Nanoro (CRUN) for processing within 4 h. Peripheral blood was collected post-partum by finger-prick from each infant visiting the health facilities with presence of fever or history of fever in the previous 24 h, and used for RDT, blood smear, and spots on filter paper (Whatman 3MM).

Toll-like receptors stimulation assay

TLRs stimulations of cord blood mononuclear cells were performed using fresh whole cord blood samples. Briefly, cord blood samples were diluted 1:1 with RPMI 1640 (1X, Gibco) and five aliquots of 200 μl were prepared. One aliquot was left unstimulated and the other four were stimulated either with the synthetic analog of

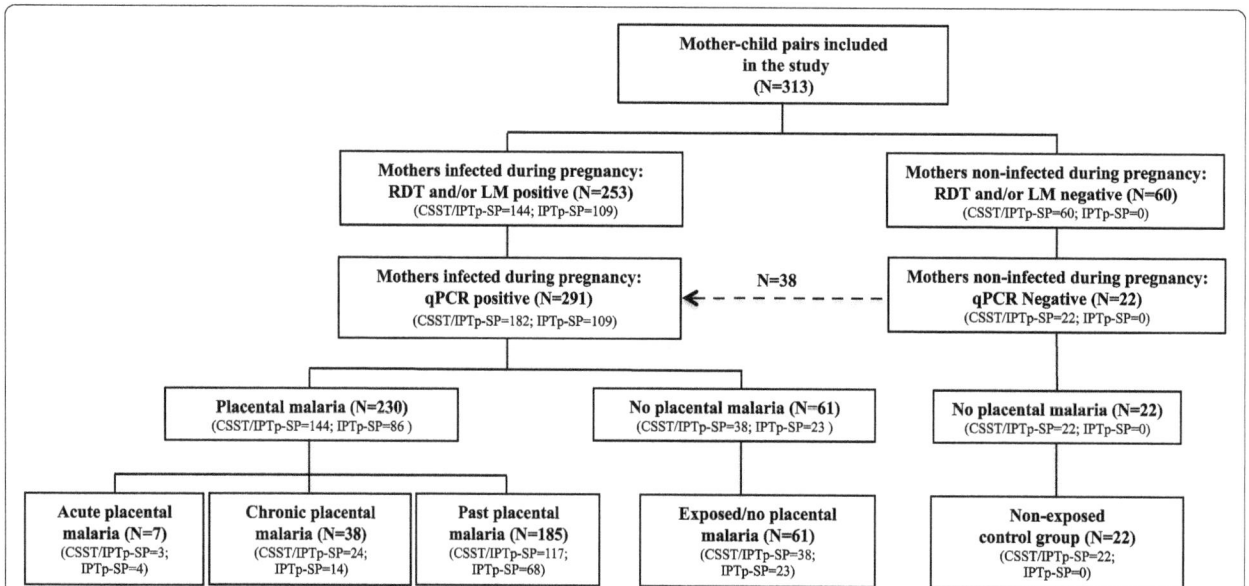

Fig. 1 Categories of prenatal malaria exposure (PME). Pregnant women infected during pregnancy with placental malaria (PM; acute, chronic, or past) or without PM (exposed/no PM) were recruited from both COSMIC study arms [37]. Pregnant women included in the non-exposed control group were only recruited among the CSST/IPTp-SP intervention arm: all of them had negative RDT/LM results for malaria infection in monthly screenings and at antenatal care visits that were later on confirmed by qPCR and, with no evidence of placental malaria

dsRNA-PolyI:C (TLR3 ligand; 10 μg/mL; InvivoGen, San Diego, USA), imidazoquinoline (R848, TLR7/8 ligand; 10 μg/mL; InvivoGen, San Diego, USA), the synthetic type B unmethylated CpG dinucleotide (ODN2006-1, TLR9 ligand, 5 μM; InvivoGen, San Diego, USA) or with a mixture of phorbol myristate acetate (PMA), and ionomycin as positive control (PMA 0.1 μg/mL and ionomycin 1 μg/mL; Sigma-Aldrich, Schnelldorf, Germany). After 24 h of incubation at 37 °C in 5% CO_2, supernatants were collected following a centrifugation at $500g$ for 5 min, then frozen at − 80 °C. Culture supernatants were subsequently shipped frozen to ISGlobal (Barcelona) for cytokines, chemokines, and growth factors measurement.

Cytokines, chemokines, and growth factors quantification

Supernatants were thawed at room temperature, centrifuged at $1000g$ for 10 min and then diluted in a ratio of 1:5 in RPMI 1640 (1X, Gibco). Cytokines, chemokines, and growth factors levels were determined using a fluorescent bead-based multiplex immunoassay (Human Cytokine Magnetic 30-Plex Panel kits, Novex®, Life Technologies™, USA). Twenty-five microliters of each supernatant were tested in single replicates applying a modification of the manufacturer's protocol, which implies using half the volume of each reagent except for the washing buffer. The 30-Plex panel kit includes the following: interleukin (IL)-2, IL-4, IL-5, IL-6, IL-7, IL-8, IL-10, IL-13, IL-15, IL-17, IL-1β, IL-1RA, IL-2R, IL-12(p40/p70), tumor necrosis factor (TNF), interferon (IFN)-γ, IFN-α, IFN-γ inducible protein 10 (IP-10), monocyte chemottractant protein (MCP)-1, macrophage inflammatory protein (MIP)-1α, MIP-1β, eotaxin, RANTES, monokine-induced by IFN-γ (MIG), vascular endothelial growth factor (VEGF), hepatocyte growth factor (HGF), epidermal growth factor (EGF), fibroblast growth factor (FGF) basic, granulocyte-colony stimulating factor (G-CSF), and granulocyte-macrophage colony stimulating factor (GM-CSF). Samples were acquired on a Luminex® 100/200™ instrument using Xponent 3.1 software. Median fluorescent intensity (MFI) data was analyzed using the drLumi 0.1.2 R package [42], in which concentration of each analyte was determined by interpolating the MFI to a standard curve (plotted using a 5- or 4-parameter logistic function) of twofold 16 serial dilutions prepared from a reference sample provided by the manufacturer. The limits of quantification (lower, LLOQ and upper, ULOQ) for each analyte and plate were obtained applying the 20% coefficient of variation method [43–45] in drLumi. Any analyte with a value below the LLOQ was given a value of half the LLOQ for that analyte, and any analyte with a value above the ULOQ was given a value of two times the ULOQ of that analyte.

Malaria detection and definitions

SD-Bioline malaria antigen P.f® test (05FK50, Standard Diagnostics, Inc., Korea) detecting PfHRP2 was used for malaria RDT according to the manufacturer's instructions. The microscopic examination of thick blood smears stained with Giemsa (10%) was performed according to standard procedures [46]. Dried blood spots on filter paper were used for DNA extraction (QIAamp 96 DNA blood kit, Qiagen, Germany) and, *P. falciparum* detection of *Pf*-varATS by qPCR, as previously described [41]. Data on past history of malaria infections during pregnancy and histological examination of placental tissues were obtained from the COSMIC trial [37]. A clinical malaria episode was defined as the detection of *P. falciparum* parasites by qPCR and presence of fever. PM infections were defined by histological examination as follows: (i) acute infection (parasites present, malaria pigment absent), (ii) chronic infection (parasites and malaria pigment present), (iii) past infection (parasites absent but pigment present), and (iv) no infection (both parasites and malaria pigment absent). PME was categorized based on placental infection (past, chronic, acute) and maternal peripheral infection as shown in Fig. 1. The non-exposed control group was composed of pregnant women only recruited among the CSST/IPTp-SP intervention arm who had negative RDT/LM and qPCR results at each screening and ANC visit and negative placental histology.

Statistical analysis

Statistical analysis was performed using R statistical package version 3.2.3 [47]. Cytokine concentrations (both crude and ratios between stimulated and unstimulated samples) were log_{10}-transformed after assessing the distribution of each cytokine using normality plots for each cytokine across TLR stimulations. To explore sample clusters by TLR stimulation, data were plotted by using principal component analysis (PCA) and the first two components were used to show associations.

To assess the effect of PME on TLR-mediated cytokine responses, ANOVA test was used to compare the mean of cytokine responses between groups of PME for significant variance among the mean of cytokine responses. Benjamini-Hochberg method was applied to adjust p values for multiple comparisons [48]. Maternal- and infant-related co-variables including gravidity, low birth weight (LBW), birth season, newborn sex, and ethnicity were used to adjust the effect of PME on cytokine responses in linear regression models.

The association between TLR-mediated cytokine responses at birth and the risk of clinical malaria during the first year of life was assessed in univariable and multivariable Cox proportional-hazard models. Proportionality of hazards assumption and functional form of each variable adjusted in the Cox models was examined using

Schoenfeld residuals analysis and p-splines, respectively. Secondary variables that showed significant association with malaria during the first 12 months of life were determined in Kaplan-Meier survival analyses (log-rank test P value < 0.05) and included in the Cox proportional-hazard regression models. A P value < 0.05 was considered statistically significant.

Results
Characteristics of study participants
The characteristics of the participants included in this study are presented in Table 1. The mean age of pregnant women at enrollment was 26.1 years, and the majority of them were multigravida (63%). More than two thirds of deliveries (77.6%) occurred during the malaria high-transmission season (July–December). The mean birth weight of the newborns was 3009 g, while 9.6% had a low birth weight (LBW). In total, 291 newborns (93%) were exposed to malaria parasites and/or antigens in utero. The majority of the newborns were born to mothers with past PM (59.1% [185/313]) followed by those born to mothers who had either clinical malaria ($N = 6$) or asymptomatic infection ($N = 55$) during pregnancy but with no evidence of PM at delivery (19.5% [61/313]). Few infants were born to mothers with acute PM at delivery (2.2% [7/313]). There was a higher but non-significant proportion of females than males among the newborns ($P = 0.158$).

TLR-mediated cytokine responses
Overall variance of cytokine responses between subjects and stimuli is shown in Fig. 2 by PCA. PC1 and PC2 contribute to explain 59.2% and 5.2% of the variance, respectively. Overall, the responses to TLR3 and TLR9 clustered together with the unstimulated samples in contrast to distinct clustering of TLR7/8 responses, suggesting that TLR3 and TLR9 ligands did not induce—or induced low responses—for most of the analytes. This pattern is further illustrated by $\log_{10}$ of ratios of stimulated and unstimulated samples for each TLR agonist (Additional file 1: Figure S1 and S2), which show that few cytokines were produced above the background level following stimulations of TLR3 or TLR9. Compared to unstimulated samples, IP10 was the only analyte significantly induced by the TLR3 agonist (ANOVA, $P < 0.001$), while those significantly induced in response to TLR9 included IFN-α, IL-1RA, MCP-1, and IP-10 (ANOVA, $P \leq 0.006$). For TLR7/8 stimulation, all analyzed cytokines (with the exception of eotaxin, $P = 0.319$) had a significantly higher concentration than that of unstimulated samples (ANOVA, $P < 0.05$).

PME and cytokine responses at birth
Variation in cytokine production by PME category is shown as boxplots in Additional file 2: Figure S3–S6.

Results indicate that PME modifies innate immune responses to TLR stimulations at different magnitudes, depending on the PME category. The main effect was observed in responses to TLR7/8 stimulation (Additional file 2: Figure S5), being past PM more frequently associated with a significantly higher production of cytokine levels (i.e., IFN-α, IL-2, MIP-1α, RANTES, FGF, G-CSF, GM-CSF) compared with the non-exposed control group (ANOVA, $P < 0.05$). As expected, there was little variation in cytokine levels according to PME category following stimulations by TLR3 or TLR9, as these PRRs ligands induced very low cytokine production. The concentrations of cytokines in unstimulated samples also differed between PME categories. Overall, there was a tendency of lower cytokine levels among infants prenatally exposed to malaria (any category) than in non-exposed infants (Additional file 2: Figure S3). The significant variations were mostly observed with past PM on IL-1β, TNF, IL-7, IL-15, IL-2, IL-4, G-CSF, GM-CSF, HGF, and VEGF and with chronic PM on IL-7, IL-15, IL-2, IFN-γ, IL-17, and GM-CSF (ANOVA, $P < 0.05$). The comparison of biomarker levels in unstimulated samples from the exposed infants did not show a significant difference between PME groups. However, the trend analysis revealed a significant trend towards decreasing production among unstimulated samples from infants born to mothers with peripheral infection to those born to mothers with PM (past, chronic, and acute, respectively) for some biomarkers including IL-10 (P for trend = 0.024), IL-12 (P for trend = 0.042), and GM-CSF (P for trend = 0.032).

Innate immune response to TLR stimulation by PME was further investigated using multivariable linear regression models. The co-factors, besides PME, affecting cytokine responses in each stimulation assessment used in subsequent models are listed in Additional file 3: Table S1. The confounding factors, including gravidity, ethnicity, birth season, LBW, and newborn sex, were controlled for in subsequent models. Results confirmed that following stimulation with TLR7/8 agonist, infants born to mothers with past PM produced a significantly larger breadth of analytes compared to non-exposed individuals (17 cytokines related to all the functional classes analyzed, except anti-inflammatory and Th17-related cytokines) (Table 2). Significant differences were also observed in infants born to mothers with chronic PM (i.e., MIP-1α, MIP-1β, FGF, G-CSF, and GM-CSF) ($P < 0.05$, Table 2). In the case of infants born to mothers with acute PM, only two growth factors (FGF and GM-CSF) had significantly higher mean ratios compared to non-exposed infants, whereas only GM-CSF was higher in infants born to mothers infected during pregnancy but with no PM at delivery. Stimulation of TLR3 resulted in higher IP-10 responses among infants born

Table 1 Characteristics of study participants

Characteristics	Overall cohort (N = 313)	Non-exposed (N = 22)	Exposed no PM (N = 61)	Past PM (N = 185)	Chronic PM (N = 38)	Acute PM (N = 7)	P value
Maternal characteristics							
Age (years, mean ± SD)	26.1 ± 6.2	28.4 ± 6.4	27.7 ± 6.0	25.5 ± 6.0	23.8 ± 5.7	28.3 ± 7.2	< 0.001
Gravidity (N (%))							< 0.001
Primigravida	58 (18.5)	1 (4.5)	2 (3.3)	40 (21.6)	15 (39.5)	0 (0.0)	
Secundigravida	58 (18.5)	2 (9.1)	10 (16.4)	38 (20.5)	7 (18.4)	1 (14.3)	
Multigravida	197 (63.0)	19 (86.4)	49 (80.3)	107 (57.9)	16 (42.1)	6 (85.7)	
ITN use (N (%))	219 (70.0)	19 (86.4)	47 (77.0)	128 (69.2)	21 (55.3)	4 (57.1)	0.061
MiP preventive strategy in COSMIC trial (N (%))							< 0.001
Standard IPTp-SP	109 (34.2)	–	23 (37.7)	68 (36.8)	14 (36.8)	4 (57.1)	
CSST/IPTp-SP	204 (65.2)	22 (100.0)	38 (62.3)	117 (63.2)	24 (63.2)	3 (42.9)	
SP doses uptake (women who received ≥ 2 doses, N (%))	293 (93.6)	21 (95.5)	55 (90.2)	178 (96.2)	32 (84.2)	7 (100.0)	0.055
AL treatment (women treated at least once, N (%))	67 (21.4)	–	7 (11.5)	43 (23.2)	14 (36.8)	3 (42.8)	0.002
Gestational age at enrollment (median (IQR), weeks)	20 (19–22)	20 (18–26.5)	20 (20.5–25.5)	20 (19–21)	20 (16–21)	20 (20–25)	0.445
Infants characteristics							
Sex (females, N (%))	169 (54.0)	7 (31.8)	36 (59.0)	105 (56.8)	19 (50.0)	2 (28.6)	0.110
Birth season (malaria high-transmission season, N (%))	243 (77.6)	14 (63.6)	44 (72.1)	141 (76.2)	37 (97.4)	7 (100.0)	0.002
Birth weight (g, mean ± SD)	3009 ± 429.6	3119.1 ± 441.7	3041.5 ± 360.5	2988.2 ± 439.1	2967.1 ± 499.8	3169.3 ± 228.4	0.470
LBW (< 2500 g) (no. (%))	30 (9.6)	1 (4.5)	3 (4.9)	20 (10.8)	6 (15.8)	0 (0.0)	0.371
Ethnicity (N (%)							0.017
Mossi	276 (88.2)	21 (95.4)	55 (90.1)	164 (88.6)	31 (81.6)	5 (71.4)	
Gourounsi	34 (10.8)	1 (4.6)	4 (6.6)	21 (11.4)	7 (18.4)	2 (28.6)	
Fulani	3 (1.0)	0 (0.0)	2 (3.3)	0 (0.0)	0 (0.0)	0 (0.0)	
Follow-up time (total time at risk, person-months)	2782.6	175.1	544.7	1664.1	330.4	68.3	
Clinical malaria episode (N (%))	189 (60.4)	11 (50.0)	37 (60.7)	113 (61.1)	24 (63.2)	4 (57.1)	0.872
Time to first clinical malaria episode (median, months)	10.3	10.2	10.6	10.2	10.5	11.4	0.990

PM placental malaria, *SD* standard deviation, *LBW* low birth weight, *ITN* insecticide-treated net, *IQR* interquartile range, *MiP* malaria in pregnancy, *COSMIC* community-based scheduled screening and treatment of malaria in pregnancy: a cluster randomized trial, *IPTp-SP* intermittent preventive treatment during pregnancy with Sulfadoxine-pyrimethamine, *CSST/IPTp-SP* community-based scheduled screening and treatment of malaria in combination with the standard IPTp-SP, *AL* artemether-lumefantrine

to mothers with past and chronic PM ($P = 0.026$ and $P = 0.008$, respectively), but lower IL-5 responses ($P = 0.046$ and $P = 0.033$, respectively). Finally, TLR9-mediated FGF and G-CSF responses were found to be significantly higher in infants born to mothers with past PM compared to the control group ($P = 0.028$ and $P = 0.016$, respectively), whereas IL-5 responses were significantly lower in infants born to mothers with chronic PM compared with those in the non-exposed control group ($P = 0.009$).

Results from the multivariable models confirmed decreased levels of cytokines in unstimulated samples from infants prenatally exposed to malaria compared to the non-exposed control group: lower cytokine responses were found in past PM exposed group (20 cytokines from all the functional classes analyzed), chronic PM (10 cytokines from all the functional classes, except proinflammatory cytokines), acute PM (IL-7 only), and for peripheral infections during pregnancy (IL-7, IL-15, IL-13, IL-17, HGF, VEGF).

TLR-mediated cytokine responses and risk of clinical malaria during the first year of life

Data on malaria incidence and prevalence among the overall birth cohort has been described elsewhere [39].

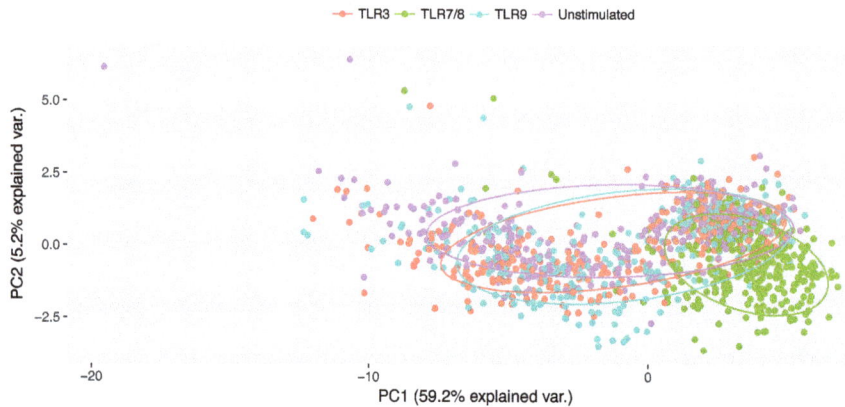

Fig. 2 Principal component analysis of cytokine responses to TLR agonists. PCA showing the variance in cytokine responses to the three TLR agonists and unstimulated samples. Ellipses represent the clusters estimated based on principal components 1 and 2

In the subgroup of infants included in the present analysis, malaria incidence was 60.4% (189/313) with a median survival time of 10.3 months (Table 1). Among the potential confounding factors analyzed (i.e., gravidity, PME, LBW, birth season, newborn sex, ethnicity, insecticide-treated net (ITN) usage by mothers), PME (Fig. 3) and LBW (Fig. 4) were found to be significantly associated with the risk of clinical malaria and, thus, were included in the Cox multivariable regression analyses. In particular, we found that infants born to mothers with PM had a significantly lower risk of clinical malaria during the first 6 months of life, while they were at higher risk of clinical malaria from age 6 to 12 months, compared to infants born to mothers with no PM. In addition, infants born with LBW had a significant shorter time to first clinical malaria episode than those born with a normal birth weight. Although birth season was not significantly associated with the risk of clinical malaria (Fig. 5), it was included in the models using an interaction term with the timing of clinical malaria to account for differences in the risk of infection between infants due to the high seasonality in malaria transmission in Burkina Faso.

Using crude concentration of cytokines, we found that higher concentrations of eotaxin (in both unstimulated and TLR7/8-stimulated samples), IL-7 (in TLR3-stimulated samples), GM-CSF (in TLR7/8-stimulated samples), and IL-1β (in TLR9-stimulated samples) in the cord blood at birth were significantly associated with an increased risk of subsequent clinical malaria episodes during the first year of life (Table 3). In contrast, an increase in the concentration of IP-10 in TLR3 and TLR9 stimulations was associated with a decreased risk of clinical malaria occurrence in early infancy. When considering biomarkers ratios, increases in TLR3-mediated IL7 response were predictive of an increased risk of clinical malaria attack, while higher TLR9-mediated eotaxin responses and TLR7/8-mediated

IL-1RA and IL-12 responses had a protective effect against developing a malaria episode during the first year of life (Table 3). Remarkably, TLR-mediated responses of some biomarkers, which showed a significant prediction of malaria protection/risk during the first 12 months of life (i.e., IL-12 TLR7/8 ratios, IL-1RA TLR7/8 ratios, GM-CSF TLR7/8 crude, IP-10 TLR3 crude), were significantly influenced by in utero exposure to malaria parasites (Additional files 2 and 3) indicating the clinical relevance of the modulation of newborn's innate immune responses by PME.

Discussion

In this study, we investigated the impact of different manifestations of malaria in pregnancy on both spontaneous and TLR-mediated cytokine production by cord blood cells at birth and we assessed whether these cytokines predicted malaria risk/protection in infancy. Overall, we found that PME has a profound effect on the fetal immune system and that the differential modulation of infants' innate immune responses by PME could have important implications with regards to malaria susceptibility in infancy. Indeed, we observed that spontaneous cytokine, chemokine, and growth factor production were all significantly lower in samples from exposed versus non-exposed infants. However, following TLR7/8 stimulation, cord blood cells from mothers with past PM (pigment only) were hyper-responsive in comparison to those without evidence of prenatal exposure. Importantly, we identified some responses (both spontaneous and following TLR stimulation) associated with differential malaria risk in infancy.

To our knowledge, this study reports for the first time the effect of these categories of PME on TLR-mediated innate immune responses, as previous studies have focused on the overall effect of PM and/or other types of PME on PRR-mediated cytokines responses [9, 29, 30, 49]. It has been shown that malaria pigment in the

Table 2 Multivariable linear regression analyses assessing the effect of prenatal malaria exposure (PME) categories on TLR-mediated cytokine responses at birth

Cytokines*		Exposed/no PM vs non-exposed		Past PM vs non-exposed		Chronic PM vs non-exposed		Acute PM vs non-exposed	
		Coeff (SE)	P	Coeff (SE)	P	Coeff (SE)	P	Coeff (SE)	P
TLR7/8 responses using $\log_{10}$ of ratio cytokines concentrations									
Pro	IFN-α	0.15 (0.08)	0.079	0.19 (0.08)	0.018	0.09 (0.09)	0.359	0.08 (0.15)	0.591
	IL-1RA	0.15 (0.12)	0.223	0.22 (0.11)	0.049	0.15 (0.14)	0.263	0.22 (0.22)	0.308
	IL-1β	0.13 (0.20)	0.522	0.36 (0.18)	0.049	0.32 (0.22)	0.140	0.11 (0.35)	0.765
	TNF	0.28 (0.24)	0.238	0.55 (0.22)	0.013	0.31 (0.26)	0.229	0.36 (0.42)	0.387
Th1	IL-12	0.18 (0.16)	0.259	0.34 (0.14)	0.015	0.30 (0.17)	0.074	0.30 (0.27)	0.276
	IL-2	0.12 (0.07)	0.092	0.15 (0.06)	0.019	0.14 (0.08)	0.081	0.09 (0.12)	0.448
	IL-2R	0.16 (0.10)	0.103	0.23 (0.09)	0.012	0.19 (0.11)	0.081	0.15 (0.18)	0.398
	IFN-γ	0.18 (0.12)	0.137	0.29 (0.11)	0.008	0.25 (0.13)	0.056	− 0.03 (0.21)	0.898
Th2	IL-13	0.14 (0.13)	0.272	0.25 (0.12)	0.031	0.25 (0.14)	0.079	0.26 (0.22)	0.237
Chemokines	MIP-1α	0.47 (0.27)	0.085	0.72 (0.25)	0.004	0.59 (0.30)	0.049	0.57 (0.48)	0.237
	MIP-1β	0.36 (0.25)	0.143	0.56 (0.22)	0.013	0.52 (0.26)	0.049	0.54 (0.43)	0.214
	RANTES	0.17 (0.10)	0.097	0.23 (0.09)	0.015	0.21 (0.11)	0.062	0.07 (0.18)	0.697
Growth factors	EGF	0.10 (0.06)	0.087	0.12 (0.05)	0.017	0.09 (0.06)	0.125	0.09 (0.10)	0.360
	FGF	0.16 (0.09)	0.069	0.22 (0.08)	0.005	0.23 (0.09)	0.017	0.32 (0.15)	0.037
	G-CSF	0.18 (0.13)	0.170	0.35 (0.12)	0.004	0.29 (0.14)	0.047	0.38 (0.23)	0.099
	GM-CSF	0.34 (0.16)	0.033	0.53 (0.14)	< 0.001	0.36 (0.17)	0.032	0.64 (0.27)	0.020
	HGF	0.08 (0.06)	0.151	0.11 (0.05)	0.029	0.06 (0.06)	0.299	0.04 (0.10)	0.676
TLR9 responses using $\log_{10}$ of ratio cytokines concentrations									
Th2	IL-5	− 0.08 (0.07)	0.283	− 0.11 (0.07)	0.008	− 0.20 (0.08)	0.009	− 0.14 (0.13)	0.267
Growth factors	FGF	0.08 (0.07)	0.231	0.14 (0.06)	0.028	0.15 (0.07)	0.050	0.14 (0.12)	0.234
	G-CSF	0.11 (0.08)	0.187	0.17 (0.07)	0.016	0.15 (0.09)	0.082	0.09 (0.09)	0.505
TLR3 responses using $\log_{10}$ of ratio cytokines concentrations									
Th2	IL-5	− 0.06 (0.06)	0.392	− 0. 12(0.06)	0.046	− 0.15 (0.07)	0.033	− 0.02 (0.11)	0.841
Chemokines	IP-10	0.13 (0.11)	0.222	0.22 (0.10)	0.026	0.32 (0.12)	0.008	0.10 (0.19)	0.584
Unstimulated samples using $\log_{10}$ of crude cytokines concentrations									
Pro	IFN-α	− 0.11 (0.07)	0.154	− 0.14 (0.07)	0.038	− 0.15 (0.08)	0.069	− 0.01 (0.13)	0.948
	IL-1RA	− 0.24 (0.12)	0.055	− 0.23 (0.11)	0.040	− 0.23 (0.14)	0.086	− 0.37 (0.21)	0.084
	IL-1β	− 0.35 (0.24)	0.152	− 0.58 (0.22)	0.008	− 0.50 (0.26)	0.057	− 0.62 (0.42)	0.142
	TNF	− 0.40 (0.26)	0.117	− 0. 61(0.23)	0.009	− 0.49 (0.28)	0.079	− 0.47 (0.45)	0.296
Anti	IL-10	− 0.22 (0.32)	0.485	− 0.60 (0.29)	0.041	− 0.45 (0.35)	0.204	− 0.92 (0.56)	0.105
	IL-7	− 0.34 (0.10)	< 0.001	− 0.40 (0.09)	< 0.001	− 0.35 (0.11)	< 0.001	− 0.40 (0.17)	0.021
Th1	IL-15	− 0.39 (0.16)	0.015	− 0.52 (0.14)	< 0.001	− 0.52 (0.17)	0.003	− 0.36 (0.28)	0.190
	IL-2	− 0.15 (0.08)	0.064	− 0.16 (0.07)	0.032	− 0.18 (0.09)	0.053	− 0.12 (0.14)	0.382
	IFN-γ	− 0.14 (0.08)	0.094	− 0.17 (0.07)	0.023	− 0.21 (0.09)	0.024	− 0.10 (0.14)	0.494
Th2	IL-13	− 0.25 (0.12)	0.038	− 0.22 (0.11)	0.042	− 0.32 (0.13)	0.014	− 0.12 (0.21)	0.056
	IL-4	− 0.27 (0.14)	0.057	− 0.40 (0.13)	0.002	− 0.26 (0.15)	0.096	− 0.07 (0.25)	0.769
Th17	IL-17	− 0.13 (0.07)	0.046	− 0.15 (0.06)	0.016	− 0.17 (0.07)	0.017	− 0.18 (0.12)	0.128
Chemokines	MIP-1α	− 0.29 (0.28)	0.297	− 0.56 (0.25)	0.029	− 0.50 (0.31)	0.102	− 0.37 (0.49)	0.453
	RANTES	− 0.23 (0.12)	0.050	− 0.25 (0.11)	0.023	− 0.28 (0.13)	0.029	− 0.19 (0.21)	0.371
Growth factors	EGF	− 0.11 (0.07)	0.106	− 0.12 (0.06)	0.047	− 0.15 (0.07)	0.049	− 0.09 (0.12)	0.446
	FGF	− 0.12 (0.08)	0.151	− 0.15 (0.08)	0.049	− 0. 17(0.09)	0.070	− 0.17 (0.15)	0.244

Table 2 Multivariable linear regression analyses assessing the effect of prenatal malaria exposure (PME) categories on TLR-mediated cytokine responses at birth *(Continued)*

Cytokines*	Exposed/no PM vs non-exposed		Past PM vs non-exposed		Chronic PM vs non-exposed		Acute PM vs non-exposed	
	Coeff (SE)	P	Coeff (SE)	P	Coeff (SE)	P	Coeff (SE)	P
G-CSF	− 0.21 (0.17)	0.229	− 0.37 (0.15)	0.019	− 0.37 (0.15)	0.045	− 0.33 (0.30)	0.276
GM-CSF	− 0.36 (0.19)	0.058	− 0.59 (0.17)	< 0.001	− 0.60 (0.21)	0.004	− 0.59 (0.33)	0.079
HGF	− 0.19 (0.07)	0.008	− 0.20 (0.06)	0.002	− 0.19 (0.08)	0.015	− 0.15 (0.12)	0.221
VEGF	− 0.45 (0.22)	0.041	− 0.59 (0.20)	0.003	− 0.43 (0.24)	0.070	− 0.35 (0.38)	0.356

PM placental malaria, *Coeff* coefficient, *SE* standard error, *Pro* proinflammatory cytokines, *P* p value, *Anti* anti-inflammatory cytokines, *Th1* Th1-type cytokines, *Th2* Th2-type cytokines, *Th17* Th17, type cytokines. *Only cytokines whose concentrations are significantly modified by categories of PME are presented. Non-exposed category was used as reference in each model. Significant results are shown in italic

placenta is associated with the maturation of cord blood myeloid and plasmocytoid DCs (innate immune cells triggered by TLR7/8 agonists [11, 30]), which may explain why cytokine responses to TLR7/8 stimulation were significantly enhanced in past PM (as well as in chronic PM, although with modest significance possibly due to the smaller sample size) compared to the other PME categories. A number of studies have also explored the effect of in utero malaria exposure on cord blood immune cell populations including dendritic cells (DCs), γδ T cells, CD4$^+$ T regulatory, and effector cells [10–15]. Interestingly, all revealed a varying effect of PME categories on cord blood mononuclear cells, thus ultimately demonstrating inter-individual variation in immune responses following different types of PME. Consequently, the differential admixture of cell types across PME

categories may be explanatory of the observed differences in cytokine production in the present study. In addition, there is increasing evidence that the innate system has immunological memory [50–54] and that innate stimulations can lead to sensitization to following pathogen exposure, a process termed trained innate immunity [53]. Therefore, in utero exposure could affect TLR responses of cord blood cells through the development of trained immunity.

While TLR7/8 stimulation induced robust cytokine responses, overall cytokine responses induced by TLR3 and TLR9 stimulations were low with limited variations between PME categories, consistent with previous investigations in African children [30, 55, 56] and non-African children [57, 58]. Although TLR3 and TLR9 are endosomal PRRs like TLR7/8, they differ in their responses depending on the cell populations, which may

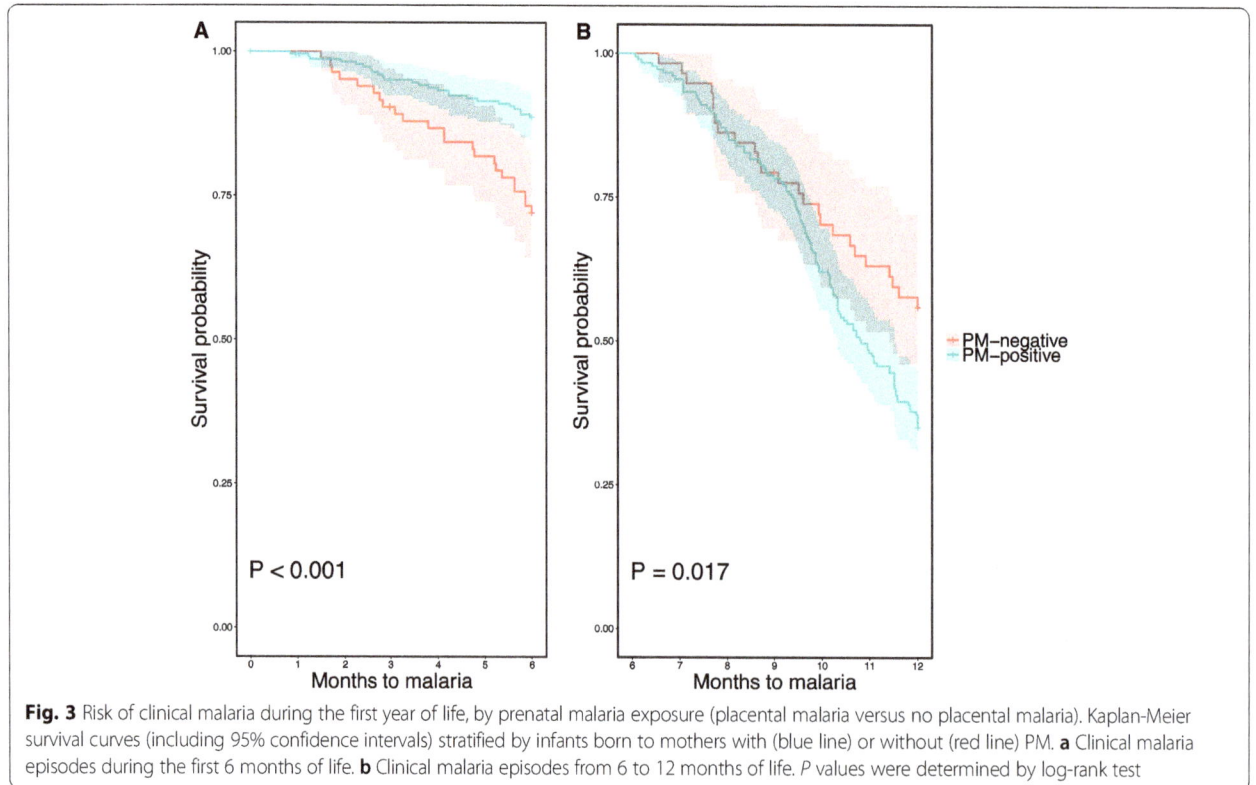

Fig. 3 Risk of clinical malaria during the first year of life, by prenatal malaria exposure (placental malaria versus no placental malaria). Kaplan-Meier survival curves (including 95% confidence intervals) stratified by infants born to mothers with (blue line) or without (red line) PM. **a** Clinical malaria episodes during the first 6 months of life. **b** Clinical malaria episodes from 6 to 12 months of life. *P* values were determined by log-rank test

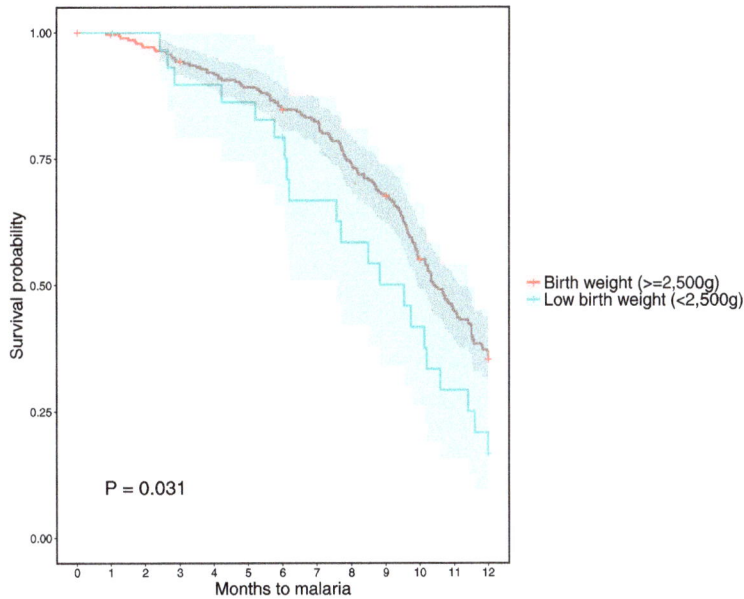

Fig. 4 Risk of clinical malaria during the first year of life, by birth weight. Kaplan-Meier survival curves (including 95% confidence intervals) stratified by infants born with a birth weight ≥ 2500 g (red line) and with a birth weight below 2500 g (low birth weight, blue line). P value was determined by log-rank test

explain differences in their inducible capacity of cytokine responses. Importantly, spontaneous cytokine production by cord blood cells in unstimulated samples also displayed significant variations between PME groups, with a trend towards decreased baseline levels in infants born to mothers with peripheral infection to those born to mothers with PM (past, chronic, and acute PM, respectively). Altogether, our findings are consistent with the hypothesis that PME results in a downregulation of cytokines production that can affect all the important functional classes of cytokines, but followed by a hyper-responsiveness to particular PRR agonists, such as TLR7/8 agonist, as compared to that in non-exposed infants.

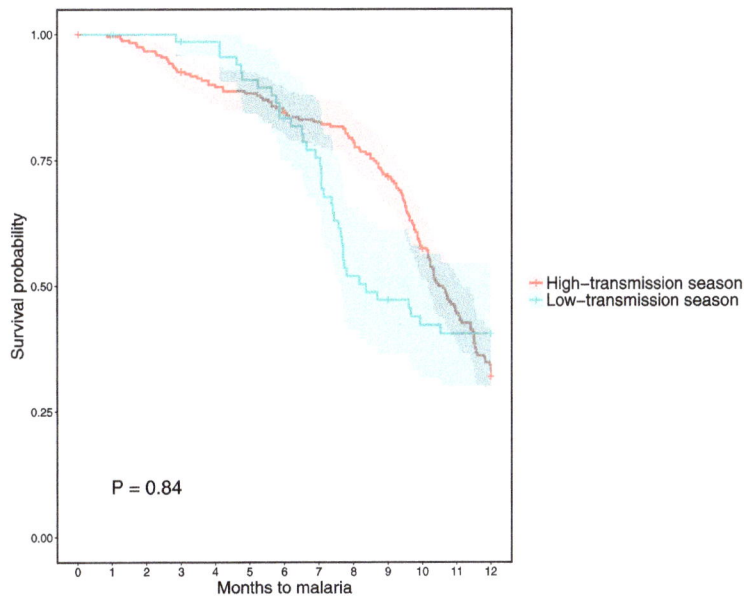

Fig. 5 Risk of clinical malaria during the first year of life, by birth season. Kaplan-Meier survival curves (including 95% confidence intervals) stratified by infants born during malaria high-transmission season (July–December, red line) and low-transmission season (January–June, blue line). P value was determined by log-rank test

Table 3 Cox proportional hazards analyses assessing the association between TLR-induced cytokine responses and the risk of malaria during the first year of life. Adjusted hazard ratio and 95% CI for each model is shown

Cytokines**		Unstimulated	TLR3 responses		TLR7/8 responses		TLR9 responses	
		Crude	Crude	Ratios	Crude	Ratios	Crude	Ratios
		AHR (95% CI)	AHR (95% CI)	AHR (95% CI)	AHR (95% CI)	AHR (95% CI)	AHR (95% CI)	AHR (95% CI)
Pro	IFN-α			0.24 (0.05–1.10)				
	IL-1RA*				0.61 (0.36–1.03)	*0.70 (0.50–0.98)*		
	IL-1β	1.16 (0.98–1.37)	1.15 (0.97–1.36)				*1.18 (1.01–1.39)*	
	TNF							
Anti	IL-10		1.12 (0.99–1.25)					
	IL-7		*1.80 (1.26–2.58)*	*1.54 (1.11–2.15)*				
Th1	IL-15						1.22 (0.96–1.54)	
	IL-12*	1.28 (0.97–1.69)	1.26 (0.95–1.68)	0.27 (0.07–1.15)		*0.76 (0.59–0.98)*		0.46 (0.20–1.04)
	IL-2							
	IL-2R							
	IFN-γ							
Th2	IL-13							
	IL-5							
	IL-4							
Th17	IL-17							
	IL-6							
Chemokines	IL-8							
	IP-10*	0.64 (0.38–1.08)	*0.66 (0.46–0.93)*				*0.75 (0.59–0.96)*	
	MCP-1							
	MIG							0.77 (0.56–1.05)
	MIP-1α						1.13 (0.97–1.31)	
	MIP-1β							
	RANTES							
	EOTAXIN	*1.83 (1.11–3.01)*	1.60 (0.99–2.58)	0.19 (0.03–1.14)	*1.72 (1.01–2.94)*			*0.46 (0.24–0.86)*
Growth factors	EGF				0.29 (0.08–1.07)			
	FGF		1.63 (0.91–2.93)					
	G-CSF	1.24 (0.97–1.57)						
	GM-CSF*					*1.28 (1.01–1.15)*		
	HGF							
	VEGF							

HR hazard ratio, *CI* confidence interval, *Pro* proinflammatory cytokines, *Anti* anti-inflammatory cytokines, *Th1* Th1-type cytokines, *Th2* Th2-type cytokines, *Th17* Th17-type cytokines. **Only results of cox proportional analysis for cytokines with P value (*P*) ≤ 0.100 are presented. *Cytokines whose levels were significantly modified by prenatal malaria exposure categories. Significant results are shwon in italic

Innate immune activation plays a crucial role in host protection as well as pathogenesis during malaria infection [59, 60]. Therefore, the second important aim of our study was to determine the predictive value of cytokines that were significantly influenced by PME for clinical malaria occurrence during the first year of life. Of note, we have shown that PME has a clinical impact on the risk of malaria among the study population. Indeed, we observed that infants born to mothers with PM had a lower risk of clinical malaria during the first 6 months of life, in contrast to

that reported in several epidemiological studies [2, 4, 5, 7]. This paradoxal finding may be at least partially explained by the protective effect of maternal antibodies and the strong malaria seasonality of the study area [39], which may make PME dynamics different from other sites. However, we cannot exclude a confounding or explanatory effect of other factors not assessed in this study.

Notably, we observed that some cytokines, which were associated with PME, were independent predictors of malaria risk or protection, demonstrating the clinical relevance of the modulation of infants' innate immune responses by PME. However, few studies have investigated the predictive value of cytokines, measured at birth either in unstimulated samples [49, 61] or upon stimulation with TLR [30], on the risk of clinical malaria during infancy. Those studies showed a protective prediction of high proinflammatory cytokine levels in unstimulated samples (TNF, TNF-RI, IL-1β), while high levels of anti-inflammatory cytokines such as IL-10 (upon TLR3 and TLR7/8 stimulations) predicted an increased risk of clinical malaria in early childhood [30, 49, 61]. Here, we found that Th1 cytokines and chemokines (IL-12 TLR7/8 ratio and IP-10 TLR3 crude) and cytokines induced upon inflammation (IL-1RA TLR7/8 ratio) were associated with a decreased risk of clinical malaria during the first year of life. These results are in agreement with a key role of IL-12 in the induction of a Th1-type protective immunity against malaria mediated by IFN-γ, TNF, and nitric oxide productions [62–66] and the inhibiting effect on disease severity of IL-1RA on IL-1A and IL-1β (through binding to IL-1 receptors) [67]. For IP-10, a cytokine belonging to the CXC chemokine family that induces chemotaxis, apoptosis, cell growth, and angiostasis, the association with malaria protection observed in this study is in agreement with studies in the murine model [68], although in contrast with others that have shown an association with clinical malaria and disease severity [69–72]. Among biomarkers that were significantly associated with PME, GM-CSF TLR7/8 crude was associated with a risk of developing clinical malaria during the first year of life, which is in contrast with previous observations [73–75], but in agreement with others [76]. These conflicting findings could be related to the fact that cytokines promoting a protective inflammatory environment during malaria infection could become harmful if exaggerated and act in favor of disease manifestation [77–79]. Overall, these results suggest that PME has an impact on malaria risk and that the effect is at least partially mediated by the modulation of TLR and the consequent cytokine responses. Given that past PM, which potentially occurs early during pregnancy, has a profound effect on fetal immune system, a strategy based on screening and treatment of malaria during pregnancy that we proved to benefit infants [40] should be implemented as early as possible during the first trimester.

In this study, two main limitations should be noted. First, some of the PME groups including acute PM and non-exposed groups were small in comparison with others. Therefore, we cannot exclude an underestimation of the effect of acute PM on innate immune responses measured. However, this number reflects the prevalence of PM categories in the main COSMIC trial as most of malaria infections in the placenta were past or chronic PM (95.5%). The relatively limited number of non-exposed controls is due to the high malaria transmission in the study area and the strict definition and recruitment that we applied to this group, where pregnant women had negative RDT/LM and qPCR results at each screening and ANC visit, in addition to negative placental histology. Second, in this study, the measurement of white blood cells population and lymphocyte subsets in cord blood at delivery was not performed while there is evidence that PME can alter myeloid subsets abundance and thus influence TLR-mediated innate immune responses. Therefore, the lack of these information has eventually limited the interpretation of our data.

Conclusions

In conclusion, despite these limitations, our findings indicate that the various PME categories have different effects on innate immune responses of the newborn at birth, which might drive variation between individuals to malaria susceptibility during the first year of life. The differential alteration of TLR-mediated immune responses by PME categories may have profound implications on immune responses to other infections as well as to vaccines formulated with TLR-based adjuvants in infants prenatally exposed to malaria.

Additional files

Additional file 1: Boxplots showing variation in cytokine responses by stimulation. **Figure S1.** Boxplots generated using $\log_{10}$ of crude concentrations (pg/mL). **Figure S2.** Boxplots generated using $\log_{10}$ of ratios (TLR/unstimulated). (PDF 287 kb)

Additional file 2: Changes in cytokine responses according to prenatal malaria exposure categories. **Figure S3.** Boxplots generated using $\log_{10}$ of unstimulated crude concentrations (pg/mL). **Figure S4.** Boxplots generated using $\log_{10}$ of TLR3/unstimulated ratio. **Figure S5.** Boxplots generated using $\log_{10}$ of TLR7/8/unstimulated ratio. **Figure S6.** Boxplots generated using $\log_{10}$ of TLR9/unstimulated ratio. Non-expo, non-exposed; expo-no-PM, exposed/no placental malaria; past PM, past placental malaria; chronic-PM, chronic placental malaria; acute PM, acute placental malaria. (PDF 350 kb)

Additional file 3: **Table S1.** Variables included in the linear regression models assessing the effect of prenatal malaria exposure on TLR-mediated cytokine responses at birth. (PDF 88 kb)

Abbreviations

AL: Artemether-lumefantrine; ANC: Antenatal care; COSMIC: Community-based scheduled screening and treatment of malaria in pregnancy: a cluster randomized trial; CSST/IPTp-SP: Community-based scheduled screening and treatment of malaria in combination with intermittent preventive treatment with sulfadoxine-pyrimethamine; EGF: Epidermal growth factor; FGF: Fibroblast growth factor; G-CSF: Granulocyte-colony stimulating factor; GM-CSF: Granulocyte-macrophage colony stimulating factor; HGF: Hepatocyte growth factor; IFN: Interferon; IL: Interleukin; IP: IFN-γ-inducible protein; IPTp-SP: intermittent preventive treatment during pregnancy with sulfadoxine-pyrimethamine; ITN: Insecticide-treated net; LBW: Low birth weight; LM: Light microscopy; MCP: Monocyte chemottractant protein; MIG: Monokine induced by IFN-γ; MIP: Macrophage inflammatory protein; MiP: malaria in pregnancy; PAMPs: Pathogen-associated-molecular patterns; PM: Placental malaria; PME: Prenatal malaria exposure; PRRs: Pattern recognition receptors; qPCR: Quantitative real-time polymerase chain reaction; RDT: Rapid diagnostic test; TLRs: Toll-like receptors; TNF: Tumor necrosis factor; VEGF: Vascular endothelial growth factor

Acknowledgements

We are sincerely grateful to the mothers and their offspring for participating into this study. We are indebted to nurses, field workers, field supervisors, data managers, and laboratory workers at the Clinical Research Unit of Nanoro (CRUN) in Burkina Faso for their valuable contribution to the successful completion of the study. We also acknowledge the research teams at the Malariology Unit, Institute of Tropical Medicine (ITM; Belgium), the Immunology Laboratory at the Manhiça Health Research Center (Mozambique), and the malaria laboratory at ISGlobal, Spain.

Funding

The study was supported by the Belgium Directorate General for Development Cooperation (DGD) through the collaborative framework agreement 3 (FA3–DGD programme) between CRUN (Burkina Faso) and ITM (Belgium); the COSMIC project funded by European Union Seventh Framework Programme (FP7/2002-2016) under grant agreement no. 305662–COSMIC); the Research Foundation-Flanders (FWO) long (V4.675.15N) and short (K2.090.17N) stay abroad travel grants. HMN holds a PhD fellowship funded by DGD.

Authors' contributions

HMN, GM, ERV, CD, and ARU conceived and designed the study. HMN, HSo, MTC, MAS, SS, and IV supervised the data and samples collection in the field. HMN, HSo, MTC, and MAS supervised the malaria diagnosis and management of malaria patients in the field. HMN performed the TLR-mediated stimulation assay and Pf-varATS qPCR experiments. HMN and RA performed the cytokines quantification experiments. IV, PFM, HDFHS, HT, LK, CD, and ARU contributed for the reagents/materials/analysis tools. HMN, HSa, GM, ERV, RA, CD, and ARU analyzed and interpreted the results and were the major contributors in writing the manuscript. All authors read and approved the final manuscript.

Competing interests

The authors declare that they have no competing interests.

Author details

[1]Department of Biomedical Sciences, Institute of Tropical Medicine, B 2000 Antwerp, Belgium. [2]Unité de Recherche Clinique de Nanoro, Institut de Recherche en Sciences de la Santé, BP218, Nanoro, Burkina Faso. [3]Department of Biomedical Sciences, University of Antwerp, B 2610 Antwerp, Belgium. [4]Barcelona Institute for Global Health (ISGlobal), Hospital Clinic – Universitat de Barcelona, Carrer Rossello 132, E-08036 Barcelona, Catalonia, Spain. [5]Department of Epidemiology and Population Health, London School of Hygiene and Tropical Medicine, London WC1E7HT, UK. [6]Department of Medical Microbiology - Parasitology Unit, Academic Medical Centre, Amsterdam 1105, AZ, The Netherlands. [7]Centre Muraz, BP390, Bobo Dioulasso, Burkina Faso.

References

1. Le Hesran JY, Cot M, Personne P, Fievet N, Dubois B, Beyemé M, et al. Maternal placental infection with Plasmodium falciparum and malaria morbidity during the first 2 years of life. Am J Epidemiol. 1997;146:826–31.

2. Le Port A, Watier L, Cottrell G, Ouédraogo S, Dechavanne C, Pierrat C, et al. Infections in infants during the first 12 months of life: role of placental malaria and environmental factors. PLoS One. 2011;6:e27516.

3. Malhotra I, Dent A, Mungai P, Wamachi A, Ouma JH, Narum DL, et al. Can prenatal malaria exposure produce an immune tolerant phenotype? A prospective birth cohort study in Kenya. PLoS Med. 2009;6:e1000116.

4. Mutabingwa TK, Bolla MC, Li J-L, Domingo GJ, Li X, Fried M, et al. Maternal malaria and gravidity interact to modify infant susceptibility to malaria. PLoS Med. 2005;2:e407.

5. Schwarz NG, Adegnika AA, Breitling LP, Gabor J, Agnandji ST, Newman RD, et al. Placental malaria increases malaria risk in the first 30 months of life. Clin Infect Dis. 2008;47:1017–25.

6. Rachas A, Le PA, Cottrell G, Guerra J, Choudat I, Bouscaillou J, et al. Placental malaria is associated with increased risk of nonmalaria infection during the first 18 months of life in a Beninese population. Clin Infect Dis. 2012;55:672–8.

7. Sylvester B, Gasarasi DB, Aboud S, Tarimo D, Massawe S, Mpembeni R, et al. Prenatal exposure to Plasmodium falciparum increases frequency and shortens time from birth to first clinical malaria episodes during the first two years of life: prospective birth cohort study. Malar J. 2016;15:379.

8. Broen K, Brustoski K, Engelmann I, Luty AJF. Placental Plasmodium falciparum infection: causes and consequences of in utero sensitization to parasite antigens. Mol Biochem Parasitol. 2007;151:1–8.

9. Ismaili J, Van Der Sande M, Holland MJ, Sambou I, Keita S, Allsopp C, et al. Plasmodium falciparum infection of the placenta affects newborn immune responses. Clin Exp Immunol. 2003;133:414–21.

10. Engelmann I, Santamaria A, Kremsner PG, Luty AJF. Activation status of cord blood gamma delta T cells reflects in utero exposure to Plasmodium falciparum antigen. J Infect Dis. 2005;191:1612–22.

11. Fievet N, Varani S, Ibitokou S, Briand V, Louis S, Perrin RX, et al. Plasmodium falciparum exposure in utero, maternal age and parity influence the innate activation of foetal antigen presenting cells. Malar J. 2009;8:251.

12. Flanagan KL, Halliday A, Burl S, Landgraf K, Jagne YJ, Noho-Konteh F, et al. The effect of placental malaria infection on cord blood and maternal immunoregulatory responses at birth. Eur J Immunol. 2010;40:1062–72.

13. Prahl M, Jagannathan P, McIntyre TI, Auma A, Farrington L, Wamala S, et al. Timing of in utero malaria exposure influences fetal CD4 T cell regulatory versus effector differentiation. Malar J. 2016;15:497.

14. Brustoski K, Mo U, Kramer M, Petelski A, Brenner S, Palmer DR, et al. IFN-g_ and IL-10 mediate parasite-specific immune responses of cord blood cells induced by pregnancy-associated Plasmodium falciparum malaria. J Immunol. 2005;174:1738–45.

15. Breitling LP, Fendel R, Mordmueller B, Adegnika A a, Kremsner PG, Luty AJF. Cord blood dendritic cell subsets in African newborns exposed to Plasmodium falciparum in utero. Infect Immun. 2006;74:5725–9.

16. King CL, Malhotra I, Wamachi A, Kioko J, Mungai P, Wahab SA, et al. Acquired immune responses to Plasmodium falciparum merozoite surface protein-1 in the human fetus. J Immunol. 2002;168:356–64.

17. Metenou S, Suguitan AL, Long C, Leke RGF, Taylor DW. Fetal immune response to Plasmodium falciparum antigens in a malaria-endemic region of Cameroon. J Immunol. 2007;178:2770–7.

18. Xi G, Leke RGF, Thuita LW, Zhou A, Leke RJI, Mbu R, et al. Congenital exposure to Plasmodium falciparum Antigens: prevalence and antigenic specificity of in utero-produced antimalarial immunoglobulin M antibodies. Infect Immun. 2003;71:1242–6.

19. Dent A, Malhotra I, Mungai P, Muchiri E, Crabb BS, Kazura JW, et al. Prenatal malaria immune experience affects acquisition of Plasmodium falciparum Merozoite surface Protein-1 invasion inhibitory antibodies during infancy. J Immunol. 2006;177:7139–45.

20. Malhotra I, Mungai P, Muchiri E, Ouma J, Sharma S, Kazura JW, et al. Distinct Th1- and Th2-type prenatal cytokine responses to Plasmodium falciparum erythrocyte invasion ligands. Infect Immun. 2005;73:3462–70.

21. Maródi L. Innate cellular immune responses in newborns. Clin Immunol. 2006;118:137–44.

22. Levy O. Innate immunity of the newborn: basic mechanisms and clinical correlates. Nat Rev Immunol. 2007;7:379–90.

23. Staros EB. Innate immunity: new approaches to understanding its clinical significance. Am J Clin Pathol. 2005;123:305–12.

24. Takeda K, Akira S. Toll-like receptors in innate immunity. Int Immunol. 2005;17:1–14.

25. Iwasaki A, Medzhitov R. Toll-like receptor control of the adaptive immune responses. Nat Immunol. 2004;5:987–95.

26. Maródi L. Neonatal innate immunity to infectious agents. Infect Immun. 2006;74:1999–2006.

27. Erdman LK, Finney CAM, Liles WC, Kain KC. Inflammatory pathways in malaria infection: TLRs share the stage with other components of innate immunity. Mol Biochem Parasitol. 2008;162:105–11.

28. Angulo I, Fresno M. Cytokines in the pathogenesis of and protection against malaria. Clin Diagn Lab Immunol. 2002;9:1145–52.

29. Adegnika AA, Köhler C, Agnandji ST, Chai SK, Labuda L, Breitling LP, et al. Pregnancy-associated malaria affects toll-like receptor ligand-induced cytokine responses in cord blood. J Infect Dis. 2008;198:928–36.

30. Gbédandé K, Varani S, Ibitokou S, Houngbegnon P, Borgella S, Nouatin O, et al. Malaria modifies neonatal and early-life toll-like receptor cytokine responses. Infect Immun. 2013;81:2686–96.

31. Coban C, Ishii KJ, Kawai T, Hemmi H, Sato S, Uematsu S, et al. Toll-like receptor 9 mediates innate immune activation by the malaria pigment hemozoin. J Exp Med. 2005;201:19–25.

32. Gazzinelli RT, Kalantari P, Fitzgerald KA, Golenbock DT. Innate sensing of malaria parasites. Nat Rev Immunol. 2014;14(11):744–57.

33. Zhu J, Krishnegowda G, Gowda DC. Induction of proinflammatory responses in macrophages by the glycosylphosphatidylinositols of *Plasmodium falciparum*. J Biol Chem. 2005;280:8617–27.

34. Eriksson EM, Sampaio NG, Schofield L. Toll-like receptors and malaria – sensing and susceptibility. J Trop Dis. 2014;02:126.

35. Esposito S, Molteni CG, Zampiero A, Baggi E, Lavizzari A, Semino M, et al. Role of polymorphisms of toll-like receptor (TLR) containing adaptor protein (TIRAP) and FCGR2A genes in malaria susceptibility and severity in Burundian children. Malar J. 2012;11:196.

36. Omar AH, Shibata H, Yasunami M, Yamazaki A, Ofori MF, Hirayama K, et al. Toll-like receptor 9 (TLR9) polymorphism associated with symptomatic malaria: a cohort study. Malar J. 2012;11:168.

37. Scott S, Mens PF, Tinto H, Nahum A, Ruizendaal E, Pagnoni F, et al. Community-based scheduled screening and treatment of malaria in pregnancy for improved maternal and infant health in the Gambia, Burkina Faso and Benin: study protocol for a randomized controlled trial. Trials. 2014;15:340.

38. Derra K, Rouamba E, Kazienga A, Ouedraogo S, Tahita MC, Sorgho H, et al. Profile: Nanoro health and demographic surveillance system. Int J Epidemiol. 2012;41:1293–301.

39. Natama HM, Vallbona ER, Somé MA, Zango SH, Sorgho H, Guetens P, et al. Malaria incidence and prevalence during the first year of life in Nanoro, Burkina Faso: a birth-cohort study. Malar J. 2018;17:163.

40. Natama HM, Rovira-Vallbona E, Sorgho H, Somé MA, Traoré-Coulibaly M, Scott S, et al. Additional screening and treatment of malaria during pregnancy provides further protection against malaria and nonmalarial fevers during the first year of life. J Infect Dis. 2018;217:1967–76.

41. Natama HM, Ouedraogo DF, Sorgho H, Rovira-Vallbona E, Serra-casas E, Somé MA, et al. Diagnosing congenital malaria in a high-transmission setting: clinical relevance and usefulness of *P . falciparum* HRP2-based testing. Sci Rep. 2017;7:2080.

42. Sanz H, Aponte J, Harezlak J, Dong Y, Ayestaran A, Nhabomba A, et al. drLumi: an open-source package to manage data, calibrate, and conduct quality control of multiplex bead-based immunoassays data analysis. PLoS One. 2017;12:e0187901.

43. Defawe O, Fong Y, Vasilyeva E, Pickett M, Carter D, Gabriel E, et al. Optimization and qualification of a multiplex bead array to assess cytokine and chemokine production by vaccine-specific cells. J Immunol Methods. 2012;382:117–28.

44. Gottschalk P, Dunn J. Determining the error of dose estimates and minimum and maximum acceptable concentrations from assays with nonlinear dose-response curves. Comput Methods Prog Biomed. 2005;80: 204–15.

45. Reed G, Lynn F, Meade B. Use of coefficient of variation in assessing variability of quantitative assays. Clin Diagn Lab Immunol. 2002;9:1235–9.

46. World Health Organization. In: WHO, editor. Basic malaria microscopy: part I. Learner's guide. 2nd ed; 2010. https://www.who.int/malaria/publications/atoz/9241547820/en/. Accessed 10 Oct 2017.

47. R Core Team. R: a language and environment for statistical computing. R Foundation for statistical computing, Vienna. 2016. https://www.r-project.org/. Accessed 3 Nov 2015.

48. Benjamini Y, Hochberg Y. Controlling the false discovery rate: a practical and powerful approach to multiple testing. J R Stat Soc. 1995;57:239–300.

49. Kabyemela E, Gonçalves BP, Prevots DR, Morrison R, Harrington W, Gwamaka M, et al. Cytokine profiles at birth predict malaria severity during infancy. PLoS One. 2013;8:e77214.

50. Netea MG, Quintin J, Van Der Meer JWM. Trained immunity: a memory for innate host defense. Cell Host Microbe. 2011;9(5):355–61.

51. Aaby P, Kollmann TR, Benn CS. Nonspecific effects of neonatal and infant vaccination: public-health, immunological and conceptual challenges. Nat Immunol. 2014;15:895–9.

52. Levy O, Wynn J. A prime time for trained immunity: innate immune memory in newborns and infants. Neonatology. 2014;105:136–41.

53. Blok BA, Arts RJW, Van CR, Benn CS, Netea MG. Trained innate immunity as underlying mechanism for the long-term, nonspecific effects of vaccines. J Leukoc Biol. 2015;98:347–56.

54. Bauer M, Weis S, Netea M, Wetzker R. Remembering pathogen dose: long-term adaptation in innate immunity. Trends Immunol. 2018;39:438–45.

55. Burl S, Townend J, Njie-Jobe J, Cox M, Adetifa UJ, Touray E, et al. Age-dependent maturation of toll-like receptor-mediated cytokine responses in Gambian infants. PLoS One. 2011;6:e18185.

56. Smolen KK, Ruck CE, Fortuno ES, Ho K, Dimitriu P, Mohn WW, et al. Pattern recognition receptor-mediated cytokine response in infants across 4 continents. J Allergy Clin Immunol. 2014;133:818–26.

57. Levy O, Suter EE, Miller RL, Wessels MR. Unique efficacy of toll-like receptor 8 agonists in activating human neonatal antigen-presenting cells. Blood. 2006;108:1284–90.

58. Levy O, Zarember KA, Roy RM, Cywes C, Godowski PJ, Wessels MR. Selective impairment of TLR-mediated innate immunity in human newborns: neonatal blood plasma reduces monocyte TNF-alpha induction by bacterial lipopeptides, lipopolysaccharide, and imiquimod, but preserves the response to R-848. J Immunol. 2004;173:4627–34.

59. Frosch AEP, John CC. Immunomodulation in *Plasmodium falciparum* malaria: experiments in nature and their conflicting implications for potential therapeutic agents. Expert Rev Anti-Infect Ther. 2012;10:1343–56.

60. Dobbs KR, Embury P, Vulule J, Odada PS, Rosa BA, Mitreva M, et al. Monocyte dysregulation and systemic inflammation during pediatric falciparum malaria. JCI Insight. 2017;2:e95352.

61. Brickley EB, Wood AM, Kabyemela E, Morrison R, Kurtis JD, Fried M, et al. Fetal origins of malarial disease: cord blood cytokines as risk markers for pediatric severe malarial anemia. J Infect Dis. 2015;211:436–44.

62. Stevenson MM, Tam MF, Wolf SF, Sher A. IL-12-induced protection against blood-stage Plasmodium chabaudi AS requires IFN-gamma and TNF-alpha and occurs via a nitric oxide-dependent mechanism. J Immunol. 1995;155:2545–56.

63. Yoshimoto T, Yoneto T, Waki S, Nariuchi H. Interleukin-12-dependent mechanisms in the clearance of blood-stage murine malaria parasite *Plasmodium berghei* XAT, an attenuated variant of *P. berghei* NK65. J Infect Dis. 1998;177:1674–81.

64. Boutlis CS, Lagog M, Chaisavaneeyakorn S, Misukonis MA, Bockarie MJ, Mgone CS, et al. Plasma interleukin-12 in malaria-tolerant Papua New Guineans: inverse correlation with *Plasmodium falciparum* Parasitemia and peripheral blood mononuclear cell nitric oxide synthase activity. Infect Immun. 2003;71:6354–7.

65. Sarangi A, Mohapatra PC, Dalai RK, Sarangi AK. Serum IL-4, IL-12 and TNF-alpha in malaria: a comparative study associating cytokine responses with severity of disease from the coastal districts of Odisha. J Parasit Dis. 2014;38:143–7.

66. Luty AJF, Perkins DJ, Lell B, Schmidt-Ott R, Lehman LG, Luckner D, et al. Low interleukin-12 activity in severe *Plasmodium falciparum* malaria. Infect Immun. 2000;68:3909–15.

67. Berg A, Patel S, Gonca M, David C, Otterdal K, Ueland T, et al. Cytokine network in adults with falciparum malaria and HIV-1: increased IL-8 and IP-10 levels are associated with disease severity. PLoS One. 2014;9:e114480.

68. Armah HB, Wilson NO, Sarfo BY, Powell MD, Bond VC, Anderson W, et al. Cerebrospinal fluid and serum biomarkers of cerebral malaria mortality in Ghanaian children. Malar J. 2007;6:147.

69. Jain V, Armah HB, Tongren JE, Ned RM, Wilson NO, Crawford S, et al. Plasma IP-10, apoptotic and angiogenic factors associated with fatal cerebral malaria in India. Malar J. 2008;7:83.

70. Liu M, Guo S, Hibbert JM, Jain V, Singh N, Wilson NO, et al. CXCL10/IP-10 in infectious diseases pathogenesis and potential therapeutic implications. Cytokines Growth Factors Rev. 2011;22:121–30.

71. Hunt NH, Grau GE. Cytokines: accelerators and brakes in the pathogenesis of cerebral malaria. Trends Immunol. 2003;24:491–9.

72. Prakash D, Fesel C, Jain R, Cazenave P-A, Mishra GC, Pied S. Clusters of cytokines determine malaria severity in *Plasmodium falciparum*-infected patients from endemic areas of Central India. J Infect Dis. 2006;194:198–207.

73. Riopel J, Tam M, Mohan K, Marino MW, Stevenson MM. Granulocyte-macrophage colony-stimulating factor-deficient mice have impaired resistance to blood-stage malaria. Infect Immun. 2001;69:129–36.

74. Weiss WR, Ishii KJ, Hedstrom RC, Sedegah M, Ichino M, Barnhart K, et al. A plasmid encoding murine granulocyte-macrophage colony-stimulating factor increases protection conferred by a malaria DNA vaccine. J Immunol. 1998;161:2325–32.

75. Moncunill G, Mpina M, Nhabomba AJ, Aguilar R, Ayestaran A, Sanz H, et al. Distinct helper T cell Type1 and 2 responses associated with malaria protection and risk in RTS,S/AS01E vaccinees. Clin Infect Dis. 2017;65:746–55.

76. Ringwald P, Peyron F, Vuillez JP, Touze JE, Le Bras J, Deloron P. Levels of cytokines in plasma during *Plasmodium falciparum* malaria attacks. J Clin Microbiol. 1991;29:2076–8.

77. Clark IA, Budd AC, Alleva LM, Cowden WB. Human malarial disease: a consequence of inflammatory cytokine release. Malar J. 2006;5:85.

78. Lyke KE, Burges R, Cissoko Y, Sangare L, Dao M, Diarra I, et al. Serum levels of the proinflammatory IL-8, IL-10, tumor necrosis factor alpha, and IL-12 (p70) in Malian children with severe *Plasmodium falciparum* malaria and matched uncomplicated malaria or healthy controls. Infect Immun. 2004;72:5630–7.

79. Mbengue B, Niang B, Niang MS, Varela ML, Fall B, Fall MM, et al. Inflammatory cytokine and humoral responses to *Plasmodium falciparum* glycosylphosphatidylinositols correlates with malaria immunity and pathogenesis. Immunity Inflamm Dis. 2016;4:24–34.

18

The arrhythmogenic cardiotoxicity of the quinoline and structurally related antimalarial drugs

Ilsa L. Haeusler[1,2†] [iD], Xin Hui S. Chan[2,3,4†], Philippe J. Guérin[1,2] and Nicholas J. White[2,3,4*]

Abstract

Background: Several quinoline and structurally related antimalarial drugs are associated with cardiovascular side effects, particularly hypotension and electrocardiographic QT interval prolongation. A prolonged QT interval is a sensitive but not specific risk marker for the development of Torsade de Pointes—a potentially lethal polymorphic ventricular tachyarrhythmia. The increasing use of quinoline and structurally related antimalarials in mass treatments to eliminate malaria rapidly highlights the need to review their cardiovascular safety profiles.

Methods: The primary objective of this systematic review was to describe the documented clinical and electrocardiographic cardiovascular side effects of quinine, mefloquine, lumefantrine, piperaquine, halofantrine, chloroquine, sulfadoxine-pyrimethamine, amodiaquine, and primaquine. Trials in healthy subjects or patients with *Plasmodium falciparum* or *P. vivax* infection were included if at least two ECGs were conducted during the trial. All trial designs were included except case reports and pooled analyses. Secondary outcomes were the methods adopted by trials for measuring and reporting the QT interval.

Results: Data from trials published between 1982 and July 2016 were included. A total of 177 trials met the inclusion criteria. 35,448 participants received quinoline antimalarials in these trials, of which 18,436 participants underwent ECG evaluation. Subjects with co-medication use or comorbidities including cardiovascular disease were excluded from the majority of trials. Dihydroartemisinin-piperaquine was the drug most studied (5083 participants). Despite enormous use over the past 60 years, only 1076, 452, and 150 patients had ECG recordings reported in studies of chloroquine, amodiaquine, and primaquine respectively. Transiently high concentrations of quinine, quinidine, and chloroquine following parenteral administration have all been associated with hypotension, but there were no documented reports of death or syncope attributable to a cardiovascular cause, nor of electrocardiographic recordings of ventricular arrhythmia in these trials. The large volume of missing outcome information and the heterogeneity of ECG interval reporting and measurement methodology did not allow pooled quantitative analysis of QT interval changes.

Conclusions: No serious cardiac adverse effects were recorded in malaria clinical trials of 35,548 participants who received quinoline and structurally related antimalarials with close follow-up including 18,436 individuals who underwent ECG evaluation. While these findings provide further evidence of the rarity of serious cardiovascular events after treatment with these drugs, they also underscore the need for continued strengthening of pharmacovigilance systems for robust detection of rare drug adverse events in real-world populations. A standardised approach to measurement and reporting of ECG data in malaria trials is also needed.

(Continued on next page)

---

* Correspondence: nickw@tropmedres.ac

†Ilsa L. Haeusler and Xin Hui S. Chan contributed equally to this work.

[2]Centre for Tropical Medicine and Global Health, Nuffield Department of Medicine, University of Oxford, Oxford, UK

[3]Mahidol-Oxford Tropical Medicine Research Unit (MORU), Faculty of Tropical Medicine, Mahidol University, Bangkok, Thailand

Full list of author information is available at the end of the article

(Continued from previous page)

Trial registration: PROSPERO CRD42016036678

Keywords: Systematic review, Malaria, Antimalarials, Quinolines, Piperaquine, Electrocardiogram, QT, Arrhythmia, Torsade de pointes, Mass drug administration

Background

Quinoline antimalarials and structurally related compounds have long been known to cause cardiovascular side effects. Many of these antimalarial drugs cause hypotension, partly through alpha blockade, and they affect both depolarisation and repolarisation of cardiac and skeletal muscle [1]. The dangers of rapid intravenous injection of quinine, the marked prolongation of the electrocardiographic (ECG) QT interval caused by quinidine, and the lethality of chloroquine in overdose have each caused considerable concern over their use in the treatment of malaria. The discovery in 1993, after its registration, that halofantrine was associated with marked QT prolongation and sudden death augmented these concerns [2]. More recently, there has been uncertainty over the potential risks associated with the QT prolongation following use of piperaquine and the fixed-dose combination dihydroartemisinin-piperaquine (DP), the latest addition to the artemisinin-based combination therapies (ACTs) recommended for treatment of malaria by the World Health Organization (WHO) [3]. While the European Medicines Agency has approved DP, it called for more data to substantiate the cardiac safety of DP and its effect on the QT interval, particularly in children [4]. Consideration of this well-tolerated antimalarial drug for use in intermittent preventative therapy (IPT) and in mass drug administration (MDA) as part of malaria control interventions underlines the urgent need to clarify the cardiovascular safety profile of DP and structurally related antimalarials [5].

Characterising the electrophysiological effects of a drug, particularly during the treatment of acute illness, is not straightforward. It is not a problem unique to antimalarials and is a major consideration during drug development. A prolonged QT interval, reflecting a delay in ventricular repolarisation, is a sensitive but not specific risk marker for ventricular tachyarrhythmia development, notably Torsade de Pointes (TdP) [6]. This rhythm if sustained can degenerate into ventricular fibrillation and result in sudden cardiac death. The relationship between QT prolongation and the risk of developing ventricular tachyarrhythmias is incompletely understood, although many factors are known to contribute. These include the presence of underlying genetically determined QT prolongation, electrolyte abnormalities, structural heart disease, female gender, and co-administration with other drugs which also prolong the QT interval or increase drug levels [6]. Without detailed investigation, it is therefore difficult to assess an individual's risk of a drug precipitating life-threatening ventricular tachyarrhythmias.

Acute malaria illness itself has significant effects on the QT interval [1]. Prior to treatment, patients are usually febrile, anxious, tachycardic, and often anorexic and nauseated. The sympathetic nervous system is activated, and the QT interval shortens. As the patient recovers, often supine in bed, the fever settles, appetite returns, and the heart rate declines. The QT interval lengthens. The difference between the pre-treatment shortened interval and the third day normalised value (which often coincides with peak antimalarial drug concentrations) is often misattributed to a drug effect [1]. If there is a drug effect, then it may be compounded by this systemic physiological response to recovery.

The only previous systematic review on antimalarial cardiotoxicity analysed case reports of deaths secondary to possible halofantrine-related cardiotoxicity [7]. To clarify the cardiovascular safety profile of DP and structurally related antimalarials, we assessed, by systematic review of published clinical trials, the frequency of reported clinical and electrocardiographic cardiac adverse effects after use of quinoline and structurally related antimalarials for malaria-related indications, with a focus on QT interval prolongation.

Methods
Eligibility criteria

The nine antimalarial drugs included in this review were quinine, mefloquine, lumefantrine, piperaquine, halofantrine, chloroquine, sulfadoxine-pyrimethamine (SP), amodiaquine, and primaquine. SP, a non-quinoline containing combination antimalarial, was included in the review as a negative control as it has negligible effects on the QT interval. Trials which administered these drugs as antimalarials to patients with *Plasmodium falciparum* or *P. vivax* mono- or mixed infections or to healthy participants, and in which at least two systematic electrocardiograms (ECGs) were performed, were eligible for inclusion. All trial designs except case reports and pooled analyses were included. Conference abstracts were excluded. All ages and populations, including children and pregnant women, were included. There was no restriction of date of publication or language of article. This review conformed to the PRISMA statement and has been registered in the PROSPERO database (CRD42016036678).

Search strategy and study selection

Articles were identified between October 2015 and July 2016 through electronic searches of the MEDLINE, Embase, and Global Health databases (Additional file 1) and by using reference lists of relevant articles. Records were deduplicated using Mendeley (Mendeley Ltd., Version 1.17.8). Abstracts were reviewed to assess eligibility; the full article was obtained for assessment if there was doubt as to the relevance of an article. Unpublished literature was not included, and abstracts were excluded if the full-text article could not be obtained.

Data extraction and review outcomes

Data were extracted into a structured database. Variables included study year and location, trial design, population demographics, drug(s) assessed, ECG measurement methodology and timepoints, drug measurement and pharmacokinetic analysis methodology, and clinical and electrocardiographic cardiovascular adverse events (Additional file 2). Patient series were compared with those of other included articles to minimise data duplication. Primary outcomes were the number and character of clinical cardiovascular adverse events (palpitations, syncope, or sudden cardiac death) and ECG-documented arrhythmias (including ventricular tachycardia, ventricular fibrillation, and TdP). Additional primary outcomes included the mean QT interval corrected with Bazett's formula at baseline, 4 and 24 h, and 7 days after drug administration and the proportion of patients who developed a prolonged QT interval during the trials. Secondary outcomes were the features of ECG methodology and QT interval analysis adopted (Additional file 3).

Risk of bias

A standard set of criteria were used to assess bias in each study (Additional file 4). This included assessment of blinding of participants, study personnel, and ECG readers; selective outcome reporting and completeness of outcome data; and method of electrocardiographic interval measurement. The proportion of studies with a low, unclear, or high risk of bias for each criterion was calculated per drug.

Results

In total, 177 articles (Fig. 1, Additional file 5) enrolling a total of 39,960 participants were included in the review. Of these participants, 35,448 received at least one of the drugs relevant to this review and 18,436 underwent ECG evaluation (Table 1).

Quinine, mefloquine, and lumefantrine were the most intensively studied drugs by number of published studies

(51, 45, and 39 studies respectively), whereas piperaquine and lumefantrine had the largest number of participants undergoing ECG investigation (5083 and 4787 participants respectively). Despite vast use of chloroquine over the last six decades (hundreds of tonnes consumed annually), only 1076 participants in 17 studies of chloroquine underwent ECG investigation. Amodiaquine and primaquine have been the least intensively investigated (10 and 7 studies respectively) with 452 and 150 participants respectively undergoing ECG investigation. Fifty-nine studies included children, most of which were trials of quinine, mefloquine, or lumefantrine. Seven trials enrolled pregnant women (1232 participants).

Study characteristics

Overall, articles were published between 1982 and 2016 (Table 2).

Most quinine, mefloquine, piperaquine, chloroquine, and primaquine trials were conducted in Thailand, and the majority of halofantrine trials were reported from France. Although African countries are underrepresented (Additional file 6), the majority of lumefantrine and amodiaquine trials were conducted in countries throughout sub-Saharan Africa.

Sixty-eight of the 177 trials (38%) were open-label randomised control trials, 41/177 (23%) were non-comparative trials, and 26/177 (15%) were double-blind randomised control studies. Only 29/177 trials (16%) specified that their primary aim was to investigate cardiovascular safety, and 15/177 trials (8%) were designed to investigate pharmacokinetic-pharmacodynamic relationships. For halofantrine, 9/22 trials (41%) had investigation of cardiovascular safety as the primary aim, with only 3/24 (13%) for piperaquine.

The total number of participants included in each trial ranged from 7 to 10,925. Lumefantrine trials had the largest median number of participants per trial ($n = 165$) followed by piperaquine ($n = 130$), and the fewest participants were in primaquine trials ($n = 16$).

Patient characteristics

Trial populations were young with mean ages in the 20s (range 19.9 [halofantrine] to 33 years [primaquine]), although there was a large proportion of missing data (Table 3). The numbers of male and female participants were not reported in 27/177 (15%) of trials. In the other trials, there were a total of 14,921 males and 8502 females.

Malaria patients

Seventy-two percent (127/177) of trials included participants with *P. falciparum* mono- or mixed infection. Sixteen trials included patients with *P. vivax* infection

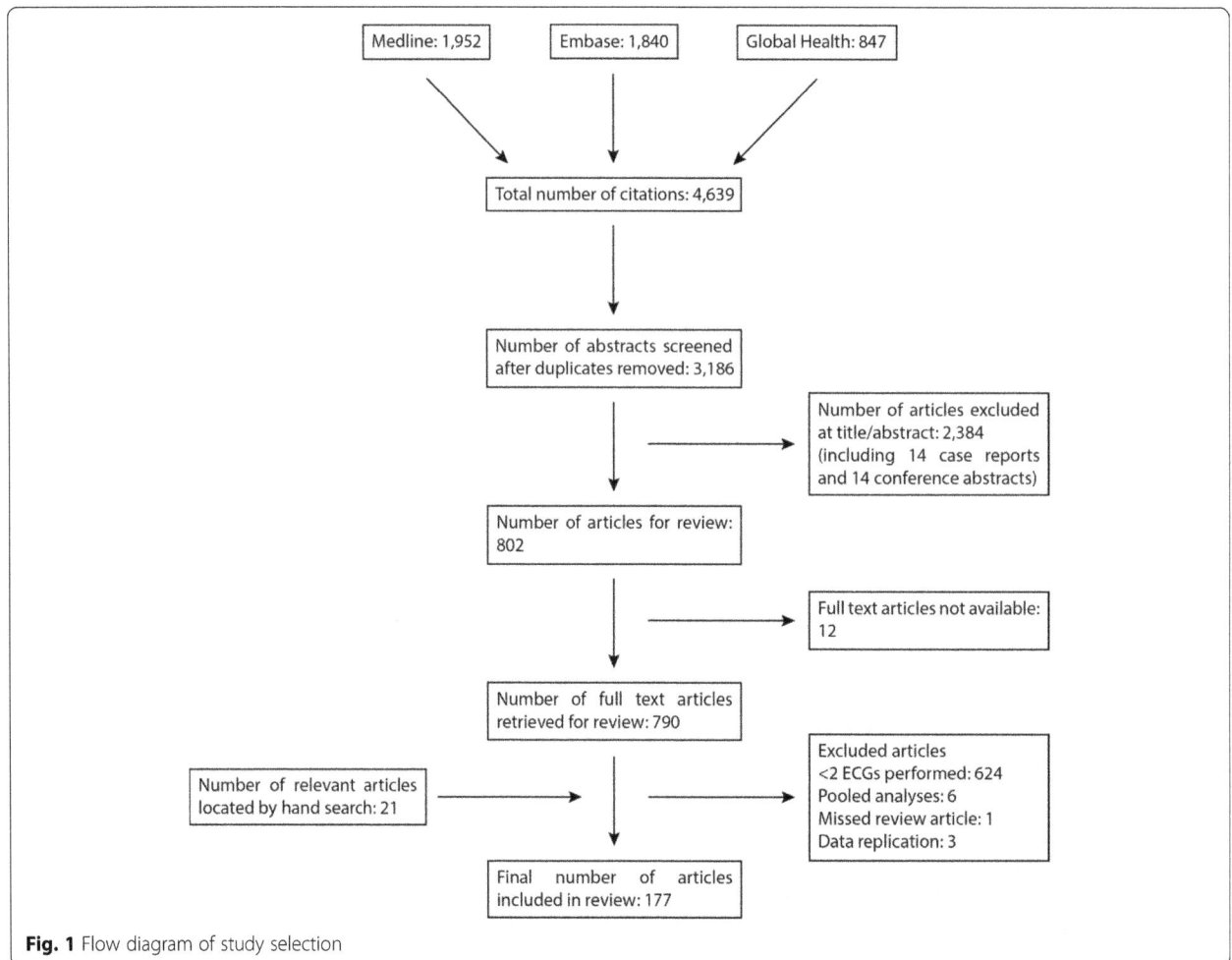

Fig. 1 Flow diagram of study selection

Table 1 Total number of studies and participants per antimalarial drug, with number of studies including children and pregnant women

Drug	Total number of studies	Total number of participants who had drug	Total number of participants who had ECGs	Total number of studies which included children	Total number of studies which included pregnant women	Total number of studies which included pharmacokinetic analysis
Quinine	51	2611	2320	18	1	19
Mefloquine	45	7874	3099	13	2	19
Lumefantrine	39	5703	4787	19	3	19
Piperaquine	24	15,224	5083	7	1	12
Halofantrine	22	822	774	7	0	10
Chloroquine	17	1207	1076	6	0	10
Sulfadoxine-pyrimethamine	14	1288	695	4	2	5
Amodiaquine	10	569	452	2	1	8
Primaquine	7	150	150	0	0	4

Forty-nine studies evaluated more than one of the drugs included in this review. These articles have been included under each of the appropriate drugs for analysis

Table 2 Summary of study characteristics for each antimalarial drug

	Quinine (51 studies)	Mefloquine (45 studies)	Lumefantrine (39 studies)	Piperaquine (24 studies)	Halofantrine (22 studies)	Chloroquine (17 studies)	SP (14 studies)	Amodiaquine (10 studies)	Primaquine (7 studies)
Range of dates studies were published	1982–2014	1983–2012	1997–2014	2003–2016	1993–2004	1983–2014	1983–2015	1987–2014	1992–2015
Countries where studies were most frequently conducted in (% of studies)	Thailand (43%) Vietnam (8%) Myanmar (8%)	Thailand (54%) Brazil (11%)	Thailand (23%) Kenya (13%)	Thailand (25%) Cambodia (17%)	France (32%) Nigeria (18%)	Thailand (41%) India (24%)	Brazil (36%) Thailand (21%)	No majority (each trial in different country)	Thailand (71%)
Median (range) number of participants	59 (7–561)	94 (8–3673)	165 (12–1553)	130 (12–10,925)	38.5 (8–120)	58 (11–456)	99 (20–3673)	32 (10–336)	16 (8–329)
% (number) of studies OLRCT	43 (22)	56 (25)	36 (14)	54 (13)	18 (4)	18 (3)	50 (7)	40 (4)	14 (1)
% (number) of studies DBRCT	6 (3)	24 (11)	18 (7)	8 (2)	9 (2)	35 (6)	36 (5)	0 (0)	14 (1)
% (number) of studies OLRCTX	0 (0)	2 (1)	10 (4)	8 (2)	14 (3)	6 (1)	0 (0)	40 (4)	57 (4)
% (number) of studies non-comparative	29 (15)	9 (5)	21 (8)	13 (3)	45 (10)	6 (1)	0 (0)	10 (1)	14 (1)
% (number) of studies primary outcome CV safety	20 (10)	13 (6)	13 (5)	13 (3)	41 (9)	18 (3)	14 (2)	20 (2)	0 (0)
% (number) of trials PK or PK/PD primary aim	26 (13)	24 (11)	26 (10)	21 (5)	27 (6)	53 (9)	7 (1)	60 (6)	71 (5)
% (number) of papers PK/PD primary aim	6 (3)	9 (4)	10 (4)	4 (1)	13 (3)	18 (3)	0 (0)	10 (1)	0 (0)

SP sulfadoxine-pyrimethamine, *OLRCT* open-label randomised control trial, *DBRCT* double-blind randomised control trial, *OLRCTX* open-label randomised control crossover trial, *CV* cardiovascular, *PK* pharmacokinetic, *PD* pharmacodynamic

Table 3 Summary of patient characteristics for each antimalarial drug

	Quinine (51 studies)	Mefloquine (45 studies)	Lumefantrine (39 studies)	Piperaquine (24 studies)	Halofantrine (22 studies)	Chloroquine (17 studies)	SP (14 studies)	Amodiaquine (10 studies)	Primaquine (7 studies)
Median of mean age (years)	25.6	26	26	23.4	19.9	20.8	–	22.1	33
% missing data for mean age	55	80	64	38	41	71	93	60	57
Median of median age (years)	16.4	24	25	23	23.8	–	–	–	–
% missing data for median age	93	96	85	88	91	94	100	100	100
Age range (years)	0.3–90	0.4–88	0.2–75	6–65	0.25–84	1–74	12–62	0.8–65	16–74
Total number of males	2571	5137	5226	4522	684	1052	723	287	373
Total number of females	1141	1848	4233	2682	256	422	377	519	118
% (number) trials including healthy participants	14 (7)	22 (10)	28 (11)	29 (7)	18 (4)	35 (6)	14 (2)	40 (4)	71 (5)
% (number) trials including P. falciparum infection	88 (45)	78 (35)	72 (28)	71 (17)	77 (17)	41 (7)	86 (12)	60	14 (1)
% (number) trials including P. vivax infection	4 (2)	0 (0)	5 (2)	17 (4)	14 (3)	29 (5)	7 (1)	0 (0)	14 (1)
% (number) trials including uncomplicated malaria infection	45 (23)	69 (31)	72 (28)	71 (17)	77 (17)	35 (6)	71 (10)	60 (6)	29 (2)
% (number) trials including complicated or severe malaria infection	51 (26)	4 (2) (both studies also trialled quinine)	0 (0)	0 (0)	0 (0)	12 (2) (1 study just chloroquine, the other also trialled quinine)	0 (0)	0 (0)	0 (0)
% (number) trials excluding any medical comorbidities	31 (16)	58 (26)	62 (24)	71 (17)	68 (15)	65 (11)	57 (8)	90 (9)	86 (6)
% (number) trials specifically excluding cardiovascular comorbidities	12 (6)	16 (7)	49 (19)	38 (9)	46 (10)	41 (7)	14 (2)	60 (6)	57 (4)
% (number) trials excluding any co-medication use	65 (33)	53 (24)	62 (24)	42 (10)	54 (12)	71 (12)	57 (8)	100 (10)	86 (6)
% (number) trials excluding co-medication with antimalarials	57 (29)	44 (20)	39 (15)	13 (3)	36 (8)	24 (4)	50 (7)	80 (8)	43 (3)
% (number) trials excluding drugs which interfere with cardiovascular system	6 (3)	2 (1)	23 (9)	13 (3)	18 (4)	12 (2)	0 (0)	30 (3)	0 (0)

Unavailable data is indicated by '–'
SP sulfadoxine-pyrimethamine

specifically, and only 4 of these investigated participants with *P. vivax* mono-infections (3 trialled chloroquine and 1 trialled halofantrine) [8–11]. The majority of studies were of patients with uncomplicated malaria (106/177, 60%), and 15% were of severe or complicated malaria (27/177).

Healthy subjects
Forty-seven of the 177 trials (27%) included healthy participants. Such trials were generally pharmacokinetic studies or trials of intermittent preventative therapy.

Exclusion criteria
Overall, 34/177 studies (19%) did not detail any exclusion criteria. In 103/177 studies (58%), participants with at least one medical comorbidity were excluded. In the remainder of trials, it was not specifically mentioned if medical comorbidities were excluded. In 29% of trials (52/177), cardiovascular comorbidities were stated to have been excluded, with only three trials specifically detailing that cardiovascular comorbidities were not excluded. Similarly, in 63% (112/177), participants who had co-medications (most commonly other antimalarials and other drugs which interfere with the cardiovascular system) were excluded and only one trial did not exclude participants with co-medications. Seventy-nine of the 177 trials (45%) excluded participants with both comorbidities and co-medication use, and there were no trials which included both groups of participants.

Primary outcomes
There were no reports of death attributable to a cardiovascular cause in any trial included in this review. There were no electrocardiographic recordings of ventricular tachycardia, ventricular fibrillation, or TdP. Other ECG abnormalities were described, the most common of these being bradycardia and first-degree atrioventricular block (Additional file 7).

Bradycardia
Bradycardia was reported in 3.9% of 3099 participants after mefloquine [2, 12–16], 1.6% of 774 after halofantrine [2, 17], and 10.8% of 452 after amodiaquine [18, 19]. Although nausea and vomiting are common in malaria, particularly in children, and may be provoked by antimalarial drugs, the association with nausea was not reported.

Atrioventricular block
Halofantrine was associated with atrioventricular block: 25 episodes of first-degree block were reported of 774 participants who had ECGs (3.2%) [2, 17, 20], while two children had second-degree Mobitz type 1 (Wenkebach)

block after treatment for falciparum malaria [2, 21]. Following quinine, amodiaquine, and mefloquine (with SP), 2.5% (57/2320), 0.4% (2/452), and 0.2% (7/3099) respectively of participants with ECG recordings developed first-degree heart block [13, 15, 22–24].

Others
Other ECG abnormalities were described in patients undergoing treatment for cerebral malaria although investigators attributed these to severity of malaria illness rather than drug treatment [12, 25, 26]. A 20-year-old male developed Wolff-Parkinson-White syndrome following piperaquine which was not detected on baseline ECGs [27]. The significance of this apparent revelation of an accessory conduction pathway is uncertain.

QT assessment
Due to the heterogeneity of ECG methodology, analytical techniques and reporting, as well as the large volume of missing reported information, it was not possible to perform the planned analysis to quantitate the antimalarial drug effects on the QT interval. The mean maximal change from baseline (Bazett's corrected QT interval, QTcB) and the individual maximum QTcB or QTcF (Fridericia's corrected) values were the most frequently detailed outcomes but were insufficient to perform a quantitative analysis.

Analytical and reporting heterogeneity included using different measures of central tendency (mean or median), reporting the QT interval corrected for heart rate variation by different methods, reporting absolute values at different time points (as ECGs were performed at various time points across studies), or changes from a certain time (most often the baseline) either as an absolute value or a proportion. Many studies, despite performing ECGs as part of the trial, either did not report ECG findings or only stated that none were clinically relevant.

Secondary outcomes
Additional file 8 shows the summary of secondary outcomes for each drug.

Assessments of the temporal relationship of ECG changes to drug concentrations
In total, 87 studies included pharmacokinetic data. Quinine, mefloquine, and lumefantrine have undergone the most PK evaluations, each with 19 trials measuring drug concentrations. Overall, 74 of 177 trials (41%) specified food intake of participants around the time of drug dosing.

Apart from baseline ECGs taken before administration of the first dose of drug, the overwhelming majority of trials did not specify whether subsequent ECGs were taken before drug administration (likely to be trough level of drug) or following drug administration (higher drug levels, which could include peak drug levels). Only one trial of primaquine specified that all ECGs were taken in the morning to minimise the effects of diurnal variation of the QT interval [28].

QT interval measurement method
Overall, 118 of 177 trials (67%) did not specify the method of ECG reading (manual or automatic). Nineteen percent ($n = 34$) of trials reported manually reading ECGs, 3% ($n = 6$) used only automatic readings, and 11% ($n = 19$) used both. van Vugt and colleagues included both manual and automatic measurements and found automatically measured values were generally higher than manually measured values, and this difference was greater at larger QTc values [29]. A piperaquine trial was stopped prematurely on the basis of electronic measurements of the QTc because the machine measured the QU interval as the QT, despite correct manual readings on the same traces [30]. Some more recent trials used electronic rulers for manually reading the QT interval [30–32]. In total, there were five trials which sent their ECGs to a centralised ECG laboratory for assessment, each of which investigated piperaquine [32–36].

QT rate correction
The majority of trials did not specify which QT correction formula was used, although every trial reporting QT intervals reported corrected QT values. Fifteen trials used two or more correction formulae. Twenty-seven percent ($n = 48$) of trials used Bazett's formula alone. Bazett's and Fridericia's were both reported in 10% ($n = 12$) of trials. Five trials [18, 31, 37–39] used alternative formulae, including Wernicke et al.'s [40], Hodges' and Karen [41].

Criteria for QT prolongation
There were many definitions used (Additional file 9), specified in only 64 of 177 studies (36%). Definitions included absolute values with thresholds between 420 and 470 ms, with many trials using different values for men and women, such as > 430 ms (males) and > 450 ms (female). Other definitions included a proportional increase, commonly 25% increase from baseline, or an absolute increase, such as > 30 or > 60 ms from baseline. Most trials used the QT corrected using Bazett's formula for these definitions.

Risk of bias
Additional file 10 shows the assessment of methodological quality of individual studies, and Additional file 11 summarises the risk of bias for each criterion per drug. In the majority of trials, neither the participants nor the investigators (especially ECG readers) were blinded to treatment allocation. Most trials did not specify cardiovascular or ECG outcomes. Many studies were limited by incomplete reporting of ECG methodology.

Discussion
This systematic review assessed available published prospective trials to determine the incidence and severity of clinical and electrocardiographic cardiovascular adverse effects of antimalarial drugs. The primary focus was QT prolongation and related arrhythmic cardiotoxicity after use of the quinoline and structurally related antimalarials for malaria. There were no sudden deaths attributed to cardiac arrhythmias recorded in the > 35,000 individuals who received the quinoline and structurally related antimalarials in the 177 clinical trials included in this review. Among the > 18,000 subjects who underwent ECG evaluation, a variety of generally non-serious self-limiting cardiac rhythm abnormalities were described usually without contextual information, making interpretation of causation difficult. Balanced against the clear life-saving benefits of giving effective antimalarials promptly in malaria, with the exception of halofantrine, concerns over cardiotoxicity have not limited the current use of the quinoline and structurally related antimalarial drugs.

These findings provide further evidence of the rarity of serious cardiovascular events after treatment with the quinoline and structurally related antimalarials, although the precise estimation of risk is limited, because of this rarity, by the total size of the source data available despite an inclusive search strategy. In this review, the median number of participants per trial ranged from 16 to 165 among the nine antimalarials studied. Such individual study sample sizes are designed to evaluate drug efficacy and are too small, even when pooled, to characterise the risk of very rare (< 1/10,000) drug adverse events such as Torsade de Pointes [42, 43]. The representativeness of the clinical trial population of potential recipients of population-based drug administration, e.g. in terms of age, gender, ethnicity, and cardiovascular risk factors, is another potential limitation. Fifty-eight percent (103/177) and 63% (112/177) of included studies listed medical comorbidities and co-medications as exclusion criteria, while healthy volunteer studies, often of adult males from non-malaria endemic countries, comprised 27% (47/177) of the included studies.

The importance of robust detection and evaluation of extremely rare and serious adverse events such as sudden unexplained death in real-world populations and the implications of such findings for population-based drug administration strategies underscore the need for ongoing synthesis of all available clinical evidence.

Post-marketing pharmacovigilance approaches such as spontaneous individual case safety reporting are especially important in signal detection of very rare adverse events despite challenges in assessing causality [43]. For example, the two sentinel cases of sudden death and collapse with extreme QTc interval prolongation after halofantrine given for the treatment of clinical malaria were important in stimulating the accumulation of further evidence which confirmed the arrhythmogenic effects of the drug [2, 7]. The findings of this review should therefore be interpreted in the context of this wider evidence base and the intended treatment indication(s) for each antimalarial.

The quinoline antimalarials have antiarrhythmic effects, best illustrated by quinidine, the D-diastereomer of quinine. Quinidine has been used mainly as an antiarrhythmic and it can cause TdP. It produces substantially greater QT prolongation than quinine. Quinidine and quinine are now used mostly in the treatment of severe falciparum malaria which itself has a significant risk of mortality. The benefit of effective treatment of malaria where these are the only parenteral drugs available outweighs the potential risks of cardiotoxicity [3].

Chloroquine is the most widely used antimalarial drug in history. It has a terminal elimination half-life of one month and an annual consumption of hundreds of tonnes for over 50 years, so it may be the drug to which humans have been exposed to most [1]. Despite producing consistent QT prolongation, the only case reports of TdP and sudden death have been for its use for non-malaria indications such as systemic lupus erythematosus or rheumatoid arthritis, where high doses are used for much longer than in malaria treatment, or in overdose [44].

Halofantrine is the only antimalarial drug considered to have an unacceptable arrhythmogenic risk when used for malaria indications [44]. The earliest report of its cardiotoxicity provided evidence of both extreme QT prolongation, conduction delay, and clinical cardiovascular adverse effects [2]. A 2009 review of the published literature and the GlaxoSmithKline Global Safety Database found 35 cases of fatal cardiotoxicity after halofantrine use between 1988 and 2005 [7]. Of the 35 cases, 26 had one or more risk factors for cardiotoxicity, including underlying cardiovascular disease or other comorbidities, concomitant use of a drug which can cause QT prolongation, administration with food, and higher than recommended doses given. As for other drugs, females were at greater risk; 70% of the patients who died were female. In all five paediatric deaths, either there was a contraindication to halofantrine use, or a higher dose was given in error.

DP is the most recent ACT to be recommended by WHO as first-line treatment of malaria. Its registration coincided with increased regulatory scrutiny of drugs which prolong the QT interval (most of the older antimalarials were introduced before awareness of the arrhythmogenic risk associated with this effect). This review identified 24 trials of piperaquine with systematic ECG assessment, with 7 trials including children and one including pregnant women. Of the 8 trials which included healthy participants, 2 trials investigated DP for use as IPT, 5 were PK trials in healthy participants, and 1 was a PK trial in healthy participants and participants infected with *P. falciparum*. In these 24 studies, there were no reports of sudden death suggestive of a fatal arrhythmia nor of any other major cardiovascular adverse outcomes following piperaquine use. A systematic review and meta-analysis was recently published (after the period of this review) of nearly 200,000 DP-treated individuals, including over 150,000 individuals in unpublished studies of mass drug administration in which exclusion of TdP risk factors was not possible [45]. The review reported one case of sudden death following DP use in MDA of a previously healthy 16-year-old female in Mozambique who developed palpitations after her second dose of DP, then collapsed, and died on the way to hospital (no ECG or autopsy was performed). This case of sudden unexplained death was considered possibly drug-related by cardiology and pharmacology experts at the WHO Evidence Review Group on the Cardiotoxicity of Antimalarials (there are also non-drug-related and non-cardiogenic causes of sudden unexplained death) [44]. The subsequent meta-analysis found that the risk of sudden unexplained death within 30 days of taking DP was no higher than the baseline risk of sudden cardiac death over the same period [45]. In addition, despite millions of doses having been distributed, there have been no cases of TdP after DP reported to global pharmacovigilance databases [44].

Pyronaridine is structurally related to the quinoline antimalarials, and its effect on the QT interval has been investigated in clinical trials of antimalarial efficacy. Artesunate-pyronaridine is a highly effective antimalarial drug which has been studied in > 3500 individuals in both pre- and post-registration studies [9, 16, 28, 46–49]. The most extensive of these studies has recently been reported after the period of this review [46]. This included a total trial population of nearly 5000 people, of whom 1342 received artesunate-pyronaridine. Of the other trials, all but one included other antimalarials included in this review [48]. There have been no marked ECG changes and no cardiovascular adverse effects attributed to artesunate-pyronaridine reported in any of these trials.

The QT interval is the most frequently used clinical biomarker for assessing the potential for the development of ventricular tachyarrhythmias and thus risk of sudden cardiac death. However, it is a surrogate marker, which while sensitive, has limited specificity. Its interpretation is further compromised by the extensive heterogeneity of the methods used in its measurement and reporting. Also, many factors affect the QT interval. These include patient factors such as age, gender, genetic predisposition, and comorbidities such as myocardial ischaemia and electrolyte disturbances [6]. The time of day the recording is made (the effects of circadian rhythm), position of the patient, food intake (independent of the effect of food on drug pharmacokinetics), and drug-drug interactions (with drugs which prolong the QT or increase drug concentrations including traditional medicines) also affect the QT interval. These variables are very difficult to control, particularly in the context of clinical trials involving patients with acute malaria infection.

Acute malaria infection is associated with disease factors such as fever, sympathetic activation, and tachycardia which can affect the QT interval; they are therefore confounders. These effects of malaria (particularly recovery from malaria) and other covariates and their effect on the QT interval have not been characterised adequately. Studying healthy controls allows a pure assessment of drug effects but does not allow characterisation of a disease-drug interaction. Comparing pre-dose versus post-dose ECGs which are recorded at the same times as plasma concentration measurements reduces the effects of these confounders, but there are relatively few such data. More comprehensive reporting of food intake and time of ECG measurement relative to drug intake as well as characterisation of antimalarial drug absorption profiles would improve assessments in future studies, with peak rather than trough drug levels being of greater relevance in the evaluation of potential cardiovascular toxicity.

This work has highlighted important methodological issues which confounded a standardised assessment of the cardiovascular effects of the quinoline and structurally related antimalarial drugs. There is considerable variation in the recording and measurement of the QT interval in antimalarial drug trials. The QT interval is technically difficult to measure, even by experts, and the process of measurement introduces further confounding factors and systematic error [50]. There is also substantial variation in the interpretation and reporting of the QT interval in a clinical context.

Automated measurements are considered not as accurate or reliable compared with manual measurements [51]. Many machines have problems with identifying U waves which can be mistaken for the T wave: a recent trial assessing high-dose DP was stopped because of apparent QT prolongation when the machine read the QU interval as the QT interval [30]. T and U wave morphology can be difficult to identify even manually, and readings are subject to a high degree of inter-user variability [50]. For paper recordings, a slower speed of recording, at 25 mm/s rather than 50 mm/s, makes the interval more difficult to measure if manual readings are employed. Some recent studies have used computer-aided ECG interpretation by specialist personnel at centralised laboratories. Whilst some investigators take multiple QT interval measurements across different leads and calculate an average, there is no agreement over this method. There are also many definitions of the end of the T wave used by trials.

Another source of potential confusion is the heart rate correction. This is necessary because the QT interval has an inverse relationship with heart rate. Several correction formulae are used, but the choice of the best formula is the subject of ongoing debate. The most widely used are Bazett's and Fridericia's formulae. In a healthy population, Bazett's formula overestimates at higher heart rates (lengthens the QTc interval) and underestimates at lower heart rates (shortens the QTc interval). In healthy subjects, Fridericia's provides better, although still imperfect correction at heart rates < 60 and > 100 beats per minute [6]. Where possible, the QT correction formula used should be derived for the study population, but this requires a large study and sufficient variation in heart rates [52].

Interpretation of the QTc interval in a clinical context is difficult because different populations have different normal QTc ranges. There are broadly accepted 'normal' QTc values, but many different values of 'abnormally long' exist and are used, ranging from > 420 to ≥ 500 ms in this review. This reflects uncertainty over the relationship between degree of prolongation and risk of arrhythmia development although a QT/QTc interval of > 500 ms is generally accepted to be a threshold for clinical concern [53].

More specific alternatives to evaluation of QT/QTc prolongation for determination of drug TdP risk are being developed, including through the Comprehensive in vitro Proarrhythmia Assay (CiPA) initiative, a multi-stakeholder global effort among regulators, industry, and academia. CiPA proposes a mechanistic-based, four-component approach coupling in vitro assessment of drug effects on multiple ion currents with an in silico computational model of the human ventricular cardiomyocyte for predicting proarrhythmic risk. These assessments would be followed by confirmatory in vitro studies on human stem cell-derived cardiomyocytes and in vivo phase I ECG safety evaluation. A validation programme is ongoing, and if successful and adopted by regulators, a CiPA evaluation demonstrating low arrhythmogenic risk could potentially obviate the need for intensive ECG monitoring in clinical phase III trials of QT/QTc prolonging drugs.

Conclusions

Several of the quinoline and structurally related antimalarial drugs are associated with electrocardiographic QT prolongation, but the only drug clearly associated with harm when used for the treatment of malaria is halofantrine. There have been no reports of death or syncope attributable to a cardiovascular cause nor electrocardiographic traces recording ventricular arrhythmia captured during malaria clinical therapeutic trials of other quinoline or structurally related antimalarial drugs which included systematic ECG assessment. While these findings add to existing evidence from individual case report databases in supporting the rarity of these adverse events, they also underscore the need for continued strengthening of pharmacovigilance systems for robust detection of such rare drug adverse events in real-world populations. The variable definitions, procedures, and analytical methods employed precluded systematic analysis of the QT interval. Pooled analyses of individual patient clinical trial data including from IPT and MDA studies are important next steps to determine the effect of the quinoline antimalarials on the QT interval. A standardised approach to measurement and reporting of ECG data in malaria trials is also urgently needed.

Additional files

Additional file 1: Search strategies from Ovid MEDLINE, Embase, and Global Health. (DOCX 25 kb)

Additional file 2: Complete list of variables extracted from articles. (DOCX 15 kb)

Additional file 3: List of primary and secondary outcomes. (DOCX 14 kb)

Additional file 4: Criteria used for assessment of risk of bias of individual studies. (DOCX 17 kb)

Additional file 5: List of references included in the review. (DOCX 28 kb)

Additional file 6: Number of studies conducted in each region, for each drug. (DOCX 14 kb)

Additional file 7: Other cardiovascular events observed, organised by arrhythmia. (DOCX 17 kb)

Additional file 8: Summary of secondary outcomes, for each drug. (DOCX 17 kb)

Additional file 9: List of definitions of prolongation used per drug. (DOCX 18 kb)

Additional file 10: Assessment of risk of bias for individual studies. (DOCX 26 kb)

Additional file 11: Risk of bias for each criterion per drug. (PDF 621 kb)

Abbreviations

ACTs: Artemisinin combination therapies; DP: Dihydroartemisinin-piperaquine; ECG(s): Electrocardiogram(s); ICH: International Conference on Harmonisation of Technical Requirements for Registration of Pharmaceuticals for Human Use; MORU: Mahidol-Oxford Tropical Medicine Research Unit; PD: Pharmacodynamic; PK: Pharmacokinetic; PRISMA: Preferred Reporting Items for Systematic Reviews and Meta-analyses; QTc: Heart rate-corrected QT interval; QTcB: Bazett's formula-corrected QTc; QTcF: Fridericia's formula-corrected QTc; SP: Sulfadoxine-pyrimethamine; TdP: Torsade de Pointes; WHO: World Health Organization; WWARN: WorldWide Antimalarial Resistance Network

Acknowledgements

We would like to thank the team at the WorldWide Antimalarial Resistance Network (WWARN) for their help throughout this work as well as Dr. John Reynolds and Dr. Charles Woodrow for their advice. We would also like to thank Shona Kirtley (EQUATOR Network, Oxford) for her assistance with the literature search, as well as Dr. Yan Naung Win and Dr. Shu Kiat Chan for additional research support.
XHC is supported by the Wellcome Trust [106698/Z/14/Z], the Medical Research Council of the United Kingdom [MR/N013468/1], and the Jill and Herbert Hunt Travelling Scholarship of the University of Oxford. NJW is a Wellcome Trust Principal Research Fellow [107886/Z/15/Z].

Funding

The authors received no specific funding for this work.

Authors' contributions

ILH, PJG, and NJW conceived and designed the experiments. ILH performed the experiments. ILH and XHC analysed and interpreted the data. ILH, XHC, PJG, and NJW wrote the paper. All authors read and approved the final manuscript.

Competing interests

The authors declare that they have no competing interests.

Author details

[1]WorldWide Antimalarial Resistance Network (WWARN), Oxford, UK. [2]Centre for Tropical Medicine and Global Health, Nuffield Department of Medicine, University of Oxford, Oxford, UK. [3]Mahidol-Oxford Tropical Medicine Research Unit (MORU), Faculty of Tropical Medicine, Mahidol University, Bangkok, Thailand. [4]Oxford University Hospitals NHS Foundation Trust, Oxford, UK.

References

1. White NJ. Cardiotoxicity of antimalarial drugs. Lancet Infect Dis. 2007;7: 549–58.
2. Nosten F, ter Kuile FO, Luxemburger C, Woodrow C, Kyle DE, Chongsuphajaisiddhi T, et al. Cardiac effects of antimalarial treatment with halofantrine. Lancet. 1993;341:1054–6.
3. World Health Organization. Guidelines for the treatment of malaria. Third edition. 2015. http://apps.who.int/iris/bitstream/handle/10665/162441/9789241549127_eng.pdf;jsessionid=FF86896C56304582909FE8E5C71BB30A?sequence=1. Accessed 18 Oct 2018.
4. European Medicines Agency. Eurartesim - summary of product characteristics. 2011. http://www.ema.europa.eu/docs/en_GB/document_library/EPAR_-_Product_Information/human/001199/WC500118113.pdf. Accessed 18 Oct 2018.
5. Gutman J, Kovacs S, Dorsey G, Stergachis A, Ter Kuile FO. Safety, tolerability, and efficacy of repeated doses of dihydroartemisinin-piperaquine for prevention and treatment of malaria: a systematic review and meta-analysis. Lancet Infect Dis. 2016;17:2095–128.

6. Yap Y, Camm J. Drug induced QT prolongation and Torsades de Pointes. Heart. 2003;89:1363–72.

7. Bouchaud O, Imbert P, Touze JE, Dodoo ANO, Danis M, Legros F. Fatal cardiotoxicity related to halofantrine: a review based on a worldwide safety data base. Malar J. 2009;8:289.

8. Llanos-Cuentas A, Lacerda MV, Rueangweerayut R, Krudsood S, Gupta SK, Kochar SK, et al. Tafenoquine plus chloroquine for the treatment and relapse prevention of Plasmodium vivax malaria (DETECTIVE): a multicentre, double-blind, randomised, phase 2b dose-selection study. Lancet. 2014;383:1049–58.

9. Poravuth Y, Socheat D, Rueangweerayut R, Uthaisin C, Pyae Phyo A, Valecha N, et al. Pyronaridine-artesunate versus chloroquine in patients with acute Plasmodium vivax malaria: a randomized, double-blind, non-inferiority trial. PLoS One. 2011;6:e14501.

10. Na-Bangchang K, Limpaibul L, Thanavibul A, Tan-Ariya P, Karbwang J. The pharmacokinetics of chloroquine in healthy Thai subjects and patients with Plasmodium vivax malaria. Br J Clin Pharmacol. 1994;38:278–81.

11. Khan SJ, Munib S. Efficacy of halofantrine hydrochloride in vivax malaria. J Postgrad Med Inst. 2005;19:276–80.

12. Win K, Than M, Thwe Y. Comparison of combinations of parenteral artemisinin derivatives plus oral mefloquine with intravenous quinine plus oral tetracycline for treating cerebral malaria. Bull World Health Organ. 1992; 70:777–82.

13. Harinasuta T, Bunnag D, Vanijanond S, Charoenlarp P, Suntharasmai P, Chitamas S, et al. Mefloquine, sulfadoxine, and pyrimethamine in the treatment of symptomatic falciparum malaria: a double-blind trial for determining the most effective dose. Bull World Health Organ. 1987;65:363–7.

14. Karbwang J, Bangchang KN, Bunnag D, Harinasuta T. Pharmacokinetics and pharmacodynamics of mefloquine in Thai patients with acute falciparum malaria. Bull World Health Organ. 1991;69:207–12.

15. Bunnag D, Karbwang J, Viravan C, Chitamas S, Harinasuta T. Clinical trials of mefloquine with tetracycline. Southeast Asian J. trop. Med. Public Health 1992;23:377–382.

16. Tshefu AK, Gaye O, Kayentao K, Thompson R, Bhatt KM, Sesay SSS, et al. Efficacy and safety of a fixed-dose oral combination of pyronaridine-artesunate compared with artemether-lumefantrine in children and adults with uncomplicated Plasmodium falciparum malaria: a randomised non-inferiority trial. Lancet. 2010;375:1457–67.

17. Karbwang J, Na Bangchang K, Bunnag D, Harinasuta T, Laothavorn P. Cardiac effect of halofantrine. Lancet. 1993;342:501.

18. Adjei GO, Oduro-Boatey C, Rodrigues OP, Hoegberg LC, Alifrangis M, Kurtzhals JA, et al. Electrocardiographic study in Ghanaian children with uncomplicated malaria, treated with artesunate-amodiaquine or artemether-lumefantrine. Malar J. 2012;11:420.

19. Ngouesse B, Basco LK, Ringwald P, Keundjian A, Blackett KN. Cardiac effects of amodiaquine and sulfadoxine-pyrimethamine in malaria-infected African patients. Am J Trop Med Hyg. 2001;65:711–6.

20. Lavallée I, Marc E, Moulin F, Treluyer JM, Imbert P, Gendrel D. Cardiac rhythm disturbances and prolongation of the QTc interval with halofantrine. Arch Pédiatrie. 2001;8:795–800.

21. Sowunmi A, Falade CO, Oduola AM, Ogundahunsi OA, Fehintola FA, Gbotosho GO, et al. Cardiac effects of halofantrine in children suffering from acute uncomplicated falciparum malaria. Trans R Soc Trop Med Hyg. 1998; 92:446–8.

22. Miller RS, Wongsrichanalai C, Buathong N, McDaniel P, Walsh DS, Knirsch C, et al. Effective treatment of uncomplicated Plasmodium falciparum malaria with azithromycin-quinine combinations: a randomized, dose-ranging study. Am J Trop Med Hyg. 2006;74:401–6.

23. Sabchareon A, Chongsuphajaisiddhi T, Sinhasivanon V, Chanthavanich P, Attanath P. In vivo and in vitro responses to quinine and quinidine of Plasmodium falciparum. Bull World Health Organ. 1988;66:347–52.

24. Liu Y, Hu C, Liu G, Jia J, Yu C, Zhu J, et al. A replicate designed bioequivalence study to compare two fixed-dose combination products of artesunate and amodiaquine in healthy Chinese volunteers. Antimicrob Agents Chemother. 2014;58:6009–15.

25. Karunajeewa H, Lim C, Hung TY, Ilett KF, Denis MB, Socheat D, et al. Safety evaluation of fixed combination piperaquine plus dihydroartemisinin (Artekin) in Cambodian children and adults with malaria. Br J Clin Pharmacol. 2003;57:93–9.

26. Bethell DB, Phuong PT, Phuong CX, Nosten F, Waller D, Davis TM, et al. Electrocardiographic monitoring in severe falciparum malaria. Trans R Soc Trop Med Hyg. 1996;90:266–9.

27. Gargano N, Ubben D, Tommasini S, Bacchieri A, Corsi M, Bhattacharyya PC, et al. Therapeutic efficacy and safety of dihydroartemisinin-piperaquine versus artesunate-mefloquine in uncomplicated Plasmodium falciparum malaria in India. Malar J. 2012;11:233.

28. Jittamala P, Pukrittayakamee S, Ashley E, Nosten F, Hanboonkunupakarn B, Lee S, et al. Pharmacokinetic interactions between primaquine and pyronaridine-artesunate in healthy adult Thai subjects. Antimicrob Agents Chemother. 2015;59:505–13.

29. van Vugt M, Ezzet F, Nosten F, Gathmann I, Wilairatana P, Looareesuwan S, et al. No evidence of cardiotoxicity during antimalarial treatment with artemether-lumefantrine. Am J Trop Med Hyg. 1999;61: 964–7.

30. Manning J, Vanachayangkul P, Lon C, Spring M, So M, Sea D, et al. Randomized, double-blind, placebo-controlled clinical trial of a two-day regimen of dihydroartemisinin-piperaquine for malaria prevention halted for concern over prolonged corrected QT interval. Antimicrob Agents Chemother. 2014;58:6056–67.

31. Roggelin L, Pelletier D, Hill JN, Feldt T, Hoffmann S, Ansong D, et al. Disease-associated QT-shortage versus quinine associated QT-prolongation: Age dependent ECG-effects in Ghanaian children with severe malaria. Malar J. 2014;13:219.

32. Baiden R, Oduro A, Halidou T, Gyapong M, Sie A, Macete E, et al. Prospective observational study to evaluate the clinical safety of the fixed-dose artemisinin-based combination Eurartesim (dihydroartemisinin/piperaquine), in public health facilities in Burkina Faso, Mozambique, Ghana, and Tanzania. Malar J. 2015;14:160.

33. Bassat Q, Mulenga M, Tinto H, Piola P, Borrmann S, Menendez C, et al. Dihydroartemisinin-piperaquine and artemether-lumefantrine for treating uncomplicated malaria in African children: a randomised, non-inferiority trial. PLoS One. 2009;4(11):e7871.

34. Valecha N, Phyo AP, Mayxay M, Newton PM, Krudsood S, Keomany S, et al. An open-label, randomised study of dihydroartemisinin-piperaquine versus artesunate-mefloquine for falciparum malaria in Asia. PLoS One. 2010;5(7): e11880.

35. Mayxay M, Keomany S, Khanthavong M, Souvannasing P, Stepniewska K, Khomthilath T, et al. A phase III, randomized, non-inferiority trial to assess the efficacy and safety of dihydroartemisinin-piperaquine in comparison with artesunate- mefloquine in patients with uncomplicated Plasmodium falciparum malaria in southern Laos. Am J Trop Med Hyg. 2010;83:1221–9.

36. Darpo B, Ferber G, Siegl P, Laurijssens B, Macintyre F, Toovey S, et al. Evaluation of the QT effect of a combination of piperaquine and a novel anti-malarial drug candidate OZ439, for the treatment of uncomplicated malaria. Br J Clin Pharmacol. 2015;80:706–15.

37. Krudsood S, Looareesuwan S, Wilairatama P, Leowattana W, Tangpukdee N, Chalermrut K, et al. Effect of artesunate and mefloquine in combination on the Fridericia corrected QT intervals in Plasmodium falciparum infected adults from Thailand. Trop Med Int Heal. 2011;16:458–65.

38. Mytton OT, Ashley EA, Peto L, Price RN, La Y, Hae R, et al. Short report: electrocardiographic safety evaluation of dihydroartemisinin piperaquine in the treatment of uncomplicated falciparum malaria. Am J Trop Med Hyg. 2007;77:447–50.

39. Ogutu B, Juma E, Obonyo C, Jullien V, Carn G, Vaillant M, et al. Fixed dose artesunate amodiaquine - a phase IIb, randomized comparative trial with non-fixed artesunate amodiaquine. Malar J. 2014;13:498.

40. Wernicke JF, Faries D, Breitung R, Girod D. QT correction methods in children and adolescents. J Cardiovasc Electrophysiol. 2005;16:76–81.

41. Price RN, Nosten F, White NJ. Letters to the editor. Am J Trop Med Hyg. 1998;59:504.

42. World Health Organisation. Definitions by WHO. 2003. http://www.who.int/medicines/areas/quality_safety/safety_efficacy/trainingcourses/definitions.pdf. Accessed 18 Oct 2018.

43. Evidence synthesis and meta-analysis: report of CIOMS Working Group X. Council for International Organizations of Medical (CIOMS). 2016.

44. WHO Evidence Review Group. The cardiotoxicity of antimalarials. 2017. http://www.who.int/malaria/mpac/mpac-mar2017-erg-cardiotoxicity-report-session2.pdf. Accessed 18 Oct 2018.

45. Chan XHS, Win YN, Mawer LJ, Tan JY, Brugada J, White NJ. Risk of sudden unexplained death after use of dihydroartemisinin – piperaquine for malaria: a systematic review and Bayesian meta-analysis. Lancet Infect Dis World Health Organization. 2018;3099:1–11.

46. Sagara I, Beavogui AH, Zongo I, Soulama I, Borghini-Fuhrer I, Fofana B, et al. Pyronaridine–artesunate or dihydroartemisinin–piperaquine versus current first-line therapies for repeated treatment of uncomplicated malaria: a randomised, multicentre, open-label, longitudinal, controlled, phase 3b/4 trial. Lancet. 2018;391:1378–90.
47. Rueangweerayut R, Phyo AP, Uthaisin C, Poravuth Y, Binh TQ, H. T, et al. Pyronaridine-artesunate versus mefloquine plus artesunate for malaria. N Engl J Med 2012;366:1298–1309.
48. Morris CA, Lopez-Lazaro L, Jung D, Methaneethorn J, Duparc S, Borghini-Fuhrer I, et al. Drug-drug interaction analysis of pyronaridine/artesunate and ritonavir in healthy volunteers. Am J Trop Med Hyg United States. 2012;86: 489–95.
49. Kayentao K, Doumbnao OM, Kimani J, Tshefu AK, Kokolomami JHT, Ramharter M, et al. Pyronaridine-artesunate granules versus artemether-lumefantrine crushed tablets in children with *Plasmodium falciparum* malaria: a randomigobara K Pénali, Louis K Offianan, André T Bhatt, Kirazed controlled trial. Malar J. 2012;11:364.
50. Viskin S, Rosovski U, Sands AJ, Chen E, Kistler PM, Kalman JM, et al. Inaccurate electrocardiographic interpretation of long QT: the majority of physicians cannot recognize a long QT when they see one. Hear. Rhythm. 2005;2:569–74.
51. Isbister GK. How do we assess whether the QT interval is abnormal: myths, formulae and fixed opinion. Clin Toxicol. 2015;53:189–91.
52. Malik M, Färbom P, Batchvarov V, Hnatkova K, Camm AJ. Relation between QT and RR intervals is highly individual among healthy subjects: implications for heart rate correction of the QT interval. Heart. 2002;87:220–8.
53. International Conference on Harmonisation of Technical Requirements for Registration of Pharmaceuticals for Human Use (ICH). ICH Topic E 14 The Clinical Evaluation of QT / QTc Interval Prolongation and Proarrhythmic Potential for Non-Antiarrhythmic Drugs (CHMP/ICH/2/04). 2005. http://www.ema.europa.eu/docs/en_GB/document_library/Scientific_guideline/2009/09/WC500002879.pdf. Accessed 18 Oct 2018.

Permissions

All chapters in this book were first published in MEDICINE, by BioMed Central; hereby published with permission under the Creative Commons Attribution License or equivalent. Every chapter published in this book has been scrutinized by our experts. Their significance has been extensively debated. The topics covered herein carry significant findings which will fuel the growth of the discipline. They may even be implemented as practical applications or may be referred to as a beginning point for another development.

The contributors of this book come from diverse backgrounds, making this book a truly international effort. This book will bring forth new frontiers with its revolutionizing research information and detailed analysis of the nascent developments around the world.

We would like to thank all the contributing authors for lending their expertise to make the book truly unique. They have played a crucial role in the development of this book. Without their invaluable contributions this book wouldn't have been possible. They have made vital efforts to compile up to date information on the varied aspects of this subject to make this book a valuable addition to the collection of many professionals and students.

This book was conceptualized with the vision of imparting up-to-date information and advanced data in this field. To ensure the same, a matchless editorial board was set up. Every individual on the board went through rigorous rounds of assessment to prove their worth. After which they invested a large part of their time researching and compiling the most relevant data for our readers.

The editorial board has been involved in producing this book since its inception. They have spent rigorous hours researching and exploring the diverse topics which have resulted in the successful publishing of this book. They have passed on their knowledge of decades through this book. To expedite this challenging task, the publisher supported the team at every step. A small team of assistant editors was also appointed to further simplify the editing procedure and attain best results for the readers.

Apart from the editorial board, the designing team has also invested a significant amount of their time in understanding the subject and creating the most relevant covers. They scrutinized every image to scout for the most suitable representation of the subject and create an appropriate cover for the book.

The publishing team has been an ardent support to the editorial, designing and production team. Their endless efforts to recruit the best for this project, has resulted in the accomplishment of this book. They are a veteran in the field of academics and their pool of knowledge is as vast as their experience in printing. Their expertise and guidance has proved useful at every step. Their uncompromising quality standards have made this book an exceptional effort. Their encouragement from time to time has been an inspiration for everyone.

The publisher and the editorial board hope that this book will prove to be a valuable piece of knowledge for researchers, students, practitioners and scholars across the globe.

List of Contributors

Ross A. Chesham, Emma L. Sweeney, Gemma C. Ryde, Trish Gorely, Naomi E. Brooks and Colin N. Moran
Faculty of Health Sciences and Sport, University of Stirling, Scotland FK9 4LA, UK

Josephine N. Booth
Institute of Education, Community and Society, Moray House School of Education, University of Edinburgh, Scotland EH8 8AQ, UK

Trish Gorely
Present address: School of Health, Social Care and Life Sciences, University of the Highlands and Islands, Centre for Health Sciences, Old Perth Road, Inverness IV2 3JH, UK

Zobair M. Younossi, Azza Karrar, Aybike Birerdinc, Maria Stepanova, Dinan Abdelatif, Fanny Monge, Lakshmi Alaparthi and Zachary D. Goodman
Betty and Guy Beatty Center for Integrated Research, Inova Health System, 3300 Gallows Rd., Falls Church, VA, USA

Zobair M. Younossi, Azza Karrar, Maria Stepanova, Zahra Younoszai, Thomas Jeffers, Sean Felix and Vikas Chandhoke
Department of Medicine, Inova Fairfax Hospital, Falls Church, VA, USA

Zobair M. Younossi, Dinan Abdelatif, Fanny Monge, Lakshmi Alaparthi and Zachary D. Goodman
Center for Liver Diseases, Inova Fairfax Hospital, Falls Church, VA, USA

Kianoush Jeiran, Alex Hodge, Weidong Zhou and Vikas Chandhoke
Center for Applied Proteomics and Molecular Medicine, School of Systems Biology, George Mason University, Manassas, VA, USA

John R. Williams
Department of Infectious Disease Epidemiology, School of Public Health, Faculty of Medicine, Imperial College London, St Mary's Campus, Norfolk Place, London W2 1PG, UK

Piero Manfredi
Dipartimento di Economia e Management, University of Pisa, via Ridolfi 10, 56124 Pisa, Italy

Alessia Melegaro
Dondena Centre for Research on Social Dynamics and Public Policy and Department of Social and Political Science, Bocconi University, Via Roentgen 1, 20136 Milan, Italy

Winnie Lau, David Forbes, Sean Cowlishaw, Dzenana Kartal and Meaghan O'Donnell
Phoenix Australia, Melbourne, Victoria, Australia

Winnie Lau, David Forbes, Sean Cowlishaw, Dzenana Kartal and Meaghan O'Donnell
Department of Psychiatry, University of Melbourne, Melbourne, Victoria, Australia

Derrick Silove
Liverpool Hospital, Sydney, NSW, Australia
School of Psychiatry, University of New South Wales, Sydney, NSW, Australia

Ben Edwards
ANU Centre for Social Research and Methods, Australian National University, Canberra, Australian Capital Territory, Australia

Richard Bryant and Angela Nickerson
School of Psychology, University of New South Wales, Sydney, NSW, Australia

Alexander McFarlane and Miranda Van Hooff
Centre for Traumatic Stress Studies, University of Adelaide, Adelaide, SA, Australia

Zachary Steel
Black Dog Institute, Sydney, NSW, Australia

Zachary Steel
St John of God Hospital Richmond, Sydney, Australia

Kim Felmingham
Melbourne School of Psychological Sciences, University of Melbourne, Melbourne, Victoria, Australia

Sean Cowlishaw
Population Health Sciences, Bristol Medical School, University of Bristol, Bristol, UK

Nathan Alkemade
Monash Health, Melbourne, Victoria, Australia

Christopher Burton
Academic Unit of Primary Medical Care, University of Sheffield, Samuel Fox House, Northern General Hospital, Sheffield S5 7AU, UK

Alison Elliott and Amanda Cochran
University of Aberdeen, Aberdeen, UK

Tom Love
University of Otago, Wellington, New Zealand

Alison Elliott
Abertay University, Dundee, UK

Jenni Burt and Natasha Elmore
THIS Institute (The Healthcare Improvement Studies Institute), University of Cambridge, Cambridge Biomedical Campus, Clifford Allbutt Building, Cambridge CB2 0AH, UK

Stephen M. Campbell
NIHR Greater Manchester Patient Safety Translational Research Centre, Division of Population Health, HSR & Primary Care, School of Health Sciences, Faculty of Biology, Medicine and Health, University of Manchester, Manchester, UK

Sarah Rodgers
Division of Primary Care, University of Nottingham, Room 1312, Tower Building, University Park, Nottingham NG7 2RD, UK

Anthony J. Avery
Division of Primary Care, School of Medicine, University of Nottingham, Dean's Office, B Floor, Medical School, Queens Medical Centre, Nottingham NG7 2UH, UK

Rupert A. Payne
Centre for Academic Primary Care, Population Health Sciences, Bristol Medical School, University of Bristol, Canynge Hall, 39 Whatley Road, Bristol BS8 2PS, UK

Freya J. I. Fowkes, Kerryn A. Moore, D. Herbert Opi, Freya Langham and James G. Beeson
Burnet Institute, Maternal and Child Health Program, Life Sciences and Public Health, Melbourne, VIC 3004, Australia

Freya J. I. Fowkes and Freya Langham
Department of Epidemiology and Preventive Medicine, Monash University, Melbourne, VIC 3008, Australia

Freya J. I. Fowkes, Kerryn A. Moore and Julie A. Simpson
Centre for Epidemiology and Biostatistics, Melbourne School of Population and Global Health, The University of Melbourne, Melbourne, VIC 3010, Australia

Freya J. I. Fowkes and James G. Beeson
Department of Infectious Diseases, Central Clinical School, Monash University, Melbourne, VIC 3004, Australia

D. Herbert Opi
Department of Immunology, Monash University, Central Clinical School, Melbourne, VIC 3004, Australia

Danielle I. Stanisic
Institute for Glycomics, Griffith University, South Brisbane, QLD 4101, Australia

Alice Ura and Peter M. Siba
Papua New Guinea Institute of Medical Research, Goroka, EHP, Papua New Guinea

Christopher L. King
Center for Global Health and Diseases, Case Western Reserve University, Cleveland, OH, USA

Ivo Mueller
Walter and Eliza Hall Institute of Medical Research, Parkville, VIC 3050, Australia
Department of Parasites and Insect Vectors, Institut Pasteur, 75015 Paris, France

Stephen J. Rogerson and James G. Beeson
Department of Medicine (RMH), The University of Melbourne, Parkville, VIC 3010, Australia

Alison F. Crawshaw, John Were and Hilary Kirkbride
Travel and Migrant Health Section, National Infection Service, Public Health England, 61 Colindale Ave, London NW9 5EQ, UK

Manish Pareek
Department of Infection, Immunity and Inflammation, University of Leicester, Leicester, UK

Steffen Schillinger and Kolitha P. Wickramage
International Organization for Migration (IOM), Citibank Center, 28th Floor, 8741, Paseo de Roxas, Makati, 1200 Metro Manila, Philippines

Olga Gorbacheva
International Organization for Migration (IOM), 17 Route des Morillons, 1218 Grand-Saconnex, Switzerland

Sema Mandal
Immunisation, Hepatitis and Blood Safety, National Infection Service, Public Health England, 61 Colindale Ave, London NW9 5EQ, UK

Valerie Delpech and Noel Gill
HIV and STI Department, National Infection Service, Public Health England, 61 Colindale Ave, London NW9 5EQ, UK

Dominik Zenner
TB Screening Unit, National Infection Service, Public Health England, 61 Colindale Avenue, London NW9 5EQ, UK
Institute for Global Health, Faculty of Population Health Sciences, University College London, Gower Street, London WC1E 6BT, UK

M. E. Murphy, S. Murthy, A. L. C. Bateson, R. D. Hunt and T. D. McHugh
UCL Centre for Clinical Microbiology, Division of Infection and Immunity, University College London, Royal Free Campus, Rowland Hill Street, London NW3 2PF, England, UK

G. H. Wills, A. J. Nunn, S. K. Meredith and A. M. Crook
MRC Clinical Trials Unit at UCL, Institute for Clinical Trials and Methodology, Aviation House, 125 Kingsway, London WC2B 6NH, England, UK

C. Louw
Madibeng Centre for Research, Brits, South Africa
Department of Family Medicine, School of medicine, University of Pretoria, Pretoria, South Africa

M. Mendel and M. Spigelman
Global Alliance for Tuberculosis Drug Development, New York, NY 10005, USA

S. H. Gillespie
School of Medicine, Medical and Biological Sciences Building, University of St Andrews, North Haugh, St Andrews KY16 9TF, Scotland, UK

Myrela O. Machado
Department of Clinical Medicine and Translational Psychiatry Research Group, Faculty of Medicine, Federal University of Ceará, Fortaleza, CE 60430-140, Brazil

Nicola Veronese
Institute for Clinical Research and Education in Medicine (IREM), 35128 Padova, Italy
National Research Council, Neuroscience Institute, Aging Branch, 35128 Padova, Italy.

Marcos Sanches
Biostatistical Consulting Unit, Centre for Addiction and Mental Health (CAMH), Toronto, ON, Canada.

Ioanna Tzoulaki
Department of Epidemiology and Biostatistics, School of Public Health, Imperial College London, W2 1PG, London, UK
MRC-PHE Centre for Environment, School of Public Health, Imperial College London, London W2 1PG, UK.
Department of Hygiene and Epidemiology, University of Ioannina Medical School, Ioannina, Greece

John P. A. Ioannidis
Department of Medicine, Stanford University, Palo Alto, CA 94305, USA
Department of Health Research and Policy, Stanford University, Palo Alto, CA 94305, USA
Department of Statistics, Stanford University, Palo Alto, CA 94305, USA
Department of Meta-Research Innovation Center at Stanford (METRICS), Stanford University, Palo Alto, CA 94305, USA

André F. Carvalho
Department of Psychiatry, University of Toronto, Toronto, ON, Canada
Centre for Addiction & Mental Health (CAMH), 33 Russel Street, room RS1050S, Toronto, ON M5S 2S1, Canada

Liriye Kurtovic, Gaoqian Feng, Linda Reiling, Freya J. I. Fowkes and James G. Beeson
Burnet Institute, Melbourne, Australia

Liriye Kurtovic and James G. Beeson
Department of Immunology and Pathology, Monash University, Melbourne, Australia

Marije C. Behet and Robert W. Sauerwein
Department of Medical and Microbiology, Radboud University Medical Center, Nijmegen, The Netherlands

Kiprotich Chelimo
Kenya Medical Research Institute, Kisumu, Kenya

Arlene E. Dent
Center for Global Health and Diseases, Case Western University, Cleveland, USA

Ivo Mueller
Division of Population Health and Immunity, Walter and Eliza Hall Institute, Melbourne, Australia
Department of Parasites and Insect Vectors, Institut Pasteur, Paris, France

Freya J. I. Fowkes
Department of Epidemiology and Preventative Medicine and Department of Infectious Diseases, Monash University, Melbourne, Australia
Centre for Epidemiology and Biostatistics, Melbourne School of Population and Global Health, The University of Melbourne, Melbourne, Australia

James G. Beeson
Department of Microbiology, Monash University, Clayton, Australia
Department of Medicine, The University of Melbourne, 185 Commercial Road, Parkville, Australia

Debebe Shaweno and Romain Ragonnet and Emma S. McBryde
Department of Medicine, University of Melbourne, Melbourne, Victoria, Australia

Debebe Shaweno, Malancha Karmakar, James M. Trauer and Justin T. Denholm
Victorian Tuberculosis Program at the Peter Doherty Institute for Infection and Immunity, Melbourne, Victoria, Australia

Malancha Karmakar and Justin T. Denholm
Department of Microbiology and Immunology, University of Melbourne, Melbourne, Victoria, Australia

Kefyalew Addis Alene
Research School of Population Health, College of Health and Medicine, The Australian National University, Canberra, Australia

Institute of Public Health, College of Medicine and Health Sciences, University of Gondar, Gondar, Ethiopia

Romain Ragonnet
Burnet Institute, Melbourne, Australia

Archie CA Clements
Curtin University, Bentley, Western Australia, Australia

James M. Trauer
School of Public Health and Preventive Medicine, Monash University, Melbourne, Australia

Emma S. McBryde
Australian Institute of Tropical Health and Medicine, James Cook University, Townsville, Queensland, Australia

Dara O'Neill
CLOSER, Department of Social Science, Institute of Education, University College London, London, UK

Annie Britton and Diana Kuh
Research Department of Epidemiology and Public Health, University College London, London, UK

Mary K. Hannah
MRC/CSO Social and Public Health Sciences Unit, Institute of Health and Wellbeing, University of Glasgow, Glasgow, UK

Marcel Goldberg
Inserm UMS 011, Villejuif, France and Paris Descartes University, Villejuif, France

Diana Kuh
UK MRC Unit for Lifelong Health & Ageing at UCL, London, UK

Kay Tee Khaw
Cambridge Institute of Public Health, University of Cambridge, Cambridge, UK

Steven Bell
Department of Public Health and Primary Care, University of Cambridge, Cambridge, UK

Florian Büttner, Stefan Winter , Matthias Schwab and Elke Schaeffeler
Dr. Margarete Fischer-Bosch Institute of Clinical Pharmacology, Auerbachstrasse 112, 70376 Stuttgart, Germany

Florian Büttner, Stefan Winter, Matthias Schwab and Elke Schaeffeler
University of Tuebingen, Tuebingen, Germany

Steffen Rausch, Jörg Hennenlotter, Stephan Kruck and Arnulf Stenzl
Department of Urology, University Hospital Tuebingen, Tuebingen, Germany

Marcus Scharpf and Falko Fend
Institute of Pathology and Neuropathology, University Hospital Tuebingen, Tuebingen, Germany

Abbas Agaimy and Arndt Hartmann
Institute of Pathology, Friedrich-Alexander University Erlangen-Nuernberg, University Hospital Erlangen-Nuernberg, Erlangen, Germany

Jens Bedke and Matthias Schwab
German Cancer Consortium (DKTK) and German Cancer Research Center (DKFZ), Heidelberg, Germany

Matthias Schwab
Department of Clinical Pharmacology, University Hospital Tuebingen, Tuebingen, Germany
Department of Pharmacy and Biochemistry, University of Tuebingen, Tuebingen, Germany

Yu-Tzu Wu, Linda Clare, John V. Hindle, Sharon M. Nelis and Anthony Martyr
The Centre for Research in Ageing and Cognitive Health, St Luke's Campus, University of Exeter Medical School, Exeter EX1 2LU, UK

Fiona E. Matthews
Institute of Health and Society, Newcastle University, The Baddiley-Clark Building, Richardson Road, Newcastle Upon Tyne NE4 5PL, UK

Yu-Tzu Wu
Health Service and Population Research Department, Institute of Psychiatry, Psychology and Neuroscience, King's College London, David Goldberg Centre, De Crespigny Park, Denmark Hill, London SE5 8AF, UK

Nicholas L. Syn, Andrea Li-Ann Wong, Soo-Chin Lee, LM Poon, Patrick Marban and Boon-Cher Goh
Department of Haematology-Oncology, National University Cancer Institute, Singapore, Singapore

Nicholas L. Syn, Andrea Li-Ann Wong, Soo-Chin Lee and Boon-Cher
Cancer Science Institute of Singapore, National University of Singapore, Singapore, Singapore.

Hock-Luen Teoh and Raymond CS Seet
Division of Neurology, Department of Medicine, National University Health System, Singapore, Singapore

Wee Tiong Yeo, William Kristanto and James Wei Luen Yip
Department of Cardiology, National University Heart Centre, Singapore, Singapore

Ping-Chong Bee
Department of Medicine, University of Malaya Medical Centre, Kuala Lumpur, Malaysia

Tuck Seng Wu
Department of Pharmacy, National University Hospital, Singapore, Singapore

Michael D. Winther
Genome Institute of Singapore, Agency for Science, Technology and Research, Singapore, Singapore

Liam R. Brunham
Translational Laboratory in Genetic Medicine, Agency for Science, Technology and Research, Singapore, Singapore
Department of Medicine, Centre for Heart Lung Innovation, University of British Columbia, Vancouver, Canada

Richie Soong
Department of Pathology, Yong Loo Lin School of Medicine, National University Health System, Singapore, Singapore

Bee-Choo Tai
Saw Swee Hock School of Public Health, National University of Singapore, Singapore, Singapore

Boon-Cher Goh
Department of Pharmacology, Yong Loo Lin School of Medicine, National University Health System, Singapore 119228, Singapore

Raymond CS Seet
Department of Medicine, Yong Loo Lin School of Medicine, National University of Singapore, Singapore, Singapore

Hamtandi Magloire Natama, Eduard Rovira-Vallbona and Anna Rosanas-Urgell
Department of Biomedical Sciences, Institute of Tropical Medicine, B 2000 Antwerp, Belgium

Hamtandi Magloire Natama, Hermann Sorgho, Maminata Coulibaly-Traoré, M. Athanase Somé, Innocent Valéa and Halidou Tinto
Unité de Recherche Clinique de Nanoro, Institut de Recherche en Sciences de la Santé, BP218, Nanoro, Burkina Faso

Hamtandi Magloire Natama and Luc Kestens
Department of Biomedical Sciences, University of Antwerp, B 2610 Antwerp,
Belgium.

Gemma Moncunill, Héctor Sanz, Ruth Aguilar and Carlota Dobaño
Barcelona Institute for Global Health (ISGlobal), Hospital Clinic – Universitat de Barcelona, Carrer Rossello 132, E-08036 Barcelona, Catalonia, Spain

Susana Scott
Department of Epidemiology and Population Health, London School of Hygiene and Tropical Medicine, London WC1E7HT, UK

Petra F. Mens and Henk D. F. H. Schallig
Department of Medical Microbiology - Parasitology Unit, Academic Medical Centre, Amsterdam 1105, AZ, The Netherlands

Halidou Tinto
Centre Muraz, BP390, Bobo Dioulasso, Burkina Faso

Ilsa L. Haeusler and Philippe J. Guérin
WorldWide Antimalarial Resistance Network (WWARN), Oxford, UK

Ilsa L. Haeusler, Xin Hui S. Chan, Philippe J. Guérin and Nicholas J. White
Centre for Tropical Medicine and Global Health, Nuffield Department of Medicine, University of Oxford, Oxford, UK

Xin Hui S. Chan
Mahidol-Oxford Tropical Medicine Research Unit (MORU), Faculty of Tropical Medicine, Mahidol University, Bangkok, Thailand

Xin Hui S. Chan and Nicholas J. White
Oxford University Hospitals NHS Foundation Trust, Oxford, UK

Index